American Journal of Obstetrics and Gynecology, Volume 3

You are holding a reproduction of an original work that is in the public domain in the United States of America, and possibly other countries. You may freely copy and distribute this work as no entity (individual or corporate) has a copyright on the body of the work. This book may contain prior copyright references, and library stamps (as most of these works were scanned from library copies). These have been scanned and retained as part of the historical artifact.

This book may have occasional imperfections such as missing or blurred pages, poor pictures, errant marks, etc. that were either part of the original artifact, or were introduced by the scanning process. We believe this work is culturally important, and despite the imperfections, have elected to bring it back into print as part of our continuing commitment to the preservation of printed works worldwide. We appreciate your understanding of the imperfections in the preservation process, and hope you enjoy this valuable book.

THE AMERICAN JOURNAL OF OBSTETRICS AND GYNECOLOGY

ADVISORY EDITORIAL BOARD

CHANNING W. BARRETT
C. L. BONIFIELD
J. WESLEY BOVÉE
W. W. CHIPMAN
JOHN G. CLARK
H. S. CROSSEN
THOMAS CULLEN
EDWARD P. DAVIS
J. B. DELEE
ROBERT L. DICKINSON
PALMER FINDLEY
ROBERT T. FRANK

GEORGE GELLHORN
ALBERT GOLDSPOHN
WILLIAM P. GRAVES
HERMAN E. HAYD
BARTON C. HIRST
E. J. ILL
J. C. LITZENBERG
F. W. LYNCH
FRANKLIN H. MARTIN
C. JEFF MILLER
GEORGE CLARK MOSHER
HENRY P. NEUMAN

GEO. H. NOBLE
REUBEN PETERSON
JOHN OSBORN POLAK
F. F. SIMPSON
HENRY SCHWARZ
HOWARD C. TAYLOR
THOMAS J. WATKINS
B. P. WATSON
GEORGE GRAY WARD, JR.
J. WHITRIDGE WILLIAMS

OFFICIAL ORGAN OF
THE AMERICAN GYNECOLOGICAL SOCIETY
THE AMERICAN ASSOCIATION OF OBSTETRICIANS, GYNECOLOGISTS, AND ABDOMINAL SURGEONS
THE OBSTETRICAL SOCIETIES OF NEW YORK, PHILADELPHIA, BROOKLYN

Editor, GEORGE W. KOSMAK
Associate Editor, HUGO EHRENFEST

VOLUME III
JANUARY, 1922—JUNE, 1922

ST. LOUIS
C. V. MOSBY COMPANY
1922

COPYRIGHT, 1922, BY C. V. MOSBY COMPANY

Press of
C. V. Mosby Company,
St. Louis.

The American Journal of Obstetrics and Gynecology

Original Communications

END RESULTS OF AMPUTATION OF THE CERVIX AND TRACHELORRHAPHY*

By REGINALD M. RAWLS, M.D., F.A.C.S., NEW YORK, N. Y.

IT IS a far cry from the crude amputation of the cervix, with the ecraseur, to the finished surgical procedure devised by Sims and perfected by Emmet and the conservative trachelorrhaphy of Emmet. The technic of these masters has survived for a little over a half century and during this time there has arisen a considerable literature *pro* and *con*. Some writers refer to trachelorrhaphy as "uterine tinkering" and others hold that subsequent to amputation there is a high percentage of sterility and if by chance pregnancy occurs it is likely to end in abortion or premature labor or if it should go to term there will be more or less dystocia. A few even contend that, after amputation of the cervix, elective cesarean section is indicated in subsequent pregnancies. Such sequelae are unquestionable if cervix operations are performed without proper technic or indications.

Almost fifty-nine years ago Emmet[1] performed his first trachelorrhaphy, as he believed amputation of the cervix unnecessary except for removal of a cauliflower growth, malignant disease or excessive hypertrophy sometimes several inches in length. But after thirty-five years' experience with the operation, he states "for many years I held the opinion that it was possible, in almost every instance, by careful local and general treatment to restore in time the lacerated tissues to so near the normal condition that, when the operation (trachelorrhaphy) had been properly performed complete restoration would eventually take place with the result of bringing about involu-

---

*Read in abstract at the Forty-Fourth Annual Meeting of the American Gynecological Society, June, 1921, Swampscott, Mass.

NOTE: The Editor accepts no responsibility for the views and statements of authors as published in their "Original Communications."

tion of the uterus. But I am now of the opinion that there are exceptions to this rule, when it is better surgery to amputate a portion or the whole of the cervix provided the diseased tissues are completely removed and the wound treated in the manner I shall describe." This quotation gives us the indication for cervical repair of a quarter of a century ago as recognized by the originator of trachelorrhaphy and the man most capable of carrying out the technic.

Hirst,[2] Crossen,[3] Eden and Lockyer,[4] Anspach,[5] and Graves,[6] all agree on the indications for trachelorrhaphy but Anspach limits amputation to women past the childbearing period and Graves to procidentia. Others, including Sturmdorf,[7] question the efficacy of either procedure.

The most recent statistics of the postoperative results of amputation of the cervix and trachelorrhaphy are those of Leonard[8] which are based on replies to circular letters received from 128 of 400 cases of amputation of the cervix, performed during the preceding twenty years, and from 39 of the cases of trachelorrhaphy, performed during the preceding ten years, in the Gynecological Clinic of the Johns Hopkins Hospital. The method of operation in this series of cases was either "almost without exception, a high amputation . . . from 2.5 to 3 cm. of the cervix above the external os being removed" or the classical trachelorrhaphy of Emmet. The indications governing the selection of the method of operation was almost invariably to amputate a cervix badly infected or one showing multiple lacerations and to use trachelorrhaphy in those cases presenting one or two more or less discrete lacerations and without a marked endocervicitis. Sturmdorf, after giving a summary of Leonard's conclusions says, "accepting these data from authoritative sources, as a correct exposition of facts, the obvious deduction is, that with chronic endocervicitis as the recognized pathologic indicator, trachelorrhaphy is an inadequate, and cervix amputation an injurious, operation."

To me it seems unfair to condemn the old and tried methods of cervical repair of Sims and Emmet and to recognize the newer and less tried tracheloplasty methods as a specific in all cervical disease. Especially is this true if we accept the statistics of Leonard for high amputation and apply them to all degrees of amputation. Thus the time seems ripe to study another series of cases of cervical operations and to compare the postoperative results of amputation of the cervix and trachelorrhaphy.

At the Woman's Hospital from January 1, 1916, to January 1, 1919, there were admitted approximately 6503 gynecological patients and alone or combined with other operative procedures 11 per cent had cervical operations. Amputation of the cervix was performed 461 times and trachelorrhaphy was performed 232 times. Two-thirds of the amputations and seven-eighths of the trachelorrhaphies were done on women under forty years of age, and were about equally combined with vaginal plastic and abdominal operations. This series is composed of 305 private cases and 394 ward cases performed by 41 individual operators. Two hundred eleven, or approximately 30 per cent, have been followed from one to five years. The technic of, and indications for, operation were those of Emmet more or less faithfully carried out, namely, to excise the diseased cervical tissue by a low, median or high amputation or to perform the classical trachelorrhaphy.

PLAN OF STUDY

To classify the cases and to find the immediate results the individual hospital records of the 693 cases were carefully gone over. The remote or end results were obtained, from the ward cases, by writing to each patient to report to their follow-up clinic and when they did not report, a questionnaire was sent requesting that it be filled out and returned to the Record Department of the hospital. For the private cases, questionnaires were sent to their surgeons who were asked to return their end results with the privilege of using them in this report. In this manner 67 ward cases were re-examined by ten examiners and 75 returned complete questionnaires two and one-half to five years after operation. Among the private cases, 69 were re-examined by 17 operators from one to five years after operation. Combining these returns we have 136 cases re-examined from one to five years and our end results based on letters in only 75 ward cases. Included in these 211 cases, there were 132 amputations of the cervix and 79 trachelorrhaphies. Amputation was done in 81 patients under forty years of age and in 51 patients over forty years of age. Trachelorrhaphy was done in 74 under and in 5 over forty years of age. Seventy-three amputations and 33 trachelorrhaphies were done alone or were combined with other vaginal plastic operations, 56 amputations and 45 trachelorrhaphies had in addition some form of conservative abdominal operation, and three amputations and one trachelorrhaphy accompanied a bilateral salpingectomy. Approximately 64 per cent of the cases were re-examined, one to five years subsequent to operation. The personal equation of the author has been eliminated as he is merely the tabulator, in the great majority of the cases, of the findings recorded by a number of examiners. Further but 35.5 per cent of our end results are dependent upon answers to circular letters, as compared to 100 per cent in Leonard's series.

PATHOLOGY OF CERVICAL TISSUE REMOVED

About 67 per cent of the specimens of cervical tissue removed at operation was subjected to a microscopic examination including about

92 per cent removed by amputation and about 18 per cent removed by trachelorrhaphy. Approximately 76 per cent of the tissue specimens examined, showed cervical changes other than simple lacerations. This was present in cases of amputation in about 76 per cent and in cases of trachelorrhaphy in about 71 per cent. These changes, in their order of frequency were erosion, cervicitis, hyperplasia, endocervicitis, circulatory disturbance, precancerous changes, and carcinoma. It is most interesting to note that in 466 cases in which the tissue was examined microscopically, there was but one case each of precancerous change and carcinoma.

I. IMMEDIATE RESULTS

1. *Secondary Hemorrhage.*—There were 8 cases of secondary hemorrhage, or 1.2 per cent in our series. In none of these cases was it necessary to resort to resuturing and in but one case was it necessary to use a vaginal pack, and in all but three of these cases there was subsequent primary union. Hemorrhage occurred on the second day in 2 cases, the sixth day in 1 case, the ninth day in 2 cases, and the twelfth day in 3 cases. Thus less than ½ per cent of the amputations (2 of 461) and about 2.5 per cent of the trachelorrhaphies (7 of 232) were complicated by secondary hemorrhage. The percentage of hemorrhage, but not the degree conforms with the earlier reported cases following trachelorrhaphy of Goodell and Emmet[9] rather than the more recent cases reported by Leonard. The latter in his study found six of 128 amputations severe enough to require resuture, or 4.7 per cent, and two of 39 cases of trachelorrhaphy which were controlled by vaginal pack, or 5.1 per cent. The low percentage for amputation in our series as compared to Leonard's, is possibly due to two factors. First, high amputation was the exception rather than the rule and, second, a vaginal pack was usually placed following all cervical operations. An interesting fact in this connection is that but three of these cases, all trachelorrhaphies, were followed by secondary or partial union which would seem to indicate that the hemorrhage was due to faulty hemostasis or errors of technic in tying the sutures which caused necrosis of the tissues rather than a sepsis from existing endocervicitis.

2. *Secondary Union or Partial Primary Union.*—In addition to the three cases of secondary or partial primary union, there were five cases of secondary or partial union or a fraction over 1 per cent (8 of 693). Four occurred after trachelorrhaphy and four after amputation, about 2 and 1 per cent, respectively. Three of the four cases of secondary or partial union in trachelorrhaphy were subsequent to secondary hemorrhage, and one of the four amputations in which secondary or partial union resulted was a case in which an extensive vaginal

section was also done. In none of the cases was there a serious sepsis which in any way contributed to the mortality in this series of cases.

II. REMOTE OR END RESULTS

1. *General Health.*—The influence of cervical operations on the general health is a complex question and one that must be almost entirely analyzed from a subjective basis. This is necessarily the case as primarily the patient must be relieved of the symptoms for which she sought operation. A review of the following table shows that trachelorrhaphy alone gives a little over 16 per cent greater improvement in the general health than amputation alone. On the other hand, amputation when combined with vaginal plastic operations gives almost 21 per cent greater improvement in the general health than trachelorrhaphy combined with vaginal plastic operations. When combined with abdominal operations, the difference for the two methods is negligible as they both show improvement in over 86 per cent. The discrepancy in the end results of amputation and trachelorrhaphy alone when contrasted with the results when they are combined with vaginal plastic measures seems to be explained on the theory that in the cases requiring amputation the primary injury also caused lesions in the vagina which should have been repaired to relieve the symptoms and thus improve the general health. Thus our statistics indicate that both methods improve the general health but the greater improvement results from amputation when combined with plastic repair.

TABLE I
INFLUENCE OF AMPUTATION AND TRACHELORRHAPHY ON THE GENERAL HEALTH

OPERATION	NUMBER OF CASES	NUMBER OF CASES IMPROVED
Amputation	12	8 (66.6%)
Trachelorrhaphy	12	10 (83.3%)
Amputation and vaginal plastic operations	48	42 (87.5%)
Trachelorrhaphy and vaginal plastic operations	21	14 (66.6%)
Amputation and abdominal operations	53	47 (86.8%)
Trachelorrhaphy and abdominal operations	48	43 (89.6%)
Totals—		
Amputation	113	97 (85.8%)
Trachelorrhaphy	81	67 (82.7%)
	194	164 (84.5%)

2. *Leucorrhea.*—The most frequent cause of persistent vaginal discharge is cervical disease and in the multiparous woman the predisposing cause is cervical laceration. On this basis it is interesting to determine, in our series of cases, the occurrence of leucorrhea before operation and its degree or cure after operation (see Chart 1).

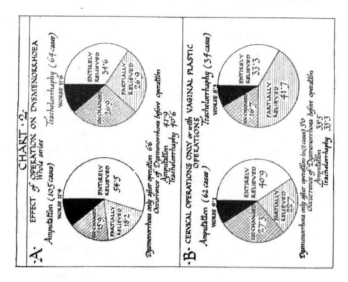

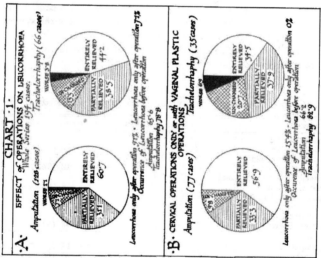

In 194 cases of cervical operations a leucorrhea more or less constant and of varying degrees occurred in 70.1 per cent, before amputation in 65.6 per cent and before trachelorrhaphy in 78.8 per cent. To determine accurately the end results for leucorrhea requires examinations made from time to time but unfortunately, in most of our cases, the end results are based on one examination made from one to five years after operation. The discharge present may be due to a reinfection of a cervix restored to the normal by operation or the discharge may have eventually disappeared notwithstanding. This applies equally to both methods of operating; it seems reasonable to assume that any difference in the end results would be due to the form of operation.

Subsequent to amputation the leucorrhea was entirely relieved in 60.7 per cent and partially relieved in 31.1 per cent as compared to trachelorrhaphies with subsequent entire relief in 44.2 per cent and partial relief in 38.5 per cent. As to the character of the existing leucorrhea after amputation it was unchanged in 7.1 per cent and worse in 1.1 per cent and for trachelorrhaphy it was unchanged in 13.5 per cent and worse in 3.8 per cent. In cases without leucorrhea before operation, it was present in 4 of 44 cases, or 9.1 per cent, for amputation and in 1 of 14 cases, or 7.1 per cent, for trachelorrhaphy.

If we exclude cervical operations combined with abdominal section which show an almost equal percentage of improvement for each method of operating (94.0 compared to 95.6), there will remain cervical operations alone or combined with vaginal plastic operations. From this series, cervical operation being the principle cause of the change in the vaginal discharge, we obtain definite end results. Therefore for amputation with existing leucorrhea in 66.2 per cent and for trachelorrhaphy with existing leucorrhea in 82.9 per cent, there was for amputation, contrasted with trachelorrhaphy, 22.4 per cent more complete relief (56.9 compared to 34.5) but 4.6 per cent less partial relief (33.3 compared to 37.9) and 10.9 per cent fewer cases in which the leucorrhea was unchanged in character. On the other hand, following amputation no cases were made worse whereas following trachelorrhaphy 2 of 35 cases, or 6.9 per cent, were worse. But 4 of 26 cases, or 15.4 per cent, of the cases subjected to amputation who were free of leucorrhea now had a mild degree of vaginal discharge.

Finally, amputation of the cervix is more efficient than trachelorrhaphy in the cure of leucorrhea, but more often than trachelorrhaphy causes a leucorrhea in cases previously free from a vaginal discharge. Such end results are not surprising even if we accept the theory that endocervicitis is the principal cause of leucorrhea. For it is unreasonable to assume that in every case of leucorrhea all the cervical glands, from the external to the internal os, are diseased. Therefore, as demonstrated by our series of cases, there is a place even in the treatment of leucorrhea for low, medium and high amputation and to a lesser degree for trachelorrhaphy. The end results further demonstrate the necessity for careful study of the indications and the performance of proper technic or too small an external os will result or some of the diseased glands will be left and the vaginal discharge will be worse in character or it will occur in cases free of leucorrhea before operation.

3. *Dysmenorrhea.*—In the nullipara, malformation or disease of the cervix is recognized as a causative factor of dysmenorrhea, but in the multipara laceration and its accompanying disease has received but scant attention as a cause of dysmenorrhea. However a review of Chart 2 of cervical operations shows an existing dysmenorrhea in 41.4 per cent; for amputation in 41.9 per cent and for trachelorrhaphy in 40.6 per cent.

Subsequent to amputation there is entire relief of dysmenorrhea in 54.5 per cent and partial relief in 18.2 per cent as compared to trachelorrhaphy with entire relief of the dysmenorrhea in 34.6 per cent and partial relief in 26.9 per cent. The degree of remaining dysmenorrhea was, for amputation, unchanged in 15.9 per cent and worse in 11.4 per cent as compared to trachelorrhaphy with the pain unchanged in 26.9 per cent and worse in 11.6 per cent. However, in cases free from monthly pain before operation it was subsequently present only after amputation in 6.6 per cent.

If we deduct the cervical operations combined with abdominal section, which give for amputation 31.8 per cent more entire and partial relief of the dysmenorrhea than trachelorrhaphy there remain cervical operations alone or combined with vaginal plastic operations. Thus for amputation contrasted with trachelorrhaphy with about an equal percentage of existing dysmenorrhea (35.5 compared to 35.3) there was for amputation 7.6 per cent more entire relief from the dysmenorrhea (40.9 compared to 33.3) but there was 19.0 per cent less partial relief (22.7 compared 41.7). Therefore while trachelorrhaphy gives more cases with an improvement of the dysmenorrhea yet amputations give more cures of this symptom. Of the unimproved cases amputation contrasted with trachelorrhaphy gives 10.6 per cent more cases with the dysmenorrhea unchanged in character (27.3 compared to 16.7) but for each operation there is about the same percentage of the cases (9.1 compared to 8.3) in which the character of the pain was worse after operation. However, only after amputation in 40 cases free from dysmenorrhea before operation it was now very severe in 2 or 5 per cent.

Finally amputation, as compared with trachelorrhaphy, is more efficient in the cure of dysmenorrhea but both operations cause the existing pain to be more severe in character in from 8 to 11 per cent of the cases and amputation alone causes subsequent dysmenorrhea in from 5 to 6 per cent of the cases previously free from menstrual pain. Thus there is the necessity for careful study of the individual case and the application of the proper operation and technic for each case or the external os may be made too small or the cervical canal may become stenosed. For amputation the increased dysmenorrhea may be due in part, as has been held by some writers, to the scar which is perpendicular to the long axis of the cervical canal and by contracting may cause a narrowing of the canal. This was probably the condition in the following history of one of the two cases of amputation in which dysmenorrhea was present only after operation.

Mrs. H. was operated upon by a divulsion and curettage, with dull curette, and the cystic portion of the cervix was excised and the raw edges were coapted with chromic gut sutures, four being used as canal sutures, uneventful recovery, no secondary hemorrhage or unusual vaginal discharge. On discharge from the hospital there was no eversion of the cervical flaps and there was primary union. Some time later, because of severe dysmenorrhea the cervical canal had to be dilated and a stem pessary introduced. Thus the dysmenorrhea was eventually cured.

4. *Sterility.*—Many factors have to be considered in determining the cause of sterility. Duncan[10] has shown that the age at marriage and the number of years married must be taken into account in our final analysis.

Unfortunately, successful operations on the cervix and vagina often produce increased voluntary sterility. The most frequent cause is the fear, held equally by the patient and her medical adviser and many times by the gynecologist and obstetrician, that labors subsequent to successful plastic operations will result in conditions as bad or even worse than those from which the patient had been relieved. This fear of bearing children, after operation, is shown in our series, as in 72 questionnaires, 84 per cent of the women stated that they were not anxious for more children, 8 per cent acknowledged the use of contraceptive measures and a few had practiced continence. Further there were three elective cesarean sections performed for indications, in part due to the fear of undoing successful repair work or the fear of dystocia due to these operations. In our final analysis of cervical operations and the bearing on secondary sterility all available facts must be taken into consideration.

Among 149 women in the childbearing period (see Chart 3) under forty years of age at time of operation and menstruating regularly for at least one year after operation, there was sterility of 72.6 per cent for 73 cases of amputation compared to a sterility of 57.9 per cent for 76 cases of trachelorrhaphy or a greater sterility following amputation of 14.7 per cent. In Leonard's series of 101 similar cases there was sterility in 80.6 per cent of 72 amputations compared with sterility of 62.0 per cent of 29 trachelorrhaphies or a greater sterility for amputation of 18.6 per cent. As my series is made up of low, medium and high amputations and there is almost an equal number of cases of amputation and trachelorrhaphy, I believe 14.7 per cent more accurately represents the increase of sterility which follows amputation of the cervix. Therefore, in all cases, where cervical

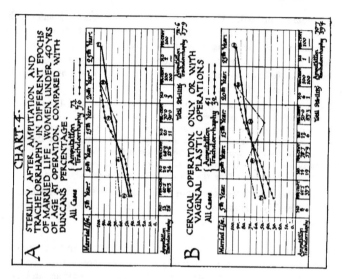

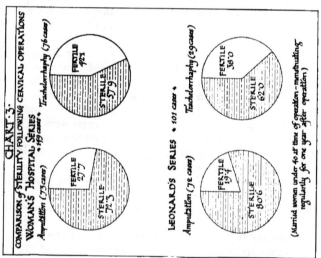

operations are used with other operations a little less than three-fourths of those subjected to amputation remain sterile whereas one and a half times more cases of trachelorrhaphy than amputation were subsequently fertile.

This increase of sterility after amputation in my series cannot be explained on the ground of the different age at marriage or the different number of years married. This is brought out in a classification of the cases which shows that the sterility for trachelorrhaphy when compared amputation is even less or more nearly corresponds to the percentages established by Duncan. This is true for cervical operations alone or combined only with vaginal plastic operations as it is for the whole series of cases. This is graphically shown, for the different epochs of married life, in Chart 4.

Women in the childbearing period, classified according to different groups of operations (Table II), show 11.3 per cent greater sterility for amputation; for the amputation and trachelorrhaphy combined with round ligament or uterosacral shortening or ventral suspension or a combination of these operations, it shows 15.2 per cent greater sterility in the cases of amputation; and in amputations and trachelorrhaphy combined with myomectomies, or resections of one or both ovaries, or salpingooöphorectomy unilateral or a combination of these operations there was 18.2 per cent greater sterility for the cases of amputation. Therefore as there is a marked influence of the intraabdominal operations it seems reasonable to exclude these cases and to base our final analysis only on cases in which cervical operations alone or in combination with vaginal plastic work have been done. Thus the increase of sterility for cases of amputation compared to trachelorrhaphy is 11.3 per cent.

TABLE II
OPERATIONS ARRANGED IN GROUPS

	NUMBER OF CASES	FERTILE AFTER OPERATION	STERILITY
A. Cervical Operations alone or with Vaginal Plastic Operations.			
Amputation	41	12	70.7%
Trachelorrhaphy	32	13	59.4%
B. Cervical Operations with Abdominal Operations for Uterine Displacement.			
Amputation	21	7	66.7%
Trachelorrhaphy	33	16	51.5%
C. Cervical Operations with Conservative Abdominal Operations.			
Amputation	11	1	90.9%
Trachelorrhaphy	11	3	72.7%
Totals—			
Amputation	73	20	72.6%
Trachelorrhaphy	76	32	57.9%

5. *Course of Pregnancies after Cervical Operations.*—To determine the cause of abortion, of premature labor, or of dystocia in women who give a history of former easy full-term labors is often a difficult task. Therefore to classify the character of the pregnancies and labors and to assign their cause to different operative procedures, of necessity in different series of women, makes the problem become even more difficult. However, if we compare pregnancies and labors before and after amputation of the cervix and before and after trachelorrhaphy, we are able in each group to establish the influence of operation on the subse-

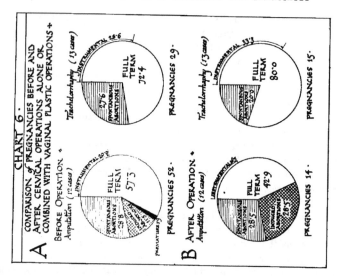

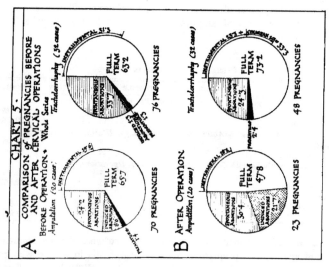

quent pregnancies and labors. Then using these facts as a check in comparing the subsequent pregnancies and labors, of necessity in a different series of cases, should give fairly accurate facts as to the occurrence of abortion, premature labor and dystocia as a result of amputation of the cervix or of trachelorrhaphy.

(a) *Premature Labor and Abortion.*—Comparing pregnancies before and after amputation (Chart 5), we find, after amputation, 17.9 per cent fewer full-term labors, and 6.2 per cent more spontaneous abortions. Of the remaining pregnancies interrupted before term there were, after amputation, no premature labors as compared to 1.4 per cent before operation but there was an increase of two and a half times the number of induced abortions. Comparing the pregnancies before and after trachelorrhaphy we find a 10.0 per cent increase of full-term pregnancies and a decrease of 9.4 per cent in the spontaneous abortions, but twice as many premature labors (1.3 compared to 2.4). Thus in like groups of cases amputation decreases and trachelorrhaphy increases the number of full-term labors while the opposite is true for spontaneous abortions. But premature labor which occurred in an equal percentage (1.3) before operation recurred only after trachelorrhaphy.

With these facts established let us contrast, of necessity in different series of cases, the pregnancies following amputation with those following trachelorrhaphy. There were 25.4 per cent fewer full-term labors, and 6.1 per cent more spontaneous abortions but no premature labors for amputation as compared with trachelorrhaphy which had 2.4 per cent premature labors.

To obtain more accurate statistics let us contrast, in the same way, cervical operations alone or combined with vaginal plastic operations (Chart 6). Comparing the pregnancies before and after amputation we find for the latter cases 14.4 per cent fewer full-term labors and about an equal number of spontaneous abortions. Of the remaining cases interrupted before term we find no premature labors after operation as compared to 1.9 per cent before operation but an increase after operation of over twice as many induced abortions. Comparing the pregnancies before and after trachelorrhaphy we find 7.6 per cent more full-term labors and a decrease of 7.6 per cent of spontaneous abortions. Thus in the same series and like groups of cases amputation decreases and trachelorrhaphy increases the number of full-term labors but while trachelorrhaphy decreases the number of spontaneous abortions amputation has but little effect one way or another, but it is followed by more cases of induced abortions.

Now let us contrast the pregnancies following amputation with those following trachelorrhaphy. There were, for amputation, 37.1 per cent fewer full-term pregnancies and 8.5 per cent increase in the spontaneous abortions and 28.5 per cent of induced abortions with none following trachelorrhaphy. Finally, taking all facts under consideration, amputation of the cervix is more often than trachelorrhaphy followed by the interruption of labor before term, but is no more likely than trachelorrhaphy to be followed by premature labor. While the final analysis of cervical cases alone or with vaginal plastic operations showed for amputation practically no increase of spontaneous abortions yet trachelorrhaphy showed a slight reduction of spontaneous abortions. This confirms the well accepted fact of cervical laceration as a cause of abortion and the reason it does not apply to amputation is in proportion as high amputations occur in the series. While we lack definite records of our high amputations it is reasonably certain that of eleven full-term pregnancies but one followed high amputation and of five spontaneous abortions, with no contributing cause, two of them followed high amputation. This fact is substanti-

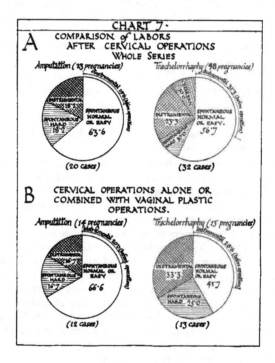

ated by Leonard's series of high amputations, which showed the interruption of pregnancy before term in 64.0 per cent of which 45.0 per cent were abortions.

(b) *Dystocia.*—In labors before cervical operations our only available data of dystocia are the use of forceps. Comparing labors before and after amputation, there is present about the same percentage of instrumental deliveries and the labors after trachelorrhaphy show a slightly higher percentage of instrumental deliveries than before operation. The three elective cesarean sections must be included in this end result as there was an apparent if not an actual dystocia—the "cervices showing no prospect of safe dilatation."

Comparing labors before and after cervical operations alone or combined with vaginal plastic operations we find after amputation a slight decrease of instrumental deliveries and after trachelorrhaphy a slight increase of instrumental deliveries. Note that in this series there were no cesarean or other operative cases.

For spontaneous labors we have definite data for dystocia only as it occurred after operation. Thus for amputation we find a slightly higher percentage of labors classified as spontaneous, normal, or easy. However, after amputation, compared to trachelorrhaphy, there are about 8.0 per cent more cases classified as hard spontaneous labors but a little more than half as many operative deliveries.

Comparing subsequent spontaneous labors after cervical operations alone or combined with vaginal plastic operations, we find, after amputation as compared to trachelorrhaphy almost 25 per cent more spontaneous easy or normal labors with 8.3 per cent fewer cases classified as hard spontaneous labors and about half as many instrumental deliveries.

Therefore considering dystocia from the data at hand, it is more frequent after trachelorrhaphy than after amputation and I feel it is at its minimum for trachelorrhaphy, as some of the cases classified as spontaneous, normal, or easy deliveries would have shown dystocia but for a laceration of the cervix before full dilatation and for amputation this occurrence was less frequent.

(c) *Relaceration of the Cervix.*—Our statistics are incomplete as to relaceration of the cervix in labors following cervical operations. However, of cases of amputation examined after spontaneous labors 2 of 5 cases, or 40.0 per cent, showed relaceration and for trachelorrhaphy, under similar conditions, 6 of 12 cases, or 50 per cent, showed relaceration.

A review of the following abstracts of pregnancies and labors before and after amputation of the cervix and after trachelorrhaphy will, I believe, substantiate my analysis for dystocia.

CASE REPORTS ILLUSTRATING CASES OF LABOR BEFORE AND AFTER
CERVICAL OPERATIONS

I. Amputation of the Cervix.

1. *Forceps Deliveries in Subsequent Labors.* (2 of 11 full-term deliveries or 18.2 per cent)

CASE 1.—Mrs. G., twenty-two years of age, married six years. Two full-term labors, first, instrumental in 1911. A 10 pound living child. Second, three years later delivered of a living baby by breech extraction. Unsuccessful perineorrhaphy after first delivery, fever following each delivery.

Amputation of cervix, repair of cystocele and pelvic floor. In the subsequent labor the first stage lasted 11 hours and 35 minutes, with moderate pains, regular, but infrequent. Second stage 2 hours and 44 minutes, pains, strong, regular, frequent but ineffectual. Third stage 6 minutes. Total duration of labor, 14 hours and 25 minutes. Position, L. O. A., at outlet O. A. Complication, prolapsed cord, narrow bi-ischial diameter.

After fourteen hours of labor the head deeply engaged and greatly moulded but there was no progress for two hours although there had been hard pains and the baby was passing some meconium. High median forceps applied and head extracted with great difficulty, median episiotomy on account of scar tissue in the perineum which was beginning to split. Male baby 9 pounds in weight.

NOTE: Dystocia was not due to the amputation of the cervix but to the large size of the child and to pelvic contraction as her previous labors were hard, first instrumental and second a breech, and there was a distinct narrowing of the bi-ischial spines.

CASE 2.—Mrs. N., 26 years, married 6 years, two children, no abortions or miscarriages. First labor, 1914, dry, spontaneous, 9½ hours, with male child, 7 pounds, 12½ ounces. Second labor, 1916, dry, spontaneous, 9 hours, male child, 8 pounds and 15 ounces. Operation, January 26, 1917, median amputation of cervix, repair of pelvic floor, Alexander's operation.

Subsequent dry labor with no real pains until the end of 14½ hours, when the cervix was fully dilated. Position L. O. P., converted and after pituitrin 1 c.c. and strychnine 1/20 by hypodermic, the pains became regular, frequent and effectual. Later, after an interval of three and a quarter hours there was no advance of the labor and low forceps were applied and a male child, 9 pounds and 14 ounces, was delivered. Total duration of labor, 18 hours and 3 minutes. First degree perineal tear.

NOTE: This labor was twice as long as either previous delivery due to the L. O. P. position, large baby and the lack of real labor pains but the cervix was not the cause of dystocia as it was fully dilated without effectual pains and without the aid of the bag of waters.

2. *Hard Deliveries in Subsequent Labors.* (2 of 11 full-term deliveries or 18.2 per cent)

CASE 1.—Mrs. McK., thirty-four years, admitted August 27, 1917. Married three years, never pregnant. Chief complaint, procidentia and cervical growth. Operation for cystocele, median amputation of cervix, transposition of uterosacral ligaments (Jellet's Operation) and repair of pelvic floor. Result partially satisfactory. Readmitted four months later because of retroversion of uterus and vaginal prolapse. Second operation for cystocele, Alexander's for retroversion and repair of pelvic floor.

Subsequent labor, 2½ years after last operation. Membranes ruptured spontaneously and labor lasted 10 hours and 40 minutes. In three hours and fifteen minutes from the beginning of labor, the cervix was dilated three fingers. Pituitrin M 10 at end of second stage and a female child, 7 pounds and 6 ounces, was delivered. Immediately following birth of head there was a sudden gush of blood, inspection revealed lacerations of anterior and right lateral walls of vagina; as well as around the urethra, posterior wall intact. The laceration of anterior wall about 3 inches in length. Lacerations sutured and vaginal pack placed.

Readmitted to hospital on September 21, 1920, and a vaginal hysterectomy, with over-lapping of broad ligaments and the fascia of anterior wall and a repair of pelvic floor was done.

NOTE: The unhappy sequelae in this case were not due to the amputation of the cervix but to the extensive and frequent operations and possibly to the injudicious use of pituitrin.

CASE 2.—Mrs. P., twenty-seven years, married 3 years, two spontaneous, hard labors, no abortions or miscarriages. Operation, 1918, amputation of cervix and repair of pelvic floor. Subsequently she had what she terms a hard full-term spontaneous delivery.

NOTE: Unfortunately this case was followed up only by a questionnaire, but as there is subjective evidence of the nature of her labors, it is reasonable to assume the hard labors before operation, and the hard labor subsequent to operation were due to the same cause and not to amputation of the cervix.

3. *Easy Deliveries in Subsequent Labors.* (7 of 11 full-term deliveries or 63.6 per cent)

There were seven full-term deliveries in which the subsequent labors were classified as normal or easy. In three of these cases there were previous operative deliveries. In one of these with two previous forceps operations of long duration, the subsequent delivery was spontaneous and two hours in duration. At the ninth month the cervix admitted one finger and at the onset of labor the cervix was three fingers dilated. Of the two others with previous single full-term deliveries, both instrumental, one had a subsequent delivery at full term of nine hours' duration and the other an easy subsequent full-term delivery.

Of the four remaining cases with spontaneous labors before and after operation we have the following: In two there were premature labors at the seventh month and in one the subsequent labor was easy, of fifteen hours' duration and in the other there was a subsequent precipitate labor. In the remaining two cases, one with three previous spontaneous normal labors of an average duration of twenty-four hours each with a subsequent normal labor of twelve hours and the other with seven normal previous labors with a subsequent normal labor.

From a study of subsequent labors in cases of amputation of the cervix, we must question the statistics of others who claim a high percentage of subsequent dystocia and premature labors after this operation.

II. *Trachelorrhaphy.*

1. *Forceps Deliveries in Subsequent Labors.* (7 of 30 full-term deliveries or 23.3 per cent)

CASE 1.—Mrs. R., 24 years, one instrumental full-term stillbirth. Operation, divulsion and curettage, trachelorrhaphy, repair of pelvic floor, and appendectomy. Two years after operation, delivered at full term after manual dilatation of cervix and median forceps of a living baby boy weighing 7½ pounds. Presentation vertex R. O. A.

NOTE: Both the previous and subsequent deliveries were instrumental but the latter resulted in a live baby after the dystocia of cervix was overcome by dilatation.

In six cases, with instrumental deliveries in their subsequent pregnancies, all had had full-term pregnancies, before trachelorrhaphy, terminated by instruments. In four of these there were single previous full-term pregnancies which resulted in stillbirths although the subsequent pregnancies all resulted in live babies. Of these cases but three were re-examined and two showed a relaceration of the cervix. Of the remaining cases each with two previous pregnancies, one with an instrumental and spontaneous birth with subsequent instrumental delivery and the other with previous instrumental delivery and an abortion with subsequent instrumental delivery.

NOTE: In none of these was the duration of labor or the kind of operative delivery more severe than in previous deliveries and in a few, it was less severe. However, there was slight dystocia from the repaired cervix in over 42 per cent; in one manual dilation was done and in two there was relaceration of the cervix.

1. (a) *Elective Cesarean Section in Subsequent Labors.* (3 of full-term deliveries or 10 per cent)

CASE 1.—Mrs. D., twenty-six years, one full-term pregnancy, baby delivered by a forceps operation of long duration. Operation, divulsion and curettage, trachelorrhaphy, repair of pelvic floor, shortening of round ligaments and appendectomy. Two years later patient delivered, at term, by cesarean section because of extensive perineal and cervical repair following previous labor. The cervix showed no prospect of safe dilatation and there was a large unengaged head. Living male baby weighing 8 pounds and 11 ounces.

CASES 2 and 3.—These two sections were in successive pregnancies in the same patient. Mrs. A., thirty-four years, married ten years. Four full-term, normal deliveries. Operation, trachelorrhaphy, repair of pelvic floor, resection of left ovary and appendectomy. In the following three years patient was delivered twice, at term, by elective cesarean section for a large baby and a cervix which did not promise satisfactory dilatation and also to avoid possible extensive injury to the small parts.

NOTE: In all three of these cases there was an apparent dystocia due to the trachelorrhaphy.

2. *Hard Deliveries in Subsequent Labors.* (3 of 30 full-term labors or 10 per cent)

CASE 1.—Mrs. E., thirty-four years, married eighteen years. Four spontaneous full-term children and two abortions. Last child seven years ago and last abortion four years ago. Operation, divulsion and curettage, trachelorrhaphy and repair of pelvic floor. Subsequent labor was at full term and patient reported in her questionnaire that it was a "hard labor."

CASE 2.—Mrs. L., thirty years, married seven years. Four years ago a full-term 7 pound baby delivered by a spontaneous easy labor of two hours' duration. Operation, divulsion, curettage and trachelorrhaphy. Three years later or seven years after first pregnancy delivered of a 7½ pound baby by a long labor of twenty hours due to slow dilatation of cervix which was slightly lacerated.

CASE 3.—Mrs. C., twenty-two years, married four years, two full-term, normal spontaneous labors, last two years ago. Operation, curettage, trachelorrhaphy and removal of urethral caruncle. One subsequent full-term labor referred to by the patient as a "hard slow labor."

NOTE: Thus in the three cases in which previously only normal labors occurred there were subsequent hard labors. This was unquestionably due to a prolonged first stage due to slow dilatation of the cervix. In two a trachelorrhaphy alone was done and in the third a trachelorrhaphy and repair of pelvic floor.

3. *Easy Deliveries in Subsequent Labors.* (17 of 30 full-term deliveries or 56.7 per cent)

CASE 1.—Mrs. M., thirty-two years, married seven years. One full-term labor terminated by a hard instrumental delivery resulting in extensive cervical laceration and complete tear through the sphincter. During early months of her pregnancy the uterus was prolapsed. Subsequently patient had two abortions the last one followed by curettage. Operation, divulsion and curettage, repair of complete laceration of pelvic floor and trachelorrhaphy. Three years later delivered of male child weighing 7 pounds and 14½ ounces. Membranes ruptured spontaneously one hour before pains were established. Duration of labor two hours and thirty minutes.

Hemorrhage, sixteen ounces in amount, immediately after third stage. Inspection revealed a right lateral laceration of the cervix extending up into broad ligament, which necessitated immediate suturing with three chromic gut sutures to control the hemorrhage.

CASES 2 AND 3.—Both of these subsequent normal labors occurred in the same patient. Mrs. C., twenty-six years, married three years. One full-term labor of forty-eight hours' duration, which was terminated by forceps. This was followed by four spontaneous abortions. Operation, trachelorrhaphy, repair of pelvic floor, shortening of round ligaments and appendectomy. In the following five years there were two full-term labors. The first was normal and spontaneous but was followed by relaceration of the cervix. The second was a breech extraction of a 6 pound 2 ounce female baby. Duration of labor, 8 hours and 13 minutes.

NOTE: Of the above three subsequent deliveries the easy and short duration can be accounted for in the first by the relaceration instead of dilatation of the cervix, and the same thing can be said for the first labor of the second case. As to the third case the cervical repair had given away in the previous labor. Therefore it seems to me that there was dystocia due to the trachelorrhaphy.

Five of the remaining cases with instrumental deliveries in previous labors had subsequent easy or normal deliveries as follows: (a) Previous operative delivery, with stillbirth, and subsequent easy labor; (b) previous 27-hour instrumental delivery with subsequent 7- or 8-hour normal labor with relaceration of cervix; (c) previous instrumental delivery with a subsequent easy, normal labor; (d) previous instrumental delivery of 10 hours' duration and a premature, 8 months' baby, with a labor of 1 hour; subsequently a full-term spontaneous delivery of 2 hours' duration; (e) previous instrumental delivery of 24 hours' duration and a second pregnancy ending in an abortion with a subsequent premature delivery at the thirty-seventh week of gestation. Nine of the remainder of the seventeen cases had previous and subsequent normal or easy deliveries but one of these cases should be excluded as there had been a failure of the trachelorrhaphy due to secondary hemorrhage and secondary union.

NOTE: Of the 17 subsequent labors, one a premature following trachelorrhaphy, there is definite information in regard to relaceration in but 7, or 41.1 per cent. However, from this I am inclined to believe that the dystocia may not be apparent but that if all trachelorrhaphy cases were examined after subsequent easy labors, laceration would be more often found.

CONCLUSIONS

1. Amputation of the cervix and trachelorrhaphy are effectual and adequate operations and have a definite place in the gynecology of today.

2. Secondary hemorrhage and secondary union occur more often after trachelorrhaphy and are due rather to faulty technic than infection.

3. Improvement in the general health occurs in over 82 per cent of the cases for each operation but it is greater after amputation of the cervix.

4. Amputation of the cervix is more efficient than trachelorrhaphy in the cure of leucorrhea and dysmenorrhea but is more often the cause of these symptoms in cases previously free of vaginal discharge and menstrual pain.

5. Voluntary sterility is increased by cervical and vaginal plastic operations, but, all things being equal, there is 11 per cent greater sterility after amputation of the cervix than after trachelorrhaphy.

6. Amputation of the cervix is more often than trachelorrhaphy followed by interruption of labor before full term but is no more liable to end in premature labor than trachelorrhaphy. Abortion is more frequent after amputation in proportion to the number of high amputations.

7. Dystocia is greater after trachelorrhaphy both as to the number of operative deliveries and of difficult spontaneous labors.

8. With proper indications and technic, low, or medium amputation is as applicable as trachelorrhaphy to women in the childbearing age.

REFERENCES

(1) Emmet, T. A.: Am. Jour. Obst., February, 1869; ibid., November, 1874; ibid, November, 1897. (2) Hirst, B. C.: Atlas of Operative Gynecology, p. 85. (3) Crossen, H. S.: Operative Gynecology, 1920, ed. 2, p. 251. (4) Eden and Lockyer: New York, ed. 2, p. 819. (5) Anspach, B. H.: Gynecology, 1920. (6) Graves, W. P.: Gynecology, 1920, ed. 2, p. 599. (7) Sturmdorf, A.: Gynoplastic Technology, 1919, pp. 28-31. (8) Leonard, V. N.: Surg., Gynec. and Obst., 1913, xvi, 390; 1914, xviii, 35. (9) Goodell and Emmet: See Leonard: Surg., Gynec. and Obst., 1914, xvii, 35. (10) Duncan, Matthew: Sterility in Women, London, 1919.

350 WEST EIGHTY-EIGHTH STREET.   (*For discussion, see vol. ii, p. 652.*)

DIABETES AND PREGNANCY*

BY JOHN N. BELL, M.D., F.A.C.S., DETROIT, MICH.

THE subject, diabetes and pregnancy, is brought before the Association for discussion in the hope that we may arrive at some more definite conclusions regarding the prognosis and treatment.

INCIDENCE

If we are to judge from what appears in the standard textbooks on obstetrics relative to this subject, pregnancy complicating a true diabetes is a rare condition, Williams in 1909 being able to collect only 66 cases in the medical literature. It is quite conceivable, however, that many cases may have died in coma supposedly uremic, when, in reality, the condition was an unrecognized diabetic coma, since a hyperglycemia may exist with a high renal threshold and no glycosuria. Most textbooks dispose of this subject by stating that it is a very grave complication of pregnancy and give a gruesome picture with a maternal mortality of approximately 30 per cent and a fetal mortality of 50 per cent or higher.

The writer believes these figures, with our present understanding

---
*Read at the Thirty-Fourth Annual Meeting of the American Association of Obstetricians, Gynecologists and Abdominal Surgeons, St. Louis, Mo., September 20-22, 1921.

and treatment of this condition, must be materially modified, as these percentages were based on the old time treatment of diabetes when no blood chemistry tests were made. It is my purpose to discuss more especially the true diabetes of pregnancy or, perhaps, it might be better to say pregnancy complicating a true diabetes, and to cite two cases occurring in my practice recently in which the outcome illustrates quite clearly the importance of the modern treatment of true diabetes. In order to arrive at a clear understanding of what constitutes a true diabetes in a pregnant woman, a brief discussion of the different types of glycosuria may not be amiss at this time.

Lactosuria, as is well known, is a condition in which milk sugar is found in the urine and is due to resorption of milk from the breasts and its excretion by the kidneys. It can be distinguished from grape sugar by the fact that Fehling's solution can be reduced after the fermentation test has been applied.

Alimentary glycosuria is a condition sometimes called "physiologic glycosuria" where grape sugar is found in the urine especially in the latter months of pregnancy, but the characteristic symptoms of a true diabetes, such as furuncles, pruritus, thirst, etc., are absent. It is due to an excessive ingestion of starches and sweets in the diet and disappears promptly when these are withheld.

Renal diabetes is a condition where there exists: I. A fairly constant glycosuria not affected by carbohydrate intake, thus distinguishing it from alimentary glycosuria. II. Absence of symptoms of diabetes. III. A *normal* blood-sugar content. In these cases glycosuria is more or less constant in each pregnancy, but the sugar disappears promptly from the urine after delivery.

Diabetes mellitus is differentiated from the other types of glycosuria in that a hyperglycemia is present together with the characteristic symptoms of true diabetes—thirst, pruritus, etc., thus distinguishing it from the so-called renal diabetes.

Obviously, therefore, when confronted with a glycosuria in a pregnant woman our first concern should be to determine whether or not we are dealing with a hyperglycemia. This may be done by a careful inquiry into the patient's family and personal history, applying the regular tests for the milder forms of glycosuria and a careful blood-sugar estimation, in order to determine if the renal threshold has been passed and sugar is being poured out in the urine.

If it is found that we have one of the milder forms of glycosuria to deal with, we may rest assured the case will terminate favorably with the ordinary attention to diet, and, in the renal type, an occasional blood ratio test. Should, however, the case prove to be one of hyperglycemia, the question then arises: Shall we terminate the gestation or attempt to carry the patient to term by instituting the Allen-Joslin treatment or some modification?

I desire to report the two following personal cases, of which the first illustrates a decidedly happy outcome for both mother and child; while in the second, death of the child occurred *in utero* at term.

CASE 1.—Was that of a young woman, age twenty-six, primipara, weighing 140 pounds, apparently in perfect health, five months pregnant, personal history negative, except for childhood diseases. About the sixth month of her gestation she developed a glycosuria. On careful inquiry it was found that her father was a diabetic and that the patient had shown a trace of sugar in her urine when about seventeen years of age. This, however, had disappeared and she was in excellent health up to the time of her marriage. The glycosuria did not respond readily to the withholding of the carbohydrates and she was placed in the hospital under the care of a competent internist.

Unfortunately the blood-sugar ratio was not determined until she had been three days in the hospital. It was then .165 per cent. Following three days' starvation treatment the glycosuria dropped from a 4+ to 1+ and on the twelfth day the blood sugar was .12 per cent. After about three weeks green vegetable and fat treatment with an occasional allowance of oatmeal, she reached a tolerance of 1333 calories and was allowed to go home, but was requested to report daily the condition of her urine and to adhere rigidly to the modified diet. She entered the hospital again at term feeling perfectly well, with a trace of sugar in the urine and a 2+ albumin. Blood sugar .15 per cent. Labor was induced by the administration of 1½ ounces of castor oil. She was delivered under gas-oxygen anesthesia, low forceps and mediolateral episiotomy. At no time after delivery did she show any signs of coma and both mother and child made a normal recovery, except that the mother has a persistent mucoid vaginal discharge which resists all treatment. The urine (5 months after delivery) is free from sugar and she has lost about 10 pounds in weight. At birth, the baby's blood and urine were negative for sugar and now, at five months, she is a perfectly normal child. It seems fair to presume this to be a case of pregnancy complicating a mild diabetes mellitus. This patient had shown grape sugar in the urine prior to her marriage and there may have been an inherited tendency toward diabetes; her father being a true diabetic for many years.

The favorable outcome in this case, I am inclined to believe, was due to careful supervision and modern treatment. The case is reported with the hope that obstetricians may be led to take a more optimistic view of this complication of pregnancy and report their experiences, so that in the future we may be able to have sufficient data on which to base a more definite and encouraging prognosis. It will be noted on referring to the accompanying chart that the urine sugar was + when the blood sugar was .165 and did not decrease when the blood sugar was .12, thus suggesting a low renal threshold.

CASE 2.—Is quite another picture. A primipara, age thirty-seven, weighing 180 pounds, of full habit, consulted me in her eighth month of gestation; she gave a negative history, except for childhood diseases. Urine free from sugar and albumin up to within three weeks of term, at which time she developed a trace of sugar. Supposing it to be an alimentary glycosuria, I placed her on a restricted diet, eliminating the carbohydrates. She responded promptly, and the next specimen of urine was free from sugar. She remained on the restricted diet, but one week before term the sugar reappeared in the urine. A blood sugar estimation was now made and it was found she had a mild hyperglycemia, 138 mg. to the 100 c.c. Her urine at this time showed .432 per cent sugar. Patient felt perfectly well; the child was

BELL: DIABETES AND PREGNANCY

CHART OF CASE 1.

DATE	C.C. VOL.	SP.GR.	REACT.	ALB.	SUGAR	GR. NH₃	SUGAR	N.C.N	URIC	FAT	WGT.	B.P.	CARB.	PROT.	FAT	CALOR
													House diet			
1- 8-21	1018	Alk.	****							142	124/76					
1- 9-21	1020	Ampho	Tr.										5%	23	18	285
													Starvation			
1-10-21	1020	Acid	—	***	.25							10.5	31.5	29	420
1-11-21	1018	Acid	—	**								72.5	57	29	775
1-12-21	1019	Acid	—	(—)	.46	.165	25	4.3	.857	138½		72.5	57	29	775
1-16-21	1017	Acid	—	**	.32					140½		64	52	29	915
1-17-21	1020	Acid	—	*	.44	.12	20			139⅔		72.5	50.5	52	1133
1-21-21	1019	Acid	—	*	.46							57	50.5	70	775
1-23-21	1018	Acid	—	*								60	60	80	1133
1-27-21	1020	Acid	—	**	.24					138½		70	69.5	90	1260
1-29-21	1016	Acid	—	**								65	70	90	1333
1-30-21	1013	Acid	—									65	70	90	1333
2- 1-21	1014	Acid	—	—								65	70	90	1333
2- 2-21	1014	Acid	—	—			Return to Hospital									
							20				120/87	77	38	24	674
4-20-21	360	1012	Acid	**	*		Day following delivery					64	26	20	540
4-22-21		1020	Acid	**	Trace	.15	21				140/90	74	58	73	1183
4-27-21	1024	1020	Acid	—	—	.15				.70		66	45	96	1330
5- 1-21	1728	1020	Acid	—	Trace	.38						74	53	102	1420
5- 4-21	1696	1020	Acid	—	Trace	.21	Home					89	74	92	1615
5- 6-21																

Delivery—Gas Oxygen—Low Forceps—Medio-lateral episiotomy. Baby's urine neg. for sugar.

living and active. She reported again at term, feeling in the best of spirits, but on auscultation and palpation it was found the child was dead *in utero*. Labor was induced with Voorhees' bag, the patient making an uninterrupted recovery. The urine still shows a marked trace of sugar. On more careful inquiry into her history before marriage it was found that she had, at times, been troubled with a vulvar pruritus and thirst; but she had never consulted a physician.

This case, I believe to have been one of a long standing mild hyperglycemia with a high renal threshold as it was an easy matter to render the urine free from sugar by simply withholding the carbohydrates, and a more favorable outcome might have resulted had the true condition been determined and proper treatment instituted earlier in her pregnancy.

In conclusion permit me to suggest: 1. That a more careful prenatal history be taken in all obstetric patients. 2. That a blood-sugar estimation be made in all cases in which symptoms of diabetes are present regardless of the presence or absence of glycosuria. 3. That a fair trial of the newer forms of treatment of diabetes be instituted before terminating the pregnancy.

The writer is indebted and deeply grateful to Dr. O. C. Foster, Chief Resident in Obstetrics, Harper Hospital, for valuable assistance in the preparation of this paper.

1149 DAVID WHITNEY BUILDING. (*For discussion, see p. 77.*)

HEART DISEASE IN PREGNANCY[*]

By W. G. DICE, M.D., F.A.C.S., TOLEDO, OHIO

JUST as the examination of thousands of men for the army revealed, as never before, the presence of heart murmurs that did not mean organic disease of the heart, so the careful examination of women during pregnancy shows that many women have or are developing murmurs which are not dependent on heart lesions.

There are certain changes that take place within the heart and circulation during pregnancy which are familiar to all: In the early months, the quickening of the pulse; by the sixth month, the shortness of breath on exertion; and by the seventh or eighth month, the encroachment of the enlarging uterus upon the diaphragm alters the shape of the chest, broadens it out at the lower rib edge, and with the widening of the chest circumference, the heart is displaced upwards, frequently to an inch beyond the nipple line, and the apex is pushed up to the fourth interspace. At this period, also, the pressure of the heavy uterus sometimes gives rise to more or less extensive edema and varicosities of the legs. Formerly we were taught that the heart hypertrophied during pregnancy; but more careful observations and study with x-rays disprove this.

---

[*]Read at the Thirty-Fourth Annual Meeting of the American Association of Obstetricians, Gynecologists and Abdominal Surgeons, St. Louis. Mo., September 20-22, 1921.

With all these changes there arise physiologic or functional murmurs in 40 per cent of pregnant women; and, unless properly interpreted, they may lead to undue anxiety on the part of the physician and, consequently, unwise advice to the patient. No cardiac irregularity or murmur is, of itself, an evidence of heart disease.

Newell states that valvular lesions, the result of chronic endocarditis, can be demonstrated in from 1.5 to 2.5 per cent of all pregnant women, the percentage varying according to the interpretation put upon the presence of murmurs.

The mortality from the various heart lesions differs greatly: Mitral stenosis gives the highest mortality, 50 per cent; uncompensated aortic disease, which is rare in pregnancy, 25 per cent; while mitral regurgitation, with no previous break in compensation, shows an almost negligible mortality under proper care in young and vigorous patients. However, the actual mortality does not tell the whole story in these cases with true organic lesions; for, whereas the patient may survive the pregnancy and labor, the extra strain thrown upon the heart during gestation, is often the beginning of years of invalidism, or the heart is left so crippled that the patient succumbs to later intercurrent disease from which she otherwise might have recovered.

An acute endocarditis arises rarely in pregnancy as the result of some septic process, such as acute articular rheumatism, influenza, tonsillitis, or other infectious disease; but when it does occur, it is always a serious complication; occurring late in pregnancy it may prove fatal; or, if it happens early, will lead to an abortion. Late in pregnancy, as a result of toxemia, an acute dilatation of the right heart may take place, where in addition to the increased blood pressure and albuminuria, there are added edema of the lungs, cyanosis, and valvular murmurs.

In a recent case, seen in consultation, this condition occurred and the patient, at the time, was *in extremis*. She weighed 230 pounds, had a blood pressure of 160, pulse was irregular and rapid; she was unable to lie down for the previous two weeks; she was cyanosed and gasping for breath. A cesarean section was quickly performed under gas and oxygen, with the patient in a semireclining position. A living child was delivered. The mother was in a critical condition for several weeks, but ultimately made a good recovery. She now does her usual work and no murmur can be heard.

More frequently there come to us patients with a history of a heart murmur, or some form of heart trouble, the result of a previous infection. Every one of these cases requires the most painstaking examination, along lines that will later be explained, to determine the efficiency of the heart and the actual condition present. In taking the history of every obstetrical patient, careful inquiry should be made as to any past infection which may have damaged the heart valves or muscle, and yet show no symptoms during ordinary life, but which might give rise to symptoms later under the burden of pregnancy and labor. Pregnancy imposes more work on the heart in maintaining the placental and the general circulation against the increased intraabdominal pressure and the augmented body weight (20 to 50 pounds), which the ordinary patient puts on during gestation. It is this which reveals the myocardial inefficiency during the later months of pregnancy.

Patients with a history of heart murmur or cardiac disease, come to consult us, occasionally, as to the advisability of marriage and childbearing; but more frequently they come after marriage, already pregnant, and with a history of previous heart trouble. Even when they have consulted a physician as to childbearing, they are often ill advised; the physician making only a cursory examination, not appreciating all the dangers ahead in certain lesions. A case, now under observation, came after the fourth month of pregnancy with beginning decompensation from mitral stenosis; yet, she had been advised that she might have two or three children if she so desired.

One should remember that a sound heart may have a murmur; it may be physiologic or functional and, therefore, innocent; but it is important for the patient's peace of mind, as well as our own, that we carefully differentiate the harmless from the dangerous murmurs. The significance of a murmur is based on the functional efficiency of the heart and on the presence or absence of other symptoms of cardiac disturbance. Detection of a mitral systolic murmur or any other murmur, a mitral being the most frequent, should cause us to consider carefully the pulse rate, its rhythm, and the size of the heart; if the response of the heart to effort is good and the size of the heart is not increased, then the murmur is of no significance; and if the heart is enlarged and there is good response to effort, then pregnancy may be allowed. If the heart is hypertrophied and the response to effort is limited, pregnancy requires most careful watching. If there is any question in regard to the advice that should be given, a competent heart specialist should be consulted.

Physiological heart murmurs, according to MacKenzie, are always systolic in time, and it is impossible to tell the origin of most of them; they may be louder at the apex, base, or midsternum, and may vary with respiration or posture; sometimes they are heard when lying down and disappear when rising, or *vice versa*. As a rule functional murmurs are systolic in time and are heard with equal clearness over different parts of the heart. The murmur is usually soft and blowing; there is no accentuation of the second pulmonic sound; they may increase or decrease during pregnancy, or may come and go.

A rough murmur, especially if accompanied by a purring tremor or a musical note, is indicative of a valve lesion; the transmission of the murmur is important; in actual organic murmurs, the smaller the leak, the louder the murmur. Bearing all these things in mind, the physician, in advising a cardiopath as to marriage and childbearing, should make certain that the heart is defective and should then endeavor to determine the efficiency of the heart. Every case of heart disease should be painstakingly studied and treated on its own merits.

Burckhardt and others have called attention to the importance of a continuously low blood pressure, or pulse pressure, as a symptom of an inefficient heart muscle; a muscle that is able to meet the demands of ordinary life, may give way under the strain of labor.

Webster has said that it is a safe generalization that a woman with a chronic cardiac lesion, i.e., valvular or myocardial degeneration has, *ceteris paribus*, a shorter life expectancy if she becomes pregnant than if she does not, and the risk increases with successive pregnancies. One sees, occasionally, a patient with a definite organic heart lesion go through one, or several, pregnancies with no more discomfort than the average patient.

Heart failure is a question of myocardial efficiency. The force of the heart is of two kinds, rest and reserve force. The former is the force of the heart when the individual is at rest; the reserve force is called into play when effort is made. Heart failure begins by a diminution of the reserve force, and shows itself by a limitation of the power of the heart to respond to effort. The first sign of heart failure is the patient's consciousness that efforts, formerly made with ease and comfort, now cause distress. As has been said above, during pregnancy a healthy heart may show such a symptom from the burden of pregnancy, the encroachment of the uterus upon the diaphragm, the increased body weight, etc.; but, usually, there is not much danger, unless there is some previously unrecognized myocarditis. But this symptom, when due to heart failure, does not subside as quickly as when the heart is normal.

In beginning heart failure from organic disease the patient is apt to notice first, as MacKenzie puts it, "breathlessness with its associated phenomena in consequence of the stimulation of the respiratory reflex, and she complains next of pain and its associated phenomena in consequence of exhaustion of the heart muscle." The breathlessness is due to the failure of the heart to supply sufficient blood to the respiratory center, while the pain is due to the insufficient blood supply to the heart muscle.

Any woman who has suffered from these two symptoms during ordinary life should be advised against childbearing; or, if pregnant, it is advisable to empty the uterus early in most instances, otherwise she will more than likely abort, and her heart will be left in still worse condition; or, if allowed to go on, and decompensation occurs, she is apt to lose her life.

If a patient with definite heart lesion has never had failure of compensation, and if her age is such that she is apt to have good recuperative powers in the event of possible decompensation, and if the lesion is a mitral regurgitation and not a stenosis, she may be permitted to become pregnant, or, if pregnant, may be allowed to continue; but she should be told the whole story of the importance of taking care of herself and of keeping under careful supervision, not only throughout the pregnancy, but for some time thereafter. Therefore, the valvular lesions of themselves do not constitute a bar to pregnancy, but rather the manner in which the circulation is and has been maintained.

Every patient with a history of cardiac trouble should be most painstakingly examined before and after exercise; she should also be examined in the morning after a night's rest before rising, so as to determine whether there are signs of passive congestion at the base of the lung on the side upon which she has been lying. If there are some subcrepitant râles audible in this region, and these râles disappear after one or two deep inspirations, they are of no significance; but if the râles persist, and there is a change in the percussion note of that side, it is an evidence of inefficient heart muscle, and pregnancy should be forbidden, or, if present, it should be interrupted. Many heart cases will do fairly well until the sixth or seventh month of pregnancy; then, when digestive disturbances and abdominal distention give rise to pressure, or toxic symptoms set in, the heart is embarrassed.

Other factors also enter into the question of allowing pregnancy, or the continuation of a pregnancy, in these cases. As intimated above, the valve involved and the condition of the heart muscle are of importance; also the patient's general health, habits, and social status must be considered in determining the course to be pursued.

If the patient is poor and unable to have sufficient help with her work, or if she has other children to care for, the strain of pregnancy will be greater than if she is able to enjoy ease and comfort. One of the greatest difficulties with which the physician has to contend, is to make cardiopaths realize that they are cripples, more so than if they were minus a leg and compelled to use a crutch or cane. Because the symptoms are more or less subjective, they do not appreciate that they come from overtaxing the heart, and so are rebellious at the restrictions we put on their efforts.

During pregnancy a cardiopath requires more careful watching than a normal case, for the patient is more prone to toxemia and the digestive functions are more easily disturbed; she requires plenty of fresh air, a restricted diet, and most careful supervision of bodily exercise, so that she may not overtax her heart. One must be ever on the alert, especially in the later months of pregnancy, for the first symptoms of impending heart failure. If inefficiency of the heart muscle is evident, the patient should at once be put to bed and every effort made to restore the circulation. If the pulse rate is much increased digitalis in sufficient dosage to slow the pulse should be given. In auricular fibrillation the best results are obtained from digitalis, for here the heart failure is associated with rapid pulse rate, and many of the beats are inefficient.

While digitalis slows the heart, the individual beats are stronger and more effective. One should give sufficient dosage to obtain results. In a recent case one dose of 60 minims was given, followed by 30 minims every three hours until the pulse fell to 80, and was then stopped on account of nausea, to be resumed as soon as possible in smaller doses. Usually, one needs to give only 15 to 20 minims every three or four hours, for from four to seven days, to bring the pulse down to 60 or 70 per minute. Symptoms of overdose of digitalis are nausea, vomiting, and diarrhea, with a feeling of tightness across the chest and a drop in the pulse rate. Patients should avoid everything that might throw a strain on the heart, like mental worry, straining at stool, digestive disturbances, etc. They should also have small frequent meals, and mild hypnotics for sleep, if needed.

The course for further action, must depend on the period of pregnancy and whether there is a history of past broken compensation. If early in pregnancy, as soon as compensation has been reestablished the uterus should be emptied, unless the heart responds promptly to treatment. If the patient realizes the risk of continuing the pregnancy and can take the best of care of herself, and is willing to take the chance, then pregnancy may be allowed to continue, though frequently the child is lost anyhow through prematurity. If there is a history of previous decompensation, the outlook for going through the pregnancy safely is bad. If the lesion is a mitral stenosis or a chronic myocarditis, the chances of the heart bearing the strain of the later months of pregnancy and labor is small. In mitral stenosis the termination of pregnancy is indicated when edema of the lungs persists in spite of sitting up in bed, or if the pulse remains over 100 with palpitation on effort.

As stated above, mitral stenosis is the most serious heart lesion; it is usually due to rheumatic endocarditis, and is not often noticed during the acute stage of the illness, because the stenosis does not begin until cicatrization has narrowed the orifice, and because the lesion is progressive.

If in any heart lesion decompensation occurs late in pregnancy, and if, by careful treatment and nursing, there is hope of securing a viable child, pregnancy may be allowed to continue; but as soon as labor begins, everything must be done to reduce muscular strain. The treatment to be adopted will depend upon whether the patient is a primipara or a multipara, the condition of cervix and perineum, and the size of the child. If she be a primipara, a cesarean section will prove the best procedure. When heart failure is so pronounced as to threaten life, immediate intervention is necessary. If premature labor does not set in, and even this is dangerous, a prompt hysterotomy will often save the life of both mother and child. In these extreme cases the heart failure is shown by the dropsy, enlarged liver, edema at the base of the lungs, and cyanosis. Each day the pregnancy continues is fraught with danger. The patient's condition is desperate whether the pregnancy continues or not.

Ether is not a safe anesthetic. One should choose between gas and oxygen or a local anesthetic, as advocated by Webster. In any case in which a cesarean is done, sterilization should be performed to prevent subsequent pregnancy. In a case with a definite heart lesion, without broken compensation, one must realize that labor may bring on heart failure, and labor must be so conducted as to save the heart in every way. Morphine and scopolamine should be given during the first stage to quiet the patient and assist in dilatation of the os. As soon as the cervix is dilated or dilatable, a version should be performed, or the forceps applied, to shorten the second stage.

Death of the mother may occur after the delivery of the child, or during or after the third stage of labor, from the change in the intra-abdominal pressure and consequent overdistention of the right heart. To forestall this, some have advised the gradual removal of the placenta, thus allowing a rather free loss of blood. Unless the loss of blood is too free, one should avoid the use of pituitrin and ergot. The use of sandbags weighing from 25 to 50 pounds has been advocated in order to maintain the intraabdominal pressure; but, at all events, a tight abdominal binder and compress should be applied and the patient most carefully watched after she is returned to bed.

During the puerperium prolonged rest in bed, with appropriate medication, is indicated. The patient's activities for weeks must be carefully supervised. The question of nursing the child will be determined by the patient's general condition, especially the condition of the heart and her natural recuperative powers. Patients who have gone through with no break in compensation are usually able to nurse, while those who have had decompensation will be better off when relieved of this added strain.

CONCLUSIONS

During pregnancy no cardiac murmur or irregularity is of itself an evidence of heart disease.

Pregnancy lessens the life expectancy of any woman with a chronic valvular or muscular lesion.

Valvular lesions of themselves do not constitute a bar to pregnancy; but the manner in which the heart does its work is all important.

Every cardiopath is a cripple, and her treatment throughout pregnancy and labor must be such as to spare the heart in every way.

Cesarean section gives the best results in uncompensated cases and in those cases where heart failure threatens during labor.

240 MICHIGAN STREET. (*For discussion, see p.* 78.)

THE BREAST PHYSIOLOGICALLY AND PATHOLOGICALLY CONSIDERED WITH RELATION TO BLEEDING FROM THE NIPPLE*

By Gordon K. Dickinson, M.D., F.A.C.S., Jersey City, N. J.

THE breast is the most restless and susceptible of organs, being influenced by hormones, toxins and the psyche, intended by Nature to functionate in a cycle as a secondary sexual organ. It is composed of converted dermal basal cells, supported by a soft hyaline connective tissue.[1]

Hyperemia is induced monthly by the ovarian secretion, and, if pregnancy ensues, the hormones, sent out from the placenta, activate the gland to further growth[2] and the formation of colostrum, which has, according to Robertson,[3] the same effect when reabsorbed as the secretion of the hypophysis, determining the time of labor. With weaning, the breast returns to a quiescent state, but not as before.

It might be said that the breast yearns for normal function, that every bosom will tend to pathologic states of the tumor type, as will also the uterus and ovary, if the natural cycle be interfered with. If, perchance, abortion occurs, particularly the self-induced, the tissues of the breast are shocked, and a woman who has suffered repeated abortions has a breast more prone to the formation of tumors with malignant tendencies, for she who suppresses or defies Nature is penalized.[4]

In certain people suppression of the menstrual flow may produce an active congestion of the breasts with pain, tenderness, and sometimes bleeding. In my early practice I can recollect a woman, well

---

*Read at the Thirty-Fourth Annual Meeting of the American Association of Obstetricians, Gynecologists and Abdominal Surgeons, St. Louis, Mo., September 20-22, 1921.

nourished, and not of the neurotic type, whose flow was suppressed for some unknown reason. Her bosoms were large, overhanging, and there was excoriation of the skin underneath. At the time she should menstruate there would be an oozing of blood from this excoriation and, occasionally, a discharge of blood from the nipple. After a year or so the menses were reestablished and the phenomenon ceased. This case was in the dim past when notes were not taken, but the mental recollection is, I think, accurate. Literature ascribes to dysmenorrhea the same condition of bleeding, which we believe to be a fiction.

It is recorded that there is also a response in conditions of metritis, parametritis, and ovarian tumors. Lane[5] claims that the breast, particularly the upper outer lobe, will harden when there is present what he calls "fecal blood." Lockwood[6] has had a similar condition in a case of infective vaginitis and another in cholecystitis, the hyperplastic process in the bosom disappearing with relief of these conditions.

The instability of the breast is also seen as the woman ages, the breast of puberty passing over to the full-formed condition of adolescent life, then with menopause there is recession, more or less complete, with increased tendency towards pathologic changes. With the psychic states of love and its expressions in prolonged courtship, the breast often responds with alteration in its tissue substance. So we see that this organ responds, normally and abnormally, to diverse conditions with a low margin of normality.

Before thirty-five years of age the most common tumor found in the breast is the fibroid, which is an overgrowth of the hyaline connective tissue, discreet, movable under the skin and, occasionally, accompanied by slight but sharp pain. It is considered benign. We have had one case in which its irritation was sufficient to produce a bloody discharge from the nipple. These fibromas sometimes seem to be neuropathic, for we have known them to disappear when the exciting cause, psychopathic or otherwise, passed away. They then soften and become a natural part of the bosom.

After thirty-five years of age, the fibrous tissue grows into and includes areas of the breast substance. These tumors are in the periphery, often slightly tender, occasionally associated with pain, and if they remain benign, they are not apt to grow. In a somewhat larger percentage of cases than the fibroid, irritation and hyperemia are sufficient to produce a blood-stained discharge. We have had several instances of this.

Occasionally the lining of the ducts will proliferate and form papillomas. They are always well supplied with blood and the normal movements of the breast will rub off the surface and produce hemorrhage. This type of growth is the most common cause of bleeding from the nipple. It is to the duct what warts are to the skin, and may exist for many years, bleeding without becoming malignant. According to Bloodgood,[7] it would be inferred that the tendency to malignancy is slight enough not to be seriously considered, while Rodman[8] claims the dangers of malignant changes are great. We have had a number of cases of this type, and, in the majority of them, the microscope has shown that the cells at the base had begun to wander and other evidences of malignancy were demonstrable.

Sometimes the ducts will become occluded by constriction and distended with a clear serous fluid. It is often difficult to differentiate between a cyst and a fibroadenoma. Tapping will establish a diagnosis. These cysts are prone, however, to have small papillomas on the surface which, not being rubbed or irritated, are not given to hemorrhages. They possess the same tendency to malignancy as the first-mentioned type, which occurs nearer the nipple.

It is now believed by pathologists that tumor formation in the mammae is a type of chronic inflammation. We know that the breast excretes germs from the blood and also that germs can pass up through the ducts of the nipple and into the tissues of the breast. We have referred to the findings of Lockwood, where vaginitis and cholecystitis were associated with temporary hyperplasia of the mammary substances. Lane's investigations also tend to confirm this.

Curiously, the upper outer lobe, the left one in particular, is the portion more apt to be hardened and multicystic and the site of chronic interstitial change which, eventually, passes through the bosom and is known as chronic cystic mastitis. Why this particular lobe should be selected cannot be explained on embryonal or histologic grounds; but it seems to us possible that there is some correlation with the long-lost axillary breast, which comparative anatomy shows once existed, and which we now find occasionally as an anomaly; that the forces which led to the disappearance of this gland are acting upon the lobe which extended out toward it. This may be an idle opinion of the writer, nevertheless, it is the portion of the breast first affected. If we can discover and eliminate the cause, we may have recovery; if not, we have tissue changes where the basal cells are prone to go wild, lose their centresomes, undergo active mytosis irregularly, and escape through the poorly resisting hyaline connective tissue and develop carcinoma. Applegate[9] claims carcinoma is preceded by abnormal involution.

The wandering cell acts very much as a parasite, producing local inflammatory reaction, with formation of fibrous tissue. If the glandular substance be in excess, we have a soft cancer; if the fibrous, the scirrhus type, both equally malignant. We have noted hemorrhages from the nipple in both soft and hard types, but the blood is always mixed with serum so that the discharge is more sanious than bloody.

We feel that gratitude should be extended to the pathologists for the work done in the study of the breast; but, like all specialists, from a clinical viewpoint they have exceeded themselves in nomenclature, obscuring the clinical condition by the various names given to each pathologic stage. Not until Warren,[10] in 1905, simplified the classification of tumors was the clinician and the average surgeon able to grasp the subject intelligently. The register of the American College of Surgeons includes the names of several thousands of this cult, and we fear some may not think in terms of pathology; therefore, if we are to fight cancer and comprehend so-called precancerous conditions or, better stated, conditions which often develop into or are followed by carcinoma, we should give to those who operate a ready means for diagnosis by simplifying terminology.

Every surgeon hesitates to mutilate a woman, and particularly this organ, but every surgeon with a conscience will attack that which is or may become cancer. Benign means "born good," but all tumors of the breast, which have this title, are apt to go bad and are not to be trusted. As to their innocence there is no reliable sign or symptom. Bleeding from the nipple we see associated with them all at times, as well as with functional conditions, and we cannot always tell by naked eye appearances what we may find after removal. Sad experience has taught us to be prompt and thorough in operation.

Neither is there a reliable sign as to malignancy or beginning malignancy. The benign condition is apt to be but temporary. We see that blood coming from the nipple is neither diagnostic nor prognostic. We know from experience that the touch cannot differentiate between adenoma and beginning carcinoma. For frank malignancy Dr. Willy Meyer, in 1894, gave us a technic which has satisfied the time test; but for tumors only "born good," we have not as yet a definite plan of attack. Some surgeons resect in part; some do a complete plastic subcutaneous resection, and others a radical removal. Can we today say who does wisely?

REFERENCES

(1) *McCarthy*: Mayo's Clinics, 1915. (2) *Schaefer*: Endocrine Organs, 1916. (3) *Robertson*: Principles of Bio-Chemistry, 1920. (4) *Bryant*: Cyclopedia of Obstetrics and Gynecology, ix, 1887. (5) *Lane*: Personal Communication. (6) *Lockwood*: Diseases of the Breast, 1913. (7) Jour. Am. Med. Assn., Dec., 1913. (8) *Bodman*: Diseases of the Breast, 1908. (9) Sajou's Encyclopedia, 1921. (10) Jour Am. Med. Assn., July, 1905.

280 MONTGOMERY STREET. (*For discussion, see p. 78.*)

THE SLAUGHTER OF THE INNOCENTS*

By Palmer Findley, M.D., Omaha, Neb.

THE medical profession would do well to consider, seriously, some of the phases of the subject of criminal abortion. We should know what constitutes a criminal abortion in contradistinction to therapeutic abortion; we should inquire as to the extent of this nefarious practice; we should ask ourselves who are the offending parties; we should know how best to protect ourselves against unjust accusation when called upon to treat these cases after they have passed from the hands of the abortionist; and, finally, we should inquire into the responsibility of the profession in view of the widespread prevalence of this social plague.

The civil law clearly recognizes the right to interrupt pregnancy before the period of viability when the life of the mother is jeopardized by the continuation of pregnancy. To interrupt pregnancy prior to the period of viability for any reason other than to safeguard the life of the mother is a moral, ethical and legal crime. Yet in spite of all civil and ecclesiastical law this heinous crime has stealthily increased from the dawn of civilization to the present time.

We are told that one in five or six pregnancies ends in abortion, and that 50 per cent of all abortions are criminal. It has been estimated that in New York City alone there are 80,000 criminal abortions annually. The practice exists in all parts of the globe and infests all grades of society. Indeed, it would appear that this social plague is more prevalent in the higher classes of society. Women of keen moral sensibilities either commit the act themselves or seek aid from others with little knowledge of the dangers involved and with conscience undisturbed. This is so because of ignorance. They know little of the pitfalls involved in the undertaking and they are possessed of the sentiment, prevalent among the laity, that there can be no life until fetal movements are felt. To illustrate how difficult it is to convince the lay public that life begins at the moment of impregnation, the eminent German naturalist, Ernest Haeckel, relates how he once made this assertion to an eminent jurist only to be laughed at. We often find women of unquestioned moral standing bitterly resenting their state of pregnancy, and who are determined to put an end to the whole affair; yet, when the date of quickening arrives and they are conscious of sheltering and nourishing a human life, their viewpoint

---
*Read at the Thirty-Fourth Annual Meeting of the American Association of Obstetricians, Gynecologists and Abdominal Surgeons, St. Louis, Mo., September 20-22, 1921.

is completely changed, and from that moment to the date of birth they live in happy expectation.

But what of the professional abortionist who, for a few paltry dollars, will destroy a potential human life and place the life and health of a mother in grave danger? The woman abortionist, who plies her trade under the guise of a midwife, the charlatan, who covertly or openly advertises in the daily press, and the physician of high or low degree, who prostitutes his profession, all alike ply their nefarious trade unabashed and unrestrained; for not one in a thousand is ever held accountable for the crimes he commits. This is largely because of the technical difficulties in getting evidence admitted in the courts; partly because of embarrassment to any individual in filing a complaint, but more than anything else, because organized medical associations have not taken definite and determined steps to rid the profession of these criminals and to educate the lay public in the dangers involved in the practice of committing abortions. Lombrosa, the great criminologist, says that "abortions in the United States have become so common that, instead of being regarded as a crime, it is a laudable and justifiable means of limiting the size of families." And Lyons says: "if concerted action be taken against these men by the profession at large the evil might easily be overcome. The most of them are arrant cowards and as soon as they realize that men of undoubted professional reputation and standing are determined that they should cease plying their nefarious calling, they will stop." Be that as it may, we must admit that the profession assumes a grave responsibility when this most universal of crimes receives from its hands little more than passive condemnation. If we are to merit the respect and confidence imposed in our profession, a determined campaign should be inaugurated by our medical organizations to the end that the ignorant may be enlightened and offenders within our ranks be brought to the bar of justice. It is futile for the profession to transfer the responsibility to our civil authorities and it is not fair to assume that it is the business of individual members of the profession to handle the situation. The civil authorities may be depended upon to do their part, and the individual member of the profession, however courageous, will find little encouragement and much embarrassment if he fights alone. The individual may be charged with ulterior motives but, when action is taken by an organized medical association of the dignity of our state and county medical societies, the affair becomes impersonal and cannot fail to impress the public and the courts with the seriousness of the charge.

Because of the grave responsibility imposed upon the induction of abortion, it is provided that one or more consulting physicians shall be employed and shall agree upon the indication for the interruption of pregnancy. This is wise not only in the interest of the patient, but for the protection of the physician on whom the responsibility rests. But what are the safeguards to be established to protect the physician who is called to attend a woman on whom a criminal abortion has been done and who may be in a critical condition? The position of the physician in these cases is disagreeable; it is embarrassing and may prove disastrous to him if he fails to fortify himself with moral safeguards. He is charged with the double responsibility of doing all that can be done for his patient and of protecting himself against unjust accusation. He cannot afford to disregard the gossip, neither should he fail to protect himself against the real offender who would eagerly embrace the opportunity of shifting the responsibility for the misdeed. To this end, it would be a good rule, in such cases, to call a consultant for the initial examination and to witness the statement of the patient. The statement of the patient should best be in writing and should comprise a recital of her known condition prior to the abortion; when the operation was performed; where it was performed; how it was done, and by whom. If the patient is unwilling to divulge this information, then the physician would be justified in declining to assume the responsibility of the case. It is common experience that the patient will tell all she knows when made to realize her danger and a double purpose is attained—the physician in charge is protected and the guilty party is revealed.

BRANDEIS THEATRE BUILDING.   (*For discussion, see p. 81.*)

LEGAL ASPECT OF ABORTION*

BY ERNEST F. OAKLEY, JR., PROSECUTING ATTORNEY, ST. LOUIS, MO.

IT IS my desire at the outset to express to your Association the appreciation I entertain in accepting the honor you conferred by inviting me to address you. My subject as assigned is "The Legal Aspect of Abortion." Much has been written and still more will be contributed by pens mightier than mine on the several phases of this subject, approaching as it does, in my opinion, more intimately into the everyday practice of the physician and surgeon than any other single element of the ethics which guide you. I say, "In my opinion," and I might add that my opinion is based on experience acquired while an assistant State's attorney assigned to the office of the Coroner of the City of St. Louis; I formed the conviction that the majority of medical men are strongly imbued with the principles of the ethics of their profession, but I was impressed, however, with their lack of practical application of the principles of ethics, due, not to their desire

*Read by invitation at the Thirty-Fourth Annual Meeting of the American Association of Obstetricians, Gynecologists and Abdominal Surgeons, St. Louis, Mo., September 20-22, 1921.

to thwart the administration of justice, but rather to their professional hesitancy to divulge, under any conditions, matters between themselves and their clients, which they held sacredly privileged.

There has existed the necessity of informing your profession in this regard, to the end that greater cooperation may exist between you and the law-enforcement officials. To what extent you are privileged and what is your particular duty under the circumstances of a case presenting evidence of abortion, I shall endeavor to present the legal side.

State v. Shields, 230 Mo. 9, defines abortion as the delivery or expulsion of the human fetus prematurely or before it is yet capable of sustaining life. The same case is authority that the terms "abortion" and "miscarriage" do not of themselves import a crime.

Abortion has been made a crime by statute. At common law it was generally recognized as no offense to produce an abortion on a woman with her consent and before she was quick with child. It was not even murder at common law to take the life of the child at any period of gestation, even in the act of delivery. Today the several states have enacted laws holding the commission of an abortion a felony and punishable as such. The reason is obvious. Regardless of the law and the attendant opprobrium and ruin of exposure, abortion in its unlawful sense is practiced extensively in our country. It is with regret and an expression of condolence to the great majority of your profession, that I state the abominable and nefarious practice is not confined to those outside your ranks. There are renegades among you—as indeed exist in all circles—who for one motive or another, lend their skill to the commission of this crime.

The Statute of Missouri may be taken as a fair example of the law of the several states on the subject, and I quote and discuss Section 3239, Revised Statutes of Missouri, 1919.

"Sec. 3239. Manslaughter—producing miscarriage. Any person who, with intent to produce or promote a miscarriage or abortion, advises, gives, sells or administers to a woman (whether actually pregnant or not), or who, with such intent, procures or causes her to take, any drug, medicine or article, or uses upon her, or advises to or for her the use of, any instrument or other method or device to procure a miscarriage or abortion (unless the same is necessary to preserve her life or that of an unborn child, or if such person is not a duly licensed physician, unless the said act has been advised by a duly licensed physician to be necessary for such a purpose) shall in event of the death of said woman, or any quick child, whereof she may be pregnant, being thereby occasioned, upon conviction be adjudged guilty of manslaughter, and punished accordingly; and in case no such death ensue, such person shall be guilty of the felony of abortion, and upon conviction be punished by imprisonment in the penitentiary not less than three years nor more than five years, or by imprisonment in jail not exceeding one year or by fine not exceeding one thousand dollars, or by both such fine and imprisonment; and any practitioner of medicine or surgery, upon conviction of any such offense, as is above defined, shall be subject to have his license or authority to practice his profession as physician or surgeon in the state of Missouri revoked, by the state board of health in its discretion."

You will note that the gravamen of the offense is the intent to produce a miscarriage or abortion by administering drugs or using instruments. Also that the acts included within the statute coupled with the intent, constitute the offense. That when either the woman or quick child dies, the party responsible is chargeable with manslaughter. That when neither dies, the crime is designated "Felony of Abortion." The punishment in the former ranges from two to ten years in the penitentiary; in the latter, from three to five years in the penitentiary. In either case, the act is a crime whether the woman is pregnant or not, and in either case, the intent to produce miscarriage or abortion must be present.

The exceptions are where it can be shown beyond a reasonable doubt that the abortion was necessary to preserve the life of the expectant mother or unborn child; (a prima facie case of nonnecessity is complete by proof of the fact that the woman was in good health or her ordinary condition of health immediately prior to the abortion); or where the act has been so advised by a duly licensed physician. To this extent, is abortion as such, lawful, and would seem to be the rule generally. The moment the womb is instinct with embryo life and gestation has begun, the crime may be committed.

A Texas case in agreement with the Missouri law, holds that it is not necessary that the means employed should produce the effect desired. A physician's testimony is sufficient to show that the means employed are capable of producing an abortion. Cave v. State, 33 Texas Crim. 335.

A New Jersey case holds in point that the intent to produce the abortion may be present without knowledge or even strong belief that the woman is pregnant. State v. Poe, 48 N. J. Law 34.

Should the woman recover, she is a competent witness against the accused. In the event of her death, her dying declaration is equally competent. In State v. Stapp, 246 Mo. 338, defendant asked for an instruction to the effect that the fact that the prosecuting witness was implicated in the alleged transaction, be taken into consideration by the jury in determining the credibility to be given her testimony. The refusal of the trial court was one of the assignments of error. The Appellate Court held this instruction should not have been given, considering such an instruction useless, containing no legal proposition, and purely a comment on the evidence.

In this connection, Bishop on Statutory Crime declares:

"An accomplice swears under the temptation of earning thereby his own immunity, while the witness does not. She discloses her own disgrace, and where no evil motive appears for it, this fact may in reason strengthen her credibility."

State v. Jones, 197 S. W. (Mo.) is authority that a woman involved in a case of this character is not an accomplice.

The Missouri law regulating the admission in evidence of dying statements, and found in Section 4034, Revised Statutes, 1919, announces the principles of the general rule.

"Sec. 4034. PROSECUTIONS FOR ABORTIONS—DYING DECLARATIONS. In prosecutions for abortion or for manslaughter occasioned by an abortion or miscarriage, or by an attempt to produce either, or attempted abortion, or for any crime of which abortion or miscarriage may be a part of the essential facts to be proven, the dying declarations of the woman whose death is charged to have been caused thereby shall be competent evidence on trial of any person charged with such crime, with like effect and under like limitations as apply to dying declarations in cases of felonious homicide: PROVIDED, that the party offering such declarations shall first satisfy the court by competent testimony that such woman was of sound mind when such declarations were made: AND PROVIDED FURTHER, that no conviction shall be based alone upon such declarations unless corroborated as to the fact that an abortion or miscarriage has taken place, and in all such prosecutions aforesaid any physician or medical practitioner who may have attended or prescribed for such woman shall be a competent witness in said cause to testify concerning any facts relevant to the issue therein, and shall not be disqualified or held incompetent by reason of his relation to such woman as an attending physician or surgeon."

A dying statement made by the deceased is competent as evidence and admissible under certain conditions.

State v. Craig, 190 Mo. 339, announcing a rule generally followed, holds it must appear that the declaration was made under a sense of impending and immediate death, and that the declarant at the time believed that she had no hope of recovery.

State v. Walter Lewis, 264 Mo. 420, follows State v. Craig, supra, holding the admissibility of the declaration is dependent upon the declarant's belief of her impending dissolution at the time it is made, and not on the length of time that intervened between its making and her death.

In the several dying statements made to me, I adopted a rule to put two questions to the declarant, in the presence usually of the nurse. "Do you know that you are about to die?" "Have you abandoned all hope of recovery?" Receiving an affirmative answer, in each instance the declaration would be taken in shorthand, immediately transcribed and read to the declarant for her approval. She would be asked if that was her statement, and if her physical condition permitted, she would sign it.

A dying declaration in proper form, supported by the autopsy physician's testimony that an abortion had been performed, and that *causa mortis* was peritonitis superinduced by the criminal operation, constitute a prima facie against the accused.

As you gentlemen well know, a statement made by deceased to one of you in your professional capacity, is not admissible as evidence in a court of law. Such a communication is held as privileged. There are well-founded reasons for the existence of this rule, and no one would wish to disturb the confidential relation which exists, and necessarily so, between the medical man and his patient.

But the physician must not consider that he is without obligation in the premises. There is incumbent on him a strong moral duty common to all good citizens—a duty to assist in the investigation and punishment of crime. When it is ascertained by the physician that an illegal operation has been performed, he should at once inform the proper authorities of his findings, to the end that a statement, competent as evidence, can be secured from the woman, and introduced at the trial of the accused, in the event she herself is not produced as a living witness.

A medical man may be a recognized expert in his own field; but when he encounters a situation that partakes of a legal nature, he is apt to seek refuge in the accepted ethics of his profession, without first considering the question and possible consequence to himself. You can readily see that this attitude may lead to grave suspicion. I have in mind the following statement of facts as an illustration.

> At an inquest into the cause of death of Mrs. ———, it developed as a finding of the postmortem doctor, that an abortion had been produced. The family physician, who was in attendance on the case testified that when he was called, the woman was running a temperature, and suffering acutely from abdominal pains. On information elicited from her in private inquiry, he diagnosed the case as "probable blood-poisoning" and prescribed accordingly. The woman did not respond to treatment and died.
>
> Asked whether or not she had told him that a criminal operation had been performed, he refused to answer. Asked whether he had determined from his own examination of her, that a criminal operation had been performed, he again refused to answer. Asked whether he had reported the case to the authorities, he replied, "Not until the woman died."

Here, you see the palpable inconsistency of the physician's position. Although he had full knowledge of the circumstances, both from the woman herself, and his examination of her, he hesitated to notify the authorities, because he feared that thereby he would be violating a professional confidence; yet, rather than certify the cause of death, actuated by the same ethics, he considered it his duty to apprise the Coroner of the case; with what results? The facts which he had in good faith suppressed were brought out and made public at the inquest; the lips of the woman sealed in death could no longer speak the name of the person criminally responsible; the verdict—"Peritonitis—resulting from abortion, at hands of parties unknown to jury."

The physician, who in his heart, despised and condemned the wrongdoer, had, in fact, protected him. Justice had not been served.

Whatever qualms or misgivings the medical man may entertain in divulging such confidences, I submit to you, they must be subordinated to his natural desire and duty to assist the State in the apprehension and prosecution of the criminal.   *(For discussion, see p. 81.)*

TREATMENT OF ABORTION*

By H. Wellington Yates, M.D., F.A.C.S., and B. Connelly, M.D., Detroit, Mich.

THE series of abortion cases upon which this paper is based was taken from records of the gynecological division of the Receiving Hospital in Detroit, admitted from April 1st to August 15th, 1921. During these four and one-half months, we had 81 abortion patients, whose histories included 256 pregnancies, making the instance of abortion 1 to 3.1. It would seem that these figures are fairly conservative from our review of the literature.

A preponderance of cases occur during the second and first half of the third month, probably on account of the nutritional changes of the fetus, rapid development of the placenta causing marked circulatory changes, radical misplacements of the uterus, and criminal interference, which probably embraces 25 per cent.

It is interesting to note the different attitudes taken by members of the profession, together with those of our own Association, in the treatment of abortion.

The success in preventing abortion depends somewhat upon its cause. But, speaking in general, our failures have far outnumbered the successes. Abortions dependent upon diseases of malnutrition, such as tuberculosis, diabetes, or anemia, would suggest rest, feeding and proper environment, with suitable reconstructive medication. Women who show an aborting habit (stock men have this phenomenon constantly before them in animals), should be given one or two years' rest before conception is permitted. Absolute rest in bed ranging from a few days to several weeks may be necessary, together with morphine. The anodyne should be stopped at the earliest possible moment. Enemas should be used, when needed, instead of cathartics.

While lues is more often the cause of abortion in the later months, occasionally its results are seen early. I had a patient who was apparently in good health, but whose husband was Wassermann positive, who had 12 abortions, all spontaneous, before her full-time child was born. She has since had three more healthy children, but between all of them she has had numerous abortions, until they totaled 27. She was never seriously ill with any of them. She desired children, and submitted to medication and confinement to bed without complaint, for long periods of time. For the most part, her abortions occurred on the seventh week. Opiates, rest and uterine sedatives were valueless.

---
*Read at the Thirty-Fourth Annual Meeting of the American Association of Obstetricians, Gynecologists and Abdominal Surgeons, St. Louis, Mo., September 20-22, 1921.

I am inclined to believe that, given a patient who is an early syphilitic, both she and her husband should have intensive treatment until they are Wassermann negative in both blood and spinal fluid. We can with some hope look forward to healthy offspring, but with the old cases where the disease has become a part of their very being, pregnancy, when it does occur, should be interrupted. Treatment is of little avail.

There are times when good treatment demands emptying the uterus, as in hypertension and nephritic cases, especially when these evince their symptoms in the early months and are uninfluenced by other treatment. Then there is hyperemesis gravidarum and early incipient tuberculosis. We believe the complete operation done at one sitting is the method of choice, by either dilating and emptying the uterus or performing hysterotomy. The use of rubber bags and bougies, with the necessity of several replacements, appears to me unsurgical and dilatory, and even then, by virtue of an incomplete abortion, often requires later exploration.

When an abortion is complete, and we can be sure of it, rest in bed for seven to ten days, with a good full tray after the third day, is all that is required. There should be no mortality except as a result of hemorrhage during the abortion.

With incomplete abortion the sooner the uterus can be emptied with safety, the better. Much difference of opinion prevails on how this may best be done.

If the cervix is open, easily admitting a finger, and there is free bleeding, my procedure is to empty the uterus by means of the gloved finger under gas-oxygen anesthesia. Provided the mass cannot be thus withdrawn, a Longyear forceps is used for this purpose. We lay great stress on having these patients prepared as for cervical and perineal repair. When once the fingers, or if necessary, the whole hand is introduced, it should not be withdrawn until its purpose is achieved. At least we endeavor to manipulate as little as possible, and seek to avoid introducing anything from below. On the other hand, if there is free bleeding and the cervix closed and not easily dilatable, the patient afebrile, we pack the cervix, if possible, with a strip of iodoform gauze, and the vagina with sterile or borated gauze forced well up to the vault and allowed to remain for twenty-four hours. When withdrawn, the cervix is likely to be open, and often the products of conception are found expelled from the uterus. We freely confess, however, our inability to say whether this uterus is free from all products of conception, and feel more satisfied in our own minds when the index finger is the judge. Signs of infection, as manifested by chill, fever and sweating, are not the only symptoms that indicate trouble. Deciduitis, endometritis, and low grade infections with their consequences, are the results of retained products of conception, and our surgical sense tells us they should be removed.

When it becomes necessary to use instrumental means for dilatation, the Hegar sounds or graduated dilators are the best, especially in the presence of sepsis. They dilate equably and without trauma. This cannot be said of the Goodale type of instrument.

Barring criminal abortion, neglected incomplete abortion is the most potent factor in sepsis. One never has trouble with therapeutic abortions because they are made complete, but when products of conception, even though small, are left in the uterus, a sapremia results which provides fruitful culture media for the growth of pyogenic bacteria. It is the smaller pieces of placental tissue which are quite large enough to produce sepsis, but are more difficult for the uterus to expel than the larger ones. We remember the protective zone of leucocytes building up its barrier of safety, but we also know that early in the process this small placental fragment furnished the necessity for this reaction and the continuation for the same. Can anything be more logical than carefully removing this exciting cause? We dilate with graduated dilators, taking plenty of time and causing as little trauma as possible. If dilatation is enough, the index finger explores the interior; if not, the curved abortion forceps will take its place. We refrain from the use of the curette, if possible. Curettes have killed more persons than they have saved. Saturated iodinized gauze is packed into the uterus with care, allowed to remain for a moment and withdrawn. We never use intrauterine douches in septic abortion. Rest in bed, opiates, enemas to empty the bowel, with abundance of good food and large hot packs over the entire abdomen, constitute our more common methods of procedure. When the peritoneum is much involved, we morphinize to tolerance, raise the head of the bed, administer hypodermoclysis, glucose and soda bicarbonate by rectum, and liquids by mouth, as soon as they can be borne. Much has been said of electrargol. We have used it in 21, and phenol moniodide in 5 cases, with varying results, sometimes almost spectacular, and again disappointing.

No mortality should occur in spontaneous cases, unless through hemorrhage or the development of chorionepithelioma. The latter eventuality should always be in our thought. The morbidity which results from all kinds of abortions is appalling. The occurrence is progressively more common in the incomplete and septic cases. Complete abortions are often followed by ill health, as a result of hemorrhages, subinvolution, protracted weakness and displacements. It is unnecessary to note that criminal abortion enormously increases both mortality and morbidity, in consequence of the delay in seeking competent advice until the symptoms become pressing, and the infection passes beyond the confines of the uterus.

Taussig, quoting from the report of Sittner's Clinic, shows that in 267 abortions, not attended by fever, only one death occurred; but from 35 septic cases, 3 fatalities ensued, while figures from Maygriers' series gave a mortality in the spontaneous cases of 0.57 per cent, while that of criminal abortion was 56.8 per cent. Undoubtedly, abortion is the most mistreated of all gynecologic conditions.

As an inhibitive measure to criminal abortion, the physician has an opportunity to acquaint the patient with the sequelae of her contemplated act, especially in regard to the wrecking of her health. If she can be made to know that even if she were not to die, a life of invalidism and operations confronted her, she might hesitate though the moral argument failed to appeal to her. We have repeatedly found this explanation to be effectual.

SYNOPSIS OF CASES ADMITTED TO THE RECEIVING HOSPITAL, DETROIT, FROM APRIL 1 TO AUGUST 15

Incomplete septic abortions, 26; incomplete abortions, 23; complete abortions, 15; threatened abortions, 4; postabortal septicemia, 4; miscarriages, 4; postabortal chorionepithelioma, 1; total, 81.

Average days in hospital, 10.7 days; shortest period in hospital, 12 hours; longest period in hospital, 30 days; average age of patients, 26 years; oldest patient, 40 years; youngest patient, 15 years.

Causes.—In the 81 cases, 25 were self-induced; others were produced by midwives or other women. Four were produced by curettement in the doctor's office or patient's home. Others by falling, lifting, etc. Many given as cause unknown were undoubtedly criminal.

Complications. Uterine fibroids, 3; acute anteflexion, 2; cervical lacerations, 2; goitre, 2; acute gonorrhea, 2; follicular tonsillitis, 2; chronic endocervicitis, 2; secondary lues, 4; pulmonary tuberculosis, 1.

1229 DAVID WHITNEY BUILDING.   (*For discussion, see p. 81.*)

ADDITIONS TO OUR OBSTETRIC ARMAMENTARIUM*

BY CHARLES EDWARD ZIEGLER, M.D., F.A.C.S., PITTSBURGH, PA.

A NEW METALLIC NIPPLE SHIELD

THE shield shown in Fig. 1 is made of commercially pure aluminum and is perforated as indicated. Its base is 2½ inches in diameter; its dome on the inside is an inch in height, an inch in diameter at the bottom and ⅞ of an inch at the top. Its base is flared to conform to the convexity of the breast and is bordered by a rolled edge.

Metallic nipple shields "for the prevention and cure of sore nipples" are not new. Perhaps the best known is the lead shield invented by Dr. Wansbrough, an Englishman, and described by him in the London Lancet under date of July, 1842. This shield has been used extensively for more than half a century and is still in use; an illustration may be seen in De Lee's Obstetrics. Marvellous curative properties

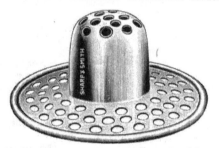

Fig. 1.

have been attributed to it. Wansbrough claimed that "its curative character consists in the nipple being immersed in a solution of lactate of lead formed by the lactic acid in the milk acting upon the metal."

It is more than likely that lactate of lead has had little to do with the good results obtained. The explanation is to be found rather in the protective character of the shield. Indispensable conditions for the treatment of the abraded, fissured, inflamed and sensitive nipple are: absolute rest of the part and its certain protection against traumatism of every sort, including that of the gown, bedclothing, binder, and occlusive dressings. These conditions the protective shield provides.

If it were possible to carry it out in practice, the "open-air treat-

---

*Read at the Thirty-Fourth Annual Meeting of the American Association of Obstetricians, Gynecologists and Abdominal Surgeons, St. Louis, Mo., September 20-22, 1921.

ment" would undoubtedly give good results. Occlusive dressings, in addition to the traumatism which they cause, favor the accumulation of moisture and maceration of the epithelium. Hardly secondary in importance, therefore, is the ventilation of the affected nipple.

Whatever differences of opinion there may be in regard to local applications to the nipples, this shield takes care of them. It effectually prevents the application from being rubbed off or absorbed by clothing or dressings and in cases where compresses are being used, the perforations in the top of the dome make it a simple matter to

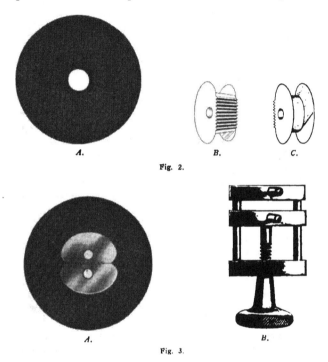

Fig. 2.

Fig. 3.

keep the compress wet (with a dropper) without the necessity of removing the shield.

The shield is kept in place by means of a properly applied binder or efficient breast suspensory, provided with an opening for the dome of the shield. The breast must be immobilized in any event, since otherwise the nipple cannot be put at rest.

For a number of years this shield has been in use in my service with gratifying results. It is presented to the profession with the hope that it may find a much larger field of application.

AN UMBILICAL CORD CLAMP

Fig 2 represents the separate parts of which the umbilical cord clamp is composed: The rubber disk (A)—the sole source of power upon which the clamp operates—is $1\frac{5}{8}$ inches in diameter, $\frac{1}{4}$ inch thick, with a $\frac{1}{4}$ inch hole in the center. The companion jaws (B and C) of the clamp are identical in every way. When their clamping surfaces are properly applied to each other, the little serrations mesh perfectly, providing compression surfaces $\frac{7}{16}$ of an inch long and $\frac{1}{4}$ inch wide. The combined thicknesses of the jaws when in contact, form between their flanges a shaft $\frac{7}{16}$ of an inch in diameter. This shaft is gripped by the rubber disk which is held in place by the flanges of the jaws. The disk is made from rubber of the very best quality obtainable for the purpose and the jaws from Monel metal—a noncorrosive nickel alloy which is in no wise affected by antiseptics, blood or other tissue substances.

Fig. 3 shows a side view of the assembled clamp (A) closed, also the retractor (B) used in opening the clamp and applying it to the cord.

Fig. 4 shows the clamp open with the retractor attached. The opening provided is $\frac{1}{2}$ inch long and $\frac{7}{16}$ of an inch wide—sufficient to receive the largest cord.

Fig. 5 shows the clamp closed upon a piece of umbilical cord, as reproduced from a photograph. Note the arteries and vein.

Fig. 6 shows the manipulation used in exposing the surfaces of the clamp jaws for purposes of cleaning—scrubbing with a brush.

The primary object of ligating or clamping the cord is, of course, to prevent hemorrhage; and while it is true that hemorrhage would rarely occur even were the cord not compressed, especially after the establishment of respiration, the fact remains that hemorrhages have occurred and even with fatal termination. In fifteen years I have had two cases of secondary hemorrhage from the cord which were all but fatal. It is likely, therefore, that some form of compression will always be regarded as necessary.

No matter at what point the cord is ligated, separation always occurs at the same place—the skin junction; and always by the same process—death of the stump and its removal by granulation tissue. Mummification or dry gangrene of the stump is of first importance, since it minimizes the chances of infection and hastens its separation. On the other hand moist gangrene, infection, and delayed separation go hand in hand. Asepsis and the elimination of moisture are therefore indispensable considerations in the treatment of the stump. If this be true, it then follows that under similar aseptic conditions that form of compression is best which most completely squeezes out the moisture from the tissues of the stump. In this respect there can be no question but that the clamp has great advantage over the ligature and that a clamp such as I am describing is far more effective than the usual artery forceps type of clamp, for the reason that there is no yielding in the compression as the tissues of the cord give way.

The serrations on the jaws of the clamp cut through the amniotic covering of the cord and thus facilitate the escape therefrom of the jelly of Wharton and other moisture. The clamp moreover fixes the

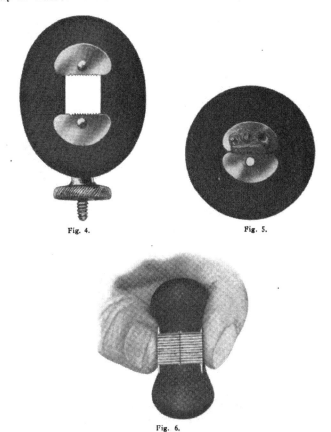

Fig. 4. Fig. 5.

Fig. 6.

stump and through the slight traction which it exerts upon it, keeps it elevated and away from the skin of the abdomen where perspiration otherwise adds to its moisture.

From what has been said it is evident that next in importance to asepsis, is the removal of all moisture as fast as it is squeezed from the stump by the clamp. This may be accomplished best by the liberal use of sterile absorbent cotton packed closely about the stump between the clamp and the skin. Gauze will not do since it is less absorbent than cotton and impossible to keep in close contact with the stump. A convenient way of utilizing cotton for the purpose is to be found in the form of a pad a half inch or more in thickness, with a small hole in its center. The pad is passed down over the cord by pulling the latter through it with an artery forceps. With the pad in place, the cotton is packed snugly about the stump with a tissue forceps. After applying the clamp to the cord close to the skin junction, the cord is cut just beyond the retractor, the retractor removed, the stump and clamp covered with a similar pad of cotton, and over all a sterile gauze binder, pinned in place.

It has been our experience that if the cord is crushed with an artery forceps before applying the clamp, the time of separation of the stump is materially shortened. Following this procedure we have invariably found the stump at the end of 72 hours either completely separated or reduced to a very thin parchment-like remnant readily twisted off by rotating the clamp.

Because of its small size, light weight and adaptable form the clamp may be incorporated into the cord dressings without discomfort to the baby and may be either left in place until the stump drops off or removed after some hours as is done with other clamps.

To those members of the profession whose custom it is to clamp the cord, this clamp will make its strongest appeal. Its simplicity, durability, compactness, strength and unyielding dependable pressure, leave little to be desired.

AN IDENTIFICATION WRISTLET FOR INFANTS

Preventing babies in a hospital nursery from "getting mixed" may not be regarded as a difficult task and yet it demands constant watchfulness. Various devices for "marking the babies" are in use and accomplish the purpose, but so far as I know an entirely satisfactory one has as yet not been announced.

The marks of identification must be in plain view or readily accessible at all times; they must be capable of instant and unmistakable interpretation; they must be proof against mutilation, soiling or other agency which may destroy them or render them indistinct; and the device which carries them must be sanitary, substantial yet simple, capable of being quickly and easily applied, free from discomfort or injury to the baby, and must be reasonable in price. To meet these requirements, the wristlet which I am presenting has been devised.

Fig. 7-1, 2, 3, 4, 5, and 6 were made from drawings of the component parts of the wristlet, and, while somewhat diagrammatic, nevertheless give correct ideas of form, relations and detail. Fig. 7-7 is an excellent reproduction from a photograph of the wristlet as it appears in use, with seal attached.

Fig. 7-*1* represents the mounting of the wristlet which has been pressed into shape from a single piece of metal. It is curved to conform to the more or less oval contour of the wrist and has two compartments—*A* and *B*: *B* to receive the rubber band (*2*) upon which it is mounted; and *A* to receive the identification label (*3*) and the celluloid shutter (*4*), which latter covers and protects the former. The mounting is ⅞ of an inch long, is ½ inch wide and made of Monel metal, a noncorrosive nickel alloy.

Fig. 7-*2* represents the rubber band which encircles the wrist of the baby and supports the mounting (*1*) described. The band which it is

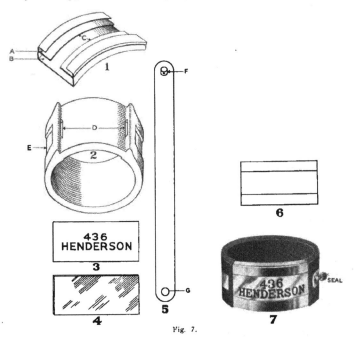

Fig. 7.

proposed to make from steel-gray rubber (not black as indicated), is ½ inch wide and ¹⁄₁₆ of an inch thick with local expansions. It has inside diameters (being oval) of ⅞ and 1⅛ inches respectively—the size which fits comfortably the arm of the average infant during the first weeks of life. A larger size will have to be provided for the very large babies.

All exposed edges of the mounting are well protected by the overlapping edges of the rubber band. The two prominent ridges or expansions running across the band on the outside, with abrupt vertical surfaces facing each other, serve the especial purpose of sealing compartment *A*, after the identification label (*3*) and the celluloid shutter (*4*) have been shoved into place. The sunken channel (*E*) encircling the rubber band on the outside, together with the openings (*D*) communicating with it, are provided to receive the flexible metal tape (*5*) to be described.

It will be seen that in order to get the rubber band into compartment *B*, it is simply necessary to stretch it until its reduced size passes the narrow rectangular opening (*C*) between the two compartments. That part of the rubber band which lies between the two expansions described, is the portion which fills compartment *B* and in length is ¼ inch shorter than the compartment. When therefore the band is released after passing into compartment *B* and regains its former size and shape, the ends of the mounting (*1*) become well embedded in rubber and compartment *A* very effectually sealed at either end.

Fig. 7-*3* represents the identification label containing the room number and name of the mother of the baby—a paper label of the thickness of ordinary writing paper used for business purposes. Because of its small size (⅞ by ½ in.) the label is trimmed after being inscribed, from a stock label (2 by 3 in.) upon which is printed the rectangular figure (*6*) outlining the exact size of compartment *A* and indicating the space available for the inscription.

Fig. 7-*4* represents the celluloid shutter of the size of *3* and of the weight and material used in automobile curtains. It serves as a transparent shutter covering and protecting the identification label (*3*) and fitting snugly into compartment *A* exernal to the label which is inserted first.

Fig. 7-*5* represents the flexible metal tape 3/16 of an inch wide, used in sealing the wristlet on the arm of the baby. It will be seen that in the assembled wristlet, the rectangular opening (*C*) beween the compartments *A* and *B* of the mounting (*1*) becomes a tunnel which opens at either end through *D* into the sunken channel (*E*) surrounding the rubber band on the outside. After the wristlet has been placed upon the baby's arm, the metal tape (with the free end containing the hole *G* in advance) is inserted into the opening *D* from one side, is pushed through the tunnel (*C*) out through *D* on the opposite side and thence along the channel (*E*) around the rubber band to the starting point where the pin (*F*) on the other end of the tape has arrived. The hole (*G*) is passed over the pin (*F*) and the tape is sealed in place by crushing a perforated shot upon the free ends of a piece of very soft copper wire passed through the hole near the top of the pin.

The Wristlet in Use.—The wristlet will be received by the hospital with the mounting (*1*) in place upon the band (*2*). All that the nurse needs to do is to take a label from the supply box, write the room number and name upon it, trim it to the size indicated and slip it into compartment *A* and over it the shutter. By pulling upon the band just beyond one end of the mounting and then turning the stretched end into the concavity of the mounting and holding it there, the corresponding end of the compartment will be fully exposed so that shoving the label and shutter into it becomes a very simple matter. The wristlet is now ready for the baby and is applied by simply stretching the band until it passes over the baby's hand and the wristlet is in place. The metal tape is next applied as above described and the seal attached. The wristlet should be gotten ready during the labor and put on before the baby leaves the delivery room.

4700 FIFTH AVENUE. (*For discussion, see p. 85.*)

TEACHING UNDERGRADUATE OBSTETRICS[*]

BY A. M. MENDENHALL, M.D., INDIANAPOLIS, IND.

DURING the last twenty years there have been a few valuable contributions to the practice and teaching of obstetrics, but no progress has been made toward reducing the total number of maternal deaths due to childbirth. Only a casual glance over the records of vital statistics in the registration areas of the United States is necessary to see clearly there has been, on the contrary, an increase in the maternal death rate.

In order that this may be proved beyond doubt, we must go back at least twenty years and note the gradual increase and not be misled by going back but three or four years and, thereby, fail to consider the fact that the years 1918 and 1919 saw a very great increase which, in reality, was largely due to influenza.

In a recent article by J. O. Polak[1] it is stated that "from 1902 to 1919 there was noted an increase to approximately three times as many deaths from sepsis, four times as many deaths from eclampsia, and twice as many deaths from other obstetric causes, besides the hundreds that die annually from indirect results of labor, as from injuries and consequent operations for repair, from nephritis originating during pregnancy, and from endocarditis aggravated by repeated labors."

By careful analysis of the records we find that, in 1916, there were approximately 16,000 deaths due to childbirth and, in 1918, 23,000, this marked increase being largely due to influenza. Nevertheless the one outstanding fact remains, that approximately 20,000 women die annually in the United States as a result of pregnancy and labor. Out of this number of deaths, approximately 28 per cent are due to sepsis alone,[2] a fact that seems but a sad reflection upon our care of the puer-

---

[*]Read at the Thirty-Fourth Annual Meeting of the American Association of Obstetricians, Gynecologists and Abdominal Surgeons, St. Louis, Mo., September 20-22, 1921.

peral patient. Also, about 20 per cent of these deaths are due to toxemia of pregnancy, although it is well known that proper prenatal care should very greatly reduce these figures.

The number of infants lost as a direct or indirect sequela to improper obstetrical care, is appalling in the extreme. If we add to this the great morbidity rates for mothers and infants, for which we have no satisfactory statistics yet very logical deductive evidence, it at once becomes apparent that we are falling short of our duty.

In other branches of medicine, almost without exception, there has been marked progress in the last two decades; but in obstetrics we have but little to which we may point with pride. And when our attention is called to these facts it seems well to pause long enough to try to find the reason.

The writer is becoming more and more convinced that one of the fundamental reasons is that there are some defects in our methods of teaching obstetrics.

We will agree in advance with all those who feel that the laity must become better educated to the fact that the process of childbearing is not a normal physiological event, and that every primipara who gives birth to a full term child has, at least, some pathologic lesion, and that this may be, and frequently is, quite serious if not fatal. We realize that if the laity could be made to thoroughly understand these facts, a great obstacle would be eliminated and much progress could be made; but this would by no means answer the whole question. And before we can hope for even a small minority of the laity to understand this, we must be sure that their instructors, the physicians themselves, are properly impressed with these facts. Rarely does the obstetrician pass a day when he does not see or hear of some practitioner who still feels that obstetrics requires but little skill and care. Hence our first and greatest defect in teaching obstetrics in the past has been that we have failed to impress our students with the seriousness of the case, when they are conducting the care of a woman through the period of pregnancy, labor, and the puerperium.

This is in part due to the fact the heads of our teaching institutions have been and still are unwilling to place the department of obstetrics on its proper level with the departments of surgery and medicine. They themselves have not been properly impressed with the importance of obstetrics and do not regard it as a definite and independent specialty and are, therefore, unwilling to give this department its proper ratio of time and equipment.

Many educators feel that we are rapidly approaching the time when the busy obstetrician, as well as other clinicians, must have compensation commensurate to the services he renders his school, else the service may become too largely delegated to assistants and more inferior teachers. Whether the head of the department of obstetrics should be a full time professor is a question which is confronting us at the present and, if this offers a real solution for the better teaching of obstetrics, it is deserving of careful consideration. But it is with conditions as they exist at present that I desire to search for weaknesses and offer remedies.

In this attempt I have sent out a questionnaire to twelve of our leading representative teaching institutions in the country with the view of determining, as nearly as possible, how the departments of obstetrics are being conducted.

The first two questions are as follows: "In what year of the medical course is obstetric teaching begun?" "Of what does the first course consist?"

The answers to these questions are quite uniform, showing that a general didactic course in embryology, and the physiology of pregnancy, labor, and the puerperium is started in the third year. In a few instances we find that didactic obstetrics is introduced in the second year. Unless the student has completed his courses in anatomy and physiology, as well as having had some training in physical diagnosis, it is very doubtful whether he is ready for didactic obstetrics; and, since these elementary and fundamental subjects are, in most instances, not completed until the end of the second year it would seem that obstetric teaching is best introduced in the third year.

The next four questions were submitted with the idea of ascertaining the relative importance given to didactic, clinical, and manikin courses, and the average length of time devoted to each of these divisions. The replies showed that 86 hours were given to didactic obstetrics, 81 hours to clinical obstetrics and 31 hours to manikin practice. There were no wide variations in these answers except that one school has as many as 90 hours of manikin practice, and another as few as 8 hours. It is doubtful whether 8 hours is more than one-fourth sufficient time for the student to have in manikin practice. If a proper demonstration is given, and then the practice on the manikin is properly supervised, there is little doubt but that 30 hours can be most profitably utilized in this method of teaching. One of the most important fundamentals in the study of obstetrics is a perfect understanding of palpation, corroborated by an actual view of the various points considered in presentation and position, and a familiarity with the various manipulations to be acquired in prolonged work over the manikin. The average student has great difficulty in memorizing from lecture notes or textbooks the many points which can be made very practical and easy for him to remember, by a properly conducted manikin course. Less than twenty-five or thirty hours spent in this work will certainly leave much to be learned.

The next question proposed was "When, in the obstetric course, is the manikin practice started?"

There was but little uniformity in the answers received, but there seemed to be very excellent reasons why this course should be delayed until late in the senior year, after the student has completed, or practically completed, the didactic lectures in obstetrics. In other words, after he has had a thorough course in the theory of obstetrics, the manikin instruction will be a supplementary, practical application of his theoretical knowledge; it will serve to emphasize by sight and touch those facts which have been presented didactically.

The next three questions were closely related and will be discussed together. They are: "On an average, how many deliveries does each student see in a hospital?" "Are these deliveries conducted by members of the staff or by internes?" "In how many hospital deliveries does each student actively assist or personally officiate?"

These questions brought out the fact, that on an average, about fifteen hospital deliveries are witnessed by each student; but some schools fall far below this average and, the most lamentable fact is that these deliveries, unless abnormal, are almost invariably conducted by internes. The average interne is but very little more skilled than the student and has, as a rule, received his training in the same imperfect way, and falls very short of the proper amount of knowledge and skill to be posing as an instructor. In no instance, probably, is the truth of the old adage so well seen as here,—"He who is teaching all he knows is teaching very poorly." In other words, the student ought to see a number of normal as well as abnormal deliveries, in a well conducted maternity, by some one who understands thoroughly the art and science of obstetrics and who has an intimate speaking knowledge of the mechanism of normal labor and the ability to demonstrate the conduct of such a delivery. When a recent graduate goes into practice, most of his cases will probably be the so-called normal labors, and it is in regard to the conduct of such cases as this that he should have been most carefully and painstakingly educated. When the chief of the obstetric department does not take sufficient interest in these cases to make sure that his students are properly instructed on this most vital part of the course, he is not only neglecting an opportunity to do a vast amount of good in a comparatively short period of time, but is falling decidedly short of his duty. It contributes strongly to a real weakness in our teaching the subject of obstetrics. In some of our maternities where there is on duty a resident obstetrician, who presumably, and usually does have, an obstetrical knowledge far in excess of the average interne, it may be right and proper to allow him to act as demonstrator in normal deliveries; but this must be left to the decision of the chief of the department. When we have educated the profession and the laity to a greater appreciation of hospitalization of obstetrical cases, and when our teaching institutions own, or control, much larger maternities than at present, we will be better able to permit students more frequently to assist or officiate in the delivery, under skilled supervision, of at least a few hospital cases, although the answer to this question shows an average of but two deliveries. Three schools reported that they make no attempt to let the student assist in labor cases.

The next four questions bear upon antepartum and postpartum care and were as follows: "How many antepartum cases are examined by each student?" "Is there a regular antepartum clinic conducted and is a member of the staff present at dispensary hours?" "Does each student have ample opportunity to see hospital postpartum care?" "Does each student have ample opportunity to see the hospital care of the newborn baby, and of premature babies?"

The answers to these questions were very gratifying. They showed that an average of sixteen complete antepartum examinations are made by each student, that every school conducts a regular antepartum clinic, and that a member of the obstetrical staff, or a resident obstetrician, is always present at the dispensary hour.

With this part of the obstetrical course so well provided for, the writer has no comment, other than to say that in obstetrics, as in other branches of medicine, diagnosis is of transcendent importance and that a well conducted large antepartum service for each student cannot fail to greatly enhance his knowledge of obstetrical diagnosis; and that prolonged service in this department will go very far toward impressing him with the great importance of prenatal care and thorough antepartum examinations, measurements, and records.

As to postpartum hospital care, it seems that all schools are availing themselves of ward work and bedside instructions to the extent of their capacity; all agree that the student should see and know as much as possible about the puerperium.

The next three questions bear upon abnormalities and are as follows: "How many forceps deliveries are observed by each student?" "Does each student assist in at least one forceps delivery?" "Does each student, under staff supervision, perform or assist in performing at least one second degree perineorrhaphy?"

The replies to these questions show that an attempt is made for all students to witness a few forceps deliveries, but very little opportunity is given for assistance. A number of students are graduated without ever having assisted at a forceps delivery or a perineorrhaphy. Whether or not this should be left until the interneship period, brings up three very important questions. First, whether right or wrong, we are confronted with the fact that there are still many graduates who go direct into practice without having served an interneship. Secondly, whether the physician in general practice should be considered competent to apply forceps may be questioned; but he is doing it and, undoubtedly, will continue to do it for a long time to come, and it certainly seems that his first experience should not be in the home of the patient and without competent supervision and assistance. Thirdly, granting that he will serve an interneship, is it right and proper that his first personal experience with the forceps should not be supervised even though it be under hospital conditions? Not long since, I saw this idea put into practice with a really very unique result. The left blade of the forceps was skillfully applied, but as the right blade was inserted it was so rotated and manipulated that it found its way to the same side of the pelvis as the left blade. Without supervision, it may have been difficult for this newly appointed interne to have discovered his error and to have properly corrected it. So long as our graduates continue to go out into practice with the mistaken conviction that they are competent to do forceps deliveries, we believe there should be a marked increase in their opportunity to obtain more training under supervision; and, certainly, no man should practice obstetrics who is not competent to repair a second degree laceration of the perineum. I do not believe he will attain this competency in any way whatsoever except by personal assistance under skilled supervision.

The eighteenth question in the questionnaire was upon the subject of outdoor obstetrics and is subdivided as follows: "(a) How long is each student on outdoor obstetric service? (b) How many cases does he deliver there? (c) To what extent is he followed up and supervised by members of the obstetrical staff? (d) Does a member of the staff see many of the outdoor cases during labor or puerperium? (e) About what per cent of the cases are thus visited?"

The average length of time spent on outdoor obstetrics was found to be eighteen days, and the average number of cases delivered was fifteen.

In one of our leading institutions the answer, as to whether a member of the staff sees many of these cases, was negative. This I know to be a frank confession, and I cannot look upon it except as a very sad commentary on pedagogical methods, as well as from a standpoint of the patient's interest.

This naturally leads to a discussion of outdoor obstetrics in general. What is to be gained by it and what are the pitfalls? It is refreshing to learn that one of our best schools has no outdoor deliveries. This school has a thoroughly supervised prenatal clinic. It is one of the schools which gives ninety hours to manikin practice, but does not feel that the outdoor deliveries can be sufficiently supervised to be worth the time and effort on the part of the student, at least if a reasonable maternity service is available. There are but two points to be gained by this so-called tenement obstetrics; the one is confidence and self-reliance, the other is an opportunity to see and examine a few women in labor. Self-reliance is desirable and should be cultivated, but it is very doubtful whether it cannot be better and more safely acquired otherwise. Confidence, in a degree is desirable, but with it comes two dangerous pitfalls. One is that the student attends a few so-called normal labors and Nature is good enough to permit the patients to survive, and the result is that the student develops very early a superabundance of confidence and begins to look upon labor as too nearly a normal physiologic process. Then, too, unless he is most thoroughly supervised and followed up, his many errors are not pointed out to him and he goes ahead fully persuaded he has been entirely right. The technic followed in most outdoor obstetric departments is crude at the best, yet the student is quite sure to decide it is good enough. If we are going to contribute our part toward reducing puerperal sepsis, we must persistently teach the most rigid labor technic, as we cannot expect the student when he goes into practice to follow a better technic than he has been taught. In fact it will usually be very much inferior. Therefore, if we permit the impressions to make headway in his mind which are, ordinarily, obtained in his outdoor obstetric work in college, they will be very likely to become permanently implanted there.

The last two questions were as follows: "How many beds have you available for obstetric teaching? Are these beds entirely under control of the school?"

It was found that an average of 46 beds was available for obstetric teaching and these were, generally, under control of the school. Hirst maintains that the school should assign more beds to obstetric teaching than to either medicine or surgery, because the average instructive capacity in each case is limited to one or two students. In this same article Hirst[3] advocates that a school having 400 students should have 100 beds available for the teaching of obstetrics, although it is to be remembered that he is a strong advocate of a combined department of obstetrics and gynecology and these figures are given on that basis. The controversy as to whether these two subjects should be combined for teaching purposes will not be discussed in this paper. The one outstanding fact is that any school pretending to educate students in obstetrics should have 50 to 100 beds available for this purpose alone, and these should be absolutely under the school's control, and not under the control of any private or city institution. In this connection I cannot do better than quote from a recent address by Polak[4]: "In order to turn out men who are even qualified to attend a primipara in labor, there must be greater clinical facilities for instruction of our students. Millions are expended every year for research and laboratories but almost nothing is given to the establishment and maintenance of properly equipped maternity hospitals. Why, if it is necessary for the American College of Surgeons to require an apprenticeship in surgery before a man can be recognized as capable of doing a surgical operation, is it not just as necessary that the man who is to deliver a woman should have sufficient training to insure a satisfactory recovery and a live baby?''

The writer would ask further: Why teach a man to practice obstetric operations in the homes of the patients and condemn him for doing an appendectomy in the same place?

CONCLUSIONS

1. A greater effort should be made to impress the student that obstetrics is a major division of the medical curriculum, and that few, if any, primiparas are ever delivered of full-sized infants and left in as perfect condition as before delivery.

2. Then, when the student goes into obstetric practice, he will carry this impression with him to the laity and do his part toward educating the public as to the importance of proper obstetric care.

3. More emphasis should be laid upon the proper management of so-called normal labor cases, and not so much of the student's time taken up in trying to teach him the various kinds of cesarean sections and other obstetric operations which should only be performed by the skilled obstetrician.

4. So-called outdoor obstetrics is, at its best, of little real value to the student, and it would be better to abandon it entirely, than to continue this sort of teaching without very thorough and continuous supervision by the teaching staff.

5. Since diagnosis in obstetrics, as in all other branches of medicine, is the real foundation for proper care and treatment, it is well to utilize every possible opportunity to teach this branch most thoroughly, and that the student's ability in this line be developed by prolonged manikin practice, by large numbers of antepartum examinations, and by wide clinical experience.

6. Teaching by internes, or by those who have but very little more knowledge, is sure to create a wrong impression as to the importance of the subject, and to fall very far short, directly and indirectly, of the result desired.

7. One of the most important ways in which we can soon obtain better results in teaching obstetrics, is to educate the laity and our hospital managers to a realization that a large and well-equipped

maternity is the best place to teach and practice obstetrics; and that this will at once contribute strongly toward a reduction in the fetal and maternal death rates in the community in which it is established, as well as in the communities where the students later go to practice.

REFERENCES

(1) Jour. Am. Med. Assn., lxxvi, No. 26, 1809. (2) Am. Jour. Hyg., March, 1921, i, 197. (3) AM. JOUR. OBST. AND GYN., Nov., 1920, i, 128. (4) Jour. Am. Med. Assn., lxxvi, No. 26, 1810.

2369 SOUTHEASTERN AVENUE. (*For discussion, see p. 86.*)

A METHOD OF DELIVERY IN NORMAL CASES*

By MAGNUS A. TATE, M.D., F.A.C.S., CINCINNATI, O.

THE average duration of a normal case of labor varies from sixteen to twenty hours in the primipara and from ten to sixteen hours in the multipara. If by aiding Nature's efforts, we can materially cut the time without harm to mother or child and make the labor less painful, we are benefiting womankind.

All obstetricians are familiar with the uncertain nagging pains accompanying the often drawn out first, and the intense suffering incident to the second stage of labor.

You are also familiar with the frequent statement of some women: "I have never been well since the birth of my baby," and we know that this is due, not alone to unrepaired lacerations, but more frequently to the long drawn out first stage of labor, followed by an agonizing second stage, which leads to physical exhaustion and, in turn, is often followed by a peculiar syndrome of the neuroses. This is manifestly too true when we encounter those cases of badly managed malpositions in elderly primipara with a slight narrowing of pelvic diameters, who are allowed to drag through a harrowing labor; as well as in those cases of hysterical and frightened primipara and neglected dry labors. Such cases you see as consultants, or as staff members of our charitable hospitals.

Many are the remedies advocated to alleviate the pains of labor. We know that most of them have been discarded with the exception of the various anesthetics, morphia and chloral.

Advancement in the obstetric art is not so much in the selection of some method of delivery, as in the adoption of prenatal care and the observance of rigid asepsis.

We follow out methods of delivery as given to us by our forefathers, because, mechanically, their deductions were usually correct.

Skill is paramount to success, and the advent of asepsis has given

*Read at the Thirty-Fourth Annual Meeting of the American Association of Obstetricians, Gynecologists and Abdominal Surgeons, St. Louis, Mo., September 20-22, 1921.

us a leeway and freedom to attempt much that, in the past, was not advisable or wise.

Accouchement forcé has met with unfortunate results because of forcible dilatation of the cervix followed by the immediate and rapid delivery of the child. There is no doubt that it has been the means of saving some lives, especially when dealing with desperate conditions, such as hemorrhage, eclampsia, edema of the lungs, and noncompensating hearts.

Accouchement forcé is a major operation. The forcible dilatation of a firmly closed os and rapid delivery of the child must, necessarily, be followed by a high maternal and fetal mortality. The dilating of an unobliterated cervix, other than by instrumental means, is a most difficult task. Forcible dilatation is rarely practiced today. It is comparatively easy to open up a soft dilatable cervix by the Harris method.

I give much credit to Potter for demonstrating and emphasizing that a vagina can be effectively dilated without injury to vaginal and muscular structures by the ironing-out process.

CASE 1.—Mrs. ————, a refined and cultured woman, multipara, aged twenty-six. Her first labor occurred at the age of twenty-two, and was twenty hours in duration; normal presentation; instrumental delivery; perineal laceration requiring two stitches. The second labor, at the age of twenty-four, was eighteen hours in duration; twin birth; perineal laceration requiring two stitches. A slow recovery occurred in both deliveries. The following year she was subjected to an appendectomy. Third labor, age twenty-six. Knowing so well of the protracted recoveries of her previous labors, and of the appendectomy one year ago, I determined to try a method of delivery that I had been contemplating for some time.

The patient entered the Good Samaritan Hospital with the os dilated to the size of a silver half dollar. She was in the best of spirits, having regular, easily bearable pains, ten minutes apart. She was prepared obstetrically and taken to the delivery room at 10:00 P.M. Ether was administered to the surgical degree; the bladder was catheterized, and the specimen sent to the laboratory. The gloved hand, anointed with sterilized vaseline, was then introduced in the vagina, one finger at a time, following the ironing-out method. The thin and easily dilatable os and vagina were thoroughly stretched by 10:30 P.M. Anesthesia was withdrawn at 10:32 P.M. The patient was allowed to recover partially from the anesthetic by 10:40 P.M. One-half of one c.c. of pituitrin was now given, and the membranes ruptured. Regular pains ensued shortly. The patient was in a drowsy state and did not seem to suffer much. The child was delivered at 11:10 P.M., just one hour and ten minutes after the patient's entrance into the delivery room. The child weighed eight pounds. There were no lacerations.

This patient could hardly realize, thinking of her two previous labors, that she had actually been delivered within one hour and ten minutes. The following day, after a good night's rest, she showed no signs of exhaustion, and described her condition as follows: "I feel like I had had some slight vaginal operation, and while I am sore, I have not the same feeling that I had with my other labors."

CASE 2.—The patient entered the Bethesda Hospital, giving the history of having had the membranes ruptured at 8 A.M. I saw her at 9 A.M. The os was not dilated sufficiently. The pains were easily bearable. Examination at 10.40 A.M. showed the os dilated to the size of a silver half dollar, and one hand presenting. The patient was taken to the delivery room at 11 A.M. She was anesthetized at 11:30 A.M. The hand was replaced. Dilatation of the os was complete at 11:50 A.M. The patient was partially out from under the anesthetic by 12:05 P.M. One-half of one c.c. of pituitrin was given. Pains were not efficient. Pituitrin was repeated at 12:25 P.M. Rapid delivery followed at 12:35 P.M. Perineal tear, requiring three stitches. The time between entering the room and complete delivery was one hour and thirty-five minutes. That afternoon the patient's condition was very different from one who had gone through the ordinary labor. In this case the second dose of pituitrin was, probably, given too hurriedly; otherwise, I do not believe that there would have been a laceration. In two cases patients did not seem to be susceptible to the action of pituitrin, so forceps were applied after waiting one hour.

CASE 3.—Patient's first labor lasted four days, midwife attending. She was rushed to a hospital and delivered instrumentally. The baby lived six days. It weighed nine pounds and six ounces. The mother was profoundly exhausted, ran a septic temperature for three weeks, and at no time did she have mammary secretion. The pelvic soft structures were like parchment, simply dried out and tore readily. The extensive lacerations of both cervix and perineum were repaired. This patient's second labor occurred under my care in the hospital. She was delivered in two hours and forty minutes. There was no perineal tear, but one side of the cervix tore, which was immediately repaired. No exhaustion, mammary secretion normal; baby weighed nine pounds.

Another case I have had was that of a hypersensitive, hysterical, neurasthenic patient. She was crying, tossing about, and "knew that she was going to die." She refused to obey any instructions or commands. She was delivered in two hours and forty minutes.

This was one of the cases where forceps were used to lift the head over the perineum. I am sure you will agree with me, that this kind of case requires much patience, tact, and ingenuity.

Another case, that of a young negress, primipara, aged eighteen, I saw with a young physician at my solicitation. Delivery was effected in one hour and forty-five minutes. The child weighed seven pounds and four ounces.

In a later case, that of a young primipara, aged twenty-one, weighing 100 pounds, there was a very bad mitral lesion. She had been under her physician's care for a period of two years. This patient was delivered in one hour and fifty minutes. No laceration, no exhaustion, and recovery was uneventful. The child weighed six pounds and six ounces. Other cases, so far attended, were uneventful, all having been delivered with safety to mother and child.

I do not report the number of cases delivered to date; they are entirely too few to be of value from a statistical standpoint. I have had, however, a sufficient number of cases to convince me that there is merit in this method of delivery. One case, a multipara (daughter of a physician), was delivered in fifty-five minutes. There were no lacerations.

SUMMARY OF METHOD

1. Patient must be in labor, cervix obliterated, and os dilated to at least the size of a silver half dollar. 2. Surgical anesthesia. 3. Bladder catheterization. 4. Complete manual dilatation of the vagina and cervix. 5. Patient allowed to regain partial consciousness. 6.

Pituitrin one-half c.c., to be repeated once if the pains are not efficient in half an hour. 7. Membranes ruptured. 8. Management of delivery of child as in usual case.

Remarks: I am taking it for granted that all physical findings, the presentation and position of the viable child have been made and recorded; that the patient has been obstetrically prepared, and that postpartum findings are also recorded; otherwise no comparison can be made as to the merits of various methods of delivery. Deep anesthesia is requisite to procure proper relaxation; but the anesthesia must not be continued beyond a certain point. An anesthetic, at this time, is safer; the woman being in a happier frame of mind than if given later when she is disturbed, apprehensive as to the outcome, or frenzied with pain. Gentleness, dilating both vagina and cervix (with a clock before your eyes), is essential to good results. Do not rupture the membranes until the patient is partially rational and a hypodermic of pituitrin has been given, as the bulging of the membranes aids materially in keeping the os stretched to it fullest degree. The membranes often rupture spontaneously, after complete dilatation, with the first pain, following Nature's efforts, as they are no longer a functionating object.

I have found that the patient will have far better and more regular pains if we wait until she has partially recovered from under the anesthetic before administering pituitrin. Patients in this half drowsy state will respond to your commands and aid delivery by using the voluntary muscles. If pains become too severe, she may need a few whiffs of the anesthetic, especially when the head is approaching and passing over the perineum.

Episiotomy may be performed if necessary, but it is usually not required if proper dilatation of the vagina has been accomplished.

Delivery is not always painless, but can be made almost so, judging from observation and the statements of patients. The shortening of the time of labor is very advantageous from all standpoints, and of remarkable benefit to the woman. If dilatation be complete, lacerations should not be more frequent than in ordinary cases.

It is assumed that in the giving of pituitrin obstetric judgment will be used, for its injudicious use is apt to be followed by serious injury to mother and child. Unfortunately there is not, at present, an exact standardization of dosage of pituitrin. Various manufacturers have given us ampules of different strength; for instance, Armour's and Burroughs Wellcome & Co. pituitrin preparations are said to be more powerful in action than that of Parke, Davis and Co. If the patient be completely under the anesthetic, it will, naturally, require a larger dose to obtain the desired results. When we stop for a moment and consider the vast number of cases in which pituitrin has been used, we find very few reports of uterine rupture and death of child. If we analyze these cases, as I have tried to do, we will find one of three things. First, the case was one in which the drug should never have been used; secondly, the dosage was too large or repeated too often, or given when the patient was deeply anesthetized; thirdly, the patient was in an exhausted or septic state.

Puerperal complications and delayed convalescence, usually, have a starting point—shock, incident to mental and physical suffering. What obstetrician has not had it brought home to him that an exhausted woman is a good subject for septic infection? What a different picture, and what a different history, is the physically well woman who rallies immediately after labor, to that of the worn-out and exhausted patient, who may run the typical febrile course. A long drawn out labor, accompanied by a hot, dry, swollen vagina, offers a fertile field for infection, and it only requires a study of governmental and health board statistics to verify the statement that exhausting labor is the prime factor of high and unnecessary mortality.

This method is not presented with the idea of supplanting well known means of delivery, as demanded when dealing with malpositions, operative conditions, or with any form of placenta previa; but it is applicable to that type, classified under the head of normal presentations, when the delivery is conducted in a hospital or in the better class of homes. I present this method to you for your earnest consideration, suggestions, criticism, or approval.

19 WEST SEVENTH STREET.   (*For discussion, see p. 89.*)

THE CHOICE OF METHODS FOR MAKING LABOR EASY*

By ARTHUR H. BILL, M.D., F.A.C.S., CLEVELAND, OHIO

IT IS very gratifying to note the efforts put forth by those interested in obstetric progress, which aim at the elimination, as far as possible, of the terrors of childbirth. The contrast between present-day methods of conducting labor and those of ten years ago is most striking. The old plan of allowing nature to take its course, even in the face of abnormalities, with the hope that eventually the abnormality might correct itself, has given way to a far more scientific and humane method of correcting abnormal conditions, and thus assisting natural forces which act best when conditions are normal. We find also a tremendous difference of opinion as regards the relief of pain. Even those who most strongly opposed the use of anesthetics and analgesics have taken their stand with those who are exerting every effort to make the labor as comfortable as possible for the patient.

---
*Read at the Thirty-Fourth Annual Meeting of the American Association of Obstetricians, Gynecologists and Abdominal Surgeons, St. Louis, Mo., September 20-22, 1921.

All these efforts are worthy of commendation, and yet we must acknowledge the danger of overstepping the limits of safety when these efforts are misdirected or when unsafe methods are used. The object of this paper is to attempt to discriminate between the safer and more conservative, and the radical methods, and to select ways of relieving the pain and the exhaustion resulting from labor to the last degree, and at the same time, keep within the limits of safety.

Emphasis should be laid upon the fact that fads and hobbies have no place in obstetric practice. Let us remember that both for the relief of pain and for the termination of labor, there are several methods; that there are, perhaps, points in favor of most of these methods in individual cases; and, on the other hand, there are contraindications to them in others. Bearing this in mind, it would seem that the obstetrician, who would do the best for his patient, will familiarize himself with all of the better methods and select them according to the case in hand, and not allow himself to apply one method to all cases, regardless of the varying conditions which surround them. My efforts have been directed toward such a selection of methods and, naturally, what is to be said in this paper is based on the results of these efforts.

The problem of making labor easy divides itself naturally into two distinct parts: (a) The relief of pain, and (b) the shortening of the second stage, or the working stage, of labor.

(a) There are two general groups of methods of relieving labor pains: analgesia and anesthesia. Analgesia adapts itself only to the first stage of labor; anesthesia to the second stage. The latter is also useful in the first stage in multiparae, and as a supplement to analgesia in the first stage in primiparae. After trying various methods of analgesia, the writer has found the morphine and scopolamine method the most satisfactory, and uses it according to the usual prescribed method of small and frequently repeated doses. The one rule, which is strictly adhered to, is that no scopolamine be given in the second stage of labor, and not within a period of three or preferably four hours of the expected birth. This rule practically eliminates its use in multiparae, and in those occasional primiparae who have very short labors, with the latter exception, the method is used as a routine in primiparae. It has been found to be perfectly safe when the above mentioned time limit is carefully observed. In multiparae and the small proportion of primiparae mentioned, the general anesthetic is used instead. The time for beginning the anesthetic or analgesic is determined by one fact, namely, the suffering of the patient. In other words, something is given for the relief of pain just as soon as the patient seems to be feeling uncomfortable, no matter how early in labor. If the scopolamine and morphine method does not appear to give sufficient relief, a general anesthetic is also given with each pain.

Of the general anesthetics commonly used, we have ether, nitrous oxide, and chloroform. All will relieve pain with equal satisfaction, although there is a difference in their safety and practicability. In our practice, chloroform is not used, not that chloroform will not give the necessary relief, which of course, it will, but because it is a far more dangerous anesthetic than the others, and gives no better results. Ether is the usual anesthetic used because of its entire practicability and safety, and the fact that it gives better relaxation, which is an important factor at the time of delivery. Nitrous oxide is used in selected cases. Aside from the fact that many patients find it more agreeable, it has one advantage in the earlier part of labor, when the pains are not very forcible, in not inhibiting the pain quite as much as ether. The latter advantage is only seen in an occasional case, however, and is best illustrated in induction of labor, in which it is our custom to use gas. This, however, is a disadvantage at the end of labor. Ether is not given by the drop method, for in the relief of a labor pain the best results come from giving a large amount in a short time. The closed cone is used as a routine. The second stage is one of general anesthesia. Morphine, scopolamine, ether and nitrous oxide are all used in our practice, the choice being made in each individual case at the time of labor and, except for following the general principles laid down, no definite choice is made in advance. Each method has its advantages and disadvantages in certain cases. In some cases, all are used.

(b) Shortening of labor. I am in hearty sympathy with the principle of shortening labor instead of allowing the patient to carry it on to completion by her own efforts. However, in following this plan, great caution must be urged. First of all let me emphasize the fact that efforts toward the shortening of labor should, as a rule, be limited to the second stage of labor. The first stage should not be interrupted unless there is a definite indication resulting from the condition of the mother, or, more often, the failure of the fetal heart. By a combination of analgesia and anesthesia, it is possible to allow the patient to complete the dilatation of the cervix with little suffering in a very large percentage of cases. It has been my practice for a number of years to shorten the second stage of labor by delivering the patient under complete anesthesia, and of correcting abnormalities of position when the patient has reached the second stage. The method used has depended upon the individual case being a forceps delivery or a version, according to the circumstances surrounding it. No decision as to the method of delivery is ever made in advance; for by doing so, the interests of the patient are not served as well as by going to the delivery with an open mind and deciding each case on its merits.

To give an idea of the results of this selection of methods of anesthesia and of delivery, I present the last 500 cases which I have personally delivered previous to September 1st, 1921, as follows:

Ether alone in	228	cases
Morphine and scopolamine, plus ether, in	192	"
Morphine and scopolamine, plus nitrous oxide in	19	"
Nitrous oxide and ether in	56	"
Nitrous oxide alone in	5	"

The methods of delivery were as follows:

High forceps	41,	inc. posterior positions conv. by forceps	32
Medium forceps	81	" " " " " "	40
Low forceps	236	" " " " " "	6
Podalic versions	71	" posterior positions	52
Breech extractions	19		130
Abdominal cesarean sections	26		
Vaginal cesarean sections	3		
Pubiotomies	3		
Craniotomy	1		
Spontaneous Births	19		
	500		

The fetal mortality in cases delivered after the sixth month of pregnancy was:

1. *Stillborn.* Nine or 1.8 per cent. Two macerated, on one of which craniotomy was performed. Three after high forceps, 1 toxemia case in which labor had been induced. One after version. Three after low forceps, after prolonged and difficult labor. Of those living and viable at onset of labor—seven, or 1.4 per cent were stillborn.

2. *Died in First Two Weeks,* Seven or 1.4 per cent. One delivered by medium forceps in case of toxemia, died during first 24 hours. No autopsy. One 6½ months' premature, lived one day. Two died suddenly on first and second days. Autopsy revealed nothing but greatly enlarged thymus in each case. One 7½ months premature with double harelip and cleft palate, lived 3 days. One anencephalic monster, lived but a few hours. One hemorrhagic baby. Autopsy showed intestines and peritoneal cavity filled with blood.

In the combined list, there were eight babies, or 1.6 per cent that died during or after the labor, and as a result of the labor. Three of these, namely, the high forceps cases, very likely, should have been delivered by cesarean section. In the case of the other five, it is not clear how the labor should have been conducted differently.

It will be noted that in 336, or 67.2 per cent of the cases presented, the head passed spontaneously through the external os while the patient was under the influence of analgesia or anesthesia. This large percentage emphasizes the success of the policy of relieving the pain, and allowing the case to take its own course to the point when the head is well within the pelvis; and, if possible, entirely through the cervical canal, unless there are indications to the contrary. To analyze the cases further, it is well to divide them into groups: (1) Those cases in which the head was at the pelvic outlet, or well within the pelvis and in a normal anterior position. (2) Those cases in which the head lay in a vertex occipitoposterior position. (3) Cases in which the head was either in the pelvic brim or above the brim at the time of delivery, and the pelvic measurements were ample. (4) The cases of breech presentation. (5) The second child in case of twin birth.

(1) There were 271 cases in this class. Many of these would in time have resulted in spontaneous births. However, the policy followed was that of delivering them with forceps under complete anesthesia, a procedure sometimes called the prophylactic forceps operation. Experience has shown that there are several advantages in this procedure: (a) The strength of the mother is saved, and her suffering diminished. (b) The danger to the child from prolonged pressure upon its head is decreased. (c) The number and extent of lacerations of the perineum are diminished. (d) Asepsis is better maintained than when the patient is thrashing about. Preliminary manual dilatation of the birth canal, which is always performed, very materially lessens the pressure to which the child's head is subjected at the end of labor, while the complete relaxation of the patient allows the obstetrician to control the birth of the head far better than when the patient is bearing down, and it is necessary to use considerable strength to hold the head back. The delivery in such cases is simple, and very little traction force is necessary. The degree of success depends upon the care and accuracy with which the forceps are used. In their use, especial stress is laid upon the following simple rules: (a) Always make an accurate cephalic application. (b) Use axis traction so that the head will follow the course which corresponds to that of the normal mechanism of labor. In this connection I would urge the more common use of axis traction forceps, even when the head is low, for with their use, there is greater accuracy than when the ordinary forceps are used with Pajot's maneuver. (c) Take far more time than is usually allowed for the delivery, that there may be an extremely gradual birth. (d) Try to see how little force may be expended in traction. (e) Promote flexion of the head. (f) Take the forceps off and shell the head out manually as soon as the chin may be felt posterior to the perineum. While it has been my practice for some years to routinely lift the head over the perineum with forceps, I have hesitated to advocate this procedure for fear of its abuse. However, the satisfactory results would seem to indicate that greater stress be laid upon the proper use of forceps, and less upon their disuse because of damage not uncommonly resulting from careless forceps work.

(2) The occipitoposterior position. This is by far the most frequent complication of obstetric practice, and causes a large percentage of

the prolonged, painful and difficult labors. In the list of cases presented, there were 130 occipitoposterior positions, or 26 per cent. In many cases the head will rotate to an anterior position spontaneously, if the labor is allowed to go on, but only after an unnecessary prolongation, amounting to many hours in some cases. Under such conditions, the patient is working under a very severe handicap, in that the head does not tend to follow the path of the normal mechanism of labor. Much suffering and exhaustion therefore results. It is the writer's policy not to wait for the spontaneous rotation, but to correct the abnormality, when there is complete dilatation of the cervix. If the head is in the pelvic cavity, this is accomplished by rotating it with forceps, using the modified Scanzoni procedure, which I have previously described before this Society. Traction is never made upon a head in an abnormal position, such as the occipitoposterior position. After the head is rotated, we have no more of a serious problem than in the cases in Group 1.

If the head is in the pelvic brim, or above it, and in a posterior position, the choice of procedure lies between the high forceps and podalic version. In the list presented, there were 84 such cases; in 52 of them version was performed, and in 32 the forceps were used to rotate and to deliver. In my experience, both procedures have their advantage in suitable cases, and the choice between them is made at the time of delivery. To illustrate: If the membranes are intact, and the patient is a multipara, the podalic version is invariably used. If the membranes have ruptured, the uterus dry and somewhat tonically contracted, I prefer to rotate and deliver with forceps. Further, if the patient is a primipara with unusually rigid soft parts, the forceps delivery has the advantage that far more time may be allowed for the delivery than is possible in the case of a breech extraction. This must materially lessen the dangers to the child and the extent of laceration to the mother. This group comprises those cases in which the head is held up at the pelvic brim solely on account of the posterior position, cases in which the head would have readily descended into the pelvis had the position been normal.

(3) Exclusive of cases in which there is an occipitoposterior position, the head may remain at the pelvic brim even though measurements are good, for example, face presentation, brow presentation, presentation of one parietal bone, and cases in which there are insufficient or misdirected pains. For the delivery of such cases, podalic version is to be preferred. In the cases of the malpositions mentioned, forceps are contraindicated; they should never be used unless an accurate application is possible, and the head can be made to descend in the manner in which it descends in conformity to the normal mechanism of labor. This is not possible in the case of the abnormal positions mentioned.

(4) Breech presentation, especially the frank breech. Too often the patient is allowed to continue for a long period in the second stage of labor in the hope that the breech will descend spontaneously. The patient may be entirely relieved of this unnecessary prolongation of labor, and nothing is to be gained by waiting for spontaneous descent. The preferable plan is to bring down the feet and extract without further delay when dilatation is complete.

(5) In twin births, the second child is immediately delivered by version. There is no excuse for the long interval sometimes occurring between the births of twins. The conditions are never more ideal for version than in the case of the second twin.

It will be noted that in the list of cases presented, there were only nine high forceps cases if we exclude the occipitoposterior positions. These were cases in which there was a moderate dystocia and indications for delivery were present. Every effort is made to reduce the use of high forceps in such cases to a minimum.

Any plan of shortening labor may be abused. The abuse lies chiefly in too early attempts at delivery. From my own experience, and from observation of the work of others, I believe that the one great cause of failure may be attributed to the cervix; that is, attempts at delivery are made when the cervix is not completely obliterated. Its resistance may be the cause of disastrous results, whether version is performed or whether forceps are used. Manual dilatation of an undilated cervix is often insufficient. Hence, the stress which I have laid upon the importance of waiting whenever possible for the head to pass through the cervical canal, or at least for the complete obliteration of the cervix.

It is possible to so simplify labor that women will not look forward to it with dread. The part which the patient takes in labor is largely a passive one, consisting chiefly of breathing the anesthetic as directed. She is seldom urged to strain or pull. Pulling straps are never used. The results of our efforts as described, as shown by the relatively low fetal mortality, furnish ample justification of these methods. The conservation of strength is a great benefit to the patient during the puerperium, while the apparent lack of fear with which they anticipate labor, materially lessens the common nervous symptoms of pregnancy including nausea and vomiting.

In conclusion, let us remember that all obstetric cases are not alike, that neither the same method of anesthesia nor the same method of delivery offers the best solution for every case. We have various methods and most of them have their peculiar advantages for individual patients. Let us become proficient in each, and be ready to use the one which best applies to the case in hand.

503 OSBORN BUILDING. (*For discussion, see p.* 91.)

REPORT OF A CASE OF HEMIMELUS OR SO-CALLED CONGENITAL AMPUTATION*

By Harold Bailey, M.D., New York City

FOR many years deformities showing absence of part of a limb have been reported as intrauterine, spontaneous or congenital amputations, but hemimelus (half-limb) is a better term; for while it discloses nothing as regards etiology, it does not perpetuate the idea that the limbs have been amputated during embryonal or fetal life. These cases are not uncommon in the minor degrees, that is, the absence of the fingers or toes, but the presence in the living child of congenital malformations involving the entire limb is sufficiently rare to demand a description with a view of determining the etiologic factors or ascertaining by the study of the associated malformations, the developmental period at which the structural defects occur.

The malformation known as hemimelus consists in the absence of one or more of the four extremities, the distal end appearing as a healed stump and simulating the result of a surgical amputation. The stump of these extremities is usually thought to contain no developmental factors of the parts below. However, in recent years our ability to obtain x-ray plates of these lesions has produced evidence that many have a portion of the bones distal to the defect.

Before we take up the description of the case at hand, we should recall that there are other congenital malformations involving the bones of the extremities. For instance, in that rare condition, phocomelus, there is an absence of the proximal bones, the hands and feet springing from the rudimentary arm or leg, or directly from the trunk. These monsters are rare but are common enough to find their way into "sideshows," and are then usually designated as the "turtle-women" and so forth.

Examination has shown that in the short stump there are often cartilaginous rudiments of the absent bones. The absence of the long bones is fairly uncommon. However, Dr. Stafford McLean has under his care at the present time in the Babies' Hospital an infant two weeks old that has the right femur absent. The x-ray shows that the bones of the lower extremity are attached directly to the pelvis. It is apparent that these malformations of the extremities, while much more frequently occurring at the distal part, may involve the proximal bones.

---

*Read at a meeting of the New York Obstetrical Society, October 11, 1921.

CASE REPORT.—(No. 16089. Manhattan Maternity Service.) The mother is Polish, thirty-six years of age and Wassermann test was negative. She had three previous normal pregnancies. The children are living and have no deformities. Labor occurred on September 12, 1921. There were slight pains at ten-minute intervals for two hours, then three stronger pains and a 7½ pound baby was born.

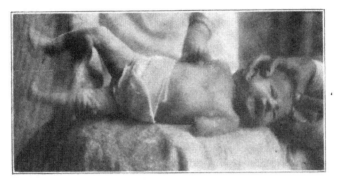

Fig. 1.—Absence of the left forearm. Note the small tab of tissue on the inner side of the stump.

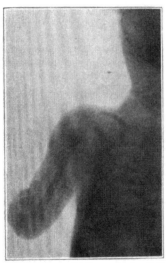

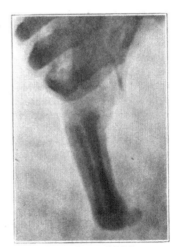

Fig. 2.—Stump of left arm showing bony growth below the elbow.

Fig. 3.—Stump of left leg.

On the arrival of the intern from the hospital, the baby and placenta were found in the bed. The placenta and membranes were apparently normal. The child had a paralysis of the left side of its face, which from the wide open eye might be considered as an external paralysis of the seventh nerve. The left arm was terminated at the elbow, with a smooth padded stump. In the tissue of the stump, the x-ray shows the evidence of bone growth which must come from the ossification centers ordinarily placed in the shafts of the ulna and radius. The olecranon and the joint ossifications do not occur at this early stage and it would appear that the bone in the stump represents rudiments of the bones of the forearm. When the child contracts its biceps, there is flexion as of a joint. There is a bud or spur of tissue attached to the inner side at the elbow joint. The left leg ends in a stump composed of the tibia and fibula. Below this is a mass of tissue somewhat resembling the heel and in the front end is a bud or spur which is like the big toe. The x-ray shows no bone below the tibia and fibula. There appear to be no other deformities. The child is a month old and gradually gaining weight. (Figs. 1, 2, 3.).

MATERNAL IMPRESSIONS

One of the older theories of these defects still held by unscientific persons is that they are the result of maternal impressions occurring at any time during pregnancy. It is interesting to note the coincidences that further such false ideas. In our case, there were family difficulties and all through the pregnancy there was discord. The husband now charges the wife with being the cause of the amputations because at one altercation while she was six months pregnant, she chased him about the house with a butcher knife. The wife does not deny this and even believes that she may have caused these deformities. The discussion ended in the Court of Family Relations.

AMNIOTIC BANDS

General credence has been given the theory that these malformations were actually amputations from the constriction by amniotic bands. There are cases in which adhesions have been found attached to the head (I have such a specimen in the Cornell Museum), to the face, and to the fingers. There are many cases with deep grooves on the limbs commonly thought to be due to constricting bands. An entire theory of teratogenesis is built upon the fact of amniotic adhesions.

There are two articles in the older literature which describe amniotic cord-like bands attaching an undeveloped foot to a stump of the limb. In the more recent literature, Fieux[1] describes the hand attached by a cord to the stump of the arm. It is possible that the maldevelopment of the extremities is the result of amniotic pressure in the first few weeks and that the bands are adhesions of the amnion to the open or inflamed area.

These grooves are in all instances located on the limbs. They are never spiral and no amniotic band has ever been found attached to them. Ballantyne[2] believes the deformities are due to a faulty development of the amnion, whereby it remains in contact with the embryo, thus producing pressure. This explanation of course refers to the first weeks of embryonic life.

A skiagraph tracing, presented by Truman Abbe, of the hands in a case of so-called intrauterine amputation shows the two stumps of the first and third fingers contain rudimentary phalanges. At the base of each short finger is a deep groove and another occurs at the level of the metacarpal bones. The x-ray proves that these fingers are not amputated but are undeveloped. The skiagraph of the apparently normal hand shows that the condition is partly bilateral for the terminal phalanx of the first and third fingers is rudimentary.

In a case reported by William Stowell[4] there was a deep circular groove on the left leg just below the knee and a shallow circular groove in the lower third of the right leg. This infant had in addition a club foot on the left side and webbing of the toes. The right hand showed amputation of the fingers and there were deep grooves about the base of the little finger constricting the soft parts nearly to the bone. The left hand had syndactylus or webbing of the fingers.

The presence of bud-like growths on the more or less conical stumps has been often noted. They are usually supposed to represent fingers or toes. In Watts'[5] case of absence of the ulna a rudimentary finger with phalangeal bones cropped out below the elbow, as if nature had attempted to complete the hand. In my case, the padded stump quite resembles the heel and the big toe.

It is evident that most of the cases have other malformations. In our case there was an external facial paralysis. As this baby had no forceps procedure and was the result of a precipitate labor, it is difficult to determine the origin of this condition. A similar condition is described by Guyl in a case of hemimelus and he attributed the paralysis to the pressure of amniotic bands upon the seventh nerve.

EXPERIMENTAL TERATOGENY

Experimental teratogeny has advanced since the time of the Saint-Hillaires until now every type of developmental defect known in the literature may be produced by experimental treatment. Stockard[6] and others have found that monsters may be artificially produced in the fish and chick embryos by changes in the moisture, temperature, oxygen supply or by the production of an excess of CO_2. The structural changes in defect or excess are due to variation in the developmental rate at a time when the organ so affected is in a rapid proliferating stage. Stockard believes that each organ or part has a distinct moment or time when it has the advantages of growth and that it actually inhibits the growth in other parts. When its own proliferating stage has passed, it does not appear again in such ascendency. If the changes in the temperature or oxygen supply cause a slowing of the rate during the embryonic phase of the organ, it is unable to make up for its loss and the resulting deformities are always secondarily due to this slow rate of development.

Such an explanation of growth and development applies to the time when the blastodermic vesicle is in the act of attaching itself to the wall of the uterus. Very considerable conformation of this general theory is evident in the human embryo. By the studies of Mall[7] of one thousand cases of anomalies of embryos from the uterus, ectopic pregnancies and stillbirths, it was found in the ectopic specimens that there were twice as many pathological as in the uterine. He believes that this is due to faulty implantation and consequent malnutrition.

HEREDITARY FACTORS

Mall states that so-called congenital amputation anomalies should be considered as a separate class, as yet unexplained, but indicating that hereditary or germ effects may have an influence in their production. Stockard believes that in these forms of amelia, the hereditary factors are involved and it is well known that one form of anomalies of the extremities, that is polydactylism, is inherited.

From this consideration of the subject, it would seem that the word amputation does not express the condition at all and that the actual state of affairs is either an inherited structural defect or one due to faulty development in the earliest embryonic period.

SUMMARY

We have definite knowledge that almost any form of monstrosity may be produced experimentally in fish and chick embryos by cutting down the oxygen supply or by some means of irritation. In the human embryo a large number of monsters have been found in ectopic pregnancies, where it is known that there is faulty implantation of the blastocyst and a resultant diminution of the oxygen supply.

As regards the extremities, the abnormality may consist of the absence of the proximal bones, the distal bones being normally formed and joined directly to the skeleton. In these so-called amputation cases where the distal extremity is absent as the forearm or foot, there are invariably other malformations. In the stump of the forearm of this case, the x-ray shows the presence of undeveloped bones arising apparently from ossification centers normally placed in the missing parts. The same condition has been noted by Truman Abbe in a case that had seeming congenital amputation of the fingers. The skiagraph shows the bones to be present but undeveloped. The bud-like spurs resembling the lost parts or portions of them may be present at the joint above as in Watts' case or may be mere projections simulating the absent soft parts as in our case. These spurs represent an apparent attempt by nature to continue the normal development.

REFERENCES

(1) *Fieux*: Rev. mens. d. gynec. obst. et paediat. d. Bordeaux, 1902, iv, 456. (2) *Ballantyne, J. W.*: Antenatal Pathology and Hygiene. The Embryo, Edinburgh, 1904, W. Green & Son. (3) *Abbe, Truman*: Am. Jour. Obst., 1916, lxxiii, 1089-1092. (4) *Howell, W. P.*: Arch. Pediatrics, 1905, xxii, 342-345. (5) *Watts, James*: Am. Jour. Anat., 1917, xxii, No. 3, pp. 386-437. (6) *Stockard, Charles R.*: Am. Jour. Anat., January 15, 1921, v, No. 2, p. 28. (7) *Mall, Franklin P.*: Am. Jour. Anat., 1917, xxii, No. 1, pp. 49-72.

22 EAST SIXTY-EIGHTH STREET. (*For discussion, see* p. 98.)

Society Transactions

AMERICAN ASSOCIATION OF OBSTETRICIANS, GYNECOLOGISTS, AND ABDOMINAL SURGEONS. THIRTY-FOURTH ANNUAL MEETING HELD AT ST. LOUIS, MO., SEPTEMBER 20, 21, AND 22, 1921

The President, Dr. Henry Schwarz, in the Chair.

Dr. John N. Bell, of Detroit, Mich., read a paper on **Diabetes and Pregnancy.** (For original article see page 20.)

DISCUSSION

DR. IRVING W. POTTER, Buffalo, N. Y.—I can report four cases of pregnancy occurring in diabetic women. The first was a woman who had undergone reverses and while three months' pregnant went into a state of coma, following a long period of mental and physical exertion. She was brought to me by a physician, and I refused to terminate the pregnancy. Possibly if I had she might have been alive. Another case came from Toronto, a distinct type who went into labor at full term and was delivered of a dead baby. She went on to recovery but still has her diabetes. Another case was a true diabetic, with a brother who was diabetic and was treated for years for the disease. She also lost her baby. The fourth case was the daughter of one of our most prominent families whose father was a diabetic, and an uncle who was a diabetic has since died of the disease, but she was carried along through the entire pregnancy, and was delivered by myself of a perfectly healthy baby at full term. She, however, shows a considerable amount of sugar in the urine and is very rarely sugar free.

DR. M. A. TATE, Cincinnati, Ohio.—Some ten years ago I presented to this Association a paper on glycosuria complicating pregnancy. One of the two greatest advances in obstetrics, as brought out by Dr. Bell, is prenatal care. Every pregnant woman when she consults a physician should receive a most careful examination, particularly of the urine. If we have a case of true diabetes, the patient having suffered for a number of years, that patient should not, in my opinion, be allowed to go on to full term. If we have a temporary glycosuria that patient can be carried through by appropriate treatment.

DR. BELL (closing).—It seems to me it is a question of just how long before term we should believe a patient could be carried to term with modern treatment. I had hoped that some of the members would discuss that point. For instance, a patient presents herself, as in my case, four or five months before term: will you, knowing she has a true diabetes, attempt to carry her to term or will you not? This case, of course, may have been an exception and had a very fortunate outcome, but I believe we should make some effort to carry these women to term in the hope that they will come through all right.

Dr. WILLIAM G. DICE, of Toledo, Ohio, read a paper on **Heart Disease in Pregnancy**. (For original article see page 24.)

DISCUSSION

DR. JOHN OSBORN POLAK, BROOKLYN, N. Y.—In the discussion of this excellent paper I wish to emphasize a few points.

First, the importance of prenatal care. In following some 5,000 cases in our prenatal clinic we found that 2 per cent presented heart lesions. In other words, there were 100 cases that had definite heart lesions. I do not believe that the internist has an appreciation of the surgical heart or the obstetric heart. It is the man who is following the case from day to day and from week to week in his prenatal work who is the best judge of the woman's cardiac force. It is not a murmur, as the Doctor has said, but the muscular force and action that must be considered in determining whether this woman is capable of going on with her pregnancy or whether it must be terminated. It is interesting that in these 100 cases there were only five that needed interference. Three had cesarean sections and two, after rest in bed with no improvement, were delivered in the early months by abdominal section, with sterilization.

We believe that section is the preferable way to empty these uteri and that these patients stand operative procedure better than they do induction of abortion, as the nervous element in all these cases is very marked. In other words, by anociassociation and plenty of morphine, scopolamin and gas, one can deliver these women at three or four months by abdominal hysterotomy, sterilize them and have better results than he can by producing abortion. That may seem odd, but it is a proved fact.

Another point is that repeated pregnancies jeopardize the patient's life and her longevity. We therefore feel that where we are able to carry a woman to term and she does not spontaneously deliver, and spontaneous labor relieved with the free use of scopolamin and morphine, supplemented with low forceps in the second stage is our choice, a cesarean section with sterilization is the safest procedure.

The next point of importance is the management in the third stage. These patients will often go through the first part of the labor and collapse in the third stage. This, I think, can be prevented by: First, use of abdominal pressure in the form of heavy sandbags; second, bleeding to relieve the right heart, and third, vigorous stimulation at that time.

Finally, these heart patients do not need as much digitalis as the internist usually thinks. They do better with rest and small doses of morphine than they do with heroic treatment.

DR. GORDON K. DICKINSON, of Jersey City, N. J., read a paper entitled **The Breast Physiologically and Pathologically Considered with Relation to Bleeding from the Nipple**. (For original article see page 31.)

DISCUSSION

DR. JAMES E. DAVIS, DETROIT, MICHIGAN.—This paper calls our attention rather directly to the etiology of cancer. It should be remembered that this gland is decidual. Its period of functioning is an active one and it is constantly subject to traumatism: therefore: inflammatory lesions very commonly develop. The connection between the functioning of the organs of gestation and the breast has been made clear in my paper. Vicarious menstruation often occurs during periods of suppression, or at least the breast is liable to show congestion, if not actual bleeding. The blood vessels about the nipple, many of them, have very thin walls, and if subjected to an active congestion it is easy to see how rupture can take place.

The cell normally has three stages to pass through: The developmental stage, the stage of maturity and the stage of senescence, and under congestion the period of development is gradually increased by the nutrition brought to the part. The growth impulse is intensified, but without adequate differentiation of cells and tissues. These cells do not all mature and the cell passes through the developmental stage directly into senescence.

In normal tissues or those with ability to return to a status of essentially normal function, a certain number of cells always fail to reach maturity. In tissues of decidual and vestigial character and in tissues undergoing the vicissitudes of inflammatory change, the number of immature cells is greatly increased. In cancer there are but few cells that reach maturity. Their number is never large enough to differentiate a tissue capable of more than very incomplete function.

DR. ROLAND E. SKEEL, LOS ANGELES, CAL.—Dr. Dickinson's paper is rather difficult to discuss in a few moments, largely because of the great number of subjects he has covered, but there are two things of which I wish to speak.

First, I wish Dr. Dickinson in closing, to say a little more about the psychic origin of any tumor. Some of us, I think, would find difficulty in subscribing to the theory that any tumor had its origin in the psychic field, although many of us are willing to believe that the psychic field has been indifferently explored as yet.

The second thing was not brought out, I think, and is really very important. Dr. Dickinson mentioned the importance of early diagnosis and of early surgical treatment of any condition producing bleeding from the breast, but the important thing about the benign tumor of the breast is that so many general practitioners advise a young patient to let a benign growth alone.

Has it not been the experience of every one in the room to have patients come to the radical operation for carcinoma who have had an adenoma for many years before? They are so accustomed to the small growth that the early development of cancer means nothing to them, and how often are we startled after removing a supposed adenoma to find that the microscope shows a beginning adenocarcinoma and our minor operation is a failure instead of a success. The woman of forty or forty-five who develops a lump in the breast, will probably consult her physician without delay, but the woman who is accustomed to the presence of her little adenoma will allow several months to elapse before doing so.

DR. AARON B. MILLER, SYRACUSE, N. Y.—A patient came under my observation with a history of bleeding from the nipple with each menstrual period. I looked over the literature and found it was very unwise to allow a condition of that kind to remain, that the probability was it would become malignant, and the thing to do was to operate early. After seeing the patient several times I found she had spent considerable time in New York City and had been shopping around the country with the advice that it should be taken care of at once, otherwise, serious conditions would probably develop. She remained under my observation for some time but continued to keep her breast, despite my advice to the contrary and she has just sailed for Europe. During each menstrual period bleeding occurs and if the breast is pressed several drops are exuded. This is merely a matter of clinical experience.

DR. CHARLES W. MOOTS, TOLEDO, OHIO.—For a number of years I have been a member of the Cancer Committee of our State Association and it has been my duty to go out into the highways and byways and talk cancer. Unfortunately, we find that the general practitioner needs educating more than the public. The public will listen and this is what occurs: the women after hearing these talks take their so-called benign tumors to their family physician and he tells them if it has never hurt them to let it alone. That is universal and I wish the men of this Association would help those of us who are working along these lines to get these men to stop that sort of advice. I am sure if we are to get anywhere in cancer we must operate on these cases in the precancerous stage. At least the patient must be put under expert service to determine whether or not the growth is cancerous.

DR. WILLIAM SEAMAN BAINBRIDGE, NEW YORK CITY.—Last year I read a paper on "Benign Mammary Tumors and Intestinal Toxemia" before this Association, and also one on "The Human Breast—A Plea for Well Directed Treatment Based on a More Accurate Diagnosis", before the Tri-State District Medical Association. The subject under discussion is so important that I feel it necessary to say a few words in emphasis of certain points.

I fully agree with the last speaker that the education is necessary not so much of the public as of the profession. I want to agree with all that has been said, but I feel it compulsory to raise a flag of caution. The layman is between Scylla and Charybdis, he has been told that every tumor is essentially malignant and should be cut out inside of forty-eight hours after its appearance. Such a statement was made before this body by one of our colleagues two years ago. Others say: "Let the tumor alone." Certainly the layman is in a difficult position. Much harm will result if there is a strict adherence to either one of these dogmas.

The examining physician must be educated to the point where he will be able to differentiate between a tumor of the breast which has become a cancer, and the "lumps" which may come from the toxemias, thyroid dyscrasia, acidosis, etc.

In my paper on "The Human Breast, etc.," I drew the following conclusions, and it may not be amiss to repeat them here:

1. The laity is coming earlier, in increasing numbers, for examination.

2. Opportunity for service, on the part of the medical profession, is being increased in proportion as the public responds to its summons.

3. The profession must develop a higher degree of diagnostic ability than in the past and possess itself of all the essential facts concerning breast conditions.

4. A judicial attitude must be maintained—careful examination with well-poised judgment.

5. Accurate diagnosis of abnormal breast conditions means and demands a careful systemic survey as well as an efficient local examination.

6. The human mamma may be the seat of changes purely inflammatory or of neoplastic nature, closely simulating malignancy.

7. The relationship between the internal genitalia and the breast has been well established. Correction of abnormal pelvic conditions may ameliorate or relieve certain mammary changes.

8. The relationship between chronic intestinal stasis and certain breast conditions seems to be proved. Toxemia from teeth, tonsils and other parts of the body may also have its effect upon the mammary gland.

9. Serious conditions are often overlooked while they are as yet amenable to the simplest measures of nonsurgical treatment.

10. The use of the terms "breast" and "mamma" as synonymous may increase the difficulties of diagnosis. The writer believes it would be helpful to confine the term "mamma" to the gland with its ducts, including its outlet, the nipple; "breast" as embracing the entire mamma with all else that surrounds it—the skin, fat, fascia, capsule, and the bed upon which the gland rests, the fascia, muscle and bone with cartilage, in juxtaposition to the mamma.

11. Any of these structures may be diseased, and multiple pathologic lesions present, rendering diagnosis more difficult.

12. Abnormal conditions, congenital or acquired, may be present in neighboring

structures, and lead to wrong diagnosis of cancer, or if malignant disease is present, lead to the diagnosis of the inoperable and incurable stage although the neoplasm is early and surgically curable.

13. In spite of present knowledge, it is impossible at times to arrive at an immediate accurate diagnosis. In justice to the patient it may be necessary to keep her under careful observation, treating general conditions, before proceeding to radical surgery. If, then, mistakes occur, it should be the earnest endeavor of the profession to make them fewer and fewer.

14. It is reasonable to assume that with the early recognition of some lumpy conditions of the breast, followed by adequate systemic treatment and mechanical support, underlying factors of malignant disease may be removed.

15. A question naturally arises: If all the foregoing is true, may it not be that in that multiplex disease grouped today under the term "cancer," there are possibly causative factors underlying malignant disease in the toxemias and the heterological activity of the endocrines? This seems to be a very promising field of research.

16. When cancer is present beyond a reasonable doubt, radical surgery is absolutely indicated.

To allow a patient to drift beyond the hope of surgical cure is a terrible tragedy; to unnecessarily and radically remove a woman's breast may be a profound calamity. With a deep sense of the limitations in the art of exact diagnosis and of the greater responsibility today in the enlarging field of service for humanity, let the profession be ever guided by the watchword, "Not Fears But Facts."

DR. DICKINSON, (Closing).—Replying to Dr. Skeel, I did not mean that the psyche made tumors, but will induce a congestion of the parts and in that way indirectly produce them.

As to Dr. Bainbridge, if you watch and wait, with all the acumen you have, you may yet be mistaken, as I was on one of my recent cases when I found that the cancer had started.

I wish to put two things on record: First, this paper was instigated by a remark of Dr. Rodman's several years ago—I respect the memory of Rodman so much that I like to mention his name. Another thing: Two years ago I developed a lump in my left breast about the size of my fingernail, psychologic, I think. (Laughter). Anyway, it came; it was tender; everything that touched it hurt it. I tolerated it for a while, then went to my local friends, who said, "Go to Deaver." I went, he examined it and told me to come back in the spring, and if it had not disappeared he would remove it. It had disappeared. It was a natural lump, without any cause apparently except that I may be unusually nervous, quick, given to emotions, and it struck me locally.

DR. PALMER FINDLEY, of Omaha, Neb., read a paper entitled **The Slaughter of the Innocents.** (For original article see page 35.)

MR. ERNEST F. OAKLEY, JR., St. Louis, Mo., read a paper on **Legal Aspect of Abortion.** (For original article see page 37.)

DR. H. WELLINGTON YATES AND DR. B. CONNELLY, of Detroit, Mich., read a paper on **Treatment of Abortion.** (For original article see page 42.)

DISCUSSION

DR. GEORGE C. MOSHER, KANSAS CITY, MISSOURI.—There are two or three things which I should like to call to the attention of the Association.

In the heart cases, I always took the position that these cases in the absence of hemorrhage or loss of weight should be kept under observation. I have in a measure changed my view in this way but still maintain that a certain number will go through pregnancy and not lose their lives.

Another thing is the symptom of pernicious vomiting as a reason for abortion. We have had seventeen cases in the last two years of which fifteen have been carried through to the termination of pregnancy.

Third, the plan of operation. In five years, from 1909 to 1914, in the Kansas City General Hospital in which I have part of the obstetric service, statistics under the use of the curette during that time showed that the average length of time of each patient in the hospital was twenty-two days. From 1914 to the present, in which period we have adopted the conservative method of treatment and the curette has not been used once, the average time in the hospital has been eight and one-third days. The average cases of complication in the old days was 70 per cent, and our average since using the modern method of treatment has been only 5 per cent.

DR. EDWARD A. WEISS, PITTSBURGH, PA.—Several years ago I presented a paper before the Association which brought forth rather violent discussions, especially by Dr. Skeel. Since then I have not changed my views, basing my beliefs chiefly on hospital work. It is rather strange that with all the advances in hospital and medical affairs we continue to stand still in the much abused and time honored so-called "therapeutic abortion." Physicians who will go almost to any limit to secure a good result in other cases, will produce an abortion on the slightest provocation. I thought that perhaps I was rather extreme on this subject, but one of my internes told me that his former teacher in obstetrics had fifteen distinct indications for therapeutic abortion, not counting many others that may be supplementary. Is it any wonder then that so many abortions are being performed by the laymen and the quacks when we, as a profession, give them so much leeway and encouragement?

I regret that papers should be read by members of the Association advocating abortions on rather restricted grounds. In twenty years I have never seen a patient die from hyperemesis gravidarum.

In a period from 1910 to 1920, some 114 cases were admitted in my hospital service for interruption of pregnancy. In not one was an abortion performed, and not one of the women died. These were not ordinary cases, such as the usual vomiting of pregnancy, but came under the classification of hyperemesis and other more or less serious conditions. So it seems to me that as a Society, composed almost entirely of teachers in medical schools, or at least heads of departments where we have a large number of internes under our care, we should be extremely careful in giving out these indications for the so-called therapeutic abortions, and further I would like to voice my emphatic protest against advocating abortion in early tuberculosis or mild heart conditions, for I have seen cases carried through, even with pyrexia and loss of weight, and go on to a happy termination and normal delivery.

DR. M. P. RUCKER, RICHMOND, VIRGINIA.—I wish to say a few words about the criminal aspect of abortion. The law is plain enough, but the trouble is, that it is difficult to apply the law in an individual case. I would like to cite an instance that occurred several years ago in Virginia. The students who saw the case first made a diagnosis of puncture of the uterine wall and sent the patient up to the hospital and immediately went up to the detective office to get to work on the legal end of the case while the hospital took care of the medical side. They finally ferreted out the woman who produced the abortion and the crochet needle she had used for the purpose. She made a confession. This happened in January and the trial was postponed until the summer. One student who lived in a distant state had to come back to the trial, at great expense and inconvenience and said he was cured of ever taking part in a criminal abortion again. The woman was bailed. She disappeared and was not produced. This is not an uncommon complication in these cases and is possibly one reason why the medical profession is so loath to take any part in them.

DR. GORDON K. DICKINSON, JERSEY CITY, N. J.—I would like to mention two points very briefly. In the literature, Myer speaks of the great prevalence of abortion in unwashed Rome. I think it has been the habit ever since. It was probably no more prevalent then than now, and it is probably no more prevalent now than it was then.

We control it in New Jersey by having the midwives licensed, and requiring them to be re-licensed every year. If we have occasion to suspect any one of them but cannot obtain full evidence to convict, the license is revoked the next year and she is put out of business.

DR. HUGO EHRENFEST, ST. LOUIS.—I wish to add a few remarks to the points brought out by Dr. Rucker. Some years ago a friend of mine was prosecuting attorney of this city and he had an idea that a group of medical men could help him in the prosecution of such cases. The result was most unsatisfactory. We were supposed to be *ex-officio* experts for the prosecutor any time he wanted us. I remember one instance when we had the midwife there, the fetus, the catheter and the patient on whom the abortion had been performed. It looked like a perfect case. I was put on the stand and the first question asked by the lawyer for the defense was: "Doctor, do you qualify as an expert in abortions?" (Laughter.) I tried to explain but was forced to answer his questions with "Yes" or "No." And so he made me confess that I had produced several abortions. I had no opportunity before cross-examination to explain that they were all therapeutic. He then asked if I had ever lost any of my abortion cases and I answered "No." He then said, "You are an expert in abortions, go ahead." (Laughter.) We had many such experiences. I have been told by an expert criminal lawyer that the average man on the jury is afraid of the accused midwife because she might know that once his own wife was helped out by her. We could work out the cases any way we wanted to, but we could not get a conviction. I would like to ask Mr. Oakley to tell us concerning the results achieved with our very excellent Missouri law. I should like to know whether there is any midwife or physician in jail in this state; whether there has been for the past ten years, and whether or not prosecutions of these criminal abortion cases do not resemble very closely those under the Volstead Act.

MR. OAKLEY, (Closing on his part).—Of course Dr. Ehrenfest could qualify as an expert on abortion in theory but not, necessarily, as an expert on abortion in practice. The doctor must distinguish between a therapeutic abortion and an abortion in its unlawful or illegal sense. The respect in which he qualified as an expert was as a therapeutic abortionist, I trust, and not in the other way.

The doctor also said something about its being difficult to secure conviction and, in that respect, I take issue. The case is very simple. All that is necessary for the State to allege and prove is the fact that the woman died from peritonitis and general blood poisoning superinduced by a criminal abortion. This must be testified to by the attending physician who was present during her illness and at her death. The other element that is necessary is that an abortion had been performed upon this woman. Although the attending physician did not perform this abortion he has to testify to the cause of death and is disposed of. The autopsy physician is the one who states under oath that an abortion has recently been performed upon the woman; that, in conjunction with the fact that she died of peritonitis, that, although the woman was pregnant, it was not necessary to operate upon her to save her life or the life of the unborn child, is enough to prove the State's case; and these three things are easily and quickly proved. I recall one case in which I had the dying statement of the woman. The general dying statement is not sufficient. The declarant must be under the impression that she is about to die. She must realize this. She must say: "Yes, I am going to die." If you gentlemen will recall this: if, in an emergency, you have any occasion to take yourselves a dying statement, base this upon that question and also upon the following question:—"Have you abandoned all hope of recovery?" and it is safe to say that there is no court in the United States that would not take your testimony. Then she names and states where she went, with whom she went, and what was done to her, and who sent her to this particular man, if a physician; or to the woman, if she be a midwife. In the particular case in which I testified, the dying statement was opposed by counsel for the defendant on the Constitutional provision that the accused must be confronted by the accuser in open court, and it was held by the Court that the accuser in this case was a dying woman, and because of that fact she could not be produced as a living witness against him. But we begged the point, and it was held that it was not the dying statement but the individual who was offering the dying statement who was the accuser, and the defendant was being confronted by the accuser inasmuch as I took the statement. I was cross-examined as to when, why and where this statement was obtained and in the various legal aspects he had offered. In that case the autopsy physician, unfortunately for the case, fell down. He was not quite sure whether or not an abortion had been performed and was the cause of the peritonitis. He did not know the date and could not tell whether it was a recent or an early affair in the life of the woman, and it was on his testimony that the case went up to the Supreme Court. That Court held that the dying statement was admissable, but that it was not according to the Missouri Constitution corroborated by the positive statement that an abortion had been performed on the woman, resulting in peritonitis and her death, and for that reason the case was remanded and sent back for retrial.

The elements constituting the criminal charge are quite simple, and you will find that no prosecutor will allow his office to issue any information in which he is not positive he can make out a *prima facie* case against the accused.

Another part of the discussion that I listened to—some of the jurors may have employed the midwife, and an aspersion was cast upon the wife of the Prosecuting Attorney in that respect. Now, gentlemen, that may be true. It is analogous in my mind with the prosecution of liquor cases and in the City of St. Louis for the State of Missouri I have the whole jurisdiction. Yesterday I obtained my second indictment, and yet I hold the record for the State of Missouri! (Laughter). They assign different reasons for the failure to convict, but the main reason is that we are all drinking men and therefore we should stand together. That is the attitude of the twelve men trying the defendant, and the physicians, I think, often hesitate, either because of their own particular interpretation of their ethics or because they are afraid of a damage suit, to divulge this information. It is not necessary for a physician to go to an attorney and say: "My patient has been operated upon and Dr. Jones did it", or "Mary E. Smith did it". No, that is not necessary. But it is his duty to go to the coroner in some jurisdictions, and to the police or sheriff in others, and inform that authority what he has found, which to his mind, speaks for abortion of a criminal aspect. That is his duty and after he has done that the authorities can go to the bedside of the patient and, if they are lucky, they will get a statement. I believe that dying statements are secured in perhaps four out of ten cases. It has been my experience that the woman, although she is at the point of death and knows it, to the very end will hold out and refuse to divulge the name of the individual who is responsible for her condition, because she looks upon that individual as her friend. I have in mind an individual who was kept alive by a physician for two weeks longer than she should have lived, but who refused absolutely to make any statement as to who was responsible for her condition, even though she knew she was going to die.

DR. CHARLES E. ZIEGLER, of Pittsburgh, Pa., presented a paper on **Additions to Our Obstetric Armamentarium.** (For original article see page 46.)

DISCUSSION

DR. EDWARD A. WEISS, PITTSBURGH, PENNSYLVANIA.—Regarding the clamp the doctor has described I will say that this is one of the appliances we have been using in our department for some time, with very satisfactory results. From the picture one would think it was rather complicated, but it is quite simple and has a great deal to recommend it. A cotton, not a gauze, pad between the clamp and the skin, it really absorbs the moisture and makes it very efficacious. The cord is mummified and drops off after seventy-two hours.

DR. JOHN O. POLAK, BROOKLYN, NEW YORK.—These devices of Dr. Ziegler's are very ingenious. Personally, I feel that the clamp is rather complicated and that it might be difficult to use. As a rule, we are all trying to make obstetrics just as simple as possible, and we have all gone through tying off the cord and burying it, as suggested by R. L. Dickinson several years ago, and have tried various ligatures, yet the fact stands out that the clamp is the most satisfactory method of treating the cord. This clamp, if it has the advantages Dr. Ziegler claims for it, certainly deserves a more extended application.

Regarding the wristlet, there is no doubt that it is very good, but there is a chain necklace on the market at present that is really so simple that we cannot see the use of a more complicated and expensive device. The baby's name is threaded in lettered beads on an ordinary trout line and the necklace is put about the neck and sealed and clamped before the child leaves the delivery room. In that way the baby's name is stationary and when the child is sent down to the office for discharge the family either buy the necklace or they cut the necklace off. Recently we have had the lettered beads painted with radium paint so that they may be seen in the dark.

DR. ZIEGLER, (closing).—I have little to add except to say that the clamp is very simple when you come to use it. Perhaps the pictures have made it appear more complicated than it really is. I am finding it very satisfactory and am never in doubt as to results.

In regard to the necklace mentioned by Dr. Polak, I am familiar with it. The principal objection to it is that the letters do not remain in alignment. The name is therefore at no time in full view and is accessible only through spelling it out by adjusting each bead in its turn. The lettered beads, moreover, are usually to be found behind the baby's neck or back.

As to the wristlet: The pictures and detailed descriptions of the parts of the wristlet, appear to have complicated it. It is in fact very simple. My own opinion in regard to the sealing device, is that in most hospitals it will likely be regarded as unnecessary. As the wristlet is put on by stretching the band, its removal requires some little trouble. Nurses and other attendants have no object in deliberately removing the marks of identification from one baby and putting it on another. However, the sealing device is there if wanted; if not, it may be left off. With the wristlet, the name is in plain view at all times. The name label being covered with the celluloid shutter and in a sealed compartment, is effectually protected against mutilation or soiling and cannot be removed while the wristlet is on the arm. Even boiling does not affect the legibility of the name; it only serves to seal the compartment the more effectually, through the expansion of the celluloid.

DR. ARTHUR M. MENDENHALL, of Indianapolis, Ind., read a paper entitled **Teaching Undergraduate Obstetrics.** (For original article see page 53.)

DISCUSSION

DR. O. H. SCHWARZ, ST. LOUIS, MO.—In this very important paper we all more or less agree with what has been brought up. It is very important that in the future if obstetrics is to keep pace with medicine and surgery so far as teaching is concerned, this branch will also have to be put on a full time basis. Such a condition will undoubtedly improve the Out-Patient Department as far as teaching is concerned. In most instances such departments do not get the proper supervision, and certainly a full time man will be able to supervise such departments better than men who are also engaged in private practice. We are now attempting to have at least an interne present at each delivery, so that he can instruct, in some measure in these cases.

The ideal thing, of course, is a maternity hospital, with a number of beds available for teaching purposes. Fifty beds would probably be more than sufficient.

I do not believe that manikin practice needs so much attention as has been pointed out. I believe individual work with the patient will do much more than the manikin practice, and I would like to know just what is carried out in 90 hours of manikin practice.

Another thing that will help in the teaching of obstetrics, particularly the abnormal deliveries, breech extraction, face presentation, etc., is the moving picture film. I have had the opportunity of witnessing the pictures taken at the Wertheim Clinic and some of these films were particularly good, especially those showing breech extraction, podalic version and face presentation. They are shown almost as well as these cases could be demonstrated in the delivery room. With the proper apparatus the pictures could be shown repeatedly and stopped at any stage in order to bring out a particular point. I believe such pictures will be of very considerable value in the teaching of obstetrics.

DR. JOHN O. POLAK, BROOKLYN, NEW YORK.—The question is, what and how much should we teach the undergraduate in obstetrics. I have taken the position for a long time that we should limit our instruction in obstetrics to teaching the management of normal obstetric cases and obstetric diagnosis. We have paid a great deal of attention to the antepartum examination. At the Long Island College Hospital each student spends four weeks in constant attendance in the antepartum clinic, and each man will make twenty-five to forty examinations, which are checked up by the man in charge, who is a part time paid instructor. We try to teach the student the aseptic conduct of labor. We know it is not possible to carry into the private home the paraphernalia so common in a maternity delivery room, and so we teach intensive asepsis,—the doctor's hands, the parts of the woman and the operative field are aseptic, and the student must use just as much care to deliver the woman as he would to open the abdomen. Then we teach him the course of labor.

From the first moment the woman falls into labor, he is in attendance and does not leave until she is delivered. He sits up with the patient and without attempting to hurry her dilatation, he records the pains and the results of his examination by rectum, listens to and records the fetal heart every half hour during the first stage. During the perineal stage the heart is studied at intervals of ten minutes.

We believe that labor is a surgical procedure, that the delivery of the primipara is just as important as the opening of the abdomen, and we tell our students that all we can teach them is diagnosis and progress of normal labor. If they want more than that we are willing to give them an internship, and if they want still more, we are willing to give them a residence if they make good. We tell them they cannot expect to go out and deliver a woman if they do not know how to repair an injury and when to interfere. All we can teach them is when to interfere; we cannot teach them how to interfere in the short time available. Here is where the manikin comes in. They can practice forceps and version and breech extractions on it and the first case they have to use forceps on they realize the benefit of this practice. The man who has never handled forceps on a manikin is absolutely at a loss. Every man will have a breech presentation sooner or later, and if he has had no practice in extraction on a manikin he is useless. We do not consider these men skilled, but they get the fundamentals during the course.

We need more hospital facilities, we need full-time men. We cannot teach obstetrics without some full-time men, and these are the facts we have to make known so that the public will give of their money and we can get the hospitals so that this work can be carried on properly.

DR. JOHN NORVAL BELL, DETROIT, MICHIGAN.—I think if they would incorporate in the Sheppard-Towner Bill a clause providing the money to pay a man to teach men how to deliver a normal case we would get good teaching. You cannot expect a man to get up in the middle of the night and go and teach students how to deliver a normal case, and that is the whole sum and substance of the thing. I believe firmly in having a full-time man, or two or three, available in the institution, but they must be men who know how to teach the students to deliver a perfectly normal case.

DR. WILLIAM H. CONDIT, MINNEAPOLIS, MINNESOTA.—I think we have struck the keynote of our future professional needs in our efforts to reduce the morbidity and mortality of the puerperal state. We have made no progress in the last twenty years. The rate of maternal mortality per 1,000 births in 1920, was 15 per cent above the rate in 1919. The United States is fourteenth of all the countries of the world. I think our weakness is in teaching students. The requirements of the students today are so advanced that by the time they are sophomores, they know all to be known in medicine. We, at the University of Minnesota, have our shortcomings, especially in regard to our personal supervision and teaching by the chiefs of the departments. We do little didactic teaching, chiefly quiz work. We have a valuable adjunct in our Fellowship coterie. We have a Fellow or two on a three year course. He has had some actual practice in general medicine and maybe in surgery. The interne is not given any actual teaching responsibility, but the Fellow under the chief is given quite a good deal of responsibility. He is in charge of the Out-Patient Department and the uncomplicated deliveries in the hospital and they are under the supervision of the instructors or of the chief himself. I think this is proving very practical; more time can be spent by him in detail technical teaching of the student. In the last year of the Fellowship he does some operative work, both in gynecology and obstetrics. We cannot help feeling that our students go out pretty well trained. There are some who should never deliver a woman. I had a junior student at the bedside very recently and the first thing he did was to begin stripping on his glove with his bare hand. Then he rushed up to cleanse the draped patient with nothing but his rubber apron on. We should not be compelled to teach a man the first principles of asepsis in his Junior year when he begins his course in obstetrics. There is evidently weakness in other departments. We cannot make experts out of poor material, but we must try to teach the student so as to prepare him for the practical, bedside, country practice. We must impress the student with the importance of this being a surgical procedure, needing probably more careful and more cleanly technic than even many surgical operations. We do not allow our students ever to make a vaginal examination. We teach the rectal examination and I think that is one of the preventives of many accidents that happen in the country practice.

DR. JAMES E. DAVIS, DETROIT, MICHIGAN.—Just a word in regard to one angle of this problem that I think has not received due attention and emphasis. After listening to the paper and discussion I could not help being impressed with the undue emphasis that has been laid upon the mechanics of this work. I, for one, do not believe that the mechanics should be overemphasized, especially with the undergraduates. Many of the best teachers are saying that the less you do in a mechanical way the better your patients are cared for. Therefore, I want to call attention to this side of the question for the undergraduate. The point I wish to make is this: If greater emphasis were laid upon the bacteriology and the pathology of the birth canal, and if the students were taught to be alert for all the conditions that may arise, I am sure they will obtain impressions that will not become easily effaced and will prove of greater value than information obtained from the manikin or from much of the outdoor clinic work, or from a certain number of cases conducted in a purely mechanical way. The examination of the placenta is also important. It is a common observation that when this organ has a dirty yellow appearance, in the majority of instances, there is infection. It is important also to know that cross sections of the placenta may reveal conditions which will postulate certain things having taken place before birth, thereby making one alert for persisting pathologic conditions in both the mother and the child. Specimens illustrating the gross and microscopic pathology are invaluable in teaching this subject.

DR. MENDENHALL (closing).—I expected more criticism and am disappointed. I believe that the out-door department must be continuously supervised. If it is so done, it is of inestimable value, but in most institutions it is not so done. Usually the student delivers the patient and does not know whether it is a posterior or anterior delivery.

Dr. Schwarz, I think, misunderstood my remarks on the manikin work. I mentioned ninety hours at one school, but recommended thirty to forty hours. I still believe that manikin work is invaluable. I agree with Dr. Schwarz that work with the patient is better if we can have enough patients. If not, the work with the manikin is second best, at least, for practical experience.

A point that Dr. Polak brought out I wish to emphasize in closing, and that is the question of diagnosis, and how much the early graduate is going to do in obstetrics. In this, I am reminded of my last lecture by Dr. de Schweinitz on diseases of the eye. He told us he was not turning us out as ophthalmologists, but hoped he had taught us enough to know when to call for help from an ophthalmologist. I hope we may teach the students enough to enable them to know when to call for consultation in obstetrics.

Dr. MAGNUS A. TATE, of Cincinnati, O., presented a paper on **A Method of Delivery in Normal Cases.** (For original article see page 61.)

DISCUSSION

DR. IRVING W. POTTER, BUFFALO, NEW YORK.—Times have certainly changed. Who ever thought, five years ago, that Dr. Tate of Cincinnati would be giving me credit for anything; and yet, today, he gave me credit for dilating the vagina; and then he goes on and messes up a beautiful labor case. Now Dr. Tate has been to Buffalo; but he didn't stay long enough to learn anything. He reminds me very much of that story of the bull in the china shop,—what he didn't spoil by breaking, he messed up, and that's the way he handled this case. Who ever heard of a patient going under an anesthetic and then waking up, being given a dose of pituitrin, and given an anesthetic again? From the very start we have tried to keep away from dilating the cervix. We have dilated and ironed out the vaginal tract with very gratifying results, but we never dilated the cervix. And why, when he had a cervix he could put his hand in, did he not go on and complete the work quickly by version instead of taking an hour and fifteen minutes to do it?

In my experience it is very dangerous teaching to advocate the use of pituitrin while the child is in the uterus. Reports of bad results have come from all over the country, and that is what we have tried to avoid. We have dilated the vaginal tract and delivered the baby; and, after the baby has left the uterus, we have given the pituitrin. After a few years Dr. Tate will do differently. He will come around to treating his cases in a clean manner. If you dilate the vaginal tract there is no occasion for an episiotomy in any case. I have never done an episiotomy in my life and would not know how to do one; but to allow a patient to have an anesthetic, then let her come out, then give her pituitrin, I do not see the necessity for such a procedure.

I am pleased to have heard this paper because it means that Dr. Tate is coming around to the point where he believes there is some discomfort to the woman in the second stage of labor. I think the first stage is very easy to manage, but it is the long drawn-out second stage that he is trying to get rid of and that we are trying to get rid of, and we feel that we have succeeded better without pituitrin and without the anesthetic by doing a clean version at the end of the first stage of labor.

DR. ARTHUR H. BILL, CLEVELAND, OHIO.—It is very hard for me to discuss a paper when I totally disagree with what has been said. Nevertheless I am afraid that is the case in the present instance. I am in hearty sympathy with anything which tends to make labor easy, but one thing I have always contended is that we should not interfere with the first stage of labor. If the pain is relieved, patients may be allowed to go through the first stage, and in the majority of cases, the head will pass spontaneously through the os. Let the first stage of labor alone and relieve the pain, no matter how long it takes. I am sorry to have Dr. Tate put the patient on a time limit basis. I think that is wrong. Ordinarily, the length of the first stage makes little difference, if the patient is comfortable.

In regard to the second stage of labor, I shall have something more to say in my paper. I wish to go on record as opposed to the use of pituitrin when the baby is in the uterus. I do not believe that all the accidents resulting from its use have been reported, including damage to the baby. We can get along without it. Whenever possible, let Nature take her course during the first stage of labor.

DR. M. PIERCE RUCKER, RICHMOND, VIRGINIA.—I agree with Dr. Bill that pituitrin is a dangerous drug. We have tried it on animals and, if you get any action at all, you get an incomplete tetanus of the uterus. I have tried it on three patients and have confirmed Dr. Haskell's experiments satisfactorily. In the tetanic contraction what are you doing? You interfere with the circulation in the uterus and produce suffocation of the baby in a great many of the cases. I went over the records of the Memorial Hospital and found the infant mortality twice that in pituitrin cases to those in which it was not given, regardless of the operators. Of course, it sometimes was not used properly, but it is mighty poor comfort to explain to the mother, who has a dead baby, by saying that she was too much exhausted, or something like that. You are just inviting trouble by giving pituitrin before the baby is out of the uterus.

DR. HENRY SCHWARZ, ST. LOUIS, MISSOURI.—I had no intention of participating in the discussion, but I cannot sit quiet and have men tell us that the use of pituitary preparations is as dangerous as they want to make us believe. It is true that you should not use pituitary preparations until you know what platform you stand on. When we, in 1912, tried all the various preparations of pituitrin in the market, when we used Armour's, Burroughs Wellcome & Company's and Parke, Davis & Company's preparations, and others, we did find exactly what you state. Armour's and Burroughs Wellcome's were twice as active as the others. We likewise found out that we must not use teaspoonful doses, cubic centimeter doses, but that we must be careful and approach the case slowly, with two or three minims at a time if need be. We found that we did not get tetanus of the uterus when it was used in that way, and the great advantage of it is that it causes contractions of the uterus which come and go, unless it is used by men who do not know how to handle it. It was first used by us, or we were one of the first, in cesarean sections because in this operation we were always afraid of hemorrhage when we had to open the uterus at a time when the woman was not in labor. In those days we usually had to wait until the woman went into labor before we could operate. Since the advent of the pituitary preparations we select our time for the operation and we have every assurance that we are safe. In the majority of operations, when we give the full dose of a pituitary preparation of some kind, we can be sure the uterus will contract on delivery of the child.

Again, we have proved, not on ten or twenty, but on hundreds of cases, that there is nothing more valuable than pituitary preparations before the baby is born. After the baby is born we want the tetanic contractions so that the uterus does not relapse and accumulate blood and create after-pains; but before the baby is born, we want the intermittent contractions. We have used it on untold cases; and they are all on record, and you are invited to come to Barnes Hospital and look at any of our case records. There are a few thousand of them, and you will find that, in the majority of them pituitary preparations have been used. You will find that in some emergency calls to the home of patients who have had several children, and who are of relaxed habit, babies are born without the assistance of the doctor; but quite often there is hemorrhage; at times inversion of the uterus. In cases in which one can feel the head in the pelvis with the membranes still intact and the cervix open, that the patient may go into labor almost at any moment, we ask them to come to the hospital and then at 7 o'clock in the morning we give them castor oil; that makes them very prone to go into labor; but to make sure of it we give them four to five minims of Armour's or Burroughs Wellcome's pituitary preparation. A doctor and a nurse remain at the bedside, and sometimes a little massage is necessary, but we keep up the pituitrin, give it every few hours in cases of relaxed habit, so as to obtain relief, avoid the danger of hemorrhage, and prevent severe after-pains which are common if the case is left to Nature. As soon as the baby is born we administer a dose of some preparation of ergot to secure tetanic contractions of the uterus.

DR. TATE, (closing).—I do not do a version on normal cases because it is wrong and I do not believe it is good obstetrics.

As to the danger of pituitrin, I have written to the various manufacturers about pituitrin, have read the literature as thoroughly as possible, have had personal experience, have tried to analyze the various papers on pituitrin; and why some few physicians will not use it, calling it a dangerous drug is beyond me. You would not say you would not use cocaine or ether because once in a while you had a death from it. I consulted Professor Jackson of the Cincinnati University as to the properties and danger of pituitrin, and he said there was no danger at all if a man understood how to use it. That is the ground which I take. The recent books on therapeutics tell you that there is no danger from pituitrin up to 1 c.c., but I never give even 1 c.c., but do give one-third to one-half of a c.c. and never repeat it but once. I have not had a death of a mother and not a death of a child so far, and cases that were from fourteen to twenty hours from the beginning of the labor pains, go three, five or six hours. The gratitude of patients is enough to make me continue this method. Within the next few years I will present my results in case reports. All that I ask is, if you have a normal case, not an abnormal one, try this method and when you have tried it and have seen how beautifully it works, and how grateful the patient is, how the hours of pain are done away with, I think you will agree with me that there is merit in it.

DR. ARTHUR H. BILL, of Cleveland, O., read a paper entitled **The Choice of Methods of Making Labor Easy.** (For original article see page 65.)

DISCUSSION

DR. IRVING W. POTTER, BUFFALO, NEW YORK.—I agree with Dr. Bill that there should be no fads or fancies in obstetrics, but I insist that the use of chloroform is not a fad or fancy. My records prove this. There should be no hurry. Not long ago I kept a woman three days after rupture of the membranes, and then I delivered her of a normal child without injury to her whatsoever.

The occipitoposterior positions occur, he tells you, in about 27 per cent of the cases. I find them in about 60 per cent. But that does not make any difference. The tissues of the primipara seem to stretch and dilate easier than those of the multipara.

In the past year I have delivered 1130 women. My fetal mortality is now about what I have been striving for, 2.3 per cent. We use chloroform; we do versions; we do not use pituitrin until after the baby is out of the uterus. We do not use pituitrin in cesarean sections until after the uterus is closed. There is no occasion for giving it before. Give it after the uterus is closed and you will have no trouble. That is what version does; it obliterates the second stage. Five years ago there was much discussion on this point. There was no shock then to these labors, and many of them lasted a week. Now we hear from many sources about eliminating the shock of the second stage. Five years ago Dr. Schwarz used to go to sleep. He told me himself that as long as the woman was groaning regularly he could snore easily. (Laughter.) Now, all is different, and we are each of us trying to relieve all the shock and suffering possible by shortening the duration of labor without injury to the mother and child.

DR. JOHN NORVAL BELL, DETROIT, MICHIGAN.—On this subject I am quite in accord with Dr. Bill. I like his attitude in the whole matter, especially when he says that we should individualize, that we must not treat these cases all along a certain way. I believe Dr. Potter does a version in all of his cases, or in the vast majority of them. I believe that this is messing it up just as much as Dr. Tate messes it up in his way. I think there is a happy medium, and that is this: to relieve the woman of suffering and get her through the labor in the easiest manner possible. We can give the patient scopolamin and morphine in the first stage. We can administer just enough to keep her comfortable until the cervix has softened up and the patient is ready for delivery. Then, instead of doing as Dr. Tate does, which is a hard thing to do, though he speaks of its being easy, but I find it difficult—do as Dr. Bill does, wait until they are dilated and then do a version if you wish. But you can anesthetize the patient, and, I think, Dr. Potter has taught us that in this way you can dilate the vagina very nicely with the gloved hand and green soap, and go ahead and deliver the child. Why do a version and get all tangled up with the cord? That is what the version usually means—not in the hands of Dr. Potter because he knows how. My method is to give the patients scopolamin and morphine up to the time the cervix is softened, then give ether, use the forceps, deliver the baby, and the patient is comfortable and happy.

DR. ARTHUR H. BILL, (closing).—Dr. Potter says that if I had stayed in Buffalo and seen all those cases, I would have changed my mind. It would not have changed my mind one iota. I know that he can do versions. We can all do versions. Version is all right in its place. There are cases in which version is advantageous and others in which other methods have greater advantage. There is no question in my mind but that the head will come down spontaneously, as I have reported in 65 or 70 per cent of the cases, in which it will either reach the pelvic floor or pass through the cervix. Thus there will be many cases in which we simply have to lift the head over the perineum, and this is so much simpler and gives so much less disturbance that it appeals to one. So far as the patient's suffering is concerned, there is no difference. The patient is relieved of pain and knows nothing about the birth in either procedure. The question under consideration is the method by which we are to deliver the baby. We are aiming at the same thing in regard to saving the patient pain, but I wish to emphasize the fact that we should choose only those methods of delivery which seem best adapted to the case in hand. I think the obstetrician should familiarize himself with all methods so that he may avail himself of the method that is best suited to the particular case.

(To be continued in February issue.)

THE NEW YORK OBSTETRICAL SOCIETY. MEETING OF OCTOBER 11, 1921

Dr. Ralph H. Pomeroy in the Chair

Dr. Franklin A. Dorman presented a report of a case of **Primary Sarcomatous Tumor of the Umbilicus**.

The patient, Mrs. T. B., was referred by Dr. John W. Stokes, of Southold, N. Y. Her mother died of intestinal cancer, her father still living and well. Eight years ago she noticed a small growth at the navel about the size of a shoe button, which slowly increased in size, causing no pain or discomfort. During the past year and a half it grew much more rapidly. In November, 1920, it began to pain and this continued at intervals until the operation. The patient lost in weight and developed a cachexia. In May, 1921, she consulted Dr. Stokes, who urged operation, which she declined. Two weeks before the operation the growth began to ulcerate. At the time of operation, July 30, 1921, the tumor was about the size of two fists, fairly symmetrical, somewhat lobulated, with a broad basal attachment about two inches wide. Some of the skin was darkly pigmented and there were two large ulcerations. A circular incision was made about an inch from the pedicle and carried down to the umbilical ring which was widely excised and removed with the tumor. Abdominal exploration revealed no other growths. The patient's recovery was uneventful. Before operation she weighed about 100 pounds, on leaving the hospital she weighed 109½ pounds and her present weight is 127 pounds. She feels well and is growing stronger.

Pathologist's Report.—Macroscopical: Specimen is an irregular, nodular growth 15 x 14 x 8 cm., covered in most of its extent except at the base by skin which shows bluish discoloration and superficial ulceration in two or three places. The base of the tumor, around the umbilicus is fatty, the rest of it consists of soft, marrow-like tissue with large areas of necrosis and hemorrhage. Firm areas can nowhere be found although the consistency of the different parts of the tumor varies somewhat in different areas.

Microscopical: Most of the sections show large areas of necrosis with areas of hemorrhage. Other firmer parts are composed of polymorphous irregular cells varying in size and in shape from round to typically spindle forms. The nuclei are dark and mitotic figures are frequent. Intercellular tissue is easily seen.

Diagnosis: Fibroblastic spindle cell sarcoma with marked necrosis.

DISCUSSION

Dr. Hermann Grad.—About eight years ago I saw a woman in whom a recurrence took place after an operation for a sarcoma of the umbilicus. The patient was brought to New York about four months later with a recurrence. The mass was about as large as a fist and it had evidently involved the entire thickness of the abdominal wall. At that time Coley's serum was in vogue and we used it together with the x-ray and the mass disappeared without any operation. She recovered completely and notwithstanding the x-ray treatment, she bore a baby about three years later. She had an amenorrhea for about a year, but this cleared up also. The patient has remained apparently well since. Perhaps these sarcoma are not as malignant as we believe them to be, although this woman had a definite recurrence after a very extensive operation. The tumor in the case I refer to was not so large as the specimen shown here tonight, being the size of a hen's egg and was thoroughly circumscribed. There was no sign of involvement of the peritoneum.

DR. FRANKLIN A. DORMAN.—Dr. Grad, I suppose that was verified by pathological report?

DR. HERMANN GRAD.—Yes.

DR. FRANKLIN A. DORMAN.—We, of course, hope this may not recur. But the chances of recurrence are probable.

There are two points of interest in this case. The first is the size of the tumor. Cullen reports one, the diagnosis of which was not verified by pathologic examination, as large as an infant's head. The second point is, this is a primary growth, of which there are apparently very few on record.

DR. O. PAUL HUMPSTONE reported **A Case of Rupture of the Uterus in a Placenta Previa.**

Mrs. M. R., Hospital 77967, was admitted to the Obstetric Service of the Methodist Hospital having been referred to me by Dr. Howard Langworthy. She was 32 years of age, married ten years. She had five previous labors, all easy, with living children. She had one miscarriage followed by curettage soon after marriage. She had been operated for pelvic plastic repair three years previously, and had one child after that operation. She had not menstruated in seven months. Her pregnancy had been without incident until the morning of her admission, when upon arising from her bed she had a profuse hemorrhage from the vagina without pain or other symptoms.

Examination showed a well built woman, weighing about 140 pounds, a trifle pale, with a pulse of 108 and a blood pressure of 110 over 80. Her blood showed 2,800,000 red cells and 40 per cent hemoglobin. Her urine was normal. The fundus measured 26 cm. and the fetal heart was 130, in the right lower quadrant.

Vaginal examination showed a very soft cervix, not shortened, admitting two fingers to impinge upon the placenta covering the internal os completely, a head presenting at the brim. She was not in labor.

Our impression was a central placenta previa in a seven months' pregnant multipara not in labor.

In the light of these facts, and considering the very slight probability of viability of the child and the evident necessity for immediate interference, after suitable preparation, a No. 3 Voorhees bag was inserted in the uterus beneath the placenta and a light pack placed in the vagina. No anesthesia was necessary. The hemorrhage was controlled and labor came on in four hours. Good pains rapidly appeared and in two hours the bag had been expelled through the cervix. The bag displaced the presenting head and it failed to advance. Profuse hemorrhage occurring, the patient was anesthetized, the long gloved arm inserted through the placenta, a foot grasped and the knee brought to the vulva, again controlling the hemorrhage. The anesthetic was discontinued and I discoursed to the staff on the danger of rupture of the lower zone of the uterus in a placenta previa by immediate extraction. After waiting 30 minutes without a pain I ordered 7 minims of pituitrin given hypodermically. Four minutes later the patient had one agonizing pain, expelled the baby, which was dead, and placenta out of the vulva and bled profusely. Examination showed a rent in the lower zone of the uterus on the right side extending half way up to the fundus and through the peritoneum. The uterine artery being torn across, I rapidly packed the uterus, filling the cavity and the rent in the broad ligament, the tear in the uterine wall and finally the vagina.

The house surgeon through the abdominal wall pushed the fundus over to the right side and down making as much pressure as possible to control the bleeding. The abdomen was rapidly prepared, the patient given an ampule of pituitrin and 1/3 grain of morphine, hypodermically and taken to the operating room. Her condition was not alarming, pulse 140, of good quality and regular. She was not in shock.

A rapid supracervical hysterectomy was done, the abdomen freed of blood clots and closed without drainage. An intravenous infusion of 1000 c.c. of salt solution was given on the table. The convalescence was disturbed by some abdominal distention with fever for five days. Her blood count the morning after the operation was 1,800,000 red cell and 40 per cent hemoglobin. The patient improved so rapidly that transfusion was not deemed necessary and she left the hospital on the 23rd day after her operation, well.

The proposals we submit for discussion in the consideration of this case are: First; That central placenta previa is a surgical disease demanding hospital treatment. Second; That central placenta previa is best managed by abdominal delivery in competent hands in all cases. Third; That pituitrin should never be employed while the baby is still in the uterus.

There is nothing new in these conclusions but increasing experience in the light of abdominal surgical treatment should have taught us that if extensive tears, rupture of the uterus and excessive hemorrhage and sepsis are to be avoided one must keep away from the lower zone of the uterus in the management of central placenta previa.

DISCUSSION

DR. G. H. RYDER.—I doubt if there is any one here who would not agree that where it is possible, all such cases are best treated in hospitals. Dr. Humpstone's second conclusion is that all severe cases of placenta previa should be delivered by Cesarean. I believe few of us will agree to this. For years, good results have been obtained in placenta previa by delivery through the vagina. The field for cesarean section in placenta previa is a limited one; usually only where the diagnosis is made early, and where there is but little dilatation, with a firm cervix. When the cervix is much dilated and soft, the vaginal route is probably safer. Again where there has already been a great loss of blood, the added shock of a section might be enough to cause death.

In the case reported, Dr. Humpstone started his operation, to my mind, in the right way. He inserted a bag and followed its expulsion by a version and pulling down of a foot and thigh into the cervix. If he will pardon me for saying it, he made three errors in judgment after having selected this method of delivery. These and not the method were responsible for the ruptured uterus. First, he used a bag of too small size. If he had used a No. 4 bag, instead of a No. 3, it would have controlled the hemorrhage as well as did the smaller one. After its expulsion the cervix would have been fully dilated and the delivery could have been effected easily and slowly without danger of tearing the cervix and rupturing the uterus. Second, having used the smaller bag and having performed the version, it would seem to me that the delivery was hurried too much, from then on. If the mother had been permitted to come out of her anesthetic and push the fetus out slowly by her own efforts, taking plenty of time, I believe there would have been no ruptured uterus. Third, I think the use of pituitrin, with an undilated cervix, friable from the low implantation of the placenta, was contraindicated, more especially in the dose given. Dr. Humpstone selected the correct method for delivery of his patient, but used faulty judgment in carrying it out. I do not think he is warranted, from this experience, in concluding that the vaginal route in previa is to be discarded altogether, and that cesarean section alone is to be used.

Dr. Humpstone's third conclusion is that pituitrin should never be used in obstetrics with the fetus *in utero*. Probably many of us will not agree to this conclusion, for some of us have so used it, over and over again, with only good results. Pituitrin, it is true, should be used with the fetus *in utero* with great care, and practically only in primary uterine inertia and in the absence of any obstruction to delivery; and even then only in small doses. In Dr. Humpstone's case I think its use was contraindicated, as I have said. There was no primary uterine inertia, or the woman would not have expelled the bag by her own efforts; and there was obstruction in the undilated and friable cervix. Moreover, the dose of seven minims given is about twice the safe dose. It does not seem convincing, therefore, to condemn the usage of pituitrin altogether with the fetus *in utero*, because of an unfortunate experience due to its misuse.

In closing, I do not want to give the idea that I am criticising Dr. Humpstone adversely for his trying experience. The complication with which he was dealing, complete placenta previa, is one of the most frightful in obstetrics. Bad results may occur in the hands of any obstetrician, and Dr. Humpstone rescued his patient from grave danger by a most brilliant operation.

DR. JOHN O. POLAK.—There has been some interesting work done by Rucker, of Richmond, in the study of pituitrin, which has been recently called to my attention. It is so graphic that I believe we should take it into consideration. Rucker studied the effect of certain drugs on patients in labor by introducing a Voorhees bag into the cervix, connecting it with a blood pressure apparatus. He tested out strychnia, ergot, morphine, quinine, castor oil and pituitrin. The interesting point in all of these graphs is that while morphine actually increased the strength and length of the contractions, it was followed by uterine relaxation, the smallest dose of pituitrin never permitted a cessation of uterine contractions, the uterus was constantly in spasm from the time that the pituitrin was given. This spasmodic contraction was augmented from time to time by a strong labor pain, but the uterus was never relaxed. That is something which I think we do not realize in the use of pituitrin. Personally, I lost a number of babies in former days in cases in which pituitrin was administered, after the child had passed out of the uterus into the vagina, when the uterus is closely wrapped around the body of the child and the uteroplacental circulation is interfered with. For until we realized just what this placental compression meant and just what it did to the fetal heart, we lost some babies and these deaths must be attributed to pituitrin. I have had two instances where the placenta has been shaken loose in the early stage of labor by the use of pituitrin. These patients had accidental hemorrhage, and death of the fetus occurred in the first stage of labor. I feel more and more that in labor, pituitrin should not be used until the child is out of the uterus.

DR. G. L. BRODHEAD.—I feel that we all agree with Dr. Humpstone that placenta previa cases should be treated in a hospital. In central placenta previa beyond the seventh month I think there can be no question of the advisability of cesarean section. Cesarean section is, however, not the operation of choice in some cases of marginal placenta previa, especially in multipara. If a primipara has a marginal placenta previa and cesarean section is done, it may be that cesarean section will have to be done the next time but we have known normal delivery to follow cesarean section for placenta previa. While the immediate result for the mother and child in placenta previa might be best obtained by cesarean section, personally I do not believe every case of placenta previa demands cesarean section.

As to pituitrin, we should begin with not more than 3 or 5 minims. We have all seen violent contractions of the uterus after 5 minims and occasionally with 3 minims. In placenta previa the lower segment of the uterus is much more likely to rupture than in a normal pregnancy. The degree of effect produced depends on the variety of pituitrin used. I believe that when infundin is used, 3 minims is enough to begin with; later 5 minims can be given if necessary.

DR. FRANKLIN A. DORMAN.—As Dr. Ryder pointed out, we succeed with some cases of placenta previa, but in other cases we do not. In such cases where we follow every precaution and avoid a rupture of the lower segment, the woman does not survive on account of hemorrhage and relaxation. The only possible conditions under which we could have saved some of the patients would have been by an abdominal operation. I personally believe that in cases of central placenta previa, where the baby is beyond seven months, I should have to have a very tempting cervix, with good dilatation, not to resort to abdominal section. The important thing before us tonight is the question of how to handle our cases of central placenta previa at term. Of course, in earlier cases it is a different situation. I would like to put on record a recent case. A patient came to me with a story of being five and a half months' pregnant. She said she had a hemorrhage while she was shopping. There was no strain at all; she was in an elevator and she simply bled. She consulted a specialist, known to all of us, and he told her that she need not pay any attention to it and that it didn't mean anything. It did stop. In a week she had another moderate hemorrhage without any exertion and she went to a general practitioner who told her she possibly had placenta previa and referred her to me. The woman being only five and a half months along, with a closed cervix, but with a story that was so suspicious, I felt it best to send her at that time to the hospital and told her my examination might result in an abortion, but that it was necessary to know the facts. She was anesthetized, the finger introduced into the cervix and it was found that there was placental material present. I put in a bag and she was subsequently delivered by Braxton-Hicks version with very little loss of blood. She had a true central placenta previa and was simply marked for trouble if it had not been recognized.

The point here is that sometimes we might, by paying attention to early hemorrhage, be able to make a diagnosis of placenta previa before the time of viability when the question of emptying the uterus is a relatively simple one.

DR. ROBERT L. DICKINSON.—I would like to ask Dr. Humpstone whether there are available any statistics of the results with cesarean section in central placenta previa, compared with the regular statistics covering results with the older methods of treatment.

DR. JOHN O. POLAK.—Is it not a fact that in central placenta previa the hemorrhage frequently does not occur until the final gush?

DR. O. PAUL HUMPSTONE, (closing).—I think that cesarean section is never indicated if a bag has been put in the cervix. I did not mean to give that impression.

I think that Dr. E. P. Davis in his description of placenta previa, or "ectopic pregnancy", as he calls it, presents probably the most valuable statistics on the success of cesarean section in placenta previa. He also, you may recall, has been very conservative as compared with Dr. Williams, of Baltimore, on the removal of the uterus in these cases as being possibly infected.

I was particularly interested in this question of pituitrin, which not many of you gentlemen referred to. I studied pituitrin during the winter of 1912 and was among the first to use it in this country. I read a paper before this Society (May 14, 1912) advocating as much as four ampoules of pituitrin at a dose, but I want to put myself on record as having changed my mind. And I want to state that I firmly believe that any man who gets up and talks about using pituitrin while the child is in the uterus has not had the proper experience. I delivered one patient three times, who had a funnel pelvis, with a resulting third degree tear. In her fourth pregnancy she had a larger baby, and when the head came through the cervix and was on the perineal floor, I gave her only 5 minims of pituitrin, and she was torn wide open, went into shock on the table, and died. I no longer use pituitrin while the baby is in the uterus.

Dr. Harold Bailey reported a **Case of Hemimelus or So-called Congenital Amputation.** (For original article see page 72.)

DISCUSSION

Dr. ROBERT L. DICKINSON.—I would like to ask whether the sulci or grooves were accounted for.

Dr. F. R. OASTLER.—I would like to ask Dr. Bailey whether he has any remarks to make about the work of Jacques Loeb, undertaken some fifteen or sixteen years ago, in which he succeeded in causing all sorts of amputations by the destruction of the chromosome bodies in the nucleus of some of the lower forms of animal life, such as mollusks. It seems to me that is probably the best explanation of these deformities that we have, and that it does not occur later on.

Dr. J. M. MABBOTT.—I would like to ask Dr. Bailey at what period of development or pregnancy the amputations were supposed to have taken place, and, secondly, whether anything representing amputated parts has ever been found in the amniotic cavity.

Dr. HAROLD BAILEY, (closing).—There is no explanation accepted by embryologists or anatomists for the formation of these grooves. It is a fact that never in those grooves has there been found a band or adhesion. However, bands and amniotic adhesions have frequently been found connecting, for instance, one of the fingers to some other part of the child's anatomy, like the leg or the body, and almost all the stories of bands or cordlike amniotic bands, relate to the older literature, strange to say, almost all before 1900. Fieux in 1902 reported a cordlike extremity to which was attached a hand and I think it has to be accepted that amniotic adhesions do occur in some of these cases. The explanation given by most anatomists who have studied this subject is that these are adhesions occurring either from inflammation of the ends of the stump (as you saw, the scar in the one child) or occurring after the injury, or rather after the deformity.

Ballantyne recites all the information about these bands and then ignores it and refers the condition to amniotic pressure in the first two or three weeks of embryologic life, before the amnion separates from the surface of the child. Of course we have all seen some forms of amnion adhesions. (I have in the Cornell Museum a specimen where the amnion is strongly attached to the entire parietal bone on one side). The nature of these grooves is uncertain. Some have referred the condition to the disease called "ainhum," occurring in Brazilian negroes. This is a disease of adult life in which the little toe is compressed by the ingrowing skin and the toe drops off without any pain or evidence of trouble. It is interesting to note that one description states that the patient was surprised to find the toe in his shoe. There have been discolorations of the ends of these stumps in the so-called congenital amputations and evidences of inflammation have been found there. I have no information about the irritation of the chromosomes. Of course, Mall, in his 1908 article said the amputations would have to be laid aside as unexplained and he felt that the frequent production of extra fingers and the absence of fingers in parent and child might indicate that it was possibly a germinal effect. However, I think that can also be laid aside because all these children have other marked malformations.

As regards time, if this occurs as a form of embryonic failure of the mesenchyme to develop into bone, it occurs before the fourth week and probably the third week of embryonic life.

In my reading I discovered one case record of a hundred years ago or thereabouts, where the leg was first delivered and then the child. I think all such records can be discounted.

Dr. WILLIAM P. HEALY reported a case of **Recovery after Postoperative Tetany Treated with Calcium Lactate**, and a case of **Sudden Death During the Preoperative Treatment of Procidentia Uteri.**

Dr. Healy referred to the fact that from time to time the occurrence of tetany has been noted following various operative procedures, more especially the removal of the thyroid or parathyroid glands, or operations upon the abdominal or pelvic viscera. The prognosis as a rule in postoperative tetany has been bad. In recent years a great deal of experimental work has been done, more especially on parathyroidectomized dogs and careful studies of the blood chemistry changes in these animals made before, during and after attacks of tetany.

Probably the most important of the earlier studies were those of MacCallum and Voegtlin. These investigators in 1908 noted that after parathyroidectomy the calcium concentration in the blood and tissues was less and in the feces and urine was greater than normal.

MacCallum and Vogel in 1913 confirmed the above findings and reported an average of 2.7 mg. of calcium per 100 gm. of whole blood in tetany as against 6.1 mg. in normal dogs. Briefly then tetany in these animals was assumed to be a result of calcium deficiency and more especially so since the administration of calcium salts was found to be most effective in relieving the symptoms.

More recently Hastings and Murray in a careful series of experiments on dogs have confirmed the above findings. They showed that the concentration of calcium in the blood decreases rapidly, beginning soon after removal of the parathyroids and they were able to demonstrate repeatedly the temporary curative power of intravenous calcium chloride injections for tetany.

During the last few years cases of tetany have been reported following the intravenous injection of sodium bicarbonate for therapeutic purposes.

In March of this year Dr. Healy reported a series of six cases of postoperative tetany, four of which resulted fatally, due to the administration of large quantities of sodium bicarbonate *per rectum*. These cases received approximately 2400 grains sodium bicarbonate *per rectum* within six hours after operation and, despite the fact that some of it was expelled, enough was retained to bring about the symptoms of tetany.

The following case is reported because a much smaller quantity of bicarbonate of soda was administered, about 600 grains. Mrs. L. P., age thirty-two, married seven years, no children, family and personal history excellent. Menstrual history normal except for severe dysmenorrhea on first and second days. Chief complaints: sterility, dysmenorrhea, severe backache, occasional attacks of dysuria. The patient was a well-developed, healthy-looking woman and the physical examination was negative except for the pelvis. The cervix was lacerated (postoperative) and the uterus was enlarged to the size of a grapefruit by two fibroids.

Operation: Nitrous oxide and ether anesthesia. Duration 1 hour 15 minutes; dilatation of cervix, tracheloplasty, multiple myomectomy and hysteropexy. There was a moderate amount of bleeding during the myomectomy but the patient was returned to bed in excellent condition with a pulse of 100, temperature 98.8°, respirations 22, at 10:10 A.M. At 10:45 morphine sulphate gr. ⅙ (hypo); 11:45 rectal enema containing 192 grains glucose, 300 grains sodium bicarbonate, 40 grains sodium bromide and 8 ounces tap water, at a temperature of 106° was given and retained; and at 3:15 P.M. the enema was repeated without the sodium bromide. At 6:00 P.M., temp. 103.4°, pulse 130, respirations 10.

The patient was conscious but her respirations were very shallow and slow, the pupils were not contracted and responded to light. She was given atropin sulphate gr. 1/150 (hypo), about 7:00 P.M. She voided 5½ ounces urine, the pulse and temperature continued to rise and at 8 P.M. were 104.8°, pulse 130, respirations 10.

Despite the high temperature, rapid pulse and slow respirations the patient did not complain. She was fully conscious and mentally quiet but rather restlessly moved her arms and legs about.

She received no further sedative and went through the night fairly well with a little disturbance from nausea until 6:45 A.M. when she suddenly complained of stiffness of her hands and a numbness and tingling of the entire body and difficulty in breathing.

The examination showed the typical bilateral tonic spasm of tetany involving both hands with also slight flexion of wrists and elbows, associated with this about every three minutes a wave of numbness would sweep over the body accompanied by rapid breathing and intense spasm of gastric and abdominal muscles with vomiting of an ounce or so of clear fluid.

The anxiety of the patient was extreme and her requests for relief were insistent.

Calcium lactate, gr. 20, with half an ounce of lime water was given by mouth every half hour for six doses, beginning at 7:30 A.M. and the greater part seemed to be retained. By 11 A.M. the spasm of the hands was much less marked but the tachycardia and attacks of numbness and rapid breathing still continued and at 11:35 an intravenous injection of 100 c.c. water with 1 gram of calcium lactate was given. The result was most striking, before the injection was finished the tachycardia and all the other symptoms disappeared and the patient became most comfortable. Thereafter the convalescence was normal.

It seemed to Dr. Healy that the symptoms of this case can be explained by a more rapid absorption of sodium bicarbonate into the blood stream than the kidneys were able to take care of by elimination because of a temporary depression from the operative procedure and this brought about a disturbance of salt metabolism especially in the balance between sodium and calcium.

This balance was restored by the administration of calcium salts and the symptoms disappeared.

The history of the case of the sudden death during the preoperative treatment of procidentia uteri, was as follows: Mrs. D. K., age thirty-three, widow, one child in 1914, instrumental delivery. Menses of the 28 day type, duration 4 days, moderate flow, no pain. Last menstruation 2 weeks ago. Complaint, prolapse of the rectum and of the womb, duration 6 years, the prolapse of the womb appeared some time before the rectal prolapse. Bowels normal and no bladder symptoms present. No subjective symptoms except the annoyance due to the protruding masses. Examination showed a well nourished, healthy-looking female of rather large frame. General physical examination negative except for pelvic lesions. Prolapse of rectum 3½x5 inches, readily reducible through a tremendously dilated and relaxed sphincter ani. Complete prolapse of uterus, adnexae and vagina forming a tumor mass

4x6 inches with extreme thickening and edema of the mucous membrane of the vagina and cervix. The prolapse was readily reducible but would promptly reappear.

The plan of treatment instituted was rest in bed, with daily vaginal douches and support of the uterine prolapse with boroglyceride and ichthyol tampons. The prolapse of the rectum was more difficult to retain as it invariably came out with each bowel movement.

It was expected by this treatment to reduce the engorgement of the prolapsed tissues and to improve the chances of an operative cure.

During the first two days in the hospital the uterus and the rectum prolapsed with each bowel movement, thereafter the former remained in place but the latter had to be replaced after each stool. There was some bluish discoloration and edema about the vulva. The patient was not allowed out of bed and by the 19th of August, two and one half weeks after admission to the hospital the edema and more or less brawny induration of the tissues about the vulva and vagina had considerably diminished, and on the morning of the 19th the patient was placed in a wheel chair and transported about twenty-five feet to the examining room and placed on the examining table, in order that we might make a careful estimate of the progress of the treatment to date and decide as to the feasibility of an early operation. As the patient was placed on the table she seemed to have a desire for a bowel movement and asked for a bedpan, which was given her, after waiting two or three minutes it was noticed that her lips were becoming cyanotic and that she was breathing rapidly, she was placed upon a stretcher and returned to bed at once, her only complaint being shortness of breath and a sense of suffocation. There was no pain at all, the pulse rate was 130, the entire body was covered with a cold perspiration, the breathing rapidly failed and within five minutes of the onset of the attack the patient was dead. There had been a careful physical examination of the patient on several occasions and the heart and lungs seemed to be quite normal.

A careful postmortem examination of the thoracic viscera failed to establish the cause of death.

DISCUSSION

DR. J. M. MABBOTT.—I have been impressed in hearing cases reported and in reading them to find how recklessly, I may say, morphine is given hypodermatically to aid the anesthesia for operations. In listening to the case of tetany, which is from my limited knowledge, a clear enough case of tetany, I was impressed by the fact that the respiration was so slow, but as I recall it, the pupils were contracted and the house surgeon treated the case with atropin, from which I assume that there might be a morphine element in the case, and it causes me to inquire as to whether Dr. Healy knows exactly how much morphine had been given to that patient, if any, in the preparation for the operation.

DR. WILLIAM P. HEALY.—There was no preoperative morphine given, Mr. Chairman, and the pupils were dilated, not contracted. One-sixth of a grain of morphine was given in one dose.

DR. WILLIAM PFEIFFER reported a case of **Intraligamentous Ectopic Pregnancy.**

Mrs. E. M., age thirty-four, white, married, entered Kings County Hospital at 4:00 P.M. September 19, 1921. Chief complaint: Abdominal pain. Had the usual diseases of childhood. Denies any venereal infection. Past history otherwise negative. Married fourteen years; husband thirty-nine years old, in good health. One child delivered by forceps thirteen years ago, a normal puerperium following. A later pregnancy terminated in miscarriage at six months, followed by two subsequent abortions of early gestations, all of these of spontaneous origin requiring no operative interference for their completion, and without sequelae. Patient noted burning on urination with frequency only during the occurrence of present symptoms; retention for part of this time before admission.

To show the worthlessness of the average history the following is noted from the record of the interne. "Menses started when fourteen years old; always regular, never painful, lasting five to six days." Date of last menstruation omitted. On close questioning after operation, the following is the correct history: Menstruation usually of thirty day type, five to six day habit, and with very little pain. Last period June 11, 1921, and typical except that it was a day or two early. At no time subsequently was there any bleeding, staining or spotting until a few days before admission to the hospital. Patient believed herself pregnant but was told by her medical adviser that the amenorrhea was due to anemia and kidney trouble, and that the uterus was empty.

On or about July 25, patient had dull sacral pain continuing for a few days, accompanied by one spell of vomiting with fainting. This was repeated one week later. Three weeks before admission or about the latter part of August, there occurred cramp-like pains over the lower abdomen and extending as described by the patient "up to the heart." These were inconstant, varying from 5 to 30 minute intervals and evidently of not severe character as they did not prevent sleep. This continued until three days before admission when pain became severe and cutting in right lower quadrant but gradually lessened and were described as "drawing," relief being obtained by local applications of cold.

Examination of upper abdomen negative. In hypogastrium was a mass extending from symphysis to one finger's breadth above the umbilicus, definitely outlined and extending somewhat higher on the right than the left. It gave a sense of fluctuation and felt more like a bladder full of urine than like a uterus. Catheterization excluded this. No fetal heart heard, or fetal movement felt or heard. Tenderness and some rigidity over entire mass especially in the right lower quadrant. No vaginal bleeding at present. Normal parous outlet. Cervix in normal vaginal axis, long and soft, with slightly restricted mobility; pressure on cervix causes pain. External os admits the finger tip. Body of uterus not definitely palpated because of rigidity. The mass above described seems to be above and behind uterus while there is nothing definitely palpable in either fornix except a sense of fullness and pain on palpation.

The uterus was the size of a three months' pregnancy and displaced to the left, a definite sulcus palpable between uterus and the mass to the right. Pressure on cervix not transmitted to the mass. Right fornix appears slightly full.

Blood examination: Red cells, 3,150,000, hemoglobin 80 per cent. White cells, 14,350, polynuclears 87 per cent, lymphocytes 12 per cent, transitionals 2 per cent, eosinophiles 1 per cent.

Urine drawn by catheter:—Amber, sp. gr. 1022, alkaline, albumin and sugar negative, amorphous phosphates many, no casts. Culture shows B. coli.

Wassermann negative. Temperature on admission 98° F., pulse 80, respirations 24. No record of blood pressure.

Provisional diagnosis: Uterine pregnancy complicated by ovarian cyst with a twisted pedicle.

Operation, September 23, 1921. Median abdominal incision from umbilicus to symphysis. On opening the peritoneum a small amount of fluid and clotted blood was found and there presented a smooth, regular mass in the midline about the size of a four months' uterine pregnancy. This was found to spring from the right side and to have displaced the uterus to the left, though that organ instead of being a three months' size was no larger than at six weeks; it was, however, soft and contracted under the hand. The mass was dark in color, soft, fluctuating, and loosely attached here and there to the surrounding coils of intestines. It was broken during the handling, causing the discharge of considerable fluid and clotted blood, followed by a fetus of about four months' development, and alive. The placenta followed without effort to remove it and it was then seen that the product of conception had come from within the folds of the right broad ligament, the upper part of which now resembled a "blowout." The bleeding was severe and was controlled by clamps placed on the base of the right broad ligament. The only part of the tube seen was a small portion about 1½ inches long at the right cornu. This was removed with the portion of the broad ligament above the clamps and the defect closed over. Right ovary not identified at any time; left tube and ovary normal. A few tabs of organized clot on the intestines from adhesions to the mass not removed. Abdomen closed in layers without drainage. Time of operation one hour and five minutes. Pulse before operation 102; after it, 120; after return to bed 98, and thereafter never rose above 100. Blood pressure one hour postoperative 110/70; one and a half hours p.o. 125/80; two hours p.o. 138/90; three hours p.o. 140/90; nine hours p.o. 145/95.

Aside from slight discomfort caused by gas, convalescence was uneventful. Sutures removed on tenth day, union primary.

On discharge October 6, 1921: Primary union in the incision, scar firm and not tender. Pelvic floor and cervix as on admission. Uterus normal in size, position and mobility, not tender. Left adnexa not palpable. There is a very small tender exudate in the culdesac.

Postoperative diagnosis: Intraligamentous pregnancy.

Conclusions: I believe that the primary rupture of the tubal pregnancy took place about the time of the first dull pain when the vomiting and fainting occurred; that there were further hemorrhages into the ligament at dates corresponding to recurrences of symptoms and that the final phenomena were the manifestation of erosion of the walls of the ligament with beginning secondary rupture found at time of operation.

DISCUSSION

DR. HERMANN GRAD.—I had an experience last summer with a woman twenty-five years old, who was still nursing her eight months' old baby, and was taken one morning with very severe abdominal pain. I saw her about three hours later, at which time a tentative diagnosis of ectopic was made, but in view of the fact that her condition was good and there were no pelvic findings, it was thought best to wait for further developments. She improved very rapidly and I saw her a week later and there were absolutely no symptoms, the blood and urinary findings were normal and there was no further pain. She was allowed to get out of bed. We were undecided as to the diagnosis of ectopic. Four weeks later she was again taken sick. She was up and about and was again seized with severe pain and was taken to another hospital, a ruptured ectopic into the right broad ligament was found at operation. There were several coils of intestine adherent to it. There was no fetus present, but the outer portion of the tube had ruptured. It was removed and the patient made a good recovery.

I believe it is very difficult to diagnose these cases because there are so very few symptoms present.

Department of Reviews and Abstracts

CONDUCTED BY HUGO EHRENFEST, M.D., ASSOCIATE EDITOR

Collective Review

THE VIEWS OF PRIMITIVE PEOPLES CONCERNING THE CARE OF THE PARTURIENT WOMAN*

BY JONATHAN WRIGHT, M.D., PLEASANTVILLE, N. Y.

WE now may turn our attention to the methods of care for the parturient woman. We have already seen that not infrequently she gets no care. Ratzel[50] says: "We are told of the Kirghises of Semipalatinsk that in extreme cases they will place the woman on horseback, with a rider, in order that a wild gallop may accelerate the operation of nature. 'Sometimes it does good, sometimes she dies.' * * * At Nij Noukha they leave a woman in childbirth to herself; among the Mussulman Georgians in the province of Zakataly * * * the poor woman, when her pains come on, is even driven from the living rooms as 'unclean,' and has to seek some stable or barn, where she must bring her child into the world without any help, nor for a period varying from five to seven days may she return to her family and go about her household affairs." "In Africa," Livingstone[51] says, "the poor creatures are often placed in a little hut built for the purpose and are left without any assistance whatever. * * * The women suffer less at their confinement than is the case in civilized countries; perhaps from their treating it, not as a disease, but as an operation of nature, requiring no change of diet except a feast of meat and abundance of fresh air. The husband on these occasions is bound to slaughter for his lady an ox, or goat, or sheep, according to his means." In Western Thibet, "the mother always goes through her time of trial alone, unless, which is frequently the case, there are other married women near by, who can conveniently attend her."[52]

While the woman is thus occasionally left alone at this moment of her extreme need, according to our notions, this is not usually the case. Help, or the attempts to furnish it, is usually at hand, but it can scarcely be doubted that much which is furnished had better be left unperformed; but the readiness to supply such as is in their power or knowledge, sharply differentiates the treatment of the human female from that of the brutes, and it is worth while to note this in studying the origin of altruistic and humanitarian practice. When a

---
*See Review of Literature on Menstruation in this Journal, January, 1921; on Conception and Puerperium, May, 1921; and on Labor, August, 1921.

child is born to an Esquimaux woman "the mother is attended by one or more of her own sex; even the husband is not allowed to be present. If it is a first child, the birth takes place in the usual tupic or igloo; if it is a second, or any other than the first, a separate tupic or igloo is built for the mother's use and to that she must remove."[53] At the Antipodes, in South Africa, the Kafir woman also used a separate hut for her confinement. Shortly before the birth of her child "she cuts grass on which to lie while secluded in her hut. * * * The husband is not allowed to be in the hut while the baby is being born, but several women act as midwives, the woman's mother being the most important person on such occasions."[54] In Polynesia "the woman is isolated in the bush in a newly built hut, a poor protection against the weather; any married woman attends her for pay—all others are excluded and the father doesn't see the child for at least fifteen days."[55] In Alaska, "in former years the universal practice was for the Thlinget[56] mother to lie outside of the house in a booth or in the bushes. A hole was made in the ground and lined with leaves or moss, and the newborn babe was deposited in it." In Central Africa "a Yao woman,—sometimes at any rate, if not always,—used to go out into the bush a few days before the birth of a child. One or two women would go with her, to put up a little grass shelter and look after her."[57] In Australia "when the time of her trouble draws nigh, some one of the old women is selected to attend her and the two withdraw from the main camp and shelter themselves in a little rudely constructed 'Miam.' "[58] "Among the Giljaka the act of parturition is looked upon as partly unclean, and cannot under any circumstances take place in the house, at the domestic hearth. Therefore, not only in summer, but even in winter, in the fiercest frost and snow storms, the women about to have children are taken into buildings for them near their dwellings. The place chosen for this purpose is, for the most part, in the private part of the grounds reserved for the women, so that it is quite plain that it is due to no reverence for the act of parturition that the women are thus isolated. The men are obliged to keep entirely away from the neighborhood."[59]

"On the Bonin Islands, as formerly in Japan, there are special lying-in-huts."[60] It is convenient to cite these two excerpts in close apposition. From what has preceded, the almost universal isolation of the parturient women, usually in a fresh hut, sometimes in the bush, we may conjecture that out of what may well have been some blood taboo, as was the case with the Giljaka, and perhaps for some similar magic reason among the Mexicans, we have arrived at a very close conformity with the best modern obstetric practice. Occasionally of course there was a faulty technic. At a much higher stage of civilization, among the ancient Mexicans, as with us, Bancroft[61] says, on the authority of de Sahagun: "The 'hour of death,' as the time of confinement was named, having arrived the patient was carried to a room previously set in order for the purpose, here her hair was soaped and she was placed in a bath to be washed." This, however, is only a flash of a suggestion of modern ideas in a civilization, doubtless much higher than we are accustomed to attribute to prehistoric Mexico. Among the Ovaherero in South Africa "immediately after a woman has given birth to a child, a small house is built for her, at the back of her own house, where she remains until the navel string has separated from the child."[62] In an Australian tribe, she remains in her husband's hut but "during her confinement her husband lives elsewhere; the neighboring 'wuurns' are temporarily deserted; and every one is sent away from the vicinity except two married women who stay with her."[63] She remains in the living hut until confined, but this is exceptional. It is interesting to see again how out of an entirely false theory grew up a practice, buttressed no doubt by the observation of favorable results, which under the limitations of the environment could scarcely be improved by a modern obstetrician. Not on account of aseptic doctrine, but because of the taboo based on the theory that the *woman* was "unclean," not the hut. On the Lower Niger women are under the care of a particular deity. "Even after confinement the greatest care is taken of the mother and infant."[64] Of asepsis and antisepsis in the strict sense of the words, there is little or no trace. In Abyssinia[65] in spite of the complete absence of aseptic precautions and of ordinary elementary cleanliness, in spite of lack of care of the linen, for on this occasion the woman puts on her oldest nightdress reserving the new for her getting up from bed, in spite of the fact that the chamber where the birth takes place is the common room, where they choose the most obscure corner, shielded by means of curtains against the light and prying eyes, in spite of the fact this common room is full of dust, of chaff and even of manure, since the mule, the goat or the sheep are often lodged beneath the same roof (true scene of Bethlehem), separated from the family sometimes only by a thin wall broken and pierced by a door—in spite of all these things, almost never does one observe any puerperal infection and still less any tetanus of the mother or of the infant through the umbilical cord.

One of the most striking things to be gleaned for the modern accoucheur, from the obstetrical practice of the primitive woman is the position assumed by her during labor. A wife of a King in Baganda "was confined in the same position as ordinary women. She was held in front by one of the midwives, while the other was behind ready to receive the child, a barkcloth only being spread on the floor for her to kneel upon. When delivered, the child was laid upon a plantain leaf, and those present waited for the afterbirth. When this came away, the umbilical cord was cut, with a bit of reed taken from the doorway, if the child was a boy, and from the fireplace, if it was a girl. The midwife washed out the child's mouth with her finger and a little water, and blew in the child's mouth for a few moments, to cause its breath to be sweet."[66] A very circumstantial account is given of the actions and customs* attendant upon childbirth in this region by the Rev. Mr. Roscoe. They concern the mother as well as the father, but they are painfully disgusting to read and without special interest which cannot be more comfortably satisfied in other ways. Curr[67] says that in Australia "aboriginal women always bear their children while they kneel; and sit back on their heels, their feet being laid on the ground, soles uppermost—a common posture always with them when sitting. One of the women attending sits behind the woman in labor, and puts both her arms around her waist, thus forming a support for her back. The other midwife will attend to her as

---

*The literature of these is of great interest and very voluminous and may be found extensively abstracted in the various volumes of the Golden Bough of Sir J. G. Fraser.

necessity requires. Parturition always takes place in this posture."[*]
Among the Melanesians and the Polynesians, Brown[68] speaks of the woman being "delivered in a squatting position, sitting like a frog." Neuhauss[69] says that in New Guinea parturition ordinarily takes place in a kneeling posture and Pilsudski[70] states that on the island of Sachalin the patient is delivered in a sitting position and is obliged, during the act, to keep herself perfectly straight. In the Andaman Islands[71] during the first two or three days the parturient woman remains in a sitting posture, propped up by articles arranged so as to form a couch. Of the Sinaugolo it is said: "Labour takes place in the bush, where the woman, half squatting on a cocoanut (to support the perineum?) grasps with her hand a young sapling or other convenient upright, or failing these, a rope hanging from the bough of a tree; should labour pains, however, come on suddenly at night the child is delivered in the house no attempt being made to convey the woman to the bush."[72] It is for the modern obstetrician to explain to us why other postures are assumed today.

The manipulations of the midwife, and it is a woman who is almost invariably in attendance, are not extensively recorded, but for the most part it is explicitly stated that the mechanics of labor are not interfered with, though we have seen the horse-back riding of the Kirghis women to produce expulsion of the fetus, which, by the way we cannot help believing is not to be looked on as routine practice. The Australian woman who receives no assistance in any way in her expulsive efforts rarely dies in childbirth.[73] It is exceptional to find primitive woman, as is related of her on the Andaman Islands, held by her husband "who supports her back and presses her as desired."[74] As we reach higher civilizations we find the ancient Mexican midwife, on the authority of Sahagun, quoted by Bancroft,[75] rubs and presses "the abdomen of the patient in order to get the child into place." This perhaps might be considered meddlesome interference, but the extent to which this might go in emergencies is illustrated in a further note. "The Teochichimes husband undertook the office of midwife when the birth took place on the road. He heated the back of his wife with fire, threw water over her in lieu of a bath, and gave her two or three kicks in the back after the delivery, in order to promote the issue of superfluous blood. The newborn babe was placed in a wicker basket, and thrown over the back of the mother, who proceeded on her journey." In some tribes on the other hand the woman receives much careful attention after childbirth. On the Niger the African woman is "washed first of all with hot water; palm oil— which is considered to be medicinal in its effects—is rubbed all over the abdomen and applied to the wounded parts, and the former is then bound very tight with a cloth by the old women midwives. A big fire is kept in the room, and the mother is fed three times a day, plenty of palm oil and pepper being put into her food. Besides this, she is washed three times a day, and spirit or palm wine, fortified by alligator pepper, is administered internally, in the belief that it warms and regulates the womb."[76] In Polynesia[77] the attendant women sometimes remove the placenta when adherent. Left to herself she adopts

---

[*]This has an interesting connotation in the most ancient Egyptian literature, (Budge, E. H. M.: Osiris and the Egyptian Resurrection, 1911) and may be found alluded to in Galen: Natural Faculties III. 3. (Daremberg's translation, vol. II p. 288.)

such measures as she can to hasten the process. Women of the Central Esquimaux "in childbirth will try to cause vomiting by tickling the throat with the finger. It is believed this will facilitate the expulsion of the afterbirth."[78] There can be no doubt this is far more efficacious than some of the magical practices, as for instance in Northern India. " 'Among the Konkan Kunbis, when a woman is in labour and cannot get a speedy delivery, some gold ornament from her hair is taken to a Rûî plant (the Dhâk Callotropis gigantea of Northern India), and after digging at its roots, one of the roots is taken out, and the ornament is buried in its stead. The root is then brought home and put in the hair of the woman in labour. It is supposed that by this means the woman gets speedy delivery. As soon as she is delivered of a child, the root is taken from her hair and brought back to the Rûî plant, and after digging at its root the ornament is taken out and the root placed in its former place.' The idea seems to be that the evil influence hindering parturition is thus transferred to the plant."[79] Again in the Mexican civilization we find advanced interference on the part of the midwife, who, de Sahagun says,[80] "was very skilful and dextrous in her duties. When she saw that the baby was dead in its mother because it did not move, and that the patient was in great pain, she then placed her hand in the parturient canal, and with a stone knife cut the body of the baby and drew it out by the feet."

BIBLIOGRAPHY

(50) *Ratzel, Friedrich*: The History of Mankind; tr. from the German by A. J. Butler, London, MacMillan & Co., 1896-98. (51) *Livingstone, David*: Missionary Travels and Researches in South Africa, 25 ed., New York, Harper & Bros., 1868. (52) *Sherring, C. A.*: Western Tibet and the British Borderland, the Sacred Country of Hindus and Buddhists, London, E. Arnold, 1906. (53) *Hall, Charles Francis*: Arctic Researches and Life Among the Esquimaux, New York, Harper & Bros., 1866. (54) *Kidd, Dudley*: Savage Childhood, London, 1906. (55) *Brown, George*: Melanesians and Polynesians, London, MacMillan & Co., 1910. (56) *Jones, Livingstone F.*: A Study of the Thlingets of Alaska, New York, F. H. Revell Co., 1914. (57) *Werner, A.*: The Natives of British Central Africa, London, Archibald Constable & Co., 1906. (58) *Smyth, R. Brough*: The Aborigines of Victoria; with notes Relating to the Habits of the Natives of Other Parts of Australia and Tasmania; Comp. for the Government of Victoria, Melbourne, 1878. (59) *Pilsudski, Bronislaw*: Schwangerschaft, Entbindung und Fehlgeburt bei den Bewohnern der Insel Sachalin (Giljaken und Ainu), Anthropos, 1910, v, No. 4, p. 756. (60) *Ratzel, Friedrich*: The History of Mankind, tr. from German by A. J. Butler, London, MacMillan & Co., 1896-98. (61) *Bancroft, Hubert H.*: The Native Races of the Pacific States of North America, New York, D. Appleton & Co., 1875-76. (62) *Callaway, Henry*: The Religious System of the Amazulu, Pt. II. Anatongo; or Ancestor Worship as Existing Among the Amazulu, in their own words, with a Translation in English, and Notes by the Rev. H. Callaway, London, Trübner & Co., 1869. (63) *Dawson, James*: Australian Aborigines, Melbourne, G. Robertson, 1881. (64) *Leonard, Arthur Glyn*: The Lower Niger and its Tribes, London, MacMillan & Co., 1906. (65) *Mérab, Docteur*: Médecins et médecine en Ethiopie, Paris, Vigot Frères, 1912. (66) *Roscoe, John*: The Baganda, London, MacMillan & Co., 1911. (67) *Curr, Edward M.*: The Australian Race, Melbourne, J. Ferres, 1886-1887. (68) *Brown, George*: Melanesians and Polynesians, London, MacMillan & Co., 1910. (69) *Neuhauss, Richard*: Deutsch Neu-Guinea, Berlin, D. Reimer, 1911. (70) *Pilsudski, Bronislaw*: Schwangerschaft, Entbindung und Fehlgeburt bei den Bewohnern der Insel Sachalin (Giljaken und Ainu, Antropos, 1910, v, No. 4, p. 756. (71) *Mann, Edward Horace*: On the Aboriginal Inhabitants of the Andaman Islands, London, Anthropological Institute of Great Britain and Ireland, 1883. (72) *Seligmann, C. G.*: The Medicine, Surgery and Midwifery of the Sinaugolo, Anthropological Institute of Great Britain and Ireland, Journal, 1902,

xxxii, 297. (73) *Dawson, James*: Australian Aborigines, Melbourne, G. Robertson, 1881. (74) *Mann, Edward Horace*: On the Aboriginal Inhabitants of the Andaman Islands, London, Anthropological Institute of Great Britain and Ireland, 1883. (75) *Bancroft, Hubert H.*: The Native Races of the Pacific States of North America, New York, D. Appleton & Co., 1875-76. (76) *Leonard, Arthur Glyn*: The Lower Niger and Its Tribes, London, MacMillan & Co., 1906. (77) *Brown, George*: Melanesians and Polynesians, London, MacMillan & Co., 1910. (78) *Boas, Franz*: The Eskimo of Baffin Land and Hudson Bay, American Museum of Natural History, Bulletin, New York. 1901, xv, pt. 1. (79) *Crooke, William*: The Popular Religion and Folk-Lore of Northern India, New ed., Westminster, England, A. Constable & Co., 1896. (80) *Sahagun, Bernardio de*: Historia General de las Cosas de Nueva Espana, Mexico, A. Valdés, 1829-30.

(*To be continued.*)

Selected Abstracts

Sterility and Sterilization

Dittler: Parenteral Injection of Semen. Muenchener medizinische Wochenschrift, 1920, lxvii, 1495.

In this work, confined to rabbits, semen was injected into the blood stream to determine whether, by a reaction akin to acquired immunity, the established affinity of sperm and ovum could be impaired, or even altogether destroyed. It had already been proved that semen parenterally acts as an antigen, developing a spermotoxic substance demonstrable in the blood stream. Can this substance be concentrated in the ovum to a degree where the latter will be able to develop an absolute resistance to the sperm? Employing corpus luteum extract has led to relative sterility in the male (apparently a "hormone reaction"). Temporary sterility in the female has been produced by parenteral injection of whole testicular extract, but these experiments were not sufficiently controlled to warrant scientific conclusions as to the nature of the reaction taking place.

In the author's research, whole, fresh, rabbit's semen (collected at copulation) was injected into the vein of the ear, and repeated 2 to 10 times at from 1 to 8 day intervals, the total semen injected varying from 2 to 5 c.c. Only such female animals were employed as had gone through at least one normal pregnancy. A part of the work was done under serologic control, i.e., the injections were continued until the blood of the animal showed definite spermotoxic properties (determined by agglutinating power as compared to a control).

In this stage, absolute sterility obtained towards the sperm of the animal whose semen had been employed for injection. Only after weeks or months did fruitful conception take place. One single (and correspondingly large) injection did not suffice to produce sterility: repeated doses at definite intervals apparently are required to produce sterility. Repeated doses of 0.2 to 1.0 c.c. did not interrupt a pregnancy already in course, which seems to indicate that the sperm quickly loses its identity and its original affinity for the sperm antibodies. In the determination of the specificity of the antisperm reaction of one species as against that of another, it was found that rabbits treated with human semen did not develop sterility. During the course of the injections laparotomies performed, frequently revealed freshly developed corpora lutea; therefore, the sterility existed in spite of a normal process of ovulation.

The author believes the resulting sterility is due to an undetermined combination of "immunity reaction" and direct hormone action, the former playing the major rôle. S. B. SOLHAUG.

Hoehne: The Physiology of Conception. Zentralblatt fuer Gynaekologie, 1921, xlv, 1047.

Hoehne studied seven tubes from patients known to have had sexual intercourse prior to operation. Examining the tubes one, two, three, and seven days after known coitus, he found one dead spermatozoon in the neighborhood of the infundibulum of the tube after a lapse of 20 hours. This contradicts the finding of Nuernberg, who had positive results 13 to 15 days after the last coitus. The question is worthy of further study. Hoehne also reported the discovery of an unfertilized human ovum obtained through irrigation of the uterine cavity. This was the result of numerous experiments made in the hope of finding an unfertilized ovum some ten days after the beginning or five days after the end of a normal menstruation. The ovum in this case was relatively small, its maximum diameter being only .07 mm. H. M. LITTLE.

Graves: The Gynecologic Significance of Appendicitis in Early Life. Archives of Surgery, 1921, ii, 315.

That the appendix may undergo considerable grades of inflammation and yet be restored to a condition of approximate normality is seemingly an established fact. That the serofibrinous exudates thrown out during an attack find their way into the pelvis is granted. That these exudates frequently lead to extensive adhesions is well known. It requires, therefore, little speculation to assume that this process not infrequently involves the adnexa of young girls following more or less acute attacks of appendicitis. The adhesions thus formed may interfere with the normal development of the ovaries or obstruct the patency of the tubes. Graves has found the adnexa so embedded in adhesions as to be indistinguishable and the uterus undeveloped, years after an attack of appendicitis in early life.

This condition is, at times, the direct cause of later dysmenorrhea and probably also of ectopic gestation later, but Graves feels that it is especially important as a cause of sterility. He, therefore, urges prompt operation in cases of appendicitis in young girls, not simply on account of the appendix, but because of the serious harm which may be done to the adnexa. He reports three cases in which there appeared to be a direct relation between the adnexal adhesions and nondevelopment, and foregoing attacks of suppurative appendicitis, for which operation had been performed in earlier life. R. E. WOBUS.

Couvelaire: Sterility in the Female. Le Progrés Médical, September 17, 1921, p. 438.

In reviewing the statistics of Paris, Berlin and Rio de Janeiro, the author finds that about 13 per cent of couples who have been married for 14 years are without children. About 60 per cent of such childless marriages are attributable to the woman, while in the remaining 40 per cent, the causal factor may be found in the male.

In this article Couvelaire deals only with the factors which cause sterility in the woman stating that they are due either to some pathology, congenital or acquired, in the genital tract, or to some functional disturbance of the individual.

The prognosis for conception in cases of congenital pathology is good when such pathology can be, and is corrected. A good prognosis also generally exists following correction of acquired pathology unless such pathology involves both tubes and ovaries.

So far as the functional disturbances are concerned, Couvelaire considers first those cases where there is a delay in the appearance of the menstrual function. He finds that 70 per cent of women in whom the menses appear between the ages of 16 and 19 years of age are capable of conception. When, however, the menses do not appear until after the nineteenth year, about 60 per cent will remain childless.

So far as amenorrhea is concerned, he states that where this condition is due to lactation, the probability of conception is lessened. There also exist those cases of unexplained amenorrhea which when the organs are normal are capable of conception.

Dysmenorrhea he considers under the head of diminished flow associated with lessened ovarian function and excessive flow associated with hyperactive ovaries. In the first case he advocates the use of ovarian and thyroid extracts together with a rigorous diet, such as the one outlined by Pinard. In the latter type he employs the use of mammary extract, claiming in both cases that the possibility of conception is greatly enhanced by such treatment.

THEODORE W. ADAMS.

Reynolds and Macomber: Diagnosis in Sterility. New York State Journal of Medicine, 1920, xx, 373.

Reynolds and Macomber condemn strongly the far too common step of persuading a woman into an operation for the correction of an abnormality on the basis that it may be the cause of sterility. Such advice can be given only by one who has taken the trouble and acquired the skill of determining with such degree of accuracy as is at present possible, whether this particular abnormality is or is not the cause of the sterility which exists between this patient and her husband.

R. E. WOBUS.

Max Huhner: Methods of Examining for Spermatozoa in the Diagnosis and Treatment of Sterility. New York Medical Journal, 1921, cxiii, 678.

The author advises examination of the cervical contents obtained by pipette as soon after coitus as possible. The presence of live spermatozoa within the cervical canal indicates that semen sufficient for impregnation has been received and that the cervical and vaginal secretions are not inimical to the vitality of the spermatozoa. Where only dead spermatozoa are found within the cervix, examination of a condom specimen is necessary to determine whether the fault lies with the husband or whether the spermatozoa have been killed by the secretions of the wife. Where hyperacidity of the vaginal secretions is suggested as the cause of death of the spermatozoa, a repetition of the first test following a sodium bicarbonate douche before the coitus will make the diagnosis and suggest the cure. Where no spermatozoa at all are found, further careful examination of both husband and wife is required to determine the cause of their absence. Examination of specimens taken from the fundus uteri demonstrate the absence of any mechanical interference with the ascent of the spermatozoa into the fundus and tubes, as well as any inimical action in the endometrium. The author gives his technic in detail. MARGARET SCHULZE.

Rubin: The Nonoperative Determination of Patency of the Fallopian Tubes. Journal American Medical Association, 1921, lxxv, 661.

A not infrequent cause of sterility is occlusion of the fallopian tubes which may occur in the absence of palpable lesions of the adnexa. An operation was formerly necessary to determine the patency of tubes. To obviate this difficulty, Rubin injects oxygen into the abdomen by means of a canula inserted into the uterus and connected to a gas tank. A manometer is connected to the line and indicates the pressure under which the gas flows. In normal cases, the gas passes through the tubes at a pressure as low as 40 mm. of mercury and usually at between 60 and 80 mm. If the pressure indicated by the manometer rises to 150 mm. or more, it is reasonably certain that both tubes are occluded. A minimum of 100 to 150 c.c. of gas are used unless it is desired to take advantage of the pneumoperitoneum produced for radiographic purposes. In this case somewhat more is required.

Under proper precautions, this method has been found to be harmless. It is indicated in all cases where it is desirable to know whether the tubes, or a remaining tube, are patent. Its only contraindications are active pelvic inflammation or infectious processes of the lower genital tract. R. E. WOBUS.

Talmey: Frigidity and Sterility in the Female. Medical Record, 1921, c, 631.

Copulation is conditioned upon three potencies and procreation requires an additional potency. There is necessary (1) the potency of voluptas or the transcendental desire of the individuals of the two sexes to unite. (2) This union must give the two parties a certain satisfaction or libido. Libido lacking, union becomes disgusting and is avoided altogether. (3) There must be facultas coeundi. For procreation must be added the facultas generandi. There must be living spermatozoa and ova and the genital tracts of both sexes must be pervious. Lacking one of the four faculties, the individuals are suffering from impotence. Impotence of voluptas or true frigidity is exceedingly rare in men or in women. The transcendental attraction between the sexes is never absent in man from infancy to old age. Inherited frigidity is occasionally found in low idiots. Impotentia coeundi, the idiopathic impotence of copulation is also a rare occurrence in either sex. But the pathologic or rather acquired impotentia coeundi is the impotence common in the male, while in the female it is rare. Painful copulation due to acute genital inflammations is not real impotence in the strict sense of the word. If the woman is willing to bear pain, copulation is possible. Idiopathic impotence of libido is very rare. It is sometimes found in men in cases of grave neurasthenia. It is a frequent anomaly in the female and is falsely named frigidity; it ought to be calidity for they are suffering either from relative or absolute orgasmus retardatus. Impotentia generandi, the idiopathic impotence of fertilization or sterility is rare in either sex, but the acquired impotence of procreation is very frequent. Half of the sterile marriages are due to azoospermia of the male as a result of gonorrhea and at least 90 per cent of the cases of sterility of the female are caused by the infection of the wife from her husband. Talmey regards electricity the best remedial agent in the treatment of endometritis, metritis, salpingitis, ovaritis, and pelvic peritonitis. Its use is strictly contraindicated where there is pus. The author believes that dyspareunia and lack of orgasm are not rarely the cause of sterility, and that electricity is of great therapeutic value in these cases. C. O. MALAND.

Nassauer: Treatment of Sterility. Muenchener medizinische Wochenschrift, 1920, lxvii, 1463.

The author briefly reviews the known causes of sterility in the female emphasizing the probable importance of the rôle played by the internal secretions and deriding simple anteflexion of the cervix, simple retroversion of the corpus uteri and especially the "stenosis of the cervix" as causes of sterility.

He holds that the nervous element as a factor in producing sterility has been overlooked and proposes it as the underlying cause for the so-called "stenosis of the cervix" which is only a temporary uterine cramp. Dilatation therefore is not indicated nor successful (because the internal os remains unaffected by this procedure). It is fair to assume that uterine cramps like those excited by the irritation of a sound, occur during coitus (a parallel is found in vaginismus).

Sterile women, by whose temperament it may be assumed that this phenomenon occurs, are treated first for their nervous condition— rest, tonic, change of surroundings, etc. Then the author employs an instrument which he calls "das Fruchtulet," an aluminum tube (sides perforated) that conforms to the size and shape of the cervical passage, extending from just above the internal os to the external os where it is joined to a doubly concave, centrally perforated button that fits the portio and also serves to gather the semen and guide it into the uterine cavity via the cannula in the cervix. It leads to an improved circulation of the uterus, the uterine contractions do not recur, and hence the instrument serves the double purpose of maintaining the passage open for semen to pass, and of preventing its expulsion after having reached the uterine cavity.

The "Fruchtulet" is inserted (repeatedly if necessary) shortly after menstruation and allowed to remain until just preceding the following menses. The woman is advised to remain quiet, with buttocks raised, for some time following insemination.

The author reports four cases where the employment of this device was followed by impregnation of patients long sterile.

E. B. SOLHAUG.

Bandler: The "Higher Up" Theory of Sterility and Its Relation to the Endocrines. New York Medical Journal, 1919, cix, 309.

After excluding gross inflammatory conditions and tumors, Bandler thinks that sterility is largely a matter of endocrine dysfunction and remediable by the administration of the proper gland extracts. He claims that corpus luteum extract aids in the implantation of the ovum in the uterine mucosa. In threatened and repeated abortions he has used for years a combination of thyroid extract, arsenic, bichloride of mercury and stypticin with good result. At present, however, his usual treatment of sterility consists in the administration of the extract of the whole ovary, thyroid and ovarian residue. To this he adds other endocrines as seem indicated. This, he thinks, should be the routine method of treatment.

In case of failure, he advises some operative measure, either in the cervix or "higher up," e.g., "curettage in cervical and uterine adenoids," and has seen pregnancy follow the resection of polycystic ovaries. If the husband is at fault, he should be fed on endocrines.

R. E. WOBUS.

Wessel: A New Method of Temporary Sterilization. Zentralblatt fuer Gynaekologie, 1921, xlv, 75.

While chronic nephritis, tuberculosis, heart disease, diabetes, certain psychoses, osteomalacia, and marked pelvic contraction, are recognized as indications for sterilization, the various methods heretofore employed for the purpose have been effective only when performed so that the result is permanent. There are certain cases, however, where temporary sterilization might be of value, as, for example, in the case of tuberculosis susceptible of cure, and for such purposes Wessel describes the technic carried out by Gutbrod on some six cases during the past two years. The technic consists in opening the inguinal canals on each side, as in the Alexander-Adams operation, passing up to the peritoneum about the round ligament, and, after depression of the ovary into the fold of this peritoneum, securing it much as the stump of an appendix is peritonized. Wessel believes that, when required, the ovary may be freed from its peritoneal covering, and that it will function as before. Unfortunately the results have not been uniform, one failure in six being attributed to too rapid absorption of the catgut. In the remaining cases the ovaries are palpable and are about the size of a walnut on each side, but the patients are without symptoms.

H. M. LITTLE.

Schiffmann: The Question of Sterilization by Means of Ligation of the Tubes. Zentralblatt fuer Gynaekologie, 1921, xlv, 464.

Sterilization by ligation of the tubes has not proved a success. The difficulty of occluding the tube by means of ligatures has long been known from animal experimentation. To four human tubes examined by him some time after this operation the author adds a fifth case: a twenty-eight-year-old woman, who had been operated upon for complete prolapse and had been sterilized by means of thin silk ligatures placed with the maximum of care. The prolapse recurred and the patient returned to the clinic seven months later. At this time the tubes were secured for histologic study. The ligatures had not produced complete occlusion of the lumen of the tubes. Schiffmann finds that the anatomic results of ligation are practically those described by Kalliwoda: Distention of the vessels, narrowing of the lumen of the tube without atresia, the appearance of flattened cubical epithelium with decrease of the infolding of the mucosa and, particularly, atrophy of the musculature. Ligation of the tube will not necessarily result in atresia and sterility. Any reliable operation on the tube depends upon resection and careful occlusion of the free ends between the leaves of the broad ligament. Resection alone is sufficient in operations such as uterine interposition. This is probably due to the pull on the ampullar end of the tube, which keeps the cut ends separated. The writer has seen no case of pregnancy in 100 cases of interposition operations in which the tubes were treated in this way.

H. M. LITTLE.

Van de Velde: The Question of Sterilization. Nederlandsch Tijdschrift voor Geneeskunde, 1921, lxv, 2920.

The cause for which a sterilization operation is performed being frequently of a temporary nature, it is desirable to have at our disposal a method for temporary sterilization. With this end in view, attention has been directed mainly at the tubes, however, it seems the less we disturb the tubes, the better. Upon this conclusion, efforts have been made to bury the ovaries in such a way that they may again functionate upon being liberated. It has been found, however, that when buried in the broad ligament, the ovary becomes so covered by connective tissue as to prevent the discharge of ova after liberation of the organ. The Alexander-Adams operation, in which the ovary is buried outside the inguinal ring, has the disadvantage that the organ so placed is subject to trauma and often becomes painful.

Van de Velde attempts to overcome these disadvantages by burying the ovaries in the vesicouterine pouch. The ovary is partly mobilized by making a small incision in the fimbria and ovarian ligaments. This is carefully enlarged without injuring any of the blood vessels. Bleeding must be carefully controlled, the blood supply not disturbed and the organs handled very gently. Taking the ovary and tube between thumb and fingers, a slit is made through both layers of the broad ligament just below the ovary and the latter pushed through this opening. The edges of the broad ligament are sewed to the mesovarium with interrupted silk sutures, care being taken to avoid leaks and not to interfere with the blood supply. The vesicouterine pouch is then obliterated by sewing abdominal to visceral peritoneum, making use of the round ligaments.

The author has performed this operation nine times and in one case had occasion to liberate the ovaries after a number of years with the result that the patient soon afterwards conceived and, in due time, gave birth to a living child. Later on she was delivered of another healthy child.

R. E. WOBUS.

Flatau: Sterilization by Knotting the Tubes. Zentralblatt fuer Gynaekologie, 1921, xlv, 467.

The author notes that Nuernberg had collected 36 methods of sterilization prior to 1917, and believes that probably half a dozen others have been described since that date. About 6.5 per cent of all cases operated on are unsuccessful, and, though this is probably a low figure, it is evident that no one operation is simple and successful. Division, incision, extirpation of the tube or its ligation with catgut or silk, have all been tried, also the compression of the tube with forceps or with the angiotribe. Flatau himself in five cases, where there had been extreme compression for five minutes, with resultant tissue-paper-like appearance of the tubes, was absolutely unsuccessful. All became pregnant later. For this reason he began to try knotting the tube. The technic is extremely simple. The tube is freed from the upper margin of the broad ligament and a true knot is made about its middle, and the incision in the broad ligament is closed by a continuous catgut suture. This has been done in six cases. The results are so far uncertain, but the operation is suggested as simple and worth a trial.

H. M. LITTLE.

Madlener: Answer to Flatau's Paper on Sterilization. Zentralblatt fuer Gynaekologie, 1921, xlv, 825.

Madlener objects to Flatau's claim that Madlener's procedure is unsatisfactory and unreliable. It consists in the crushing of the middle portion of each tube by means of a heavy forceps and placing a ligature of non-absorbable material into the pressure groove. The writer insists that his method has proved useful in his own hands.

H. M. LITTLE.

Hellendall: A New Method for Tubal Sterilization. Zentralblatt fuer Gynaekologie, 1921, xlv, 822.

There is no safe procedure of artificial sterilization available which would permit restoration of normal tubal or ovarian function if at a later date this seems desirable. Sellheim planted the fimbriated ends of the tubes extraperitoneally by drawing them into the inguinal canal. Gutbrod in a similar manner changed the position of the ovaries. But all these operations failed in certain cases to actually sterilize the patients. Pregnancies have occurred. Nuernberger pulled the fimbriated ends of the tubes into the vagina through an incision into the posterior culdesac. This leads to various disturbances. Hellendall modified this latter procedure by fixing the tubes into the abdominal incision at the occasion of a ventrofixation. H. M. LITTLE.

Hellendall: Pregnancy after Ligation of Both Tubes. Medizinische Klinik, 1921, xvii, 1116.

A forty-three-year-old woman was operated upon for inflammation of the ovary, and during the course of the operation both tubes were ligated and cut to effect sterilization. Three years later, she returned with the history of having menstruated regularly every three weeks for six days until recently, when she had been bleeding steadily for four weeks. On examination the uterus was found to be soft, the cervix closed and the uterine cavity 10 cm. long. There was slight bleeding at the time. During curettage a small piece of tissue, the size of a bean, was removed. The Pathological Institute returned a diagnosis of placental tissue. E. D. PLASS.

The American Journal of Obstetrics and Gynecology

Original Communications

THE USE OF RADIUM IN CANCER OF THE FEMALE GENERATIVE ORGANS*

BY HAROLD BAILEY, M.D., IN COLLABORATION WITH EDITH QUIMBY, NEW YORK CITY

From the Gynecological and the Physical Departments, Memorial Hospital

IN THE gynecological department cancer of the cervix is the chief lesion that calls for treatment and its varied form and development offer many problems in technic. Cancer of the body of the uterus, of the vagina and vulva, and occasionally of the ovary complete the list of malignant conditions treated on our service.

TECHNIC FOR CANCER OF THE CERVIX

Our work began in January, 1915, with a limited amount of radium so that throughout this year we were able to command amounts not greater than 50 milligrams for one dose. The Continental methods then in use were copied and consisted largely in the application of radium in heavily filtered capsules of lead. The chief factor in the technic was the application within the cervix of radium, filtered by 2 mm. of lead and a vaginal application with the lead capsule contained in a small rectangular box of tin, 3 by 2 by 1 cm. in measurement. This box was placed in the vault of the vagina and held there by a pack of gauze. In addition there were developed two methods of conveying the rays by crossfiring to the affected part. (1) A silver probe applicator was placed in the body of the uterus and held there by means of an adhesive strap band, as the wire curved over the symphysis and (2) a lead applicator was placed high within the rectum,

---

*Read at the meeting of the American Radium Society held in Boston, June 6, 1921.

NOTE: The Editor accepts no responsibility for the views and statements of authors as published in their "Original Communications."

about at the level of the uterosacral ligaments. This was held in a T-crosspiece of rubber tubing similar to the ordinary vaginal drainage tube.

While the cases falling under our care during this year were for the most part, advanced, and with very slight opportunity, in any case, of effecting a cure, the fact remains that 10 per cent of those treated are well and still free of the disease. There were many cases that passed through a period of suffering from the radium effects on the bladder and rectum and there were a considerable number that developed rectovaginal fistulae. It became evident, therefore, that the technic would have to be changed so as to protect these organs.

During the year 1916, the technic was varied with this in mind and the amount of radium at hand permitted us to use 100 millicuries of emanation. The applications by vagina and rectum were largely discontinued and three applications were made within the cervix and the neck of the uterus. For the sake of convenience these applications were placed one week apart but it was considered from the standpoint of effect as if the dose was given at one time. The filter was changed from 2 millimeters of lead to one millimeter of platinum but the real outstanding feature of the technic of this year was that no capsule was used that was not filtered by either cervical or uterine tissue. The vagina was firmly packed with gauze, thus pushing the rectum and bladder away from the cervix as far as possible.

Although the total average dose was much higher, there was a striking difference in the comfort of the patient. Proctitis and cystitis cases became fewer in number and there were few rectal fistulae developing during the year. In out-growing cancers, cauliflower type, experimental trials were made with steel needles containing about 30 millicuries of emanation.

The results obtained by Dr. Barringer with these needles plunged into the cancerous prostate would indicate that there might be a field for their use in uterine cancer. However, in the ingrowing types of cancer, the distorted anatomy, dilating and displacing the ureters and changing the position of the uterine vessels would seemingly limit the field, at least for such large doses. They cause rapid disintegration of outgrowing tumors but in most instances are accompanied by deleterious effects on the vaginal wall. It is better to burn off these outgrowths with a cold cautery before implanting the radium.

THE PERCY OPERATION

During the year 1915-1916 a Percy or modified Percy operation was performed in thirty cases. The abdomen was opened and in all instances, the burning was conducted with an assistant's hand holding the uterus. In a considerable number of cases, the vessels were tied off in addition. The operation was followed by radium, the first application usually about two weeks after the operation. The results from this procedure were not good, the majority of the cases developing rectovaginal fistulae. However, there are three cases* that have remained well up to the present. In one or two patients the results following the ligature of the vessels were disastrous, leading to a sloughing of the tissues of the pelvis.

The criticism of this work would lead to the conclusion that the blood supply should not be interfered with to the extent of tying off the vessels and further that with the abdomen open and the uterus held in the hands of an assistant, there is a tendency on the part of the operator to burn too extensively and beyond what is advisable, if radium is to be used later. In other words, the tissue sloughed away following the burning leaves a very thin wall between the cervix and

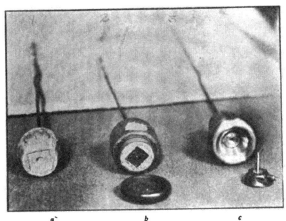

Fig. 1.—Various forms of radium applicators. a, Old lead "bomb"; b, Mercury iron filter; c, a newer mercury-iron contrivance.

adjoining parts and the slough which regularly follows radium dosage, applicable to the treatment of cancer, breaks through this thin barrier. In the latter years, this form of treatment has been modified by burning away the papillomatous parts of the lesion from below without opening the abdomen and thus creating an excavation in the cervix large enough to hold the radium capsule. The radium is applied at once and a number of good results have followed this method.

The results of the repeated doses of radium within the cervix were not very good. However, during this year the class of cases were almost all of the advanced and the advanced recurrent types. As the

---

*Two cases operated in the above manner in another hospital service and then transferred to us. All of the Percy operations were performed by Dr. George H. Mallett, at that time in charge of the service.

cervix itself could in most instances be taken care of satisfactorily, it was found necessary to use some other method of radiation to affect the tissues infiltrated by direct extension and by the lymphatic invasion of the tissues in the parametrium adjoining the cervix.

THE DEVELOPMENT OF THE "BOMB" TECHNIC

The application of radium placed in the vault of the vagina with the ordinary filter leads to irritation of the bladder and rectum, if the dose is above 1500 mc. hours. Kelly and Burnam, to overcome this difficulty, placed the radium in the vaginal vault with a cover of beaten gold. They also devised a lead cup to be placed over the

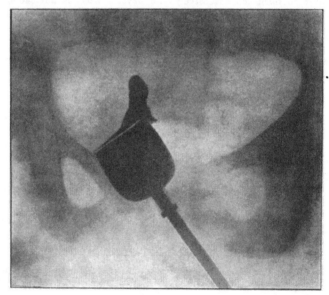

* Fig. 1—*A*.

radium capsule and by these methods they were able to filter the back and sides of the capsule so that very small amounts of radiation reached the adjoining organs.

In 1916, a lead capsule consisting of a small piece of lead pipe was fastened to a stiff rod so that the rays might be directed to various quarters. This idea was at once improved upon by making a small lead globe with a diameter of 3½ cm. with one pole sawed off and a set-in provided to hold the platinum capsule. This was applied with the capsule containing 1000 mc. of emanation. It was soon found that the cone of rays was too small and another apparatus was built which consisted of a thin capsule of iron. Into this was poured mercury

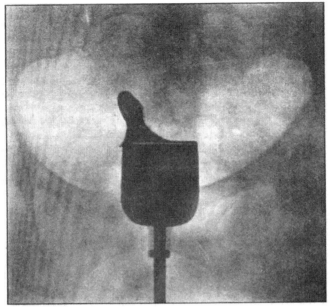

Fig. 1—B.

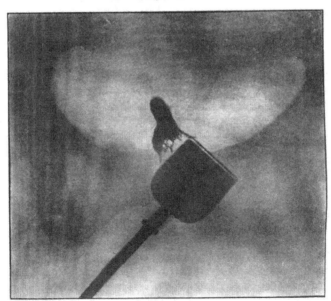

Fig. 1—C.

Figs. 1—A, B, and C.—Roentgenograms showing shadows of the bomb placed directly against the lesion in the vaginal vault and against the right and left parametrium. The cervical ulcer is packed with bismuth gauze.

to a depth of 2 cm. At the top of the apparatus was a receptacle with its sides protected by 6 millimeters of lead and in this area was placed the radium. Over this was a 1 millimeter platinum filter with a hard rubber cap. This instrument was used through the years 1917, 1918, and 1919. Radium up to 1000 millicuries was placed in the container and directed first to one side, then to the center, then to the opposite side of the vaginal vault. This has been termed the "bomb" because of its almost exact resemblance to the small hand grenades used in the war. With this instrument we have been able to give 3000 millicurie hours of radium treatment in the vaginal vault with but little irritation of the bladder and rectum. (Figs. 1, A, B, and C.)

We still had some trouble with rectal irritation because of the sagging of the pelvic floor due to the weight of the apparatus. At the suggestion of Dr. Bagg, a frame was built which is placed on the patient's bed and may be so arranged that she is in a fixed position with her legs placed in comfortable leg holders. In a track in this frame is a standard with a universal ball joint at the top which holds the entire weight of the applicator and yet enables the accurate placing of it. However, even with the aid of the above described applicator and with the radium capsule located in the cervix, the rays reaching the parametrium at a few centimeters distance are very feeble. It is necessary to reinforce them, as far as possible, by means of radium passing through the skin from several portals about the pelvis.

THE BLOCK TREATMENT

It was found by graduating the doses that 3000 millicurie hours at 4 centimeters with 2 millimeters of lead and 4 cm. of wood as a filter closely approximated the skin dose when it was applied in conjunction with the other radium. The areas selected for this type of application are directly over either groin and through the center of the symphysis on the front part of the body; against the sacrum and over either sacroiliac joint on the back. The diagram shows that each external application not only furnishes a definite radiation to a certain point in the parametrium but it is reinforced by each of the other five applications. Under such combined treatment the average case receives in all about 9000 to 18000 millicurie hours, depending upon whether the brass or lead block is used. (Fig. 2.)

In general the method outlined has been continued from 1917 to the present time, the variations being merely those of dosage rather than technic. In the latter part of 1919 and up to the present time, more and more use has been made of the direct embedding of bare glass tubes containing emanation. We have entirely confined our attempts in this direction to the small dosage, 1 millicurie being the highest used and ½ millicurie being the average strength of each tube. The method of burying emanation tubes is particularly applicable to vulval and vaginal cancers and has some value in the treatment of recurrent cancers where there are definite nodules behind the vaginal vault.

The Physical Department, under the charge of Mr. G. Failla, has been able to estimate the dosage administered by these various methods in terms of a skin dose (as used by us). They have also been able to accurately measure the dispersion of the rays from the front of the mercury "bomb" and from their computations have been able to build a new instrument of lead which correctly filters the sides and back of the radium and delivers in front a cone of rays of known extent. The most practical feature of their

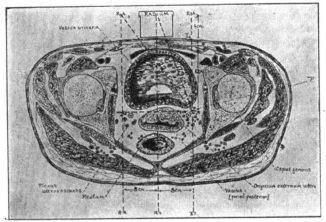

Fig. 2.—Diagrammatic horizontal cross-section of female pelvis, showing small amount of tissue through which the rays pass from surface applications on abdomen and back. Point P in the parametrium about 12 cm. from either surface.

work is the measurement of the intensity of the radiation at any point within a given area, in our case, the pelvis.

MEASUREMENT OF RADIATION

The purpose of the steel-mercury appliance was to furnish an intense beam of radiation in the forward direction and as little as possible laterally. In order to find out the actual distribution of radiation about the instrument an apparatus was constructed which gives the ionization produced by the radiation in different directions. (Fig. 3.) I is a conical lead ionization chamber, connected to a gold leaf electroscope in a lead case E, by a wire passing through the paraffin-filled tube R. The bomb is mounted at B on a support which moves on a pivot so that it can be rotated through any desired angle, which is measured on a scale S. The center of the tubes in the bomb is on the axis of the support, so that as the bomb is rotated, the radiation entering the ionization chamber passes through different thicknesses of filter. Therefore, the intensity of this radiation varies and the electroscope records this variation. Differences in intensity due to differences in distance do not enter into this experiment, since the relative positions of the source of radiation and the ionization chamber are the same throughout. Readings were taken at intervals of 10 degrees, giving a curve such as is shown in Fig. 4-A. This is for the steel-mercury bomb. The values are based on the intensity in the forward direction as 100 per cent since we are concerned only with relative values. From this curve, we see that the intensity is much greater in a forward than in a backward direction, but still 60 per cent as much comes from the sides as from the front.

Accordingly a new bomb was designed, which is shown in Fig. 1. For the protective filter lead was used, and over this a thin aluminum shell to remove the soft secondary radiation of the lead. The diameter of the bomb at the top is 3.4 cm., at the widest part 4 cm., and its total height is 4.2 cm. The rectangular pocket for the tubes is 12 mm. deep,

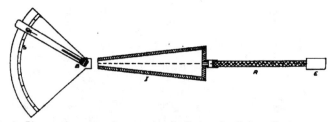

Fig. 3.—Diagram of apparatus for measuring distribution of radiation. *E*, electroscope; *R*, paraffin-filled brass tube; *I*, ionization chamber; *B*, bomb; *S*, scale.

16 × 10 mm. at the bottom and 16 × 14 mm. at the top, so that it can hold several of the enameled silver tubes ordinarily used at the hospital. The pocket is covered by a platinum plate 1 mm. thick. Therefore the filter for the useful beam of radiation is 1 mm. of platinum in addition to the silver tubes. The purpose of a rectangular pocket was to afford as much screening as possible for the lateral radiation in at least two directions. It was intended that when the applicator was in position, these two thicker sides should be toward the bladder and rectum, where it was desired to have as little radiation as possible.

The distribution curves for this applicator are shown in Fig. 4-B. It will be seen that in the direction of greater filtration, that is, toward the bladder and rectum, the intensity is 30 per cent less than from the steel-mercury bomb. This lead bomb was therefore adopted for the routine treatments.

Recent experiments have shown that it is not necessary to use such a heavy filter in order to get a sufficiently penetrating beam of radiation for deep therapy. Filtration by 1 mm. of brass plus ½ mm. of

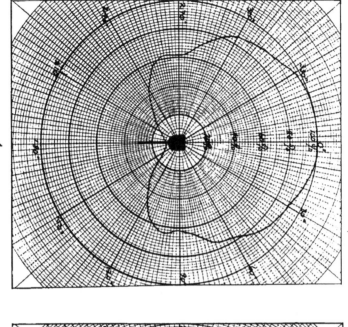

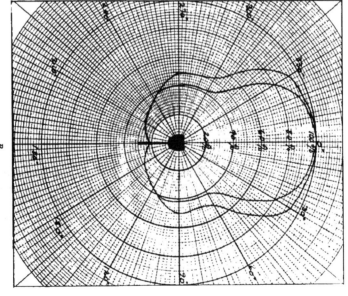

Fig. 4.—*A* and *B*.—Curves showing distribution of radiation about "bombs." The total radiation in a forward direction is 100%. *A*. Steel-mercury bomb. Too large a proportion of lateral radiation. *B*. Lead bomb, with platinum filter. This is the applicator used at present.

silver has been found sufficient.* Therefore the bomb was tested with the platinum piece replaced by 1 mm. of brass. The distribution curves for this arrangement show a gain in intensity in a forward direction of about 20 per cent for the same lateral intensity. The block has also been changed so that the filter now is 0.5 mm. of silver, 2 mm. of brass, and 1 cm. of bakelite. With this block we get just twice as much penetrating radiation as with the lead.

Distribution curves have also been obtained for the silver and platinum tubes in these treatments. One of these is shown in Fig 5.

The next step in the problem was to estimate the amount of radiation

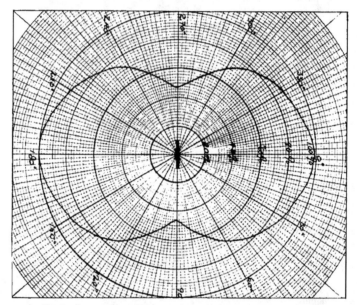

Fig. 5.—Curve showing distribution of radiation about the platinum tube.

delivered at different points within the body, due to the bomb, block and silver and platinum tubes as used in the actual treatments. The two factors which enter into the decrease in the amount of radiation are the distance from the source and the absorption by the intervening tissues. The decrease due to distance was calculated according to the inverse square law, that due to absorption was obtained experimentally, and the two combined to give the intensity at different points. The density of tissue being nearly the same as that of water, the absorption is substantially the same. Accordingly measurements

---

*Quimby, E. H.: The Effect of Different Filters on Radium Radiations. American Journal of Roentgenology, September, 1920.

were made of the absorption by different thicknesses of water of radiation from these different applicators. To calculate the amount of radiation reaching different points, the percentage transmitted by any given thickness of water was multiplied by the factor expressing the decrease due to the inverse square law. For the unit of ir-

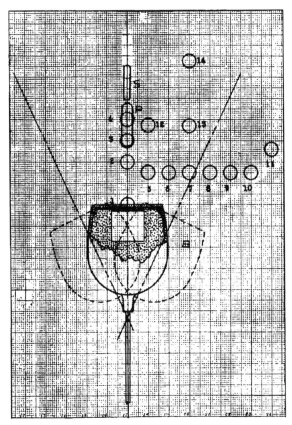

Fig. 6.—Diagram showing radium "bomb" and tubes in same relation as in vagina and uterus of patient. The figures in front of the bomb are arranged arbitrarily. Table I represents the radiation in terms of a skin dose at each of these points. B, the bomb; P, platinum tube; S, silver tube. Point 1 is on the actual surface of the bomb. Point 2 is 2 cm. above. Point 3 is 3 cm. above, but also on the surface of the platinum tube. Point 4 is 4 cm. above the surface of the bomb, on the platinum tube. Points 5 to 10 represent points 1 to 6 cm. from the median line and 1½ cm. above the surface of the bomb in its center position. Point 11 is 7 cm. from the median line and 2½ cm. above the surface of the bomb. Point 12 is 4 cm. from the bomb and 1 cm. from the platinum piece. Point 13 is 4 cm. from the bomb and 3 cm. from the platinum piece. Point 14 is 7 cm. from the bomb and 3 cm. from the silver tube.

radiation was selected the "skin dose." This is based on clinical observations of the effect on the skin of different applicators used at the hospital for the treatment of deep-seated conditions. The "skin dose" as used at the Memorial Hospital corresponds to the irradiation from a treatment of 3200 mc. hours with a filter of 0.5 mm. of silver, 2 mm. of brass and 1 cm. of bakelite in an applicator with brass sides, the radium being 4 cm. from the skin. This is more than twice as much as can be used on patients undergoing the treatment discussed in this paper, because of the additional radiation received by the skin from the other applicators,—bomb, block, tubes, etc.

Fourteen points were taken, located as shown in Fig. 6, at different positions within the pelvis, from No. 1, directly on the surface of the bomb in its median position, to Nos. 10 and 14 in the parametrium. The intensity of irradiation at each point due to each applicator, considering the bomb in three positions and the block in six, as usually used, was calculated. The results are shown in Column 6, Table I. It will be seen that the dose received by these points varies from about one-fourth of a skin dose at the most distant one considered, to several skin doses near the central applicators.

TABLE I
INTENSITIES OF IRRADIATION AT POINTS SHOWN IN FIG. 6

1	2	3	4	5	6	7
POINT	SILVER TUBE	PLATINUM TUBE	BOMB	BLOCK	TOTAL (MINIMUM)	TOTAL (NEGLECTING ABSORPTION)
1	0.06	0.14	2.73	0.06	3.03	3.27
2	0.14	0.62	0.41	0.06	1.22	1.83
3	0.28	64	0.28	0.06	65	65
4	0.66	64	0.17	0.06	65	65
5	0.13	0.53	0.61	0.07	1.34	2.33
6	0.14	0.41	0.50	0.07	1.11	1.60
7	0.12	0.29	0.36	0.06	0.85	1.11
8	0.10	0.19	0.26	0.06	0.62	0.99
9	0.08	0.13	0.17	0.06	0.44	0.71
10	0.06	0.09	0.16	0.06	0.37	0.54
11	0.06	0.07	0.01	0.06	0.26	0.45
12	0.71	5.6	0.18	0.06	6.54	7.07
13	0.31	0.55	0.16	0.06	1.08	1.44
14	0.43	0.18	0.06	0.03	0.72	1.02

These values represent the minimum amount of radiation delivered, no allowance being made for secondary and scattered radiation, which recent experiments have shown to be an important factor; making the dose much higher than that obtained by calculations such as these. Column 7 gives the theoretic maximum of irradiation, absorption being neglected and the only decrease considered being that due to the inverse square law. The actual amount of penetrating radiation reaching a given point is somewhere between these two values. However, the ionization taking place at the point and producing the therapeutic effect is greater than would be indicated by these values, on account of the soft secondary radiation generated by the penetrating radiation in the tissues.

CANCER OF THE BODY OF THE UTERUS

The technic of the radium application in the cancer of the body of the uterus depends upon whether the uterus is to be removed following the treatment. We believe, where there are no contraindications to the operation from the standpoint of the general constitution of the patient, that the removal should follow the radium treatment in all cases. The extent of the disease must remain unknown because it is in a position where neither sight nor sense of touch can aid one. However, there are certain cases where, owing to age or other disability, one has to remain content with the radium treatment.

In the first instance, where operation is to follow, radium is placed in a platinum capsule within the body of the uterus, preferably in a tandem piece, so that a large part of the organ may be radiated. The dose should be a total of 3500 mc. hours and the removal of the organ should follow at the end of six to eight weeks. We believe that there should be no earlier removal because of possible local inflammatory effects.

After the organ has been removed, external radiation should be given by the block technic. In cases where it is known that the organ is not to be removed, beside the 3500 mc. hours within the body of the uterus, the "bomb" is directed toward the parametrium on either side by one hour and in addition the block is applied to six areas about the pelvic girdle.

CANCER OF THE VAGINA AND VULVA

Cancer of the vagina and vulva are both treated by buried radium emanation. The strength of each tube is about 0.5 mc. In addition, filtered radium is administered by means of the "bomb" in the vagina or by tubes placed in dental compound if the involved area is at the entrance of the vagina or on the anterior wall. The glands of the groins in vulval carcinoma are radiated by the block method and in some instances are later removed by dissection and the open area infiltrated by bare tubes placed 1 cm. apart. In the vaginal cancer, the external radiation is given by the regular block technic through six areas.

RECURRENT CERVICAL CANCER

Recurrences are either behind the vaginal vault or by outgrowths in the vault of the vagina. Here again, the bare tubes, "bomb," and "block" are the methods selected. If there is a crater in the vault of the vagina a platinum capsule is inserted for not more than 1200 mc. hours.

Table II shows an analysis of results in 600 cases of uterine cancer and in 32 cases of vulval and vaginal cancer, followed to May 1, 1921.

TABLE II
RESULTS IN 600 CASES OF UTERINE CANCER AND IN 32 CASES OF VULVAL AND VAGINAL CANCER
(Followed to May 1, 1921)

RADIUM TREATMENT	1915	1916	1917	1918	1919	1920
Advanced Primary Cervix	15	24(1)	41	41(7)	69(23)	92(58)
Recurrent	18(1)	8(1)	26(2)	35(8)	43(17)	37(27)
Early, Operable Cervix	1(1)	3	3(2)	4(2)	9(7)	14(9)
Borderline Cervix	0	3(2)	3(2)	17(5)	10(7)	12(8)
Percy	15(2)	11(1)	3	0	0	0
Ca. Body of Uterus Prophylaxis	1(1)	1	0	7(3)	5(3)	5(5)
Following Hysterectomy	0		2	8(6)	4(3)	10(10)
Ca. Vulva and Vagina	0	1	0	6	11(4)	14(8)
	50	51	78	118	151	184

(Figures within the parentheses represent the number of cases alive May 1, 1921.)

The follow-up of these cases through the entire year 1921 will appear in the Annual Medical Report of the Hospital.

DISCUSSION OF RESULTS

From January, 1915, to January, 1921, there were 600 cases of uterine cancer and 32 cases of vulval and vaginal cancer treated with radium. The follow-up has been continued to May 1, 1921, and the figures in each group show the total number of cases treated, with the number of those alive placed in the parentheses. In the group of the first three or four years, that is from 1915 to 1918, the figures will probably remain as they are, for the cases that have lived through such a long period are presumably cured and their number will only diminish through death from intercurrent disease.

The follow-up is continued by weekly clinics, by visits of Social Service nurses and by letter. No case is discharged and those that are lost through failure to return or by change of residence are classified as dead. We find that these patients are so thoroughly impressed by their treatment that if they do not return or continue in the follow-up clinic, the reason is usually due to their ill health caused by the advancement of the disease. There have been a few who discontinued their treatment before it was completed but even these cases, since 1918, have been included in our lists because in our technic, all the treatment is given in 24 hours. In other words, they have discontinued the follow-up observations not the treatment.

We feel that the technic which has been standardized since 1918 and by means of which the parametrium is thoroughly radiated, will provide us with better results than we have had in previous years. However, the number of those alive in the 1919 and 1920 groups will drop to a considerable extent, especially in the two classes, advanced primary and recurrent cancer.

EARLY OR OPERABLE CANCER OF THE CERVIX

This group is the most important one and demands a few words of explanation. In the year 1915, the one case was a woman of about seventy years who had a very early cervical lesion but with the specimen showing epidermoid carcinoma. She has remained well. Of the 3 cases of 1916, one was operated in another clinic within a month after our treatment and died on the third day following the operation. The uterus removed showed no carcinoma. The second case died of appendicitis a few months after treatment and the diagnosis was confirmed by a visit from one of our staff. The third case, one month after treatment, had an attack of acute rheumatism and died of cerebral embolus.

Of the three 1917 cases, two are alive and the third died of cerebral hemorrhage in November, 1919, at which time there was no evidence of cancer.

Of the four 1918 cases two are alive and two died from the disease.

Of the nine cases in 1919, two are dead. One had in addition to her pelvic trouble, carcinoma of the breast and the other had a hysterectomy after our treatment was completed and died this year of recurrent carcinoma.

In 1920, there were 14 cases in all, with three deaths from the disease. One patient was lost from our records because she gave us a false address. Another died ten days after the radium treatment following a hysterectomy in another clinic performed against our advice. Of those dying from the disease, one had a hysterectomy by us about two months after her treatment and radium was inserted in the parametrium. Notwithstanding this treatment, carcinoma developed throughout the pelvis. The second patient had a general glandular metastasis with carcinoma of the neck, axillae and the groins. The third case had an attack of typhoid fever within a month after the treatment and although she recovered from this, her health never improved and she returned home to die.

Two of the fourteen cases had negative specimens but the clinical examination conducted separately by Dr. Stone on the admission of the patient and by me with the patient under an anesthetic showed all the evidences of early carcinoma. It is our contention that notwithstanding the negative specimen they should be considered as early carcinoma. In the early or operable group, there are six cases where a valid excuse occurs for their removal from our list. If these six cases remain in the list there are 34 in all for the years from 1915 to 1920 and if they are thrown out, there will remain 28 cases with 23 alive. Of course it is to be remembered that in regard to the 1919 and 1920 cases very little time has elapsed. These cases are free of clinical evidence of the disease.

BORDERLINE CANCER

Of the three cases of 1916 one is dead, although she remained well for more than four years and died of cerebral hemorrhage following an attack of pleurisy in March, 1921.

There were three cases in 1917. One died from the disease. Of the 17 cases in 1918, all but five died of the disease. Reviewing the histories of these cases it would seem that according to the classification of today, a number would not be considered as borderline but as advanced primary cases.

Of the ten cases in 1919, three are dead of cancer and seven are alive and free of evidence of the disease. One of these patients had a hysterectomy following her treatment. Of the 12 borderline cases of 1920, four are dead of the disease. One is in poor condition but the others are free of clinical signs of tumor. There is a total of 45 cases during these years, 1915 to 1920, and 24, are still alive. There are three cases of this group who are now clinically cured but who have rectal fistulae.

BODY OF THE UTERUS

The one case of 1915 is well today. One case in 1916 had her uterus removed some time after the radium treatment and carcinoma was present, the patient dying some months later. Of the seven 1918 cases only three remain alive. Of the four cases classified as dead, two dropped out of our follow-up clinic shortly after their treatment. The other two died of the disease nearly three years later.

Of the five cases in 1919, two are dead. One died from the disease and the other from pneumonia about six months after the treatment. In 1920 there were also five cases and all are alive and free of signs of disease. Of the total of 19 cases of cancer of the body that were treated throughout these years (1915-1920) 12 are alive and well.

RECURRENT CANCER

The recurrent cancer forms a large group with a very high mortality. Those cases that are alive represent the early recurrent cancer where only small areas in the vault of the vagina or in the nearby parametrium were involved. The 17 cases alive in 1919 and the 27 in 1920 will be gradually reduced in numbers at the end of a few more years for many of them still have evidences of cancer.

ADVANCED PRIMARY CANCER

Of the 80 cases treated during the years 1915, 1916, and 1917, there is but one alive. The years of 1918, 1919, and 1920, we feel will give a much higher percentage, but the 23 cases of 1919 and the 58 of 1920 that are still alive will be greatly reduced in numbers in the course of another year or two.

PROPHYLAXIS

We come now to a more hopeful group, those who had no evidence of recurrence following hysterectomy and who were treated as a prophylaxis against the return of the disease. The two cases treated in 1917 both developed cancer and died, but of the eight who were treated in 1918, six are free of the disease. Of the four in 1919, three are alive and of the ten cases treated in 1920, all are living. There are 19 cases in this group that are now free of clinical evidence of the disease.

CANCER OF THE VULVA AND VAGINA

This subject has been separately reported by us, and there are great prospects in this field through the use of bare weak tubes plus the filtered radium. Our results are encouraging, but as yet there is no surety that the disease will not recur.

SUMMARY

The full technic, using the external radiation as an aid to the capsule and bomb was not in routine use until 1918. If the advanced primary cancer and the recurrent cancer groups are taken together, there were 132 cases treated before January 1, 1918, and there are but 5 cases alive today. If these same groups are taken for 1918, there are 76 cases, and 15 are alive, for 1919, 112 and 40 are living, for 1920, 129 and 85 are still alive. While the prospects of greatly reducing these figures are present and sure, nevertheless, the indications are that in these groups we have had our greatest advance.

The follow-up of our operable and borderline classes will have to be continued through three or four more years before deductions may be made. Our present figures are remarkable and indicative.

In the prophylaxis after hysterectomy great care must be used that the tissues are not overradiated. The end results in this class are very good for the time elapsed since treatment.

We believe that these results cannot be duplicated without the use of massive doses of radium or without thoroughly radiating the parametrium.

MEMORIAL HOSPITAL.

THE ACTION OF THE COMMONER ECBOLICS IN THE FIRST STAGE OF LABOR*

BY M. PIERCE RUCKER, M.D., RICHMOND, VA.

From the Department of Obstetrics, Medical College of Virginia.

THE use of dilating bags affords us an excellent opportunity of studying the variations in pressure that take place within the uterus in the first stage of labor as the result, not only of changes in posture, respiration, vomiting, etc., but also of drugs commonly used at this time. It is to this phase of the subject that I wish to direct your attention. I can find no reference to the Voorhees bag being utilized in such a manner. Schatz,[1] 1872, obtained tracings of uterine contractions by introducing a small rubber bag, attached to the end of a stiff tube between the amnion and the uterine wall. The bag was partly filled with water and was connected with a manometer which not only measured the intrauterine pressure, but recorded it upon a moving drum. H. Hensen[2] made use of Schatz' method to investigate the influence of morphine and ether upon labor pains. In his article he states that Smolsko, (1876), found that moderate doses of quinine strengthened and lengthened uterine contractions without changing their physiologic character, and that larger doses caused the contractions to cease entirely. Rubesamen[3] criticizes Schatz' method first, because a foreign body is introduced within the uterus, which might possibly influence uterine contractions, and, secondly, because with it you are unable to investigate the third stage of labor. He used in his work a 500 gm. weight that rested upon the abdomen and was connected with a writing lever by a string and a series of pulleys. Such an arrangement would give an accurate record of the rhythm of uterine contractions in all three stages of labor and the height to which the uterus rises at each contraction, but does not measure the intrauterine pressure or the strength of the contractions, nor could it give information as to the effect of coughing, vomiting, etc. He found that quinine stimulates contractions slightly when the uterus is already contracting, but that it does not initiate them. It seems entirely inactive when used in postpartum atony.

The method that I have employed in making the tracings can, of course, be used only in the first stage of labor. In fact, towards the end of the first stage, when the bag is nearly out of the cervix, the manometer fails to register the full force of the uterine contractions,

---

*Read at the Thirty-Fourth Annual Meeting of the American Association of Obstetricians, Gynecologists, and Abdominal Surgeons, St. Louis, Mo., September 20-22, 1921.

unless a tight vagina gives the bag support. It is open to the same objection as is Schatz' method, in that a foreign body is introduced within the uterus which might have some influence upon uterine contractions. That such influence is slight, is realized when one thinks

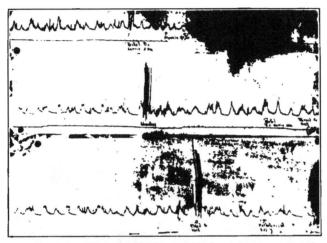

Fig. 1.—Hyoscine, gr. 1/100, administered at point indicated by arrow. Note the comparative absence of voluntary effort after this time. The record shows the effect of vomiting in the middle of the second line, and the effect of attempting to void in the bottom line. Sixteen ounces of urine were removed with a catheter five pains later. The timer marks minutes, wherever it works, in this and all subsequent records.

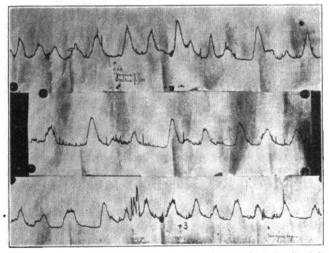

Fig. 2.—Morphine, gr. 1/6 and hyoscine gr. 1/100, were given at point in first line indicated by arrow. Note tendency to reduplication of pains. Chloroform was begun two pains before the record was stopped.

of the time it usually takes to induce labor with a bag, especially before term.

The chief advantage of this method is its simplicity. The introduction of a Voorhees bag within the cervix is often desirable and necessary upon clinical grounds. In order to observe what is taking place within the uterus, the stem of the bag is connected with a mercury manometer instead of clamping or tying it off, as is usually done. The only additional hardship imposed upon the patient is keeping her in bed. She can turn about, sit up, or use a bed pan without interfering with the working of the apparatus. There are some mechanical difficulties with the recording devices. For instance, when I used ink pencils and a continuous roll of paper, I had difficulty in

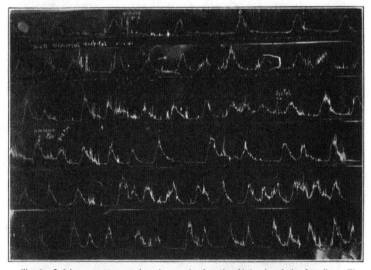

Fig. 3.—Quinine grs. 10, was given by mouth after the third pain of the first line. The effort of raising the shoulders to swallow the capsules shows on the record. There is an interval of 32 minutes between the first and second line, 75 minutes between the second and third, and 20 minutes between the fifth and sixth lines. Notice the relative smoothness of the contraction waves, after 1/100 gr. of hyoscine were given, at the apex of the second pain of the fourth line, and the reduplication of pains in the fifth and sixth lines.

keeping the timer working properly. On the other hand, when I used smoked paper on a long paper kymograph, the changing and smoking of the paper made it necessary that I be near the physiological laboratory.

At first it was thought that the cumbersome recording apparatus might alarm the patients; but, on the contrary, they took great interest in watching the record and in comparing the force of each contraction with the preceding ones.

Although experimental apparatus was used, this work is not experimental in the same sense that a pharmacologist is able to demonstrate the action of drugs by animal experiments. My work was merely observation with a more or less accurate method of recording the results. In other words, the patients received no different medication than they would have got had there been no recording apparatus. The only exception to this was when pituitrin and ergot were used and then there were extenuating circumstances. For instance, in two cases when a bag was placed on account of placenta previa before the period of viability, pituitrin was used; and once, in a full term multipara, two minims were used about the end of the first stage. Ergotol was used, in small doses, in two cases at term, once by mouth and once hypodermically. The fluid extract of ergot was used in two cases of antepartum bleeding at the sixth and the seventh month respectively.

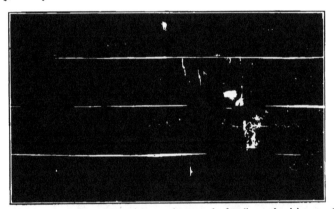

Fig. 4.—Castor oil, two ounces, was given at point *x* on the first line, and quinine, grs. 10, at the point *x* on the fourth line.

Observations were made upon twenty-one patients. Hyoscine was used in ten cases, usually with an initial dose of morphine. Quinine was used in six cases, twice hypodermically and five times by mouth; to one patient it was given both hypodermically and by mouth. Strychnine was used in one case; castor oil in one; ergotol in two cases, and the fluid extract of ergot in two cases. Pituitrin was used in three cases, twice alone and once following hyoscine. Two patients were given first quinine and later hyoscine.

Hyoscine.—There were ten patients in this group with a total of fourteen observations. Seven of these patients were given an initial dose of morphine, either $\frac{1}{6}$ or $\frac{1}{8}$ grain; two patients had quinine previously. Some received scopolamin dissolved in 10 per cent mannite, the so-called "scopolamin, stable," and some received hyoscine or scopolamin in tablet form. I could see no difference in the action of the two preparations which is in keeping with the accepted views concerning the identity of hyoscine and scopolamin.

As you see from the hysterographs, there is no very marked effect from the administration of either $\frac{1}{200}$ or $\frac{1}{100}$ grain. In some of the patients, who were showing contractions of the voluntary muscles as indicated by the perpendicular lines superimposed on the broader uterine curves, the effect was to diminish these or do away with them entirely, so that the tracing became smoother, showing only uterine contractions and some respiratory waves. In addition to this there seemed to be a tendency towards doubling or reduplicating uterine contractions as if the uterine muscle were more responsive to irritants as the result of the action of the drug. Moreover, by measuring a given number, usually ten, of uterine contractions immediately

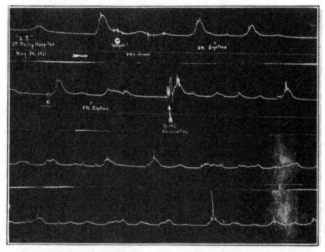

Fig. 5.—Ergotol, two minims, was given hypodermically at point *x* on the first line, and five minims at point *x* on the second line. The irregularities at *O* on the first and second lines are due to tying the stem of the bag tighter.

before and after the hypodermic injection, it is apparent that the hyoscine had a definite, although slight additional effect. In twelve out of the fourteen instances, the height of the contractions was increased, while in two instances it was decreased. One of the patients in which the strength of the contractions was diminished had no preliminary dose of morphine and the diminution of the height of the contractions was due, in part at least, to a cessation of the voluntary efforts on the part of the patient. In nine instances the duration of the pains was increased, in four it was decreased, and in one it was unchanged. The rapidity of the pains is, more or less, dependent upon the duration of the individual contractions. In nine instances there was a decrease in the rapidity of the pains; once there was no change, and once there was an increase in the rapidity of the pains. In two instances the timer was out of order so that this factor could not be determined accurately. These observations confirm the clinical impression that the first stage of labor is usually shortened by the use of scopolamin or hyoscine.

Quinine.—Six patients fall into this group. One patient was given 3 grains of quinine and urea-hydrobromide hypodermically; one was given four grains hypodermically, and later ten grains of the sulphate

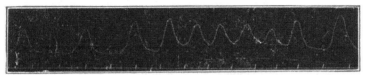

Fig. 6.—Pituitrin, two minims, was given at point indicated by arrow. Labor in this case was induced prematurely. Note that while the action is slight, the uterus does not relax completely for nine minutes.

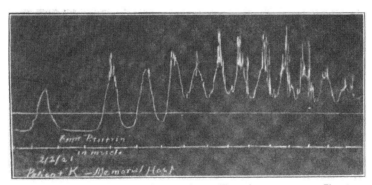

Fig. 7.—Pituitrin, two minims, was given at point *x*. The patient was at term. The uterus remained contracted 28 minutes.

of quinine by mouth; four were given 10 grains of the sulphate orally. Of the two in whom quinine was administered hypodermically, one showed a moderate increase and one a decrease in the height of the contractions. The latter showed an increase in the strength of the pains when quinine was administered orally. The length of the contractions was decreased in both instances after the hypodermic use of quinine, while the rapidity was increased in one and unchanged in another.

When quinine was given orally there was an increase in the strength of contractions four times, once quite marked, and once there was a decrease in the strength of contractions. The duration of the pains was increased once, unchanged once and decreased three times. The rapidity of contractions was increased twice, unchanged twice, and diminished at once. From this rather limited series it would seem that quinine has, sometimes, a very marked effect in strengthening uterine contractions, but that its action is variable and that occasionally it has no effect. Its action seems to be more potent when given by the mouth than when administered hypodermically.

Strychnine.—In the single instance in which strychnine was used, 1/30 grain hypodermically, there was a moderate increase in both the strength and the duration of the pains.

Castor Oil.—Castor oil was given in one case. After the administration of two ounces orally, there seemed to be no effect on either the strength, the duration, or the rapidity of the pains.

Ergotol.—The baneful effects of the use of ergot preparations before the third stage of labor were so thoroughly drilled into me in my student days, that I hesitated to try it in the first stage. I was, however, so anxious to get a tracing to compare it with some pituitrin records I had made previously, that I, finally, ventured to use minute doses on an unmarried colored girl at term. At first two minims were given hypodermically with no appreciable effect. A five minim dose was then given, and it was followed by a slight increase in the rapidity of the pains with a lessening of their strength and duration. There was no evidence of tetanic contraction, unless the first contraction after the five minim dose be so considered, which seems scarcely justifiable. Another patient at term was given ten minims of ergotol by mouth with no appreciable effect. Of course, negative findings in two cases does not mean that ergotol has no action upon the pregnant uterus. A more plausible explanation of my results, is the inertness of the preparation used.

Ergot.—The fluid extract of ergot was administered to two patients. In both patients bags were placed on account of uterine hemorrhage. One patient was in her sixth month and the other in her seventh month of pregnancy. The latter was given twenty minims orally and later one dram. The former was given a single dose of one dram by mouth. In neither case was there appreciable effect. The same explanation probably holds good here as in the case of ergotol, although the pharmacist insists that I was using the best preparation obtainable.

Pituitary Extract.—The effect of pituitrin in three cases was discussed in a previous paper by Charles C. Haskell and myself;[4] but, as our tracings were not published, I will take the liberty of showing them at this time. In two of these cases labor was induced in the seventh month, while the third was at term. In all three an incomplete tetanus followed promptly upon the administration of from two to seven and one-half minims, occurring in four minutes in the premature cases and in two minutes in the full term patient. The contraction was maintained nine, thirty-five, and twenty-eight minutes, respectively. The most marked effect followed the use of two minims in the patient at term, although it did not last quite so long as when seven and one-half minims were used in the premature labor.

CONCLUSIONS

The patient with a Voorhees bag in her cervix offers an excellent opportunity to observe the action upon the uterus of the drugs commonly used in obstetrics.

From my limited observations it would seem that hyoscine has a moderate, but rather constant, ecbolic action in the first stage of labor. The action of quinine is more variable; sometimes it markedly strengthens the normal rhythmic contractions and sometimes it shows no action whatever.

My observations upon the action of strychnine, castor oil, ergotol, and the fluid extract of ergot, are too limited to warrant even a tentative conclusion. It would seem, however, that the possibility of an inert preparation of ergotol and the fluid extract of ergot is a real one.

In the three cases in which pituitrin was used, even in minute doses, there was a continued contraction of the uterus that varied from nine to thirty-five minutes in duration. This is probably the explanation of the many disasters that have followed its use.

REFERENCES

(1) Arch f. Gynäk., iii, 1872, p. 58. (2) Arch. f. Gynäk., 1898, lv, 129. (3) Arch. f. Gynäk., 1920, cxii, 459. (4) Jr. Am. Med. Assn., May 21, 1921, lxxvi, 1390.

400 NORTH LOMBARDY STREET.   (*For discussion, see page 188.*)

TEN YEARS OF PAINLESS CHILDBIRTH*

By George Clark Mosher, A.M., M.D., F.A.C.S., Kansas City, Mo.

AT THE meeting of the British Medical Association at Birmingham, 1890, I was much impressed by an anecdote related by Alexander Simpson of Edinburgh, nephew of Sir James Y. Simpson, who in a paper on the "Management of Labor," told of a mistake made in the early years of his practice. Called to a woman in labor at some distance from his home, he found the patient having very weak pains and with evidence which he interpreted as indicating a slow delivery. Leaving several pills of ergot with directions to give one every hour until good labor had set in, he remounted his horse and returned home. On changing his clothes for dinner he found on emptying his pockets that the vial supposed to be pills of ergot did not contain ergot but pills of opium instead. Hastily returning to the house of the patient to prevent the giving of more opium he was astonished to find that the woman had fallen into a refreshing sleep after the first pill and, upon awakening, she began good hard pains which soon terminated the case. This experience set him to thinking, and he tried the experiment on subsequent occasions and usually with happy results.

On returning to America on consideration of the subject of the relief of pain in labor it occurred to the writer to try some expedient to accomplish this result since so frequently one is implored by the patient in the agony of her suffering to give her something to relieve her of pain.

To the average man the subject of pain in childbirth is a trivial matter and not longer ago than the present summer distinguished gentlemen, who are obstetricians, went on record as opposed to all drugs in labor.

Dr. Wakefield recently said that "the greatest outrage of modern civilization is the fact that, in spite of all that is recorded in medical literature, the profession and the public remain in silent acquiescence and have no regard for the suffering of women in childbirth, or make any attempt to alleviate this agony."

The twentieth century woman has by education and environment, developed into an extreme type of hypersensitiveness; she is possessed of a nervous system susceptible to impressions and feels pain more acutely; hence her physical and mental forces are easily depleted. The result is, as a general rule, she suffers under ordinary circumstances "a lack of the feeling of well-being which constitutes

---
*Read at the Thirty-Fourth Annual Meeting of the American Association of Obstetricians, Gynecologists and Abdominal Surgeons, St. Louis, Mo., September 20-22, 1921.

good health." Consequently, when she goes into labor, the modern woman cannot produce efficient .efforts, either mental or physical.

Let us consider that 20,000 women annually die from childbirth in the United States, that hundreds of thousands more are incapacitated by invalidism due to the same causes. A melancholy picture! In the chairman's address in the Section on Obstetrics of the American Medical Association, Dr. John O. Polak, 1920, disclosed the fact that the death rate in obstetrics has increased from 1901 to 1919 and this in spite of all improved hospital technic. This fact must be recognized as a reflection on the general care of women in labor. The statistics of the hospitals bear out this conclusion. As both morbidity and mortality in hospital cases are lessened, we must in some way improve the method of obstetric care of the average woman in the home to lower the mortality rate of the country at large.

In what particular is this easier than to increase her own immunity by conservation of her reserve, simply by lessening pain, fatigue, shock and exhaustion?

The effect of suffering in labor demoralizes the nervous and vital forces to such a degree that it demands recognition and cooperation.

When one studies the statistics of the alarming decrease in the size of the families in this country in the last 40 years and the alarming increase in abortion, as shown by Arthur E. Meyer in the August number of this journal, we must conclude that some reason exists for the desire to escape maternity on the part of the American women. The maternal instinct is strong in the normal woman, and there is a reason for the record of our childless homes, aside from the oft quoted "high cost of living." Every family indulges in luxuries, and even if babies were to be classed among the articles subject to war tax, people would not reject them simply because of the cost. The great bugaboo of the young wife is the fear of the suffering she must endure in giving birth to a child.

What a pity that motherhood, which is the most beautiful relation in life, should be attended by physical suffering and mental terror, when this condition may be avoided by a safe and comparatively simple method of treatment. If we are able to give assurance that pain can be lessened or prevented by any combination of drugs, which may be used without injury, we bestow a boon on our patient; we gain her confidence; later, gratitude follows her having gone through the valley of the shadow without a memory of any disturbing character.

It is but fair to state, at the outset, that the views following are based on my own experience and where they differ from those of other men, they are to be taken as drawn from cases in our own clinic.

Various methods of combination of drugs have been devised by the few investigators interested in the study of relief of pain; some of these having value, others being without virtue. As observation of one or another of these plans demonstrates to us its weak points, it has been dropped after more or less trial. For example, the tablet of hyoscine-morphine-cactin, which, after a vogue of several years has fallen into disuse, was early discovered to profoundly affect the child, and that in a most dangerous manner. This we at once discarded after a single trial. The deep narcosis of all large doses of morphine and hyoscine, or morphine and atropin was subject to the same serious objection. Scopolamin and morphine we first used in 1911, and we feel it met the indication; but the objections to it on the part of the profession have been so general, that it but slowly came into any considerable favor. It must be remembered that profound narcosis will, in greater or less degree, prevent uterine contractions, hence it is not possible to prevent pain absolutely and continuously throughout the labor.

Gauss early showed that there is a point in amnesia which falls between a simple temporary relief from pain, and absolute narcosis. This happy medium has been graphically styled, "Twilight Sleep." This term has been the subject of much opprobrium because it was formerly exploited in a popular way in articles printed in magazines for consumption by the lay public.

I believe the specific effect of the administration of scopolamin is of the greatest benefit in women of the highly organized nervous system of the cultured class. But in our experience the point at which this condition of amnesia appears is vastly different in different individuals, and must, therefore, correspond to the individual sensibility in order to avoid overdosing or fail, because of too small an amount being administered. In this individualization, as demonstrated in our own cases with the same results that have been conclusively shown by Dr. Gauss, the undesirable effect of extreme pain on the one hand, and deep narcosis on the other, are overcome.

The technic proposed by Siegel, of experimental fixed dosage, resulted in undesirable developments which I had already encountered in our early attempts to establish a fixed dosage for all patients. The sensibility of the patient is the only measure of the degree of narcosis and this can be ascertained only by observation of each patient as to the results of her treatment. If Siegel's method of the so-called "simplified amnesia" could be followed, the personal equation might be eliminated, and the care of the patient left to an intelligent nurse, except at the time of delivery; and one of the chief objections to scopolamin—the demand on the time of the physician—be thus removed. Siegel changed his technic three times; but in each method the large initial dose of scopolamin and repeated doses of narcophin of generous amount, was, to our mind, a fatal mistake. Siegel, also, in his last series, used amnesin, a combination of quinine with narcophin, for the purpose of stimulating the labor pains which are, admittedly, reduced by the large doses of scopolamin and morphine. Whether quinine will be effectual in combination with an opiate, in overcoming the reduction of the expulsive force of labor, is a question. In the individualized method this "amnesin" is unnecessary. I am not yet ready to report whether quinine will be helpful in overcoming the occasional state of excitement due to the scopolamin.

In a most elaborate study of the opium alkaloids by Dr. D. I. Macht, of the Department of Pharmacology of Johns Hopkins, as reported in the Journal of the American Medical Association and the American Journal of Medical Sciences, he demonstrates that pantopon (pantopon hydrochlorate first devised by Sahli, at the University of Zurich, 1909, which includes the chlorides of the total alkaloids of opium) acts as a stimulant to the respiratory center, and thereby obviates the objection to which morphine has been subject. All of the criticism to the use of scopolamin and morphine in labor is centered on the fetal asphyxia which followed the use of this combination in the former dosage.

The comparison of Sahli's mixture of the total alkaloids, with the administration of morphine alone, shows a remarkable result; two mgs. of morphine completely paralyzed the respiratory center in a rabbit weighing 1000 grams, while in a rabbit weighing 900 grams after 14 mgs. of the total alkaloids of pantopon, equal to 7 mgs. of anhydrous morphine, the rabbit still responded to inhalations of CO_2. Sahli's mixture of opium has the experimental value of being safe to be used in several times the amount of morphine that could be tolerated alone, and the result is more prompt and efficient; also being much less depressant. For several years it has been recognized that the great objection to morphine is the depressant sedative effect on the respiratory center. Codein, though to a less degree, has the same general effect.

The accumulation of morphine is, in our opinion, the greatest menace to the life of the fetus, as it has been shown that, while scopolamin passing into the body of the child is eliminated by the urine in twenty minutes, morphine is not so easily eliminated. We have, therefore, following these experimental discoveries coincident with our own clinical experience, in the great majority of cases, discontinued the morphine entirely, as we believe the great danger of the combination is in the use of this opiate, and morphine has practically been abandoned in favor of pantopon in our work.

We find that the other objections to morphine, nausea, vomiting, constipation, suppression of urine, and distention, are less pronounced after pantopon than morphine. However, after some experience in administration we have in our later work found it has been unnecessary to use even with the initial dose of scopolamin in many cases the pantopon. For many years we have used no opiate after the first dose. Of course, the individual cases where pantopon can be eliminated are carefully selected, the equable stable mental organization inviting the use of scopolamin alone, as these patients bear pain and respond without the necessity of the sedative before the analgesia. In other words, our personal experience has induced changes in the original detail of the administration of scopolamin, as observation demonstrates how the individual patient must be treated, rather that a fixed dose should be given to each patient, as suggested by Siegel in his experimental system, styled "the simplified method."

The question of the length of labor under scopolamin we have settled to our own satisfaction. We find that the first stage is less than in cases without the injection. The softening of the cervix in primiparae proceeds more readily than in other cases where it is not used. And this is one of the most grateful of the benefits resulting. In the second stage the duration is slightly lengthened. The average duration of labor in these cases is 10 hours and 49 minutes; in primiparae 13 hours and 20 minutes; in multigravida 7 hours 10 minutes.

We have frequently found the expulsion of the fetus expedited by ⅓ ampule of pituitrin hypodermically administered in those cases where delay is met as the head reaches the perineum and a degree of inertia prevents the forward movement of the child. The necessity for an increase in the use of forceps, is acknowledged; but with full dilatation and the head on the perineum, no harm can result from skillful application of forceps; proper care being observed to do extraction between pains, to remove forceps before the head is entirely extruded, and by pressure from below in the anal region to push the head gently through the outlet. The third stage of labor is somewhat prolonged, doubtless due to reaction after the relief from the burden of the labor ending with the expulsion of the child.

We are now trying out the procedure of giving ½ c.c. of pituitrin immediately following the expulsion of the fetus as a means of expediting the delivery of the placenta. Much of the shock, experienced in labor, is due to hurrying the placental stage before the afterbirth separates from its site in the uterine wall. As an index we clamp the cord with a hemostat at the vulva, the suggestion of Tweedy, and await the dropping of this barometer two and one-half inches before making any effort to expel the placenta. Our invariable rule is to avoid traction upon the cord, or the misapplied Credé of violent pushing against the abdomen to express the placenta.

In 1820 Charles D. Meigs said, "Show me a case of postpartum hemorrhage and I will show you a case of mismanagement of the third stage of labor." After a hundred years we are inclined to vote with

Meigs on this conclusion. At any rate, waiting for the placenta to be at the outlet, will, in the average case, diminish the tendency to postpartum shock, as well as postpartum hemorrhage. Our custom is to have the patient closely watched for two hours, cautioning the nurse as to rapid pulse, abdominal distention and free hemorrhage. We have no more tendency to hemorrhage in scopolamin cases than in those where it is not used.

All of our patients are delivered in the hospital, so that there has been no opportunity to compare the results of hospital managed cases with those confined at home. However, as there is an admitted psychic element in the success of the treatment, it would seem that an attempt to utilize this method in the bedroom of the patient at home might be disappointing, as she will be subject to disturbances from her environment. Ideal conditions in the hospital must be insured, such as absolute quiet in the delivery room and vigilant supervision on the part of the attendant. Cotton in the ears includes both suggestion and some degree of preventing disturbance by outside sounds. Since the patient in complete amnesia is likely to be unaware of the progress of the delivery, she must be watched for precipitate delivery, which is liable to occur if there is neglect of this precaution.

I believe much of the success of our method is due to using a reliable stable solution in ampules instead of the ordinary hypodermic tablet of commerce. Formerly we used a $\frac{1}{100}$ grain dose; but more recently we have depended on the $\frac{1}{200}$ grain ampule alone. Our average case has had $3\frac{1}{2}$ ampules, the largest number 12 ampules; 12 per cent of our cases have had but one ampule. Cases delivered within two hours do not respond to scopolamin and these rapid deliveries are done under ether alone, if sufficient evidence is found to base an estimate of the probable length of the labor.

Since a large number of our cases are referred, and many of these are toxemic, we have not used the gas-oxygen anesthesia. Dr. Edward P. Davis, and other observers, believe this combination of anesthesia to be dangerous in cases of maternal toxemia. While many reports are given of admirable results from those clinics where gas is used, our results have not tempted us to change our method of amnesia.

The great aim in better obstetrics is twofold; it concerns mother and child, both as to morbidity and mortality. Fortunately, the interests of the two are most frequently identical, the argument as to the mother, I have attempted to make clear. As to the child, a glance at the comparative statistics must prove conclusive, as they are most striking. Williams, of Johns Hopkins, reports a fetal mortality of 7 per cent, and Slemmons, in California, had 5 per cent, which is about the average infant death rate. Gauss, at the Freiburg Clinic, has in his last report of 500 scopolamin cases a fetal mortality of 1.89 per cent, and Polak, Brooklyn, in a series of 500 cases, reported a mortality of 4 infants, or less than 1 per cent. We have had no fetal death that could be charged to the scopolamin treatment. The fetal mortality from all causes in our last 500 cases, excluding prematurity, is 2.8 per cent. In contrast to our former experience is the fact that it has not been found necessary to tub a single scopolamin baby. Some children show an oligopnea; but none of the last series had apnea, and there were none that did not recover the respiratory rhythm after a few minutes, without more effort than allowing the mucus to be expelled from the mouth by suspending the child by the feet for a few minutes. We have, of course, no maternal mortality chargeable to scopolamin.

While no one can say what might have been the result in any case had the patient not been given scopolamin, we can only judge of the results in the aggregate of experiences compared with those delivered with this method, and those under other conditions. For instance, take the problem of occiput posterior positions of the vertex with which, unfortunately, all obstetricians are familiar. It is an axiom that given plenty of time, over 90 per cent of these cases will rotate spontaneously to an occipito anterior position; but, who has not made out the position without examination under these circumstances, by the incessant appeals for relief of pain in the back; the patient, finally, becoming exhausted by the long and tedious process of labor. These cases are admirably met by scopolamin, and the average patient comes through with a pulse under 100, and in a few hours recovers sufficiently to be asking for food.

It is only necessary to compare our experience in these cases alone, to be able to draw conclusions as to the degree of exhaustion suffered in cases with and without scopolamin. By and large our patients average a shorter convalescence and we are able to send them home earlier than under the old methods. Even in our City Hospital cases, although scopolamin has not been so satisfactory, we long ago abandoned any set day of convalescence as an indication of discharge, each woman being dismissed when the fundus of the uterus is at the symphysis and the lochia, for 48 hours, has shown no red color. In some patients this will be as early as the eighth day; ordinarily the average is the twelfth, instead of the fourteenth day, as formerly.

We find scopolamin to be of value in heart conditions, toxemia, rigid cervix, and contracted pelvis of minor degree; as the relief from agonizing pain allows for a lessening of the tension, both physical and mental, the patient recuperates for the further effort she must make for her delivery. The result is that shock is diminished, the head is more easily moulded, and the tendency to perineal laceration is diminished.

The claim that scopolamin produces a better milk supply, we have not been able to substantiate. On general principles, the less exhausted the mother the better her nursing capacity; but the question of any specific relation is still open, and must be determined by further investigation.

It is a matter of interest that in so large a degree, even the men who have not been favorably disposed toward scopolamin as an amnesic in their work, have used morphine and hyoscin, or morphine and atropin, or morphine and scopolamin, as an analgesic antecedent to an inhalation anesthetic. Various observers report between 50 and 70 per cent of perfect amnesia. In 70 per cent of our patients we have had complete amnesia. The outstanding fact, claimed by Crile, in his anoci-association in general surgery, is that, in a sense, the area of nervous irritability is blocked and the agonizing pain of the patient is thus relieved. This is the secret of the amnesia of scopolamin.

CONCLUSIONS

1. Scopolamin is both safe and efficient if intelligently managed.

2. In primiparae it is invaluable, as the moulding and rotation of the head are encouraged by its influence.

3. The technic of Gauss must be followed to insure the greatest measure of success, rather than the "simplified method" of Siegel.

4. A shortening of the time in the first stage of labor results.

5. The second stage is doubtless somewhat extended. The forceps or pituitrin may be needed at the end of the second stage of labor.

6. Patients must be constantly watched for precipitate delivery.

7. No increase in postpartum hemorrhage has occurred in our cases.

8. Shock and fatigue are diminished.

9. Perineal lacerations are greatly reduced in degree and in frequency.

10. Fetal mortality is lessened.

11. Lactation is not affected.

12. Mothers are up earlier and in more nearly physiologic convalescence than in our cases where scopolamin was not used.

605 BRYANT BUILDING.   (*For discussion, see page 188.*)

AN ANALYSIS OF THE POTTER VERSION*

By Edward Speidel, M.D., Louisville, Ky.

IT IS not necessary to explain to the members of this Association or to any one who has kept in touch with obstetric literature, what is meant by the Potter method of version. Presented for the first time five years ago, and followed up each year with an additional paper on the same method, Dr. Potter has had the gratification of seeing intense antagonism and resentment change to unqualified admiration.

Potter presented his version as a method of delivery to be used practically in all cases, with the idea of relieving the parturient woman of the discomforts and delays of the second stage of labor. He presents no indications or contraindications for the use of the version and, consequently, leaves no opening for a discussion on that point.

Having had the pleasure of a visit with Dr. Potter in Buffalo, and from a limited experience with his method in private and hospital practice, the writer would like to discuss the version from three distinct points of excellence.

First: It is such a decided improvement over all the old established procedures that it should supplant every other method of performing podalic version. Second: The delivery of the child after the version has been performed is such a marked advance over the old methods of breech delivery that it should displace that practice at once. Third: His effective treatment of the child at birth by gentle rational manipulations, is so superior to the many rough treatments to which the asphyxiated baby has been subjected heretofore, that it should induce every obstetrician to emulate them.

The writer wishes accordingly to discuss the method from these standpoints without endorsing the object for which the author presents it.

The Potter method of version, fortunately, is not solely a hospital procedure. It is easier than the older method and can be readily performed by any one at all competent to do a version. A person with a small hand is by nature especially qualified to do a version. It can be performed in the humblest home. In fact the ordinary kitchen table makes the most ideal operating table for any of the ordinary obstetric operations. The patient's head is at one end of the table convenient for the anesthetist, while the hips are at the other end with the legs upon two chairs in the modified Walcher position, which

---

*Read at the Thirty-Fourth Annual Meeting of the American Association of Obstetricians, Gynecologists, and Abdominal Surgeons, St. Louis, Mo., September 20-22, 1921.

is a feature of the technic. This position as is well known increases the true conjugate diameter about 1 cm. The vaginal outlet is drawn so far down that the angle, formed by the long axis of the uterus with that of the vagina, is diminished and the uterovaginal canal becomes less curved, approaching more a straight line and making delivery much easier. It also relaxes the perineum and so lessens the liability to laceration of that structure. This position is superior to the lithotomy position as it relieves the patient of the intense backache that often follows vaginal operations when the legs have been held up, in an unnatural manner, for some time, with the lumbar spinal curve unsupported and the patient resting upon the sacrum with the weight of the two legs superimposed. It might be worth while to try this Walcher position in some of our gynecologic operations.

It is very essential that the cervix be fully dilated and, in primiparae, Potter not only waits for full dilatation but seems to prefer partial descent of the presenting part before proceeding with his version. I venture to say that he avoids manual dilatation in primiparae if possible. In normal dilatation the cervix stretches and retracts with each pain so that, when full dilatation is attained, the cervix is obliterated. In manual dilatation the cervical tissues are simply stretched to the sides of the pelvis; there is no thinning out or retraction, and this is the cervix that catches the neck of the fetus at the crucial point of the delivery and nullifies the object of the version.

Potter prefers chloroform as the anesthetic. Many of us who remember the period of twenty-five years and more ago, when chloroform was used almost exclusively in the south, and one ounce of this drug would hold a patient in deep anesthesia for an hour or more, cannot help wondering whether an inhalation of $\frac{1}{2}$ pint or more of ether into the lungs is not more dangerous than the use of chloroform despite the findings of the anesthesia commission, that is supposed to have settled the question.

The patient is prepared as for a surgical operation, catheterized, shaved, and the parts cleansed externally with soap and water. Potter makes no mention of vaginal cleansing. Here I would like to present my own method of preparation, which I have always used in my obstetric operations. The vagina cannot be rendered sterile by letting a thin stream of bichloride or lysol solution trickle down its walls. Instead the gloved right hand of the operator holding a piece of gauze, saturated with green soap, should be used to thoroughly scrub the vagina and cervix, and this should be followed by a copious irrigation with sterile water.

In Potter's technic the right hand is not used internally throughout the precedure, consequently, it cannot contaminate the field after this preliminary cleansing. The left hand, covered with an elbow-length rubber glove, is well lubricated with green soap and introduced into the vagina. Green soap is an ideal lubricant for these passages as it is easily washed away by the secretions that pass out during and after the version. Vaseline, which is generally used for this purpose, clings to the tissues and forms the best kind of an embedding material for microorganisms.

Potter then proceeds to iron out the vagina and distends it for easy delivery of the after-coming head. His method consists in pressing downward and backward on the posterior vaginal wall from the cervix to the introitus, first with one finger, then with two, three and finally four fingers, and seems to be an advance over that advocated by Edgar, in which the fingers are inserted into the vagina to make traction on the muscular sling of the perineum for the same purpose. The left hand is then introduced through the dilated cervix, between the unruptured membranes and the uterine wall to the fundus and gently swept around in all directions, avoiding the placental site.

This maneuver is similar to the practice in cesarean section and facilitates the delivery of the placenta. The bag of waters is so elastic and the uterus so relaxed under surgical anesthesia, that the fetal parts can be readily palpated and the location of the legs determined before rupturing the membranes. By palpating the neck of the fetus one can also determine whether it is encircled by the cord. The distinctive feature of the version proper now seems to be in no wise to disturb the relation of the fetal parts before the version is completed. In this way one avoids pressure upon and entanglements of the cord, undoubtedly the most disturbing factor in determining the favorable or unfavorable outcome of a version.

Potter performs all of his versions with his left hand. It is reasonable to suppose that others, not as dexterous, might perform the operation with either hand encased in elbow length gloves and, in performing the version, follow the old rule of using the hand so that the palmer surface of it will come in apposition to the abdomen of the child. At this juncture a towel is wrapped around the left arm of the operator to absorb the liquor amnii, that gushes out with the rupture of the membranes. It seems best to break through the membranes high up near the fundus and then slide the hand down the thighs of the fetus until the feet are reached. Gentle traction, with pressure on the head in the opposite direction, will aid in readily bringing both feet out of the vagina and completing the version.

It will be remembered that in the older methods it was always demanded that only one leg be brought through the cervix, in order that a wider surface be left to dilate the cervix. The facility with which delivery can be effected when both feet are brought down shows that the older procedure was faulty. The idea that a version is dangerous if some time has passed since the rupture of the membranes and, especially, if the head has descended into the pelvis, does not hold good. The experienced obstetrician finds the uterus so relaxed and elastic under full surgical anesthesia that the head can be readily pushed up and the hand introduced for a version.

Only recently I performed a version in a head presentation bringing down both feet readily more than twenty-four hours after rupture of the bag of waters had taken place. With both feet protruding from the vagina, the final step in the procedure resolves itself into the delivery of a breech presentation. It is but fair to state that in the past, everyone has dreaded the delivery of the arms and after-coming head by the method in vogue up to recent times. The method described by Potter is so superior in every respect, that it should remove every dread of breech delivery. One need have but little trouble with the delivery of the after-coming arms, shoulders and head.

Potter makes gentle traction on the legs of the fetus, turning the back of the child up until the scapulae appear at the vulva. Then he slips a finger along the shoulder under the symphysis pubis and delivers the anterior arm. He then turns the body of the child in such a way that the posterior arm comes to rest under the symphysis pubis and delivers it in the same manner as the first shoulder. In all of my cases after delivery of the anterior arm, the posterior arm slipped out without any difficulty.

The crowning feature of the version is the delivery of the aftercoming head. It is far superior to the Smellie-Veit method and is dependent solely upon the manipulations by the operator. Potter advises against following down the fundus during the delivery; because, he claims, one creates the very condition that we seek to prevent. By pushing down on the head it sinks between the shoulders and the arms go up. Whether Potter is correct in his view, I am not prepared to say. In all of my cases the arms seemed to have been carried upward, more or less, but this made not a particle of difference in the ease of delivery.

Potter delivers the head by inserting two fingers of the left hand into the baby's mouth, the body riding astride of his left arm and then, with the right hand resting upon a sterile towel, suprapubic pressure is made downward and backward until the face distends the vulva. The feet of the child are now held high up and its throat stroked to empty the trachea, and, in many instances, the fetus will begin to breathe while in this position.

There should be no haste in forcing out the rest of the head. Instead, it may be allowed to dilate the perineum and with the ironing-out of the vagina, practiced before beginning the version, many deliveries will be completed without a laceration. Potter shows no hurry in the delivery of the child for fear of having an asphyxiated infant; and after the birth of blue babies, he quietly places them on their right side on the abdomen of the mother and allows respiration to start spontaneously. This position, of course, favors the closure of the foramen ovale. The umbilical cord is not tied until pulsation stops.

It will be remembered that the venous circulation in the cord ceases very shortly after birth in consequence of the contraction of the umbilical arteries; but the arterial circulation in the umbilical vein continues for from five to fifteen minutes adding, at least, an ounce of blood to the fetal circulation and supporting the heart of the fetus until respiration is established. It may be assumed that this is an important feature in the resuscitation.

Success seems to follow this gentle method in nearly every instance; that has been my experience. Potter's statistics show the same result. This goes to show that we can discard many of the rather rough manipulations that were practiced in the resuscitation of asphyxiated babies, without impairing our results.

In a discussion of this mode of the delivery, with Halstead of New York, it was suggested that the body of the child be allowed to come down, naturally, with the shoulders descending in the left oblique diameter at the superior strait until the scapulae appear at the vulva, then to rotate the anterior shoulder under the symphysis pubis and deliver as such. In order not to disturb the relation of the fetal parts, the posterior shoulder should then be lifted over the perineum. Theoretically, this should then leave the after-coming head in the right oblique diameter of the superior strait, consequently, the easiest delivery should be, downward pressure on the fundus with the head held in this diameter until the fingers in the baby's mouth press firmly upon the perineum, then rotation forward under the symphysis and the delivery completed as described by Potter. Potter with his enormous opportunities can quickly determine whether there is anything of value in these suggestions.

An ampule of pituitrin is injected as soon as the baby is born and serves to expedite the delivery of the placenta. It may be assumed that a uterus emptied by version, in ten to fifteen minutes, is more liable to sudden relaxation and postpartum hemorrhage than one that has emptied its contents by rhythmic contractions for an hour or more. Furthermore about 2⅓ ounces of blood are saved the mother, as has been determined by Ryder at the Sloane Hospital for Women in one hundred cases treated with pituitrin, in the third stage of labor.

With the experience gained through the Potter version the writer has solved the delivery of breech presentations for himself as follows: With full dilatation in a frank or complete breech or footling presentation, full surgical anesthesia, iron out the perineum, bring down both feet, and complete the delivery according to the Potter procedure.

Potter does not state his fetal mortality in normal cases in which he has used his version solely for the purpose of relieving the patient of the discomforts of the second stage of labor. It is surely essential that those desiring to follow that indication for the use of this version should know this.

The writer has found the version of special service in cases with apparently normal diameters but a lack of progress in labor in spite of good pains. In such instances there is generally found premature ossification and, in consequence, nonmolding of the fetal head or an overdeveloped fetal head.

Only recently the writer delivered a woman, weighing 94 pounds, of a 9½ pound baby by the Potter version, without laceration of the soft parts, after a two hour ineffective second stage of labor.

THE FRANCIS BUILDING. *(For discussion, see p. 189.)*

TREATMENT OF ECLAMPSIA; THEN AND NOW*

By JOHN F. MORAN, M.D., WASHINGTON, D. C.

ECLAMPSIA and infection are the two great scourges of pregnancy, parturition, and the puerperium. While the latter, through the introduction of asepsis, has been robbed of much of its terror and placed well within the limits of prevention, the former, because of insufficient knowledge concerning its etiology and origin, is still involved in hypothesis and theory; its treatment largely empirical and its morbidity and mortality high. Much important work, however, has been accomplished in recent years, particularly, in its pathology, which, in supporting the toxic theory, is thus contributing to a more comprehensive knowledge of the disease. That various toxemias affect alike the pregnant and nonpregnant is obvious; but the trend of opinion favors the belief that there are one or more varieties dependent on the gravid state which are, probably, the underlying causes of eclampsia, hyperemesis gravidarum, acute yellow atrophy of the liver, and many of the minor ailments and psychoses of pregnancy.

Conformable to the various views held as to the origin of eclampsia, different methods of treatment have been resorted to; but the results have remained as uncertain as the theoretic foundations on which the methods have been based. So that, at the present time, we are, unfortunately, without a rational treatment with which to combat this

*Read by invitation at the Thirty-Fourth Annual Meeting of the American Association of Obstetricians, Gynecologists and Abdominal Surgeons, St. Louis, Mo., September 20-22, 1921.

dangerous complication of pregnancy; and, in the presence of severe types of the disease, are well nigh helpless. The graver forms comprise from 3 to 5 per cent of the cases in general; they are more frequent at different periods of gestation, and they may appear in groups. These malignant cases are frequently attended with few convulsions, coma quickly supervening after the first seizure, accompanied by fever, jaundice, hemoglobinuria, or a complete suppression of urine. They are rapidly fatal.

When the writer graduated in the late eighties, the treatment included both conservative and forcible measures. The former embraced sedatives, bleeding, veratrum viride, chloroform, and elimination by purgatives and sweating; while the latter consisted of forcible dilatation of the os, or, to speak more correctly, divulsion of the cervix and the termination of the delivery of the child with forceps or version. At this time aseptic surgery was developing; its increasing brilliant results, quite naturally, brought it into competition with the conservative treatment and accouchement forcé of eclampsia. In the late nineties we were performing immediate deliveries in eclampsia by abdominal cesarean section, as recommended by Halbertsma, and later by vaginal cesarean section, as advocated by Dührssen. These operations are favored today by surgeons; but there is a growing reaction among obstetricians against such radical treatment, and obstetricians are now more in favor of medical and obstetric measures, except in cases complicated by rigid cervix, aged primiparae, contracted pelvis, or marked disproportion between the child and the mother's pelvis.

Formerly I was rightly classed as an "interventionist," being rather in favor of the cutting operations. Impressed, however, by the kindly and earnest criticism of your esteemed secretary, Dr. Zinke, who dissented from my advocacy of cesarean section in favor of the conservative treatment, I was prompted to review my surgical cases and became satisfied that some of them would have yielded favorably to more conservative measures. I have, therefore, for several years adopted a more conservative course by individualizing my cases and resorting to active, medical, or combined treatment as, in my judgment, the exigencies of the case may demand.

I wish now to invite your attention to a series of pre-eclamptic and eclamptic cases attended in consultation and in the hospital during the past four years.

The method followed is to give morphia hypodermically at reasonable intervals to reduce the respiratory movements to ten or twelve per minute; bleed, when the blood pressure is high, to reduce to 150, or thereabouts; wash out the stomach, leaving in two ounces of castor oil, irrigate the bowels and follow this with five per cent glucose and soda solution by the drip method. We feel that this method is very helpful even if, for any reason, we find it necessary to intervene surgically. In the latter emergency we would be guided by the condition of the cervix and menacing conditions as to which operation we would elect.

PRE-ECLAMPTIC TOXEMIA

CASE 1.—Mrs. S., multipara, white, aged thirty-eight. Admitted to Georgetown University Hospital. At term, headache, amaurosis, ptosis of right eyelid, blood pressure 210-132. Bag introduced. Living baby, weight, 11 pounds. Mother and child discharged in good condition.

CASE 2.—Mrs. K., white, multipara, eight months' gestation; marked toxic symptoms persisted in spite of rest, diet, etc. Blood pressure, 195. Two examinations by ophthalmologist at interval of a week; first examination negative; second, positive for retinitis. Sent to Georgetown University Hospital. Labor induced with bag. Puerperium normal. Mother and child all right.

CASE 3.—Mrs. L., white, aged thirty-seven, 4-para, seven months' gestation. Seen in consultation at Georgetown University Hospital, October 9, 1920. Patient blind and in coma. Vomiting. Treatment: Venesection, 500 c.c., replacement, glucose and soda solution. Bag inserted, but it was ineffectual. Meanwhile coma lifted and patient became rational. Labor spontaneous, complicated by prolapsed cord and transverse presentation. Version. The child succumbed prior to delivery. Mother developed pleurisy on right side. She was aspirated and made a good recovery.

CASE 4.—Mrs. H., white, aged twenty-nine, 2-para, eight months' gestation, seen in consultation, headache, insomnia, general edema, blood pressure 165-128. Removed to hospital and labor induced. Result satisfactory. Mother and child living.

ECLAMPSIA

CASE 1.—Mrs. M., white, aged nineteen, primipara, at term. Seen in consultation at Providence Hospital, June 20, 1917. In labor 24 hours. Five convulsions, morphinized, mid-forceps delivery. Mother and child living. Two births since, both normal.

CASE 2.—Mrs. K., white, primipara, at term. Seen in consultation; pre-eclamptic; had convulsion during second stage of labor; mid-forceps delivery. Mother and child living.

CASE 3.—Mrs. B., white, aged forty, primipara, at term. Seen in consultation January 26, 1917. Patient very toxic, cannot see and is markedly edematous. Advised removal to hospital at once. While being prepared for operation she had a convulsion. Cesarean section was performed shortly after admission to Columbia Hospital. Four convulsions during the following thirty-six hours, after which she regained consciousness. Mother and child living.

CASE 4.—Mrs. G., white, aged thirty-three, primipara. Seen in consultation. Admitted to Georgetown University Hospital after having had several convulsions. Coma profound, cervix intact. She was bled and morphinized; but, as the convulsions recurred together with almost complete suppression of urine, cesarean section was performed. Child weighed 6.5 pounds; lived several hours. Patient had six convulsions in the hospital; three after the operation. Recovery uneventful. She was delivered of a second child March 11, 1919. Natural labor.

CASE 5.—B. C., colored, aged twenty-five, primipara. Ward patient. Admitted to Columbia Hospital in labor with history of two convulsions, and that she had been blind a week. Marked edema. Blood pressure 180-118. Treatment: Morphinized, and labor induced with bag. Patient regained consciousness before delivery. Child stillborn, due to tetanic contraction of the uterus. Mother made uneventful recovery.

CASE 6.—Mrs. L., white, aged eighteen, secundipara. Admitted to Georgetown University Hospital, July 7, 1918, having had six convulsions before admission. Marked edema, cervix intact, not in labor. Blood pressure, 210-132. Venesection, 20 ounces. Morphinized. Convulsions recurring and coma deepening, cesarean section was performed by associate, Dr. Lowe. Living child, at term, delivered. Five convulsions after operation. Patient rational on second day after labor. Mother and child discharged in good condition.

CASE 7.—Mrs. M., white, aged twenty, primipara. Private patient. Sent to Georgetown University Hospital in labor. Protracted first stage due to premature rupture of waters. When head was on perineum patient had a convulsion. Delivered with forceps. Mother and child living. Second birth, January, 1920. Pregnancy and labor normal.

CASE 8.—Mrs. S., white, aged twenty-three, primipara, postpartum eclampsia. Admitted to Georgetown University Hospital, in labor, May 20, 1918. First convulsion fourteen hours after delivery; three seizures in all. Bled 18 ounces, and morphia was given. Mother and child living.

CASE 9.—Mrs. T., colored, aged forty-three, multipara. Admitted to Georgetown University Hospital, June 4, 1918, with history of convulsions and in profound coma. Marked edema. Blood pressure, 248-150. Bag introduced and venesection done. Owing to deep coma no sedative was given. Stillbirth. Patient left hospital in very good condition.

CASE 10.—Mrs. K., white, aged twenty-three, secundipara. Admitted to Georgetown University Hospital, March 15, 1918. Seven convulsions, edema and impaired vision. Blood pressure, 144-84. Morphine. Venesection; 1000 c.c. removed. Labor induced with bag. Child premature, lived 7 hours. Mother's recovery uneventful.

CASE 11.—Mrs. B., white, aged twenty-three, primipara. Admitted to Columbia Hospital, August 4, 1919, in coma having had three convulsions. Blood pressure, 145. Venesection, 500 c.c. Morphinized. Bougie inserted. Delivery following day. Premature child, seven months; lived seven hours. Mother living. Again pregnant. Eyes, kidneys, and blood pressure normal.

CASE 12.—Mrs. N., white, secundipara. Admitted to Columbia Hospital, August 8, 1919. Urine contains albumin and casts. Blood pressure, 198-104. Had convulsion at beginning of labor. Morphinized. Venesection, 22 ounces. Natural delivery. Stillbirth. Patient developed aspiration pneumonia, but recovered and left hospital, still anemic, but improving.

CASE 13.—Mrs. W., white, aged thirty, primipara. Seen in consultation at Georgetown University Hospital, July 31, 1918. Not in labor. Blood pressure, 142-92. Four convulsions. Morphinized. Venesection, 500 c.c. Following day, rational. Labor did not supervene for six days. Delivery natural. Mother and child living.

CASE 14.—Cr., colored, multipara. Admitted to Columbia Hospital. History of convulsions before admission; marked edema of body and vulva. Bled and morphinized. Regained consciousness and did not go into labor until three days later. Meanwhile the vulva was scarified and edema rapidly subsided. Labor and puerperium uneventful. Mother and child living.

CASE 15.—C., colored, multipara. Admitted to Georgetown University Hospital, December 9, 1919. Four convulsions. Blood pressure, 180-110. Venesection and morphine. Labor natural. Mother and child living.

CASE 16.—Mrs. C., white, aged twenty-three, primipara. Seen in consultation at Providence Hospital. Had been treated for toxemia. Flat pelvis. Seized with convulsion during trial labor. Head not fixed in pelvis. Cesarean section performed. Mother and child living.

CASE 17.—Mrs. S., white, aged thirty, primipara. Seen in consultation at Georgetown University Hospital, June 26, 1920. During tedious labor complained of diplopia and had two convulsions. Blood pressure, 198-120. Morphine given. Venesection, 600 c.c. Mid-forceps. Mother and child living.

CASE 18.—Mrs. J., white, aged nineteen, primipara. Admitted to Georgetown University Hospital, April, 1919. Blood pressure, 200-120. Two convulsions before admission to, and four while in, the hospital. Urine shows albumin and casts. Morphinized. Venesection, 500 c.c. Delivery spontaneous. Mother and child living.

CASE 19.—H., colored, aged thirty-two, primipara. Weight, 200 pounds. Admitted to Georgetown University Hospital, May 4, 1920, in labor. Blood pressure, 194-130. Urine contains albumin and casts. Had convulsion. Bled 500 c.c. Morphinized. Chill after venesection. Mid-forceps delivery. Stillbirth. Manual removal of placenta. Puerperium: Fever, maximum 101° F. Recovered. Second birth, May, 1921. Pregnancy and labor normal.

CASE 20.—Mrs. G., white, aged twenty-eight, primipara. Admitted to Georgetown University Hospital, May 24, 1920. In labor. Blood pressure, 180-130. Hot pack. Membranes punctured at 2:30 P.M. the following day. Convulsion at 3:15 P.M. Morphinized. Venesection, 500 c.c. Low forceps. Mother and child living.

CASE 21.—Mrs. S., white, aged twenty-four, secundipara. Admitted to Georgetown University Hospital, June 4, 1920. Pre-eclamptic toxemia. Blood pressure, 168-110. Urine contains albumin and casts. Left occipitoposterior position of vertex presenting. Twenty-four hours after admission she had the first convulsion. Second convulsion, 4:15 A.M., of the sixth. Bled 500 c.c. Third seizure at 6:00 A.M. Fourth and last convulsion at 3:00 P.M. In labor 62 hours. Treatment: Morphine, venesection, mid-forceps. Mother and child living.

CASE 22.—Mrs. B., white, aged twenty-six, primipara, at term. Seen in consultation. Admitted to Columbia Hospital, September 14, 1920, 4:00 P.M. In labor. Pre-eclamptic history: Headache, edema, general dimness of vision, etc.; urine contains albumin and casts. Membranes ruptured at 8:45 P.M. Pains regular. Thirteen hours after admission she had a convulsion followed by two more attacks at fifteen-minute intervals. At this time I saw the case in consultation. Examination revealed the cervix effaced and the os dilated about the size of a silver dollar. Head well engaged in left occipitoposterior position. As patient reacted well after convulsions, and labor progressed satisfactorily, conservative treatment was elected. As blood pressure had risen to 170-125, five hundred c.c. of blood was removed. Morphia was given at intervals; but the terrified nurse failed to carry out instructions to keep respirations down; so convulsions recurred, fifteen attacks in all. At 4:15 P.M., the cervix was fully dilated; forceps were applied (Scanzoni) and delivery effected. Puerperium normal. Mother and child living.

CASE 23.—Mrs. Z., white, primipara. Seen in consultation at Georgetown University Hospital. Postpartal eclampsia. Labor reported normal. Six hours after delivery she had three convulsions in 45 minutes. Blood pressure, 190. Treatment: Morphine and venesection, 1000 c.c. Mother and child excellent. Second labor, in 1920, normal.

CASE 24.—Mrs. M., white, 3-para; seen in consultation. Postpartal eclampsia. Treated for toxemia from seventh month, evidently without much relief as cardinal signs, such as headache, dimness of vision, edema, and positive urinary findings, persisted. Blood pressure varied from 140-165. On admission to hospital blood pressure was 188-110. Labor normal and four hours in duration. Six hours postpartum (3:00 A.M.) she had a convulsion, and four more before 7:20 A.M. Morphine given. Sixteen ounces of blood removed. Despite vigorous elimination and heart stimulation coma gradually deepened; she had four more convulsions on the third day, and died in coma on the fifth day. Temperature had risen to 109° F.

CASE 25.—Mrs. V., white, aged twenty-eight, secundipara. Seen in consultation at Sibley Hospital, March 26, 1921, at 10:00 A.M. Had severe hemorrhage from marginal placenta previa. Unassisted delivery at 7:20 P.M. The following morning, after a restless night, patient had several convulsions in quick succession. Blood pressure, 170. Morphine was given and venesection performed, twenty ounces of blood removed. Patient in semicomatose state until third day; then gradually lessened and was rational on fourth day. Made splendid recovery. Child living.

CASE 26.—Mrs. W., white, aged twenty-six, primipara. Seen in consultation. Admitted to Georgetown University Hospital, May 19, 1921, at 7:15 P.M. History of persistent pre-eclamptic toxemia despite treatment. In labor. At 8:25 P.M. had a convulsion, and at 10:00 P. M., a second seizure followed. Gradually deepening coma uninfluenced by removal of eighteen ounces of blood and other measures. Labor was terminated with low forceps. Stillbirth, due to toxemia. Coma never lessened and temperature rose to 109° before death took place on the third day.

CASE 27.—Mrs. R., white, aged twenty-seven, primipara; seventh month of gestation; seen in consultation. Admitted to Georgetown University Hospital, March 5, 1920, with history of vomiting extending over two weeks. Blood pressure, 130-104. Urine shows albumin and casts. The toxemia yielded to diet and elimination. Left hospital at the end of two weeks, much improved. Readmitted April 27, in labor. Had convulsion during second stage. Delivered with low forceps by attending physician. Mother and child living.

CASE 28.—Mrs. H., white, aged thirty-three, 4-para, eight months' gestation. Seen in consultation, May 11, 1921. History of several convulsions. Patient removed to Columbia Hospital for observation. Previous pregnancies and labors reported normal. Blood pressure, 128-88. Urine reveals albumin and granular casts. Treatment: Bromides and eliminants gave relief and patient was sent home on fourth day. Normal labor one month later. Mother and child living. There is, likely, a hysterical factor in this case. The physician reports that, beginning three weeks after confinement, patient had a convulsion, and that they recurred from time to time since.

CASE 29.—Mrs. Y., primipara, seventh month of gestation. Seen in consultation at Georgetown Hospital, September 12, 1921, at 10:30 P.M. Marked toxic condition extending over several weeks, which had not yielded to treatment. Labor pains began about 7:00 P. M. At 9:30 P. M. she had a convulsion and another, one hour later. Blood pressure, 170. Morphinized, and sixteen ounces of blood removed. Membranes ruptured spontaneously at 5:00 A. M. Spontaneous delivery occurred at 8:00 A. M. Child living. Mother rational and doing well.

SUMMARY

It will be noted that nearly all of the cases had suffered from pre-eclamptic toxemia. Several had been treated, but the toxemia persisted; some had been treated indifferently, and most of them not at all.

We find that morphia, if given properly, will control the convulsions. Its ease of administration and certainty of action, make it preferable to other sedatives.

Venesection we believe to be a most valuable measure. Where the blood pressure is high, with cyanosis, recurring convulsions, deepening coma and threatened edema of the lungs, it is particularly serviceable. Its beneficent effect was strikingly shown in a postpartum case, seen in consultation recently, and the writer is convinced that the bloodletting was the principal means of saving the patient.

Cesarean section was performed by election in a primipara over forty years of age; another was performed on a primipara with flat pelvis, who had a convulsion during a test of labor. The head was not engaged in the brim. In the third and fourth cases, morphinization and bleeding had been done before the cesarean section was undertaken. We believe these patients were benefited by the tranquilizing effect of the sedative and elimination obtained before operation.

All of the forceps cases were done after complete dilatation of the os in order to expedite the delivery.

Labor was induced with the bag in all of the threatened eclampsias, and in three of the actual eclampsias; the bougie was used in one case.

We do not forcibly dilate an intact or rigid cervix. It is irrational and unjustifiable. The physiologic and anatomic changes necessary to soften and unfold the cervix and dilate the os, must be borne in mind. To divulse the intact cervix in a few minutes by instrumental or manual methods, is unscientific, dangerous, and brutal. It violates Nature's law, which, under normal conditions, requires hours, thus preserving the integrity of the soft parts.

We do not give chloroform or nitrous oxide, because both induce acidosis. Ether, while not free from objection, is the least harmful anesthetic, but its administration should be restricted to the time of operative intervention.

The salutary influence of sedation and elimination was demonstrated in two of the antepartum cases; the convulsions ceased, the patients became rational, and spontaneous labor occurred several days later. Several of the intrapartum cases also regained consciousness before birth.

Of the two deaths, one at term had the first convulsion six hours after a normal delivery; the other, an antepartum case of seven months' gestation, had two convulsions and lapsed into gradually deepening coma, which continued until death took place on the third day. Both of these cases had been carefully supervised for weeks before the eclamptic seizures and the persistence of the toxemia, despite treatment, indicated that they might have been saved by induced labor.

From the foregoing data we offer the following deductions: 1. The importance of prenatal care. 2. Intermediate and conservative treatment yield lower mortality and morbidity than is obtained by surgical and forcible intervention. 3. Immediate delivery by cesarean section is rarely necessary, unless there are present indications of disproportion, rigid cervix, etc. 4. Radicalism is prompted largely by fear and expediency.

Prenatal care means careful supervision of the pregnancy, interrogating the various organs and functions from time to time. Persistent high blood pressure, resisting treatment, points to kidney insufficiency. It is here that the ophthalmoscope may reveal a developing retinitis long before the patient complains of impaired vision or the urine shows albumin and casts. The ophthalmoscope is the only means by which the earlier and relatively much less serious stages of toxemic retinal involvement can be detected. A progressive retinitis is a valuable prognostic sign for induction of labor, safeguarding vision and averting the outbreak of eclampsia. By this valuable procedure we were able to check up a developing retinitis in one of the pre-eclamptic cases, and labor was induced with gratifying results, saving both mother and child.

The blood and urinary findings, showing an increase in retention of nitrogenous products, particularly uric acid and creatinin, with changes in the ratio of urea nitrogen and nonprotein nitrogen are indicative of kidney insufficiency and give unfavorable prognosis, if the toxemia is not controlled.

The frequency of eclampsia could be greatly diminished if more careful supervision of the pregnant woman was exercised. The perfunctory examination of the urine for albumin, during the latter weeks of pregnancy, is not sufficient. The constitutional signs and symptoms should be closely scrutinized and if these persist following the use of vigorous and active measures, the safety of the mother and infant lies in the induction of labor.

The psychology in the treatment of eclampsia from the standpoint of the physician and surgeon is interesting. Analyzing my own state of mind I was dominated by subconscious fear, due primarily to want of familiarity with the disease and some unfortunate experience with accouchement forcé. Naturally the application of the cesarean section appealed to me as a saner and safer method. I therefore advocated and followed it. Upon review of my surgical work, however, I became convinced that some of the cases I had subjected to section, could have been delivered by more conservative measures, thereby preserving the integrity of the uterus. This proved to be the turning point in my attitude towards eclampsia. From then on I found myself studying each case with equanimity and deliberation and balancing action on judgment.

Fear and expediency are, I am satisfied, from experience as a consultant and from observation, potent factors in the radical treatment of eclampsia. The attending physician, unaccustomed to treating such cases, is very apt to become panicky and urge immediate delivery. The consulting surgeon, who thinks largely in surgical terms, not infrequently acquiesces and performs cesarean section.

It is easy to yield to such importunity and even a fatal result is likely to be accepted without question. It is not easy, however, for the obstetrician who elects to conduct the case along conservative lines extending over some hours. This postulates obstetric judgment and courage.

The keynote in the treatment of eclampsia is prevention. Yet either in the prevention or the treatment of actual eclampsia an even mind is essential. *"Aequam memento rebus in arduis servare mentem,"* as the old Latin bard has sung.

It was the clinical observation of Semmelweiss which led to the recognition that puerperal fever and wound infection are identical and preventable; Pasteur lifted the veil which for centuries hid the cause of disease, by exposing their microbian origin, while Lister laid the foundation of aseptic surgery with its manifold possibilities in the cure and alleviation of maladies; so may it be the good fortune of another genius to find the key that will unlock the mystery of the toxemias of pregnancy that motherhood may be immunized against this frightful scourge. May this Association be the parent of this genius.

2426 PENNSYLVANIA AVENUE.　　　　　　*(For discussion, see p. 193.)*

A STUDY OF THE ORIGIN OF BLEEDING IN ECTOPIC PREGNANCY*

By John O. Polak, M.D., F.A.C.S., and Thurston S. Welton, M.D., F.A.C.S., Brooklyn, N. Y.

THE bleeding in tubal pregnancy occurs as an early suggestive symptom in all tubal abortions, during the ovular unrest preceding tubal rupture, and, usually, at the time of the primary rupture.

To understand the mode of occurrence of this hemorrhage one must accept the analogy between uterine pregnancy and tubal gestation, with certain differences due to the morphology of the tubal mucosa. Furthermore, the mode of implantation of the ovum in the tube has a definite causative significance.

The ovum can develop only on a spot free from epithelium, sinking through the decidua to rest on the subepithelial layer of the muscularis, and producing by its presence such reaction as to provoke dilatation of the lymph spaces and edema of the myometrium and endometrium immediately surrounding the ovum.

As the ovum sinks in, the side walls of the cavity become united over the ovum by organized blood clot and fibrin and form a false reflexa. The decidual reaction in the tube is imperfect and scattered. There are cases in which no true decidua has been found (Aschoff), but where there is decidual reaction it is the same as found in the uterus; it is also noted at points in the tube, remote from the seat of the ovum implantation.

Fecundation is definitely known to take place in the tube during the passage of the ovum through the tube to the uterus. It has been shown that "in a tube, partially recovered from an inflammatory process, there may be found pockets, diverticula, and constrictions which cause the arrest of the majority of ova, and that implantation takes place at any point at which this arrest occurs." (Mall.)

This implantation may be columnar, intercolumnar or centrifugal. Columnar embedding is rare and occurs when the ovum attaches itself to one of the tree-like folds of the tubal mucosa, later it becomes attached to other folds; but at no point is it in contact with the tube wall itself. In such an implantation the ovum derives its nourishment from the blood vessels of the mucosa until the mucosa becomes eroded by the action of the syncytial cells, and then the ovum comes to lie in the tube wall when the villi penetrate the muscularis.

---
*Read at the Thirty-Fourth Annual Meeting of the American Association of Obstetricians, Gynecologists and Abdominal Surgeons, St. Louis, Mo., September 20 to 22, 1921.

In the intercolumnar form of implantation the ovum embeds itself in the cleft between the folds of the tubal mucosa and thus rests upon the surface of the tube wall, at once eroding itself into the muscular coat. In this case the mucosal folds unite over the embedded ovum and form a false reflexa.

In the centrifugal implantation, the ovum sinks into the wall of the tube and the villi invade the muscular wall and vessels, including all structures, even the serosa. The pseudoreflexa is formed by the side walls made up of the muscularis and the mucosa, into which the ovum has sunk.

The invasion of the blood vessels by the villi causes hemorrhage into the intervillous spaces. The villi may extend up to and through the

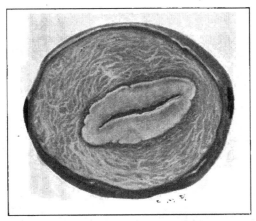

Fig. 1.—Cross section of uterus showing decidual development in a case of three months' ectopic gestation.

serosa; rupture usually takes place through penetration of the tube wall at the placental site, as a result of this erosion by the villi.

One observation has been constant, no matter what form of implantation has taken place, i.e., there is always an excessive amount of hemorrhage about the ovum, owing to the fact that there is no true decidua to protect the tubal vessels from erosion. The constant erosive action of the trophoblast causes considerable hemorrhage. Mall states that the blood in immediate apposition to the trophoblast does not clot, and thus continues to contribute towards the sustenance of the ovum.

Our observations are in accord with Mall's and Litzenberg's that, whenever we have found an early unruptured pregnancy, the ovum was very small and separated from the tubal wall by a definite layer of blood.

The tubal and uterine placenta are identical in formation. The pathologic changes which take place in tubal pregnancy are due to the thin tube walls and the absence of a true decidua serotina, which allows easy invasion by the trophoblast and syncytial cells; consequently there is no active connective tissue reaction set up by the presence of the fetal cells.

The villi rapidly penetrate the tube walls and then perforate the serosa, producing a porosity which allows blood to escape through the tube wall into the peritoneum, even before the tube wall is so weakened as to produce rupture.

Owing to these changes the tubal placenta suffers from lack of nutrition, which explains the number of pathologic embryos found in tubal pregnancies. Syncytial cells and bits of villi are often found in the tubal veins remote from the site of the pregnancy.

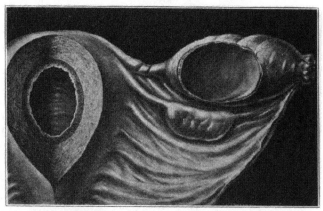

Fig. 2.—Author's specimen, showing complete decidual development in the uterus and incomplete reaction in the tube in a nine weeks' pregnancy. The imperfect reaction in the tube is the basic cause of the symptoms of tubal abortion or rupture.

Whenever an ovum implants itself in the tube wall, the gestation sac is bounded on all sides by a layer of trophoblastic cells and masses of fibrin, and a pseudodecidua reflexa is formed by trophoblastic elements and the overlying mucosa. Frequently the trophoblastic cells, owing to their erosive quality, lie between the muscle bundles; the decidual reaction is imperfect and irregular, found in remote portions of the tube, while the syncytial cells invade the blood vessels in the tube wall. The absence of a developed decidua allows excessive erosive action in the tube wall, and favors early rupture of the gestation sac.

Owing to the effusion of blood into the imperfectly formed decidua, and between the underlying tube wall and ovum and the separation of the nutritive villi from the tubal vessels, the blood accumulated about the ovum, increases the separation, stimulates peristaltic tubal contraction, and favors tubal abortion.

Whenever pregnancy occurs, no matter what its location, a decidua vera develops within the uterus. The uterus is enlarged because of the hyperemia and thickened endometrium. These changes in the endometrium are quite similar to those found in the decidua vera in early intrauterine pregnancy.

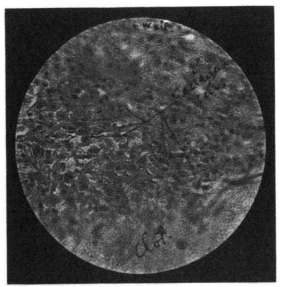

Fig. 3.—Section of tubal wall from an ectopic gestation, showing hemorrhage into the decidua at a point remote from the site of implantation of the ovum.

While tubal pregnancy is being terminated, the tube undergoes a measure of intermittent contraction, endeavoring by its peristaltic action to expel the contents; these contractions are transmitted to the uterus, which in turn contracts as in abortion, giving rise to uterine pain. The clinical expression of these uterine contractions is bleeding from the endometrium with extrusion of portions of the decidua.

Uterine bleeding indicates ovular unrest in the tube, due to hemorrhage about the aberrant ovum, and the threatened termination of the ectopic pregnancy. So long as the embryo is living and development is in progress, there is no uterine bleeding.

The uterine bleeding, which is usually small in amount, may continue for a considerable time after the attack of pelvic pain which, apparently, marks the destruction of the embryo. This is due to the fact that the termination of the tubal pregnancy is not necessarily at once complete, chorionic villi remaining alive, exerting their stimulus upon the uterus.

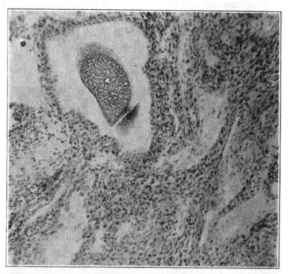

Fig. 4.—Photomicrograph of a section of uterine decidua from a case of ruptured extrauterine pregnancy at the third month, showing absence of blood in the decidual layer.

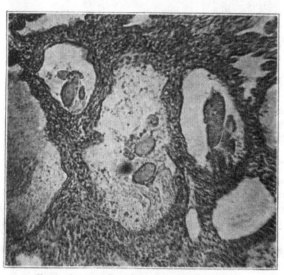

Fig. 5.—Same as Fig. 4, showing glandular structure.

Sampson found that the uterine bleeding, in all cases, was of venous origin and arose from the endometrium, and that blood did not escape from the tube into the uterine cavity. On the other hand, we have demonstrated that when the pregnancy is close to the uterus, some blood does escape through the uterine end of the tube, that the metrorrhagia has both a uterine and tubal origin, and that there is always hemorrhage into remote parts of the tube, just as there is decidual reaction at other than the seat of the ovum.

The uterine involution which takes place following the complete termination of tubal pregnancy is analogous to that following labor or abortion. When involution is delayed there is an incomplete termination of the tubal pregnancy, just as there is delayed involution when there is retained material in a uterine abortion.

The decidual cast of the uterus is passed, either *en masse*, or piecemeal, in fully 50 per cent of the recorded cases of tubal pregnancy. The pain accompanying this expulsion is nothing more than a sympathetic labor on the part of the uterus. All authorities are agreed that, in every instance where a fecundated ovum has embedded itself and developed, a uterine decidua is formed.

The ectopic cast has definite microscopic characteristics. It may be divided into a distinct compact and spongioid layer and fails to exhibit any evidences of chorionic villi. The large decidua cells with well defined nuclei, packed closely together, which make up the decidua compacta, are always characteristic proof of pregnancy.

CONCLUSIONS

(1) Our studies have shown that a decidual reaction may be found at several points in the tube in ectopic points often far remote from the seat of implantation.

(2) That coincident with the separation or death of the ovum by hemorrhage into the decidua, there is bleeding from the uterus and also bleeding from the several points of decidual reaction in the tube.

(3) That tubal peristalsis and the *vis a tergo* of the clot in the tube, expels blood from the abdominal ostium into the peritoneum, which gravitates into the culdesac.

(4) That the same factors contribute a portion of the blood, making up the bloody discharge from the uterus, which signifies the separation or death of the embryo.

20 LIVINGSTON STREET.   (*For discussion, see page 195.*)

A STUDY OF PITUITARY EXTRACT AT THE BEGINNING OF THE THIRD STAGE OF LABOR. ITS USE IN 100 CASES*

By George L. Brodhead, M.D., and Edwin G. Langrock, M.D., New York, N. Y.

IN ORDER to ascertain the effect and analyze carefully the results, we administered to 100 patients, immediately after the birth of the child, 1 c.c. of infundin hypodermically. We waited the customary 20 minutes, during which time the uterus was carefully observed and the blood loss measured; at the end of this period the placenta was expressed, if it had not been expelled spontaneously. After the delivery of the placenta all blood lost, during the succeeding hour, was measured.

There were 43 primiparae and 57 multiparae in this series. There were 96 patients at or near term. Two were between 8 and 8½ months; one was between 7 and 8 months, and one was between 6 and 7 months.

METHOD OF DELIVERY

In this series there were 87 spontaneous deliveries and 13 operative deliveries; of the latter there were 5 low forceps operations, 3 median forceps operations, 2 versions,—1 for prolapsed cord and 1 for shoulder presentation, 3 breech extractions. As a matter of interest, in the 13 operative cases in both primiparae and multiparae, the maximum total blood loss was only 390 c.c.

The placenta was expelled spontaneously in 19 cases; this may be compared with Ryder's 25 spontaneous placental expulsions in his series of 100 pituitrin cases, and may be contrasted with a total number of nine spontaneous placental expulsions in 1000 labors in which pituitrin was not used, in Williams' series. In our 19 cases in which the placenta was expelled spontaneously, the minimum time required was 4 minutes and the maximum time required was 18 minutes; the average being 10½ minutes. In 78 minutes the Credé method of expression was used. In 3 patients the placentae were manually extracted. In the first case, the Credé method was tried several times and then when the placenta was visible in the cervix at the outlet, manual extraction was easily performed.

In the second case, the Credé method was tried repeatedly and then, because of continued bleeding, the hand was passed into the uterus, where it was found that there was an hour-glass contraction; the pla-

*Read at a meeting of the New York Obstetrical Society, November 8, 1921.

centa being partly above and partly below the area of constriction. The placenta was not adherent and was very easily extracted.

In the third case, after one hour the placenta was found in the vagina and was manually removed.

Blood Loss During the Third Stage.—In 26 cases (12 primiparae and 14 multiparae) the blood loss did not exceed 30 c.c. The maximum blood loss in primiparae was 525 c.c.; in multiparae 1230 c.c. (Hemorrhage three pounds in weight.) The average blood loss in primiparae was 110 c.c.; in multiparae was 153 c.c. The average in all cases during the third stage was 135 c.c.

Blood Loss After the Third Stage.—In 77 cases (33 primiparae and 44 multiparae) the blood loss did not exceed 30 c.c. for a period of one hour following the delivery of the placenta. The maximum blood loss in primiparae was 750 c.c.; in multiparae was 800 c.c. The average blood loss in primiparae was 47 c.c.; in multiparae was 36 c.c. The average in all cases was 41 c.c.

Total Blood Loss.—The tables have been prepared to show the number of primiparae and multiparae, the duration of their respective labors, and their respective blood losses.

TABLE I
SPONTANEOUS DELIVERY

DURATION OF LABOR	NUMBER OF CASES		SUM TOTAL OF C.C. BLOOD LOSS		AVERAGE C.C. BLOOD LOSS	
HOURS	P	M	P	M	P	M
8	·5	29	990	5245	198	180
8-16	12	15	1180	3685	98	245
16-24	7	8	1000	1145	143	143
24-36	7	2	1160	110	165	55
Unknown	2		940		470	

P=Primiparae.
M=Multiparae.

TABLE II
OPERATIVE DELIVERY

DURATION OF LABOR	NUMBER OF CASES		SUM TOTAL OF C.C. BLOOD LOSS		AVERAGE C.C. BLOOD LOSS	
HOURS	P	M	P	M	P	M
8	0	1		200		200
8-16	5	1	405	390	81	390
16-24	4	0	825	0	206	0
24-36	1	1	300	120	300	120

P=Primiparae.
M=Multiparae.

The average total blood loss of all primiparae who delivered themselves spontaneously was 160 c.c. This may be compared with the average total blood loss in the 10 operative primiparae which was

153 c.c. The average total blood loss for all primiparae was 158 c.c. The average total blood loss in multiparae who delivered themselves spontaneously was 188 c.c. The average total blood loss in the operative multiparae was 236 c.c., making an average total blood loss in all multiparae 191 c.c. The average total blood loss in the complete series of 100 cases was 177 c.c.

At this point we wish to call particular attention to three cases of this series in which the blood loss was marked:

CASE 1.—Multipara, having had three previous normal deliveries. The duration of this labor at term was five hours, vertex presenting, the patient having had a few whiffs of ether and chloroform. Five hundred c.c. of blood were lost before the birth of the placenta. The Credé method was tried a number of times unsuccessfully. After waiting one hour, moderate bleeding continuing, it was decided to remove the placenta manually. An hour-glass contraction of the uterus was found, the placenta being ¾ below and ¼ above the constriction; it was easily removed, the total blood loss being 1410 c.c. In our opinion the large blood loss in this particular case was probably due to the administration of the pituitrin.

One of the writers had an experience recently, in which an hour-glass contraction of the uterus appeared in the third stage, and followed the administration of 5 minims of infundin in the latter part of the second stage. In another case where 1 c.c. of pituitrin was given after repeated attempts at Credé, the cervix was so tightly contracted that the placenta was extracted only with the greatest difficulty.

CASE 2.—Primipara, at term, was delivered spontaneously and after 25 minutes the placenta was expressed with considerable difficulty by the Credé method. During this period 80 c.c. of blood were lost. Following the birth of the placenta there was a profuse hemorrhage (750 c.c.) and the uterus was packed immediately. A fibroid, the size of an apple, was found in the lower uterine segment, and probably was responsible for at least part of the hemorrhage.

CASE 3.—Multipara, at term, delivered normally, after a 13½ hour labor. The placenta was expressed with moderate difficulty by the Credé method 30 minutes later. During this time, the woman lost 450 c.c. of blood. After the expression of the placenta there was no blood loss and the patient was taken to her bed. About 45 minutes later the uterus was soft and flabby and the woman was bleeding profusely. The uterus was packed at once. The total measured blood lost was 1250 c.c. This case emphasizes the importance of careful observation of the uterus, even though pituitrin has been given.

The average loss of blood during labor in which pituitrin is not used at the beginning of the third stage is variously estimated at 343 c.c. by Williams in 1000 spontaneous labors; 300 c.c. by De Lee; 300 to 500 c.c. by Leavitt, and 505 c.c. in 2058 cases by Ahlfeld. In contrast with these figures, Ryder states that the average blood loss in his series of 100 cases in which pituitrin was used at the beginning of the third stage was 180 c.c. This corresponds very closely with an average blood loss of 177 c.c. in our series of 100 cases. Based on these series of 200 cases,—Ryder's and the authors'—the average blood loss is materially reduced. Further, in Williams' series of 1000 cases without pituitrin there were 130 in which 600 c.c. or more of blood were lost; in contrast to these figures, Ryder in his series had no blood loss of 600 c.c. In our series we had but four.

In conclusion, we are of the opinion that in the vast majority of cases, the method as outlined is safe and valuable in minimizing blood loss. We agree with Ryder that the uterus must be observed just as carefully as when pituitrin is not given. The only drawback to the method in our small series of 100 cases, is the possibility of irregular or hour-glass contraction of the uterus which occurred in one of our series and which has occurred to the authors in several cases outside of this series where pituitrin was given. We recognize the fact, however, that this complication occurs independently of the use of pituitrin, and time only will prove and further investigation will be necessary to show whether this complication is directly attributable to the method or not.

We believe that earlier removal of the placenta would probably have reduced the blood loss in some of our cases.

REFERENCES

Williams, J. W.: Am. Jour. Obst., July, 1919, lxxx, No. 1. *Ryder*, Geo. H.: AM. JOUR. OBST. AND GYNEC., July, 1921, ii.

50 WEST FORTY-EIGHTH STREET. (*For discussion, see p. 205.*)

REPORT OF THREE CASES OF A RARE OVARIAN ANOMALY

By JAMES C. JANNEY, M.D., BOSTON, MASS.

CASLER[1] recently reported an interesting case which showed, among other things, the occurrence of uterine tissue in the ovary. Norris,[2] in the discussion of this paper, reported a similar case from his practice. At the time Casler's article appeared, I had in preparation the report of such a case and since that time have found two others, all of which I am here reporting together.

Ovarian anomalies of any sort are of sufficiently rare occurrence to be interesting. A search of the literature on the subject will show that they are not frequent, but the standard works yield a goodly array of different conditions which sometimes occur. These anomalies are of four sorts: (A) Anomalies of number; (B) Anomalies of development; (C) Anomalies of position; (D) Miscellaneous.

There are three variations of number: (1) Absence of one or both ovaries; (2) Accessory ovaries; (3) Supernumerary ovaries: all rare conditions. Accessory ovaries occur more frequently than the other variations and are usually situated very close to the "normal" ovary, sometimes being separated only by a cleft which looks like an extremely developed lobulation. The supernumerary ovary is of extreme rarity. Dudley[3] states that it has been authenticated in only one case, that reported by Winkle in Albutt and Playfair's "System of Gynecology." Absence of the ovary is usually associated with absence of the tube and uterine cornu of the same side. Absence of both ovaries has been reported, but is said to occur only in nonviable fetuses.

Anomalies of development may affect either the ovary as a whole, or may appear in isolated areas as embryonic rests. Those which affect the ovary as a whole are rudimentary conditions, congenital hypertrophy and presenile atrophy. The cases of rudimentary ovaries seem to be closely related to those which show absence of the ovary, for they too usually show underdevelopment of the follicle apparatus of the ovary and also the infantile type of uterus and tubes. This condition varies in degree and it seems likely that the cases of dysmenorrhea, irregularity, retroposition, and anteflexion with conical cervix are associated with ovaries which are underdeveloped, at least functionally. Congenital hypertrophy of the ovary is often reported as an anomaly, but some authorities (Dudley) incline to the belief that it represents, rather, the results of early inflammatory or vascular changes. Presenile atrophy of the ovary is not infrequently encountered in women of the third and fourth decades and is characterized by a sclerosis of the cortex and a marked diminution in the number of follicles. Such a condition would be normal in a woman who is close to the menopause, but not in a woman at the age of 35. It is little understood and may conceivably be either another grade of the underdeveloped ovary, or a state brought about by unknown factors in later life, possibly endocrine derangements.

The embryonic rests are the rete ovarii, egg tubes of Pflüger, either solid or tubular, remains of the Wolffian body or ducts, and possibly teratomata. These structures, with the exception of the last, are all of microscopic proportions and of little practical importance. Whether teratomata should be properly classed as embryonic rests and included among ovarian anomalies does not come within the scope of this paper, but if they be so included, they form the only group in the category which is of clinical importance and are sufficiently well known to need no further mention here.

The anomalies of position are as rare as those of number. Hernia of the ovary is described, as is the undescended ovary. Lateral and posterior descensus are also described, but here again there is a question whether these conditions ever occur except secondary to malpositions elsewhere in the genital tract.

Under the heading of "miscellaneous," are two conditions given by Veit,[4] namely, bud-like projections from the albuginea of senile ovaries and extravasations of blood about the follicles. I believe that both of these conditions are open to question as true anomalies. The former is very suggestive of fibroma of the ovary and the latter of some traumatic or infectious origin.

All of the anomalies of the ovary, then, may be said to be of academic interest only, with the exception of the teratomata and herniae of the ovary, which are of practical surgical importance, and the cases of underdevelopment, from the standpoint of endocrine therapy. It may well be that the relative infrequency of ovarian anomalies of all sorts is due in considerable degree to the concealed position of the ovary, and that if the ovary were as easily accessible as the testicle, these anomalies—some of them at least— would be of more frequent record and more importance from the viewpoint of practical therapy.

The three cases which I have to report all show the occurrence of uterine tissue in the ovary. They were found in going over a part of the pathologic collection at the Free Hospital for Women, Brookline, Mass., and occurred in a total of 4853 pathologic specimens examined. They were all discovered incidentally, the operations having been performed for other conditions which had not directed attention primarily to the ovaries.

CASE 1.—(Path. No. 2017.) Miss Mary K, aged 41, admitted to the Free Hospital for Women, February 26, 1909, with the complaint of flowing. Her family history was unimportant, as was her past history, with the exception of the menstrual

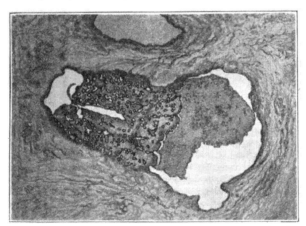

Fig. 1.—PATH. 2017, low power drawing, showing the relation of the uterine tissue to the cyst of the ovary.

condition. She had been well until the onset of the present illness, which she dates back two years.

Menstruation commenced at twelve years of age and was regular, with moderate pain the first day. Periods lasted four days, and she used seven napkins. There was no vaginal discharge between periods. Two years ago her periods lengthened to two to three weeks every month, which condition had persisted until January (the month previous to entrance). In January she skipped her period. About four weeks previous to admission she took a long walk, then a hot bath, after which she had severe hemorrhage without pain. The flowing necessitated three to ten napkins daily. She passed some clots. This condition persisted until admission.

Physical examination was negative, except for the pelvic examination, which was made by Dr. William P. Graves. Dr. Graves' note was as follows: "Uterus anteflexed and drawn back in pelvis; mass behind uterus, indefinite to touch and not very tender." This examination was confirmed under ether March 4, and operation was performed at that time by Dr. Graves. The pelvic structures were all found to be involved in an inflammatory process with many adhesions. Supravaginal hysterectomy with bilateral salpingo-oophorectomy was performed, and the patient made an uneventful recovery.

Pathologic Report: "Specimen consists of uterus with ovaries and tubes attached, vermiform appendix, and a small myoma. Uterus has been amputated at the level of the internal os and opened on its anterior surface. There are adhesions about the fundus, especially on its posterior surface. Both ovaries are much enlarged and

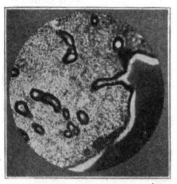 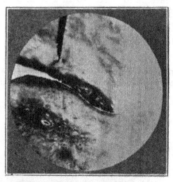

Fig. 2.—PATH. 2017, low power, showing the uterine stroma and glands, and at the right, the blood clot within the cyst cavity.

Fig. 3.—PATH. 2017, low power, showing the uterine tissue in a cleft of the ovary of the opposite side.

cystic. Fimbriated ends of both tubes closed. On opening the uterus the walls seem to be slightly hypertrophied. The endometrium is thick, about 2 mm. in depth, but there are no intrauterine polypi or other growths. Both tubes and ovaries are densely adherent and bound into one mass. The left tube is dilated and contains clear straw-colored fluid; walls are thin, forming a true hydrosalpinx."

In summary, the microscopic findings were: Chronic interstitial endometritis with hypertrophy of the endometrium, myoma uteri, hydrosalpinx, and periovaritis with evidences of still active inflammatory process.

The interesting anomaly occurred in the ovaries, both of which were involved. In one it consisted of a piece of tissue 4 x 2 mm., which appeared to be endometrium, springing from the wall of a small cyst which measured about 7.5 mm. in its greatest diameter. The cyst contained blood clot. The section of the other ovary was torn in cutting and the relations were much distorted. The uterine tissue in this ovary was not so extensive in amount and was situated on the edge of what appeared to be either a cleft or a collapsed cyst. The finding of this tissue, of course, raised the question of some strange accident in cutting and mounting. Careful examination showed that no such artefact had taken place and that the tissue was actually growing in and part of the ovary. (Figs. 1, 2, and 3.)

CASE 2.—(Path. No. 4136) Mrs. B. W., age forty-eight, entered the hospital April 14, 1913, with the complaint of having had "the womb come outside" for the past four years. Family history was unimportant as was the past history, except for nocturia, two to three times every night. Menstruation had always been normal. She had passed through the menopause nine years previously and had subsequently suffered considerably from nervousness and hot flushes for two years. These were not so troublesome at time of admission. She had had five pregnancies with normal labors. The last child was stillborn. No abortions. Present illness dates from four years ago when the uterus first began to come out. This had grown steadily worse and has caused sacral backache and a dragging feeling in the lower abdomen. Physical examination was negative, except for the local examination by Dr. Graves, which showed separation of the recti muscles, atrophy of the external genitalia, cystocele, lacerated cervix and perineum, and moderate prolapse. Operation April 16, 1913, by Dr. Graves, curettage, trachelorrhaphy, anterior colporrhaphy, perineorrhaphy, supravaginal hysterectomy, and repair of diastasis recti. Recovery was uneventful.

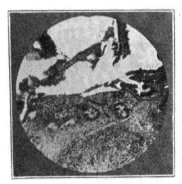
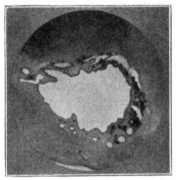

Fig. 4.—PATH. 4136, low power, showing the uterine tissue on the surface of the ovary.

Fig. 5.—PATH. 4815, 2 inch, showing the cyst lined with endometrium.

Pathologic Report: "Specimen consists of uterus with both tubes, both ovaries, and a piece of cervical tissue. Uterus measures 5 x 6 cm.; no adhesions seen. Uterine cavity is 3 cm. long, endometrium is 1 mm. thick and covered with blood. Right tube is 5.5 cm. long, very tortuous, but shows no adhesions. Right ovary is 2.5 x 1 cm., and shows nothing remarkable. Left tube is 5 cm. long; shows nothing remarkable. Left ovary measures 2x3 cm., has many adhesions on it, and contains a few small cysts."

Microscopic examination shows a good deal of connective tissue in the cortex of both ovaries. In summary, it showed interval endometrium, chronic salpingitis, bilateral. Normal ovary, right; chronic periovaritis, left; chronic cervicitis.

The uterine tissue occurs in the right ovary in this case and covers an area of approximately 2x1 mm. It is on the surface of the ovary and is not enclosed in a cyst as in the former case. (Fig. 4.)

CASE 3.—(Path. No. 4815.) Mrs. G. C., age forty-four, entered the hospital March 28, 1914, complaining of flowing. Family history unimportant. An operation was done nine years previously at Boston City Hospital for gastric ulcer. Menstruation began at 17, was regular and normal until one year ago, when present illness began. She had slight yellowish discharge. Micturition two to six times in day and one to three at night; at times has dysuria. Present illness started one year ago. Since then she has has had a backache and dull ache in both lower quadrants, worse during periods. The latter have become irregular, appearing at intervals of two to six weeks and lasting from six to twenty-one days. The flow was very profuse, necessitating twelve to fifteen napkins daily. Physical examination was negative with the exception of the pelvic examination which was made by Dr. Graves. This revealed uterus large and anteflexed, some loss of mobility, nothing definite felt on the sides, scar in posterior vaginal wall, lacerated cervix and perineum, cervical polyp. On March 31 operation was performed by Dr. F. A. Pemberton consisting of curettage, removal of cervical polyp, perineorrhaphy, and supravaginal hysterectomy. At operation the uterus was anteflexed and adhesions were found about the adnexa on both sides. The patient made a good recovery.

Pathologic Report: "Specimen consists of cervical polyp, curettings, and a uterus with two tubes and ovaries. Uterus measures 6x5 cm.; the endometrium is 3 mm. thick and smooth. There are no adhesions; tubes and ovaries look normal. On section the right ovary is found to consist of a cyst 3 cm. in diameter; no ovarian tissue was left. Left ovary is small, seems to be atrophied. Section taken of polyp, curettings uterine wall, right tube and left ovary." Histologic examination showed (in summary) interval endometrium, mucous polyp of the cervix, chronic salpingitis, bilateral, atrophy of left ovary, adenomyoma (?), retention cyst of right ovary. The microscopic note on the left ovary said: "Left ovary shows, in one place, glandular tissue surrounded by connective tissue which looks like endometrium of the uterus."

This glandular tissue in the section of the left ovary occurs in the wall of a small cyst as in the first case. It measures roughly 3x2 mm.

The more detailed histologic description of the uterine tissue in these three cases, I shall group together for the reason that the tissues are practically identical in structure. The tissue is composed of stroma and epithelial elements in about the same proportion as normal uterine mucosa. All of the cell nuclei in the stroma stain readily with hematoxylin, are regular in size and shape, and show the usual finely granular nuclear markings and a single small deeply staining nucleolus, usually eccentric. The cytoplasmic elements of the cells show a delicate reticulum, taking the acid stains. Definite mitotic figures are rare in the stroma, two only being seen. There are many irregular hyperchromatic nuclei which are apparently undergoing some change preparatory to division, but they are not characteristic mitotic figures. (Fig. 7.)

The epithelial elements are composed of columnar cells, which cover the surface fronting on the cavity of the cyst, and which line the gland spaces. The gland spaces themselves are, in places, quite irregular in size and outline, which is the main feature divergent from normal interval endometrium. These irregular glands are counterbalanced, however, by many small round glands in every way characteristic of normal uterine glands. The epithelial cells are uniform, with a good basement membrane and show no tendency to invade the deeper structures. The cell nuclei are oval and arranged near the basal end of the cells. They show numerous mitoses, as are commonly seen in the postmenstrual and interval periods of the endometrial cycle. These mitoses are very definite, showing a variety of monasters, diasters, and spindles. No ciliated epithelium was seen in the sections.

In two of the cases there were small bundles of cells on the edges of the uterine tissue which closely resembled smooth muscle. The identification of these cells could not be determined beyond question in the sections available and other sections and stains could not be made. All the sections of these cases were frozen sections and not adapted for the study of the finer cell structure. Unfortunately the gross material from the first case of the series had been destroyed so that no further sections could be made. Many sections were made of the remaining ovarian tissue of both ovaries in the last two cases but no other uterine tissue was found.

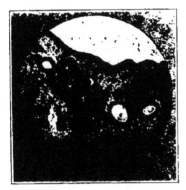
Fig. 6.—PATH. 4815, low power, showing the stroma and glands.

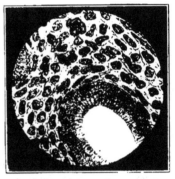
Fig. 7.—Semidiagrammatic drawing showing the characteristics of the uterine tissue found in all of the cases.

The differences between the three cases were very minor. In Case 2 the uterine tissue occurred on the surface of the ovary, while it was within the ovarian tissue in the other two cases. All of the cases showed minor histologic variations attributable to differences in the stage of the endometrial cycle, and congestion of the parts due to infection, prolapse, or accompanying conditions.

Besides those mentioned above, reported by Casler and Norris, I have been able to find only two other cases, one of which is extremely doubtful. In 1899 Russell[5] reported finding aberrant portions of the müllerian duct in the ovary. This occurred in an ovary macroscopically normal, but associated with tumor of the other ovary. The ovary contained a thick-walled cyst and in three areas in the cyst wall and solid tissue of the ovary, uterine tissue was found. It showed much the same picture that I have described, and it definitely contained smooth muscle in a relative position corresponding to the muscular coat of the uterus. The other possible case was reported by von Franqué[6] in 1898, but in such vague terms and in such a loose way that it is impossible from his article to tell whether it actually belongs to this category or not. I believe it better to omit this case from the discussion, because we have no definite facts about it to discuss.

For comparison and contrast, then, there are three cases. Of a total of six, four occurred in ovaries that were macroscopically normal and were removed incidentally in an operation directed at some other condition. Two of them were associated with tumors in the affected ovary. The interpretation of these findings must lie between teratoma, metastasis and anomaly. Casler considers teratoma long enough to discard it as a possibility, and takes the position, with which I agree, that no teratoma confined entirely to uterine glands, stroma, and muscle has been hitherto described, and that its occurrence would be extremely improbable. The possibility of metastasis must also be considered. This would demand for a premise that an analogous tumor be present elsewhere and that it be malignant. In Casler's case the uterus had been removed some years previously for an "adenomyoma, with stroma, but no glands." Here we have the tumor, and it is conceivable that it might be malignant, in which case we could explain with ease the presence in the ovary of this uterine tissue. In Russell's case also there was a tumor, an adenocarcinoma of the other ovary, but it would be very hard to explain uterine tissue, anywhere, as metastasis from an adenocarcinoma of the ovary. In one of my cases there was a myoma showing the ordinary picture of myoma uteri, and here again it would be very hard to explain on the basis of metastasis from a smooth muscle tumor (even supposing it to be malignant) the presence in the ovary of this uterine tissue, whose chief characteristic was the glandular structure. In the case reported by Norris and in my other two cases there was no tumor at all, and it seems as if the metastasis hypothesis were entirely untenable in these cases. My own belief is that all of these cases can be most rationally explained on the basis of anomaly.

When it came to an explanation of the mechanism of this anomaly, I was entirely at a loss. Two suggestions were advanced by Drs. Bremer and Begg of the Department of Embryology of the Harvard Medical School. The former believed that this might be explained on the supposition of an accessory aberrant müllerian duct bud which was included in the ovary. Accessory tubes and ducts are not infrequently recorded and accessory ostia are often seen in embryos. Admitting for the moment that this explanation is correct, the advancing or caudal end of the duct is the portion which fuses with the duct from the other side to form the uterus and vagina. If this portion were included in the ovary and continued to develop there, it would sufficiently explain the occurrence of endometrium. It is necessary to assume that this aberrant portion is an accessory duct for the reason that in each case there was a normally developed tube on the affected side. Dr. Begg suggested that the proximity of the "anlagen" of the ovary and tube in embryonic life was so great that there might be some critical period of embryonic development at which it would be possible for a tissue mixture to take place.

Casler does not advance a theory in explanation, but recapitulates that of Russell who argues that inasmuch as the epithelium of the tube and uterus and the germinal epithelium of the ovary are all originally derived from one embryologic ancestor, it is not too much to assume that tissue may develop structures in one place (namely,

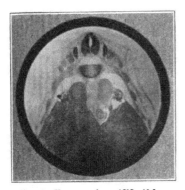

Fig. 8.—Human embryo 1597, 19.3 mm., serial section 704, 2 inch, showing the urogenital ridge on each side and the general anatomic location of all the embryologic illustrations.

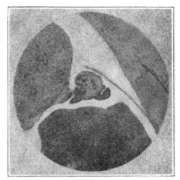

Fig. 9.—Human embryo 2044, 16.0 mm., serial section 928, right side, showing a small portion of the sex gland at the median side of the urogenital ridge and the funnel opening on the lateral side of the tubar area. The tubar and genital areas are usually separated by a cleft of considerable depth, which is absent in this section. Note the distance separating the genital from the tubar areas.

in the ovary) which its function is to develop elsewhere (in the uterus).

The only one of these theories which seems susceptible of experimental confirmation is that a tissue mixture may take place at some stage of embryonic development. With this idea in view, I have gone over the collection of human embryos at the Harvard Medical School. Of these 43 were available, ranging in size from 10 mm. to 50 mm. The others in the collection were either too young or otherwise unfit. The sex glands and ducts of the embryo are developed from the genital ridge which is on the surface of the wolffian body on either side of the midline. The genital ridge on each side is divided longitudinally by a fissure which separates the genital area from the tubar area. The genital area gives rise to the sex gland, and the tubar area to the müllerian duct. The funnel arises in the tubar area as a dimple in the celomic epithelium, from which grows backward a solid cord of epithelial cells. This cord gradually becomes tubular, thus forming the müllerian duct. Its course is at first tailward, until it gets well below the crest of the ileum, then it turns sharply toward the midline where it meets its fellow from the other side, and the two then proceed tailward together to the cloaca. The anterior portion of the müllerian duct later becomes the tube while the portion which has joined (and later fused with) the duct from the other side forms the vagina, cervix, and uterus. This development of the müllerian ducts is at first the same in both the male and female. In later stages there are slight differences in the relations of the ducts in the two sexes, but these affect the portions which are associated with the

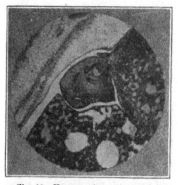

Fig. 10.—Human embryo 2155, 17.5 mm., serial section 930, left side showing the opening of the funnel on the median side of the tubar area.

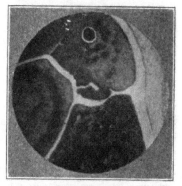

Fig. 11.—Human embryo 2155, serial section 948, right side, showing the opening of the funnel on the median side of the tubar area.

bladder or cloaca, and not the portions near the genital gland. The müllerian ducts finally atrophy in the male, with the exception of a small portion of the lower end, which opens into the urethra and forms the utriculus masculinus. (Figs. 8 and 9.)

In reviewing this series of embryos I have found cases where the funnel, instead of forming on the lateral side of the tubar area, forms on the median side, and is thereby brought into a position much closer to the sex gland, a fact which is suggestive in view of the supposition advanced by Dr. Begg.

The funnel, which is the earliest beginning of the müllerian duct, is developed usually on the lateral side of the tubar area and separated from the genital area by a fissure and the whole width of the tubar ridge, a distance of approximately 0.5 to 0.75 mm. In one case both funnels opened on the median side of the tubar area. (Figs. 10 and 11.) In two other embryos one funnel opened on the median side, and in a fourth the funnel opening seemed to extend from the lateral through to the median side of the tubar area. (Fig. 14.) This unusual median position of the funnel reduces the distance between the genital

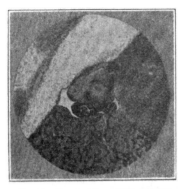

Fig. 12.—Human embryo 1913, 18.2 mm., serial section 919, left side, showing the opening of the funnel on the median side of the tubar area.

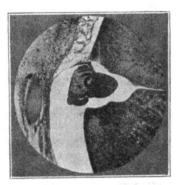

Fig. 13.—Human embryo 1597, 19.3 mm., serial section 704, left side, showing the opening of the funnel on the median side of the tubar area and its close proximity to the genital gland.

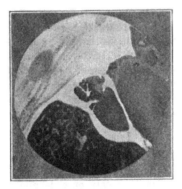

Fig. 14.—Human embryo 2042, 25.0 mm., serial section 1384, left side, showing the funnel with its tubal epithelium running through to the median surface of the tubar area.

gland and the müllerian duct very materially. In the cases which showed this variation the actual distances between the funnel and the genital gland at the nearest point were in four cases less than 0.1 mm. (about 0.0875 mm.) and in the fifth instance less than 0.2 mm. (about 0.175). It is not unreasonable to suppose that tissue mixtures between the tubal and ovarian tissue could take place in cases where the distance separating the two tissues is less than 0.1 mm.

I must note here that in the cases where this condition was present three of the embryos were too young to distinguish the sex with certainty. The genital glands were still undifferentiated. In the other two cases testes cords were present and the embryo was probably male. I do not feel that it would argue impossibility of such an explanation of uterine tissue in the ovary, had these been definitely male embryos, for there is nothing to show that such variations could not occur in the female. The most it could argue, I think, is that such an anomaly might some day be found in the testis also.

Recent experimental work in embryology has shown that certain tissues transplanted in fetal life to foreign parts of the same individual may grow and form comparatively well developed portions of their structures. Thus Lewis[7] has shown that in frogs the otic vesicle may be transplanted from one individual to another in early embryonic life and continue to grow normally, and other investigators have performed similar experiments with comparable results. We may believe, therefore, that a stray piece of uterine tissue in the ovary, even though it be eventually completely cut off from its origin, might go on and develop to a degree such as we have found in these cases.

The table shows a comparison of the six cases from various points of view. In the first place, the uniformity of age is of interest, though probably only incidental. In Russell's case the age in years is not given, but it is stated that the patient had reached the natural menopause. The gross appearance of the ovary is also worth noting. Four of the ovaries appeared grossly normal, one slightly enlarged, and one only showed gross tumor. This is interesting in view of Casler's suggestion that we might have in this anomaly another origin for tumors of the ovary. It would hardly seem, with the rarity of the condition taken into consideration, that this could be of any great practical importance in the genesis of ovarian tumor if only one in six of the cases show tumor at all. With regard to the rarity of the condition, the incidence of three cases in a series of 4853 is very high frequency for a condition that had been only once definitely described before August, 1920. I believe that it would prove more common if more searching microscopic examination of the ovaries was made in all cases, and the occurrence in most cases would probably take the form of small areas of uterine tissue in the walls of cysts. If this supposition be true, it would be an argument against Casler's idea, for many instances of this condition showing gross tumor formation cannot have been missed. It would logically mean, then, that the undiscovered cases would contain a much higher proportion of cases of harmless (if you will) uterine tissue in the ovary than of cases that have reached any clinical significance, and that the true ratio of important to unimportant should be, not 1 to 5, but rather 1 to 50 or 1 to 100.

The matter of neoplasm occurring in connection with this condition has been already partially treated. Three cases showed no tumor of any kind in the genital tract. One case had had the uterus and adnexa, except the ovary in question, previously removed because of a diffuse uterine tumor. One case had adenocarcinoma of the opposite ovary, for which the operation was performed. A third had myoma uteri.

The question of functional activity of the uterine tissue is interesting also, in that three of the cases showed undoubted signs of menstrual activity of that portion of the endometrium which lay in the ovary. Casler's case after panhysterectomy continued to menstruate for part of a day every month. After removal of the ovary in question, it was found that there was dark blood in the cyst cavity into which these uterine glands emptied. Norris' case also showed blood in the cavity of the cyst, as did one of mine. Russell made no note in his report of any findings suggestive in this respect. Closely associated with the question of functional activity is that of correspondence of this tissue with the uterine mucosa itself in the stage of the menstrual cycle. Here again Russell does not note this fact. Casler cannot note it, for the uterus was removed four years previously in his case. Norris has remarked on the correspondence of the two tissues in his case, and in all of mine there was correspondence between the two. Case 1 showed in the uterus a marked hypertrophic condition which was not reproduced in the uterine tissue in the ovary. This hypertrophy was, no doubt, largely attributable to inflammation and congestion of the pelvic organs which caused more derangement of the circulation in the uterus than in the ovary. The mitotic figures and other finer evidence of the stage of the menstrual cycle, however, showed a condition in each case conformable with the interval stage. In Case 2 the patient had passed the menopause, and the endometrium showed a moderate senile atrophy which was present, but not so marked, in the tissue found in the ovary. In the third case the endometrium showed an early atrophic condition, which was not incompatible with the history of flowing (in the presence of the cervical polyp). The uterine tissue in the ovary in this case showed distinct atrophy.

The location of the uterine tissue is of some importance in relation to the theories advanced in explanation. In four instances the tissue was found within the ovarian substance, and so far as was demonstrated it had no connection with the surface of the ovary or the germinal epithelium. In Russell's case the tissue was both on the surface and within the ovary and in one of my cases was wholly upon the surface. In Case 1, here reported, there is possibility that the

TABLE I

CASE	GROSS APPEARANCE	AGE	NEOPLASM	FUNCTIONAL ACTIVITY OF OVARIAN ENDOMETRIUM	CYCLE CORRESPONDENCE	LOCATION OF UTERINE TISSUE	COMMUNICATION WITH SURFACE
1.	Normal	41	Small subperitoneal myoma uteri	Yes	Yes	Cyst within ovary ? surface opp. side.	None found
2.	Normal	48	No	?	Yes	Surface	....
3.	Normal	44	No	No	Yes	Cyst within ovary	None found
Russell's	Normal	"Natural Menopause"	Adenocarcinoma other ovary	Not stated	?	Cyst and surface	....
Casler's	Pathological	43	Uterus prev. removed for neoplasm, also ovary in question.	Probably	Uterus previously removed	Cyst within ovary	Not noted
Norris'	Slightly enlarged	29	No	Yes	Yes	Cyst within ovary	Not noted

tissue may have occurred in a cleft, in one of the ovaries. The two cases where the tissue is on the surface seem to favor the hypothesis advanced by Russell that they arose from anomalies of growth of the germinal epithelium. In the other four cases there was no apparent connection with the germinal epithelium, and in these cases it seemed more probable that Bremer's or Begg's suggestion is correct.

In conclusion then, we are dealing with a series of cases of a rare and interesting condition whose origin, we must admit, is not satisfactorily explained. All of the theories advanced are theoretically possible and for any of them concrete proof will be next to impossible. Embryology may be suggestive but hardly conclusive, for the reason that suggestive appearances in an embryo can never be proved to be the early stages of a condition found in adults unless all of the steps can be demonstrated, which seems unlikely in a condition of this rarity. Only if we are favored, like Mark Twain, to the extent of seeing St. Peter's skull at the age of seventeen and again in another museum at the time of his death, can we hope to bring forth actual proof by the aid of embryology.

With regard to the practical importance of the condition, I think we can agree that it is interesting academically, but as yet of unknown clinical significance.

NOTE: Since the preparation of this paper, several cases of the same sort have been reported by Sampson in a paper read before the American Gynecological Society, which appeared in *Archives of Surgery*, October, 1921. The discovery of endometrium in the wall in a large proportion of the so-called "hemorrhagic cysts of the ovary" would seem to bear out the opinion expressed in this paper that the condition under discussion is not of such rare occurrence as the scarcity of reported cases would suggest.

BIBLIOGRAPHY

(1) Casler, DeW. B.: Surg., Gynec. and Obst., August, 1920, xxxi, No. 2, p. 150. (2) Norris, C. C.: Ibid., p. 158. (3) Dudley, E. C.: Principles and Practice of Gynecology, 1913 ed. 6. (4) Veit, J., and others: Handbuch d. Gynäkologie, Wiesbaden, 1907, ed. 2. (5) Russell, W. W.: Bull. Johns Hopkins Hosp., 1899, x, 8. (6) V. Franqué, O.: Sitzungsber. der Physikal Med. Gesellsch. in Würtzburg, 1898, No. 4. (7) Lewis, W. H.: Anat. Rec., vi, 141. (8) Küstner, O.: Kurzes Lehrbuch der Gynäkologie, Jena, 1904, ed. 2. (9) Gebhard, Carl: Pathologische Anatomie der Weiblichen Geschlechtsorgane, Leipzig, 1899. (10) Aschoff, L.: Pathologische Anatomie, Jena, 1911. (11) Keibel and Mall: Manual of Human Embryology, 1910, Philadelphia and London.

205 BEACON STREET.

Society Transactions

AMERICAN ASSOCIATION OF OBSTETRICIANS, GYNECOLOGISTS, AND ABDOMINAL SURGEONS. THIRTY-FOURTH ANNUAL MEETING HELD AT ST. LOUIS, MO., SEPTEMBER 20, 21, AND 22, 1921

(Continued from the January issue)

DR. M. PIERCE RUCKER, of Richmond, Va., read a paper on **The Action of the Commoner Ecbolics in the First Stage of Labor.** (For original article see page 134.)

DISCUSSION

DR. GORDON K. DICKINSON, JERSEY CITY, N. J.—In a paper which I recently read I quoted from Robertson's ''Biochemistry,'' in which he stated that the colostrum had the same effect as pituitrin. It would be well if Dr. Rucker could verify that in some of his future experiments.

DR. ARTHUR H. BILL, CLEVELAND, OHIO.—I have been much interested in this problem for some time. In the last six months, an identical series of experiments have been carried on in the Cleveland Maternity Hospital by Dr. F. S. Mowry. There is not time to discuss in detail the findings of these experiments, but I wish to emphasize the fact that experiments of this kind are extremely valuable. We have observed clinically the effect of these drugs, but to have a very accurate picture of just what they will do in labor should prove of much value to us in practice.

DR. RUCKER, (closing).—I am indebted to Dr. Dickinson for his suggestion. In the action of the ergot the interesting thing would be to see whether the ergot is properly tested, and whether it is carried to absorption. I think we are led to put more dependence in ergot than it deserves. If it does not produce uterine contractions, why use it?

DR. GEORGE CLARK MOSHER, of Kansas City, Mo., presented a paper entitled **Ten Years of Painless Childbirth.** (For original article see page 142.)

DISCUSSION

DR. WILLIAM H. CONDIT, MINNEAPOLIS, MINNESOTA.—Every new measure or method brought before the profession has gone through three stages: introduction, exploitation, and conservative application. It appears as though we were in the stage of exploitation of the methods for relief of the pain of childbirth. We cannot teach the students these extreme methods, from hypnotism to the Potter operation. We employ methods which we think strike a happy medium; treat every case for delivery as a law unto herself and use morphine when indicated. We are happy with our results from gas, with an apparatus that permits the use of ether, if necessary. We do use pituitrin, but never in more than five minim doses. We get short second stages and the patients come through with good results—we think, better statistical results—in the end. Why not take this happy middle ground instead of accepting some ground that we cannot feel absolutely sure of?

I was surprised to hear that Dr. Bill is not using nitrous oxid. We get very good results and never think of using chloroform.

DR. ROLAND E. SKEEL, LOS ANGELES, CAL.—Purely as a side issue Dr. Mosher's paper has brought out an interesting point in that he has abandoned morphine in favor of pantopon.

Shortly after Sahli made his observations upon the difference in the therapeutic effects of morphine and the combined hydrochloric acid soluble alkaloids of opium, we started on a series of clinical experiments to ascertain which was the more valuable as a surgical narcotic, inasmuch as opium had an undoubted stimulating effect upon the heart which morphine did not have. This was done by giving morphine and pantopon alternately to every operative case regardless of the nature of the operation or character of the anesthetic, and it was found that the patients having pantopon not only were more comfortable than the morphine patients but that vomiting was materially lessened after the former. In laparotomies this worked out in about the proportion of one to three, that is three times as many vomiting attacks followed the use of morphine as followed the use of pantopon as the pre-and postanesthetic narcotic. Since that time pantopon-atropine instead of morphine-atropine has been used almost without exception and if those who believe in a mixed narcosis will follow this plan in their gynecologic patients I am confident these patients will suffer less shock and have a more comfortable convalescence with much less nausea and vomiting.

DR. EDWARD SPEIDEL, Louisville, Ky., read a paper entitled **An Analysis of the Potter Version.** (For original article see page 150.)

DISCUSSION

DR. IRVING W. POTTER, BUFFALO, NEW YORK.—Dr. Speidel has discussed version from three standpoints without endorsing the procedure.

I wish he had taken another course and given his own personal experience with it and either advocated or condemned it. We know it can be performed in the house or hospital. We also know that a small hand and arm are better than a large hand and arm. We know that the position of the patient is of importance and that the modified Walcher position is the ideal one to employ. As for the anesthetic, we have concluded that chloroform is the best and see no reason to change. We use it because of the rapidity with which the patients recover and because of the complete relaxation which is necessary in doing a version.

Of course the cervix must be obliterated and the os dilated. We wait until the parts are ready, it makes no difference whether it is half an hour or three days, provided the woman is comfortable.

We have found green soap to be a splendid lubricant and a splendid cleansing agent for the vaginal canal. This makes the parturient tract about as sterile as it can be made in that length of time. With plenty of green soap and plenty of time to dilate the vaginal canal, the hand can be introduced into the vagina without any danger. Then the ironing out process is begun and version is started. I still maintain that the left hand is the proper one to use. In that way the right hand is left for outside work, and the doctor should school himself to use only one hand for the work in the uterus. When one hand has been introduced into the uterus it should not be withdrawn until the feet come along, in the average case.

There should be no time limit placed on this operation. The cord is not pulsating and has not since the baby has left the brim of the pelvis because there is pressure on it.

One of the effective points of this method consists in the delivery of the shoulders. As one of the shoulders rotates underneath the arch, the arm is being lifted up over the chest. The posterior shoulder is then brought forward by rotating the body. In that way you keep away from the rectum, avoid the tears which you formerly had, and, deliver both as anterior shoulders. What difference does it make whether the head rotates and comes through one or the other side of the pelvis? I think it is a mistake to deliver one shoulder posteriorly when it is the rectum we are trying to get away from. Another thing. These patients should not have an antepartum enema. If they do, you will have a liquid fecal matter distributed all over the field of operation, and that is wrong.

Now, who shall do versions? I do not believe the ordinary practitioner should rush in and do versions, but I think the men who are properly trained can do versions with benefit to the mother and child. I do not advocate, and never have, that the man who is seeing scarlet fever and diphtheria, and such things, should go and put his hand up in the vagina and uterus just as if he was putting it in his pocket. That is not fair to the man, the woman, or the method. I have done version in a great many cases and I have widened the field for the application of version, and I believe that I have avoided many complications by this procedure.

I work in Buffalo in many different institutions as there is no institution large enough to contain all of it. That makes my work scattered, which is unfortunate. Statistics are not reliable in all of those places. If there was but one large institution where the work could be done under the supervision of a certain set of individuals, it would be ideal. Last year I delivered over 1130 women and over 900 of them were version cases. This compares favorably with the preceding year, in which 1113 were delivered. My fetal mortality was 2.3 per cent.

I have tried for five years to bring before you a method that would stand up under opposition, and I submit to you these results. They are the best so far that I have been able to produce.

DR. M. PIERCE RUCKER, RICHMOND, VIRGINIA.—I have the honor of being one of Dr. Potter's early disciples. I started doing version, principally, because it saved the mother pain, and I became more enthusiastic because it saved the mother's perineum, and I became more enthusiastic still when I realized that it saved the babies. Men who have inquired into the deaths of babies during the first days after birth, find that a large percentage have cerebral hemorrhage, which may or may not be the cause of the death but it is a pathologic condition. Of 481 babies, 21 have come to autopsy, only 2 have shown signs of intracranial hemorrhage. One premature baby lived a few hours and died with a large intracranial hemorrhage, which, I believe, was due to pituitrin. One case had a contracted pelvis and a prolapsed hand. I did a version but had to force the head through the pelvis by brute force; that baby had a cerebral hemorrhage. The other 19 babies came to autopsy from enlarged thymus and other conditions, not intracranial hemorrhage. I think we must take this point into consideration in choosing the method of delivery. I believe if you follow up the babies for a year, you will find that the babies after easy births far surpass in their chances of survival those that have difficult deliveries.

DR. LEE DORSETT, ST. LOUIS, MISSOURI.—I had the pleasure of spending a few days with Dr. Potter and on returning home took up his method of version in some of my cases. I have not done it as a routine method of delivery, but in certain selected cases it has worked admirably. In occipitoposterior positions I think that it is the only method of delivery. I do not think that the Scanzoni or similar procedures have any place. Unless every step in Dr. Potter's technic is followed the whole method will be a failure.

It is my opinion that chloroform is the only anesthetic to be used. Ether is much slower, more of the drug is necessary, and its elimination is much slower. In abdominal cesarean sections where the resuscitation of the child is often necessary I have always noted that there is a strong odor of ether on the child's breath for some time after its delivery.

In regard to "ironing out" the vagina, Dr. Potter does not "spring" the vagina with two fingers, as some other men have taught, but inserts the whole hand within the vagina and, usually, spends from five to ten minutes in the process of dilatation.

As to bringing down both feet during extraction of the child, it has been my experience that it is often difficult to grasp both feet at the same time, so that I have been compelled to draw one foot through the cervix, then go after the other, and bring both through the vagina and vulva together.

In my work, so far, I have lost one baby in doing version. Looking back at this case now, I can readily see my mistake. The case was one of eclampsia in which labor was induced by the bag. As the patient was not doing well, having poor contractions and an alarmingly high blood pressure, I went through a partially dilated cervix and did a version; but the cervix contracted upon the aftercoming head and the baby was lost.

I have been surprised when observing the perineum in the cases after delivery, to note how readily that structure "snapped" back in place. I have examined these cases from one to two months after delivery and in all of them the perineum was intact.

DR. O. H. SCHWARZ, ST. LOUIS, MO.—I have had the opportunity of seeing Dr. Potter at work in Buffalo, and there is no question that his method of version is admirable. If one is performing his version, it must be done in the minutest detail. I think doing it as a routine procedure is entirely wrong. One must remember that where conservative obstetrics is practiced, very admirable results are obtained.

I was very enthusiastic in employing version in cases of occipitoposterior positions, but before doing this I consulted the literature on the management of occipitoposterior cases. One of the first papers I consulted was that of Plass, published in 1916, in the Johns Hopkins Bulletin. The incidence of occipitoposterior position was 11½ per cent. He explains this low percentage by the fact that many cases were not examined until well in labor, and rotation had probably occurred in many instances. Operative interference was necessary in 22 per cent of 600 cases. The mortality was 4.02 per cent, including babies of 2500 grams and up. If we employ version in such cases, we must equal or better these figures.

We employ the Potter version in occipitoposterior positions in such cases where there is no progress within a reasonable time after full dilatation of the os. We use the method in preference to Scanzoni application and to application of forceps with the occiput transverse.

DR. ARTHUR H. BILL, CLEVELAND, OHIO.—Heretofore we have discussed the question of whether version is a proper routine procedure. This morning we are to discuss the method of delivery. It seems to me to be for the most part very commendable. One or two steps which, in the hands of the average man, give trouble have not been emphasized.

In the first place, in regard to the delivery of the shoulders, I would like to suggest a slight improvement. It has been our practice to deliver the anterior shoulder first, and I think that is the proper procedure. Instead of putting the fingers in and sweeping the hand down, it is our practice to grasp the baby by the body, with its back to the front, draw it downward and outward in a direction opposite to the shoulder to be delivered, at the same time making a rotary movement. What happens is that the arm meets the resistance of the pubic arch, and is thrown across the chest, the shoulder, and usually the entire arm, being delivered by this movement without inserting the fingers into the vagina at all. Then by the same movement downward and outward in the opposite direction, the other arm is delivered. The advantage is that you do not need to insert the fingers into the vagina, and no traction is made on the arm.

Now, about delivery of the after-coming head. It has been stated that it makes no difference through which diameter of the inlet the head passes. It certainly does make a difference. I believe that many babies are lost in version because of this mistake. When the baby is delivered with its back to the front, we are drawing the occipitofrontal diameter of the child's head through the conjugate diameter of the inlet. The occipitofrontal diameter of the child's head in some cases is greater than the conjugate diameter of the pelvis, and hence there is difficulty in the extraction of the head. Before making traction on the child's head, if it lies in the anteroposterior diameter, rotate it to an oblique position, and then make traction; and, after it is through the inlet, internal rotation. Let the child's head follow the path it would follow in normal labor.

DR. SPEIDEL (closing discussion).—I am sorry to say I am not prepared as yet to follow in Dr. Potter's footsteps, by endorsing his version for every case. In a multipara with full dilatation of the os, who will easily deliver in fifteen or twenty minutes, with nitrous oxide or chloroform so there will be no discomfort in the second stage, I cannot see why such a baby should be turned, and the woman submitted to the risk of podalic version. I do say that there are indications for this version, and I cannot see why it should not be used in all face presentations. I think the majority of occipitoposterior positions should be delivered by version, and in breech presentations, the final steps should be as in the Potter version. I mentioned in my paper that the Potter version is easier than the old podalic version. But even in the hands of an expert this version is not easy. There is a decided nervous tension in such circumstances and none of us are absolutely sure that the baby is going to be born alive. The crucial point is the delivery of the after-coming shoulders and head; and Dr. Potter should be able to improve upon that.

I am glad Dr. Bill endorsed my suggestion that if the delivery is conducted according to the proper mechanism, this will make it easier. The shoulders should come down in the left oblique diameter, the head is then in the right oblique diameter and, consequently, it should be easier to deliver the shoulder and head in those diameters.

In regard to the indications: If it can be shown by postmortems that babies die of hemorrhage of the brain in normal deliveries because of a long-continued second stage of labor, then, of course, it is an indication for using this version; but if the hemorrhages only show themselves in abnormal cases it means that the version is indicated only in abnormal cases. Until you can show that these hemorrhages occur in normal cases, I am not prepared to follow Dr. Potter in using this version in normal delivery.

Dr. JOHN F. MORAN, Washington, D. C., read a paper entitled **Treatment of Eclampsia; Then and Now.** (For original article see page 155.)

DISCUSSION

DR. E. GUSTAVE ZINKE, CINCINNATI, OHIO.—I congratulate Dr. Moran not only on the splendid manner in which he presented the subject, but also upon the change which has come over him in his method of practice. I have for years held that surgery has contributed absolutely nothing to the reduction of maternal or fetal mortality in puerperal eclampsia. The old saying of obstetricians of fifty and seventy-five years ago—"treat the convulsions and let the pregnancy alone" —is a good one; but, of course, there are exceptions. I regret very much that the treatment of puerperal eclampsia by veratrum viride has received so little attention, not only by the obstetricians of this country, but by those abroad. An eclamptic woman in labor, especially if the first stage has been completed, should be delivered as soon as possible; but an eclamptic not in labor, one in whom the seizures begin perhaps during the fifth, sixth or seventh month, is an entirely different matter. I have had cases and have seen cases in the hands of other men, which were seized with puerperal eclampsia during the sixth and seventh month, have three, four or five seizures, and then the attacks would cease and the patients go to the end of term and deliver themselves without difficulty.

Veratrum viride is the remedy par excellence in the treatment of eclampsia. If it is administered properly, in antiseptic preparation, it arrests the convulsions, the woman goes on to the end of term and in nearly all instances delivers herself. Eclampsia is, in my opinion, a strictly medical disease. Cesarean section and accouchement forcé are absolutely unjustifiable in the treatment of puerperal eclampsia in the absence of other indications. This has been the position I have taken for the last fifteen years and I have seen all the varieties of puerperal eclampsia. One fact should not be forgotten: Puerperal eclampsia may be produced by three causes, the most frequent is kidney insufficiency; the second, acute yellow atrophy of the liver; the third, which is the rarest, an apoplectic seizure which cannot be cured by any means. In other words, some cases are fatal from the start; no matter what you may do, they will die.

DR. JOHN O. POLAK, BROOKLYN, NEW YORK.—In the first place it seems to me that the proper treatment of eclampsia should be the preventive treatment. No matter whether we have adopted the surgical method of delivery or the expectant plan of treatment, which we have been using for the past four or five years, we have found that there is very little difference in the actual mortality. The eclamptic patient is an exceedingly bad surgical risk. Those of you who have seen these cases and have followed them through their convulsions have noticed that at first there is an increased leucocytosis and as the convulsions increase the leucocytic count falls. Those who are very toxic never have any increase in the leucocytes, which immediately condemns them from the surgical standpoint. The temperature increases with the convulsions and that, again, condemns them from the surgical standpoint.

I was "brought up" on veratrum viride and we used it with my former chief for years, and we were losing 18 to 20 per cent, and with the morphine method about the same. We cut it down for about a year to about 15 per cent but now it is about 20 per cent again. With the surgical method we lost about 21 to 23 per cent as an average over a period of several years.

Two classes of cases come to us, one in which the toxic effect is primarily exerted on the liver and the oxidation is not complete, the toxic material enters the blood, acting as an irritant on the kidney. The other class presents a primarily sick kidney. I do not fear the latter as I do the fulminating type.

We have found that the blood pressure is the important thing in diagnosis. In making tests over many weeks we found that the hypopressure is characteristic of the normal pregnant woman. The moment there is a hypertension with relative increase, we are beginning to get into trouble, and a pressure of 130 is more dangerous and significant in the pregnant than in the normal woman. We find that the gradual increase of the blood pressure precedes by many days the toxic picture in either urine or blood. We are doing blood chemistry tests on every case, and nothing is so disappointing as this blood chemistry picture. There is nothing that gives us an early sign of what is happening in these women, so we have come to depend upon the clinical findings and the blood pressure rather than any other points.

DR. MAGNUS A TATE, CINCINNATI, OHIO.—So long as we do not know the cause, we are bound to have a variety of treatments for puerperal eclampsia. The essayist very forcibly spoke of prenatal care; and one of the most important things is blood pressure, as emphasized by the last speaker. Irving's statistics show very conclusively the value of the blood pressure, as a patient with a pressure of 180 is almost sure to have an eclamptic seizure. A valuable adjunct to the treatment of puerperal eclampsia is washing out the stomach and the flushing of the bowels, and, if necessary, repeated gavage.

I am sorry to disagree with Dr. Zinke about veratrum viride. I have tried it conscientiously for many years, but have given it up, because, I find it an extremely depressing drug, in some cases very dangerous, and the mortality from its use is very high.

I have never done an abdominal cesarean section for a case of eclampsia. I have never seen a case where I thought it was indicated. If the os is soft and dilatable, then I believe delivery should be forced. If the case be one in which the os is not dilatable but rigid, it seems to me, the expectant treatment is the best to follow.

Of drugs, morphia, in my experience, has given the best results, one-half grain to the dose, repeated as necessary.

DR. M. PIERCE RUCKER, RICHMOND, VIRGINIA.—I would like to ask Dr. Moran to tell us, in closing, if he has had any unfortunate experience with morphine. I will cite one case very briefly to illustrate what I mean.

Several months ago I had a patient who was taken with convulsions. We started morphine, stomach washing, irrigations, and so forth, and everything was going on nicely. The respirations were reduced to fourteen per minute and at 1:15 she got her last dose of ¼ grain of morphine. At 5 o'clock she suddenly stopped breathing and became livid. I pulled her over the edge of the bed and started artificial respiration and washed the stomach out again, thinking possibly some of the morphine was being reabsorbed. She became conscious and talked, but only three-quarters of an hour later had a similar attack. As soon as artificial respiration started her normal respiration I put her on the table and did a version. She woke up just as the head was being expressed and the case terminated very favorably for the mother and baby. The pulse went down to 88 or 90 although it had been around 150. The blood pressure was 130 fifteen minutes before she was taken with the attack.

Tweedy, I believe, emphasized the fact that a case of eclampsia should not be left in the charge of anyone but an obstetrician, and I think this case demonstrates that fact.

The patient received 1¼ grains in four hours. I have given as much as 5 grains in seven hours without bad effect, and would like to get Dr. Moran's idea of the cause of this reaction in this particular case.

DR. JAMES E. DAVIS, DETROIT, MICHIGAN.—I would like to ask Dr. Polak in regard to his experience with the blood chemistry findings, whether he has come to the conclusion from the negative or positive phase of the findings that blood chemistry is of no use.

He surely does not wish us to infer that when a patient in the latter months of her pregnancy changes from a normal non-protein nitrogen to 50 or 60 mgm. per 100 c.c. of blood and shows also a creatinine increase, that such a finding is not a reliable guide.

DR. POLAK (replying to Dr. Davis.)—What I meant to convey was that I expected to find a constant evidence of retention in these repeated blood chemistry examinations. Where we find an increase of creatinine or nitrogen that always indicates to us a bad prognosis. We never carry that case along, but I have been disappointed in the fact that we do not find the constant changes in the blood which correspond to the clinical picture and the blood pressure readings.

DR. MORAN (closing the discussion).—I much prefer to bleed outwardly than to bleed inwardly. Therefore, I do not use veratrum viride. I am in thorough accord with the gentleman who discussed the dangers of veratrum viride. It is a purely depressant drug and when it is once used it is hard to combat its effect. Of course, you can bleed to any point you wish and get the blood pressure down to any desired point. Our purpose in not carrying the pressure below 150 is this: If we wish to give an anesthetic or to operate we do not want it too low, so we bring the pressure to 150 or thereabouts.

As to Dr. Rucker's question about the morphine, I am rather inclined to think that the quick reaction was due to something other than the morphine. Otherwise, the patient would not have so quickly recovered. As to massive doses I am always careful in giving morphine to watch the patient and the effect. I have seen one fourth grain of morphine given without my order by an interne reduce the respirations to six, and the interne was very uncomfortable. In giving any drug we should carefully watch the effect to see just what that particular patient needs. One-fourth grain of morphine is all that is necessary for one patient, while two grains may be required for another. In cases of coma we do not need morphine at all. In conclusion, I want to emphasize again the importance of prenatal care.

As to the blood pressure, I mentioned that the eyegrounds were examined because of the increased blood pressure. I consider it the most valuable of all the signs we have. The urinary findings come late but the blood pressure is significant and on examination of the eyegrounds you will very often detect a retinitis, and that the patient is in the danger zone. In the two cases of fatality reported in the paper, I am sure if examination of the eyegrounds had been made weeks before and the blood pressure checked up it would have been of inestimable value and I believe those patients might have recovered.

DR. JOHN O. POLAK AND DR. THURSTON S. WELTON, Brooklyn, N. Y., presented a paper on **A Study of the Origin of Bleeding in Ectopic Pregnancy.** (For original article see page 164.)

DISCUSSION

DR. HERMAN E. HAYD, BUFFALO, NEW YORK.—Dr. Polak has emphasized the importance of the corpus luteum in connection with this problem. Anything that explains to us the complex and complicated methods of creation is, of course, especially interesting. The essayist has shown us how a tubal pregnancy is practically the same as a corporeal, except that in the one a better decidua is formed and better implantation; while in the tube it is distributed more irregularly. I think he is justified in the conclusions he has drawn, that the hemorrhage is consequent not only upon the peristaltic action of the tube, but also upon some endocrine influence.

Perhaps some of you have seen the reports of the work of a veterinary in Danbury, Connecticut, where there was a splendid herd of cattle on a stock farm, but only thirteen viable calves were born in a year. He found upon investigation that these cattle were infected with a virulent coccus similar to the gonococcus, and as a result there was a peritonitis and a subacute salpingitis and oöphoritis with thickened covering and as a result, the corpus luteum could not rupture. These animals did not therefore "come into heat" and no young were born. By injections into the vagina, massage and friction, he succeeded in breaking these graafian follicles, and they let loose their unabsorbed corpora lutea, and every one of these animals within eighteen to thirty hours came in heat and became impregnated. Now, when this man made a mistake and found that some of these animals he was massaging were already impregnated, he produced a terrific intraperitoneal hemorrhage or an abortion within twenty-four hours, showing that the corpus luteum had much to do in these hemorrhages.

Dr. Polak has brought out the fact that these uterine hemorrhages are a symptom, and they will continue no matter what kind of conditions are opposed to them in the way of treatment, so long as that corpus luteum exists in that ovary.

THE NEW YORK OBSTETRICAL SOCIETY. MEETING OF NOVEMBER 8, 1921

THE PRESIDENT, DR. RALPH H. POMEROY, IN THE CHAIR

DR. ONSLOW A. GORDON presented a report on a case of **Uterine Torsion in Pregnancy with Fatal Results.**

This unusual case was admitted to the Gynecological Department of Bellevue Hospital, April 28, 1921. I am indebted to Dr. Holden for the privilege of reporting this case.

History.—A. B., twenty-seven years of age, a negress, married for ten years. Her chief complaints were pain in the lower abdomen and an abdominal tumor. Her family history was irrelevant as to her present condition. Her previous history—medical and surgical—was negative. She was the mother of four children, the youngest three years old. All deliveries and puerpera were normal. There were no miscarriages. Her menstrual history began at fourteen years, was always regular every 28 days, flowing profusely for 4 days without pain. Her last regular period was in December, 1920. She was constipated, had marked frequency of urination and thought her urine contained blood.

Her present illness began several weeks prior to her admission to the hospital. She first noticed a dragging pain in the abdomen and slight vaginal bleeding. Her bleeding has not been constant. Her abdominal pain was located in both lower quadrants, was dull and continuous and had been increasing in severity for several days prior to her admission. She had noticed a gradually increasing abdominal tumor for about two months. She had considered herself pregnant but denied any intrauterine interference.

On admission, she had a profuse and foul-smelling leucorrheal discharge.

Physical Examination.—A markedly distended abdomen in a thin and emaciated patient. There is a plainly palpable tumor mass, apparently arising from the pelvis and extending several cm. above the umbilicus. This mass is regular in outline and resembles in size and shape the body of a pregnant uterus about the fifth month. There are several hard and nodular masses plainly palpable about the upper portion of this mass. The mass is only slightly tender and there is only moderate abdominal rigidity.

Vaginal examination shows a long, soft cervix dilated to about two fingers. The uterus seems to be drawn up out of the pelvis and is enlarged to about the size of a five months' pregnancy. There is no bulging in the fornices. There is a profuse and putrid bloody vaginal discharge.

A provisional diagnosis was made of pregnancy with macerated fetus and possible fibromyoma uteri.

Clinical History.—The patient presented the usual picture of puerperal sepsis. Temperature upon admission was 102.3° per rectum and pulse 130. She gradually became weaker and, on the fifth day after admission, she was transfused with 750 c.c. of blood. She died on the following day, six days after admission, presenting the usual picture of a severe puerperal sepsis with peritonitis.

Autopsy Report (Abstract).—The abdomen is very prominent. A mass is felt in the lower portion of the abdomen, extending upward to about 1 inch above the umbilicus. On section, the subcutaneous fatty layer is scant. The peritoneum is cloudy throughout. The intestines in the lower portion of the abdomen are considerably matted together and are plastered to a large tumor mass which occupies the center and lower portion of the abdomen.

The uterus is large, extends above the umbilicus and seems to be twisted on itself so that the left ovary comes around in front and is adherent to the uterine wall in the midline anteriorly; whereas the right ovary is behind the uterus and to the left. The musculature is black in color, especially near the fundus of the uterus. In this place, the walls are very thin. The cervix is considerably elongated and forms a hook-like projection below and slightly to the left side of the mass of the uterus.

On opening the uterus from the cervix, the canal goes upward to the left of the main mass of uterine tissue for about 3 inches and then turns to the right to enter the main portion of the uterine cavity.

The placenta is attached to the left inner side of the uterine wall. There are two hemorrhagic areas in the middle of the placenta, each being about 1 inch in diameter. The female fetus is about 6 inches in length and gangrenous throughout.

Conclusions.—This case presents primarily the interesting question of spontaneous torsion of the uterus. It is our opinion that this woman became pregnant, developed sepsis and peritonitis, aggravated by the spontaneous torsion of the uterus. I do not believe that the torsion of the uterus produced either the sepsis or the peritonitis.

Torsion of the uterus to a marked degree is a decidedly infrequent pathologic state. Schultze reviewed the literature prior to 1907 and found 32 cases reported of which 13 were caused by myomata, some without pregnancy and some associated with pregnancy and 17 by ovarian cysts. In 2 cases, torsion of four complete turns is recorded. There is no case on record of actual gangrene of the uterus or peritonitis, resulting solely from torsion.

Extreme torsion is nearly always associated with pregnancy which permits hypertrophy and relaxation of the round ligaments. Slight torsion is physiologic in pregnancy after the fourth month when the fundus has risen above the pelvic brim.

The rotation is only possible above the cervix because of the fascial attachments below the internal os.

The etiologic factors usually present in cases of torsion are:

1. An infantile type of uterus, giving a long cervix as an axial point about which torsion may take place.

2. A large pelvis and a partial faulty position of the uterus which may be increased by severe intestinal peristalsis.

(As I have previously stated myomata, ovarian cysts and tumors and pregnancy are usually present.)

The diagnosis of torsion is practically never made except at operation or autopsy. Intense bladder disturbances with, possibly, blood in the urine are frequently noted and may be suggestive. This is probably produced by traction upon the vesical fascia.

DISCUSSION

DR. WILLIAM M. FORD.—I would ask that Dr. Gordon suggest, in closing, what the origin of the sepsis might have been, or whether that is still an obscure cause of the rotation of the uterus.

DR. H. N. VINEBERG.—One cannot very well criticize this case although I recall a similar instance about seven or eight years ago, in which the patient with a miscarriage at four or five months, had a sloughing fibroid. She was seen by several eminent gynecologists and told that an operation would mean sure death. When I saw her she had a temperature of 105° F., a coated tongue, pulse 140 and was semicomatose, but still I thought she should be given a chance. I had the patient transferred to Mount Sinai Hospital and operated on that night. The next morning she presented an entirely different picture. She was bright, had recovered consciousness, the temperature had dropped to 102° F., and she made a good recovery. Of course that patient was in pretty good general condition. She was well nourished, and although her pulse was rapid, it was fairly good. It seems to me, on general principles, that the patient on first coming to the hospital (I understand she was there six days) should have been given a chance, because the peritonitis, I feel, was only secondary, and if the uterus had been removed early, I believe she might have recovered.

DR. EBEN FOSKETT.—The records of Bellevue Hospital will show one case of fibroid of the uterus with torsion, which also resulted in death. That was in Dr. Studdiford's service. She came in with severe shock and a distended abdomen and the case was looked on as one of an acute abdominal condition and the operation was begun. The abdomen was found full of serous fluid, which was rather dark in color. This was evidently due to the shutting off of the circulation by the torsion. The patient died on the table.

DR. ONSLOW A. GORDON, JR.—As to Dr. Ford's question about the cause of the sepsis: we quizzed the patient carefully at the time she was admitted as to any induction of abortion or interruption of pregnancy and she denied that she had had any. I presume the sepsis was spontaneous, as it may be. She had a macerated fetus in a five months' pregnancy, and many cases of spontaneous sepsis arise in that way.

As to Dr. Vineberg's question as to why we didn't operate, I would say we made a diagnosis on admission that the patient was septic and it is not our policy to operate in sepsis and remove the uterus.

DR. HARVEY B. MATTHEWS presented a case of **Bacillus Welchii Blood Stream Infection with Autopsy Report.** (Case Report to be published.)

DISCUSSION

DR. EMIL SCHWARTZ.—The cases are not very rare, but they are always very interesting. The question is as to just where the infection comes from. Dr. Matthews outlined the various habitats of the bacillus Welchii, and it is only fair to assume that a large number of them are probably from the bodies of the patients themselves, since most individuals carry the bacillus Welchii in their intestinal contents. It is just a question whether a search of the literature would not show that in practically all, or almost all of the cases there was some surgical interference. The streptococcus has been found in cases of bacillus Welchii infection. Where the case had surgical interference, it is very well possible that the patient was the carrier of the bacillus Welchii and was infected at the time of the surgical operation. Cases have been reported where a premature labor was induced under most favorable conditions in large hospitals and the gas bacillus later on killed the patients. I remember one clinic where that happened twice in six months on the induction of premature labor. In both cases gas bacillus infections occurred; so apparently it is either that the infection was taken from the floor or from the surroundings in the hospital, or that the patients were unfortunate enough to spread it into the operative cavity or otherwise.

DR. GEORGE L. BRODHEAD.—We have had two fatal cases of gas bacillus infection on the Harlem Hospital service, both after abortion (I do not know whether it was artificial or not), and the characteristic symptom in both of these cases which gave us a clue to the diagnosis, was the very intense bronzing of the skin. Both cases terminated fatally and both occurred after jaundice.

DR. J. MILTON MABBOTT.—I want to refer to a case I reported about twenty years ago before the Medical Society of the State of New York under a title that I had to coin myself of "pneumogalactocele," with an unidentified bacillus. The bacteriology was done under the supervision of Dr. Harlow Brooks, and it is a question whether there could be a localized infection by the bacillus aerogenes capsulatus in one breast only, where there were no other serious symptoms, and where, after aspiration of gas and milk, an incision was promptly followed by recovery.

DR. WILLIAM M. FORD.—May I qualify the observation made by Dr. Brodhead with my own observations in a limited number of cases of gas bacillus infection? I refer to the bronzing of the skin. Most of the cases I have had an opportunity to see, followed traumatisms involving skin wounds and had the characteristic bronzing of the skin, but it did not appear to me to be a general bronzing. It rather appeared as an extension from the site of the wound. In each instance it traveled very rapidly from the wound like an erysipelas rash. Following the bronzing of the skin, which was quite distinctly marked and limited, was the crepitation in the subcutaneous tissues. One of these infections followed an operation for inguinal hernia in which every ordinary aseptic precaution had been taken. The patient was a Greek waiter and I suppose his skin was infected from his rectum.

DR. GORDON GIBSON.—There is one thing in Dr. Matthews' paper to which I think we should take exception, and that is the treatment by expectancy. I think that is possible only if the infection is general. It is unfortunate that you cannot spot infection in the uterus unless you have a blood culture, for while the infection is in the uterus, radical operation is the only hope.

DR. RALPH H. POMEROY.—I noted Dr. Schwartz's reference to the occurrence of bacillus Welchii infection where premature labor had been induced.

Some three years ago I had a very disturbing experience with a case of that kind, in which the labor in an elderly primipara was induced in an effort to prevent her from going too far over time. After the vagina was flushed with lysol solution and with the patient under an anesthetic the membranes were stripped back through a one-finger cervix; the patient developed a gas bacillus infection, resulting in the death of the child (delivery of a dead fetus) and eventually, a week later, the death of the mother. That experience is cited just to point out the difficulties of being sure of what we can do in the way of dealing with the cervix even under conditions that we suppose are perfectly safe.

I might say that although a number of these cases have been reported, the bacteriologic diagnosis has not always been made. A clinical diagnosis is all that has been made in most instances. Dr. Brodhead did not say that he had cultured any secretions or found the Bacillus Welchii in the blood, or in the contents of the uterus.

In regard to the bronzing of the skin; I spoke of the bronze color, but thought it was better to call it a deep jaundice. The sclera of the case reported tonight was so jaundiced that you could hardly tell her eyes from the surrounding skin.

Dr. Gibson's suggestions as to the expectant treatment may or may not be well taken. His point of making a diagnosis early and doing a hysterectomy seems to me questionable because, even then, you are opening up a great many channels for infection; you are leaving blood clots in which B. Welchii thrive; there is always some, and there may be a great deal of destruction of tissue in doing a hysterectomy, and we know that these organisms grow best in dead tissue. I was in hopes I could find a case in which some one had done a hysterectomy, but they seem to be afraid to do it and in my opinion they are right.

Dr. WILLIAM SIDNEY SMITH reported a case of **Double Pyelitis Complicating Pregnancy at Sixth Month.**

This case is presented with the hope that it may provoke some discussion as to the value of catheterizing the ureters and instilling a silver salt in the kidney pelvis.

This patient was a fragile, pale primipara of twenty-eight years, with a negative past history. She came under observation during the third month of pregnancy, complaining of vomiting and loss of weight. The urine contained acetone and diacetic acid, but there was no albumin, no casts or pus. The blood pressure was low, 98/60. Appropriate treatment relieved her symptoms. The urine became normal, she was able to retain nourishment and there was a slight gain in weight.

At the end of the fourth month the patient went to the seashore and felt so well that she went in bathing. That evening she noticed some chilly feelings. During the days that followed, chilly feelings and one or two degrees of temperature occurred every afternoon. Nausea and vomiting with loss of strength again appeared. Urinalysis was reported normal.

At the beginning of the fifth month the patient again came under supervision and was sent to the Hospital, complaining of moderate nausea, with aching pain in both lumbar regions and general weakness. Heart, lungs and extremities were normal. Abdomen was slightly distended and there was tenderness in both lumbar regions. Blood pressure was 110/68 on admission, T, P, R, 99° - 100 - 20. Catheter specimen of urine showed a slight cloud, sp. gr. 1015, trace of albumin, no sugar, trace of acetone and diacetic acid. There were a moderate number of pus cells, no casts. Blood examination showed a hemoglobin 50 per cent, red cells 2,912,000, white cells 12,200, polys 89 per cent, small lymphocytes 8 per cent, large lymphocytes 2 per cent, transitional cells 1 per cent.

A diagnosis was made of pregnancy complicated by a pyelitis and toxemia. Urotropin was given and appropriate treatment for toxemia was carried out.

During the following week the patient had a chill and sweat nearly every afternoon, temperature ranged between 99° and 104°, pulse between 90 and 120. Blood pressure remained fairly constant at 110/64. In spite of treatment the gastric symptoms became worse and weakness increased. The patient looked sick. On the days when she would eat and take alkalies the acetone and diacetic acid in the urine would clear up. Casts were not present at any time and clumped pus cells with a trace of albumin were constant. The white cells increased to 17,400, with 83 per cent of polymorphonuclears. On the eighth day after admission both ureters were catheterized and cystoscopy done. The bladder mucosa was moderately congested, vault somewhat depressed by a gravid uterus, ureter orifices normal in appearance. Catheters passed readily to kidney pelvis, with free urine flowing from both pelves; on the right side the flow was intermittent and rhythmic, on the left side the flow was steady (suggesting some degree of hydronephrosis). Phthalein was recovered from the right kidney in 12 minutes and from the left in 12 minutes. Three c.c. of 25 per cent argyrol was instilled into each kidney pelvis.

The right kidney urine contained many red cells and large clumps of pus cells, no casts. Left kidney urine contained large number of clumped pus cells. No casts. Cultures of this urine reported sterile, but a culture from a subsequent catheterized specimen from the bladder showed B. coli. It was negative for typhoid bacilli. Wassermann reaction was negative. The CO_2 combining power in 100 c.c. of blood was 502; creatinine, 1.48 mg.; urea, 25.89 mg.; sugar, 127 mg.

The patient was profoundly ill, listless, abdomen markedly distended. After consultation we decided to empty her uterus. We hoped that the gastrointestinal symptoms and her general condition would improve and so give the kidney condition a better chance to clear up. I decided to have a blood transfusion done just before doing a vaginal hysterotomy.

Before operation the hemoglobin was 50 per cent, red cells 2,835,000 and white cells 26,800 with 92 per cent polymorphonuclears. Blood transfusion (citrate method) with 600 c.c. of blood and in addition 250 c.c. of normal salt solution. The operation was difficult owing to a small vagina, a long rigid cervix and a relatively good sized fetus. The patient stood the operation very well. Four hours after, her hemoglobin was 68 per cent.

The convalescence was slow, but steady and uneventful. The gastrointestinal symptoms began to improve at once. Appetite gradually returned and food was taken and retained. Chills ceased and temperature and pulse returned to normal. Strength, however, was relatively slow in returning. The acetone and diacetic acid disappeared at once after operation and the pus gradually cleared up. The patient left the hospital on the 33rd day after operation with a clear urine and feeling well except for general weakness.

DISCUSSION

DR. H. D. FURNISS.—In a great many of the cases of pyelitis there is a history of exposure to cold and chilliness, but in analyzing those cases I am in doubt whether they were chilled and had their trouble as a result of that, or whether the chill was an early evidence of the infection.

I believe a great many of these cases can be saved from hysterotomy and that they can be carried on to full term by proper treatment (pelvic lavage). This can be done as gently and with as little discomfort as an ordinary catheterization. With the use of the single catheter cystoscope there is no irritation, and very little, if any, discomfort to the patient. It is not an operating room procedure. The patient can be turned crossways in bed, put on a douche pan and the lavage done with very little trouble.

After a hysterotomy, or emptying of the uterus, a great many patients become better, but they are not necessarily cured for often they are going to be just as bad off as before.

To protect the kidneys, I think it is essential that they be properly drained and drained frequently.

In the washing out of these cases where there is hydronephrosis or hydroureter, the pelves should be thoroughly emptied and washed out with boric acid or sterile water to get rid of the urinary salts before instilling the silver nitrate.

It is also important in these cases to drain off the silver afterwards because of its caustic effect. It has recently been noted that the destructive effect of the silver on the epithelium lasted a week before new cells replaced the old.

The strength of the silver makes very little difference. The silver coagulates the albumin in the superficial layers, so 5 per cent has very little more effect than 1 per cent. Clinically, 5 per cent gives more reaction than 1 per cent. If you protect the bladder with salt solution there is no vesical irritation.

The results from pelvic lavage are so good that I feel no uterus should be emptied because of cystitis until such treatment has been tried.

DR. WILLIAM A. JEWETT.—It has always seemed to me in these cases of pyelitis complicating pregnancy that the most important thing is the question of the drainage of the kidney pelvis. In some this can be accomplished at this stage of gestation (about 6 months) by posture, having the foot of the bed elevated, and if the pyelitis is unilateral, having the patient turned to the opposite side, taking the pressure off the lower end of the ureter. We have treated some cases by washing them out with boric acid. We have also used silver nitrate. In certain cases we have used simple drainage of the kidney pelvis; that is, passing catheters on either side or on the affected side and leaving them *in situ* two, three or four hours so as to maintain drainage. In those cases we usually have a reduction in the severity of the symptoms, and there is also usually a reduction in the temperature. This procedure can be repeated at intervals, and, personally, it seems to me we get just about as good results by draining without irrigation as we do in the cases that have been irrigated.

DR. REGINALD M. RAWLS.—There is one thing which has been left out, and that is the method of treatment, and in order to make that plain I will cite a case under my care this summer in the Woman's Hospital. A woman came in five months' pregnant with apparently a surgical abdomen. The abdomen was extremely tender, the entire right side, from the umbilicus up to the point of the gall bladder, being involved. The case was running a temperature between 103° and 104°. The abdomen was very tender. The diagnosis she was sent in with was of pregnancy with acute appendicitis. The blood count showed a rather high polynuclear count. The urine was absolutely negative (bladder specimen), not a trace of pus, no albumin, no casts, normal specific gravity, reaction acid; and I was very careful to examine her for one point that I have never seen fail, and that is tenderness in the costovertebral angle. She was extremely tender on one side. She was seen in consultation by three or four men and the diagnosis ranged between ruptured appendix, or gall bladder. The patient was prepared for operation. I felt sure it was a case of pyelitis, although everything seemed against the diagnosis. She was to be operated on at 2:00 o'clock in the afternoon. About 11:00 o'clock that morning I called up Dr. Bugbee and asked him whether he would see the case. I told him I was afraid she was too ill to be cystoscoped. He saw the case with me and stated that there was no indication from her urine that she had any trouble but he decided to cystoscope her, with the result that the left kidney showed absolutely normal urine. The right kidney was entered with some difficulty and the urine returned was full of pus. He washed out the pelvis of the kidney on that side. That kidney pelvis was washed out but once and the specimen collected showed the presence of pure colon bacillus. She was at once placed in the Fowler position and given alternating doses of 10 grains of urotropin and two hours later 30 grains of monobasic sodium phosphate. The patient's temperature did not again rise above 101°, and in about five days was normal and the symptoms absolutely subsided. She was kept on urotropin in 7½ grain doses with 15 grains of acid sodium phosphate for 2 months. When I saw her last she was seven months' pregnant. She had never had a return of her former symptoms. In that particular case the washing out may have relieved the obstruction, but most of these infections, as we know, are bloodstream infections. The source of that infection was absorption from the gastrointestinal tract. By giving her acid sodium phosphate with urotropin we created a bactericide and thereby eliminated the infection.

Another case developed about the third or fourth day with high temperature and afternoon chill. She was sent to the Cystoscopic Clinic and it was demonstrated that she had a pyelitis. She was put on acid sodium phosphate and urotropin. In two days the temperature dropped to normal. In the course of time she reported again to the Cystoscopic Clinic. They are very much opposed to using urotropin and put her on methylene blue. After three days she had a recurrence of her trouble and she was put back on acid sodium phosphate and urotropin, with cessation of her symptoms.

I found by actual experiments that 50 per cent of cases in which urotropin is given alone, it is excreted as such, and that is the substance which causes the irritation. However, if you give the patient acid sodium phosphate you obviate the element of irritation. The only complication is occasionally a little diarrhea.

DR. ALBERT M. JUDD.—As I understand it, the causative factor in these cases is the colon bacillus which will develop only in an acid urine. Therefore, why would it not be just as well to alkalinize the urine so we would not have a urine in which the colon bacillus could develop? I have had cases get well under this treatment.

DR. HAROLD BAILEY.—As regards emptying the uterus, it seems to me that a woman with a pyelitis might have this done in a more simple manner, namely, by using a bag. You are going to have a pyelitis when you get through. I wonder whether it is a suitable procedure to do a hysterotomy in such cases. I noted in the paper that Dr. Smith described the cervix as long and narrow, and I think that is the reason he elected that procedure.

On the other hand, the treatment by catheterization, in speaking of which Dr. Jewett, I think, struck the keynote, although it was brought out by the reader of the paper, provides the drainage. It does not make very much difference what we irrigate with or if we irrigate with anything. As a matter of fact, no one claims that the silver kills the bacteria. It shrinks the mucous membrane and gives better drainage. There is no cleaning out of these individuals by washing out the pelvis of the kidney with 1 per cent silver nitrate. We let these cases go time and time again and the fever drops. We had a case that was seven months' pregnant with a temperature of 103°, and the moment she emptied herself the temperature dropped, but she is not well. She will probably pass out of our control and it may be three or four months before she has another attack. These patients should be turned over to the urologist for care. The mere instilling of a little silver nitrate during the acute attack does not cure the patient and only favors drainage.

DR. ALBERT M. JUDD.—May I call attention, Mr. President, to the fact that one gentleman drains his patients by raising the head of the bed and the other by raising the foot of the bed?

DR. WILLIAM S. SMITH.—This particular patient was drained by raising the head of the bed. The uterus was emptied, very largely because she was ill with her gastrointestinal symptoms. She was rapidly growing weaker. Forty-eight hours had made a very great difference in her general condition. She was not taking food, and we came to the conclusion that she could not stand it very much longer and unless we rid her of her pregnancy she would die. I did a hysterotomy rather than induce and let her have a spontaneous labor, which was discussed, because I felt that was the easiest and quickest way.

Dr. Edwin G. Langrock read a paper on **Pituitary Extract at Beginning of the Third Stage of Labor—A Report of 100 Cases.** (For original article see page 170.)

DISCUSSION

DR. GEORGE L. BRODHEAD.—When Dr. Ryder read his very interesting paper a year or so ago, Dr. Langrock and I determined to carry through a series of 100 cases to see how closely our figures would approximate those given by Dr. Ryder.

First, in regard to the method that was used: Williams in his discussion of hemorrhage in 1,000 cases of spontaneous labor placed a bed pan under the patient at the end of the second stage and kept it there until the placenta was delivered and for some little time afterwards. In our series as soon as the child was born, a basin was placed under the buttocks of the patient and was kept there until the placenta was removed, at which time another basin was placed, because we wished to ascertain the blood loss during the third stage as well as the blood loss following the birth of the placenta. The work was done a good many times under the direct observation of Dr. Langrock and myself, hence we believe that it was very carefully done and the statistics are reasonably accurate.

In our series the average blood loss was 177 c.c., which is very close to the figures of 180 c.c., given in Dr. Ryder's paper.

It is interesting to note that in the 200 cases in this and Dr. Ryder's series only four women lost 600 c.c. or more of blood, whereas, as Dr. Langrock pointed out, in the 1,000 cases reported by Williams, there was a loss of 600 c.c. or more in 130 cases, without pituitrin.

There is one point which I think we must consider. Is it possible that in giving 1 c.c. of pituitrin, if we do it often enough, we are eventually going to have a rupture of the uterus? Personally, I have not seen it, but Dr. Langrock has given me permission to report a case that I saw in consultation with him of rupture of the uterus after the birth of the placenta, apparently due to the administration of 1 c.c. of pituitrin. This patient was a multipara and Dr. Langrock reached the patient's house about thirty minutes after the birth of the child. The patient was in splendid condition. After making preparations to remove the placenta, the latter was easily expressed by Credé. He then gave her 1 c.c. of pituitrin and in a very few minutes the patient had a very sharp pain and had to have two doses of ¼ grain of morphine to quiet her. Her pulse rose to 120 or 130 and she was acutely ill. She evidently had a rupture of the uterus. When I saw her with Dr. Langrock she had a distinct mass reaching from the pelvis to the left lumbar region, apparently a very extensive hematoma. Dr. A. A. Berg who saw her later, agreed in the diagnosis of rupture of the uterus, and said that if she was operated on she would undoubtedly die. Several days later a large abscess opened in the fornix of the vagina and the patient made a slow, but complete recovery.

I see no reason why we should not in a long series of cases with a dose of 1 c.c. of pituitrin get a rupture of the uterus, although as to this I am frank to admit that I really do not know if such a thing is possible. However, this case of Dr. Langrock's, with the uterus empty, calls our attention to the possible danger from the use of pituitrin. I hope that in the course of the discussion if any one has had a rupture of the uterus in the third stage of labor (following the use of 1 c.c. of pituitrin) or knows of any, he will report it.

DR. GEORGE H. RYDER.—The series of cases in which pituitrin was given as a routine in the third stage of labor, is very interesting to me because of a similar series, tried at the Sloane Hospital, and reported by me last January.

Before speaking of this series, however, I would like to ask Dr. Brodhead a question in regard to the case that he reports, in which he says a rupture of the uterus took place after the administration of 1 c.c. of pituitrin, at the end of labor, that is, with an empty uterus. How did he make the diagnosis of the rupture? Is he sure that there was one? Is he sure that the woman did not have a pus tube that was ruptured? Up to this time, for years, it has been considered entirely safe to give pituitrin or ergot with an empty uterus; and I think we should always accept with reserve any unusual occurrence which tends to change such an idea, founded on such long and universal experience.

Referring to the series of 100 pituitrin cases reported in the paper, there are two things of which I wish to speak.

First, concerning the occurrence of hour-glass contraction of the uterus, after the administration of pituitrin in the third stage of labor. Since reporting in January the 100 cases of pituitrin in the third stage of labor, I have had an hour-glass contraction of the uterus, where pituitrin was so given. The case is interesting. The woman had what we call an irritable uterus for four days preceding labor. During all this time she was having irregular pains, which did not disturb her greatly, and which allowed her to sleep under small doses of morphine at night, and which caused practically no change in the dilatation of the cervix. At the end of this time, she went into normal labor, and was delivered by an easy low forceps operation. One-half c.c. of pituitrin was given four minutes after the birth of the baby. At the time it was given, the fundus was very hard and well contracted. Following this an hour-glass contraction of the uterus developed, and the placenta could not be expressed. Under ether it was extracted manually without difficulty. Looking back on this case, I think it was unwise to have given the pituitrin in the third stage. How much, if anything, the irritable uterus had to do with the hour-glass contraction, I do not know. At any rate, the fundus was already hard and well contracted. It seems possible that the pituitrin given with the uterus already very firm might have been responsible for the hour-glass contraction following. This experience has caused me to modify my technic in the use of pituitrin. Since then, where the fundus remains well contracted, no pituitrin is given till after the birth of the placenta. Where the fundus begins to soften and balloon or where there is hemorrhage, one-half c.c. of pituitrin is given, usually from four to five minutes after the birth of the baby, and another half c.c. immediately following the birth of the placenta. The idea is that the first dose holds the uterus firm until the second is given, and this continues the effect until the ergotole begins to exert its effect, which is not for nearly half an hour after. In this way, there is a continuous effect on the uterus to keep it contracted. Whereas if only the ergot or ergotole is given after the third stage, there is nearly half an hour elapsing before there is any such effect.

In speaking of hour-glass contraction, however, it is well to remember, as has been said, that it sometimes occurs where no pituitrin has been given. I have delivered one woman twice, at an interval of two years, and each time she had an hour-glass contraction of the uterus, with no pituitrin given. So it is not at all certain that the hour-glass contraction, in the pituitrin series, came from the pituitrin.

The second thing concerning which I wish to speak in the series reported, is that of undue hemorrhage in four cases mentioned. It seems to me that at least in one of these cases as reported, the hemorrhage might have been due to the fact that the placenta was not extracted soon enough. I think the statement was made that the doctor in charge waited an hour, with considerable bleeding taking place, and then extracted the placenta manually. I would say that this fact, and not the administration of the pituitrin was responsible for the bleeding. The other three hemorrhages may have had a similar cause. I believe a great many postpartum hemorrhages are due to this very cause—waiting too long with active bleeding before taking energetic measures to stop it. And I agree with the statement that bad postpartum hemorrhages are usually due to poor obstetrics.

It is very interesting to note that in both of these series, of 200 cases altogether, there is so little hemorrhage. But as the reader of the paper says, the giving of pituitrin in the third stage of labor, pleasing as the results may be, does not allow us to relax altogether our watchfulness of the uterus, during and after the third stage.

DR. GEORGE W. KOSMAK.—The resort to pituitrin in an attempt to cut down the amount of hemorrhage during and after labor is of some interest. Personally, I have never been able to comprehend its purpose. As I understand the physiology of the third stage, the uterus alternately contracts and relaxes until the placenta has separated, and that normal physiological contraction and relaxation, it seems to me, should not be interfered with because it provides for a proper and complete separation of the placenta. In giving pituitrin, especially in the comparatively large doses in which it has been administered in these cases, I believe we interfere with natural processes.

The amount of blood which is lost in an ordinary labor does not seem to harm the woman any and I think Williams showed very clearly in his series of cases that she could lose a comparatively large amount of blood and replenish it in a short time after delivery.

In view of the fact that pituitrin is such an uncertain thing and that different women react in different ways to the same dose, I personally believe it rather bad teaching to recommend pituitrin as a routine administration. I am very glad to hear Dr. Ryder, who has had a great deal of personal experience with these cases state that he does not administer pituitrin where the uterus is firmly contracted. I think the recommendation should be advanced with a great deal of caution, and it is a relief to hear Dr. Brodhead say that there is danger of uterine rupture where it is given, even after the child is out of the uterus.

DR. SOLOMON WIENER.—It has always been a surprise to me that any fixed amount of pituitrin should be mentioned as a dose. It has been my experience that in some patients you will get more of a reaction with 3 minims than in others to whom you give 1 c.c. You cannot tell beforehand what reaction you are going to get in a given patient, unless she has had a previous test, and it seems to me that that is one of the very important points in forestalling danger in using pituitrin. I have seen some patients who could get as much as three doses of 1 c.c. each inside of an hour with as little effect as if it were just that much water, and, as everybody knows, there are other patients who get a terrific contraction from a dose of 3 or 4 minims.

It is not a question of dosage only but also of the preparation.

The point is that it is necessary to individualize. One must begin by administering a small dose of any given preparation of pituitary extract. When one has learned the reaction of that particular patient to the preparation used, one can then if necessary proceed to give the larger doses.

DR. EDWIN G. LANGBOCK.—The patient with the rupture of the uterus was a para ii who awakened her nurse stating she had very slight pain in the back. The nurse suspected the onset of labor, and although the patient had asked her not to call the doctor, the nurse went to the phone and while she was talking to me the patient had another uterine contraction and the baby was born. It was probably thirty-five or forty minutes before I arrived.

The patient was in good condition, and the placenta was very easily removed by a Credé. I made it a routine to give 1 c.c. of pituitrin immediately after the uterus had been completely emptied. Before getting this at least three-quarters of an hour had elapsed, during which time the patient's color was good, and her general condition excellent. Immediately after the administration of the pituitrin she had a terrific pain in the left lower quadrant. I watched her for a few minutes. The pulse rate kept going up. She looked sick. She had a peculiar ashy facial expression, not a pallor. We gave her ¼ grain of morphine and in a half-hour she was given another ¼ grain. In the four or five hours following this one could map out an increasing flatness in the left flank, which suggested a retroperitoneal hemorrhage. Whether she had a rupture of a varicosity in the left broad ligament or a rupture of the uterus, I did not know. If you can get a rupture of a varicosity in the broad ligament after the administration of 1 c.c. of pituitrin, we do not advise giving it. I did not make a vaginal examination. Dr. Berg, however, did a vaginal, and felt a rent in the uterus. This hematoma finally broke down and drained through the vagina and she made a good recovery.

I stated that in all probability, had the placentae in our bleeding cases been removed sooner, the patients would have been saved some hemorrhage.

Ergot is always given to these patients as a routine.

In answer to Dr. Kosmak, I would say that we did not recommend the use of pituitrin at the beginning of the third stage indiscriminately. We are simply giving the results of what happened in our series of 100 cases.

As far as a fixed amount of pituitrin goes, I would say that what Dr. Wiener states is perfectly correct.

Department of Reviews and Abstracts

CONDUCTED BY HUGO EHRENFEST, M.D., ASSOCIATE EDITOR

Collective Review

Toxemia of Early Pregnancy: Etiology and Treatment*

Part I. Etiology

BY PAUL TITUS, M.D., F.A.C.S., PITTSBURGH, PA.

A REVIEW of the extensive literature on toxemia of early pregnancy and of the ingenious theories which have been advanced to explain toxemia occurring either early or late in pregnancy, is the best demonstration of the fact that no single idea is sufficiently comprehensive to cover this unquestionably complex matter.

For the purpose of study it has seemed advisable to divide the subject of pregnancy toxemia into two parts, thus enabling one to consider toxemia during early pregnancy first and alone. There are many reasons for such a division, chief among which are the facts that there is a distinct difference between the clinical pictures presented at these two times, as well as an actual difference in their pathology. At the same time there is a problematic relationship between toxemia early and late in pregnancy which makes an absolute separation of the one from the other a difficult if not an impossible matter. Stone, and later Ewing, advanced the idea that pernicious vomiting, acute yellow atrophy of the liver, and eclampsia originate from the same source, namely through a metabolic and pathologic disturbance in hepatic function, and that they are therefore essentially the same. Williams disagrees with this viewpoint, maintaining that metabolic study of the urine and blood, as well as histologic examination of tissues obtained at autopsy, clearly indicates that essential and characteristic differences exist between the various conditions thus grouped together. He believes that each clinical entity should be studied separately and that to group them even under such a heading as that proposed for this review serves merely to becloud the issue.

GENERALIZATION OF ETIOLOGIC THEORIES

Certain unknown toxic substances are supposed to be elaborated somewhere in the metabolism of a pregnant woman. The presence of

*Part II to be published in May issue.

these substances in the body is considered to be the cause of vomiting and the pathologic changes which result if the diseased condition is prolonged. While Zweifel has summarized fifteen different theories as to the cause of toxemia late as well as early in pregnancy, Underhill and Rand point out that there are four main theories as to the source of these toxic substances.

The first is that they are of gastrointestinal origin and akin to an ordinary autointoxication; the second, that they occur as the result of disturbances in the various glands of internal secretion, notably the ovaries; the third, that they are of fetal origin; and the fourth, that they result from disturbance in liver and kidney metabolism and function.

I. THEORY OF AUTOINTOXICATION

Dirmoser was the first to assert that these toxins were the result of intestinal putrefaction, and LeLornier elaborated this idea by the opinion that the condition is due to a placental toxemia plus a deficient bowel action. There can be no question that the bowel plays a part in toxemia of pregnancy for it is the main avenue of excretion, and while it may not have an active part in the actual production of all of the toxins, it most assuredly has a real rôle in the elimination of putrefactive poisons.

McDonald feels that the trouble originates in digestive faults in the duodenal region and employs "duodenal enemas" in its treatment. Tweedy, likewise, inclines to the view that manifestations of toxemia result from the appearance in the blood of a foreign protein which interferes with the normal food antibodies. The nausea and vomiting, he says, are Nature's attempt to get rid of food which cannot be assimilated and neutralized. In close connection with the idea that gastrointestinal autointoxication plays a rôle, there is the opinion of Albert that bacterial action as found in an infectious endometritis may produce absorbable toxins, while Talbot observes that a definite focus of infection in such places as the teeth, the tonsils, the sinuses, or the ears· is practically always to be found as an underlying cause of toxemia. DeLee agrees that some focus capable of throwing infection into the maternal blood-stream often becomes a menace to the life of the fetus, and for the past twenty years he has been suspicious that an infection will be found at the bottom of eclampsia.

II. INTERNAL GLAND SECRETION THEORY

Lange, and also Nicholson, attack the problem on the side of the glands of internal secretion and are confident that the trouble is due to the occasional failure of the thyroid to enlarge. Foulkrod, as well as Ward, claim exceptional results from the administration of thyroid extracts.

The Italian writers have done considerable work in the glandular theory, and Cerecedo, as well as Zulogoa, feel that adrenal insufficiency is the true factor in hyperemesis gravidarum, and that if this defect be remedied the condition promptly clears up.

American readers, in particular, are familiar with the group who believe that toxemia of early pregnancy results from a deficient corpus luteum secretion. This idea was expounded by Hirst and the administration of corpus luteum extract was adopted with great enthusiasm only to meet with many disappointing failures. A large number of the successful results, on the other hand, were obviously due to the psychical and suggestive effect of the treatment combined with the generally sensible management of the patient by regulation of diet and bowels, and rest in bed.

III. FETAL SOURCES OF TOXEMIA

That the toxemia is of fetal origin is plausible and has many adherents. In general, the line of reasoning has been, that such toxemia is peculiar to pregnancy, and resulting from the presence of the fetus, must therefore be due to certain unknown fetal products. These may be serologic or metabolic, according to various observers.

Many conjectures have been made on the serologic aspect of this question. Veit believes that both the transportation and the dissolution of syncytial elements of the placenta which may have made their way into the maternal blood stream, have a toxic action if they are not combated by antibodies in the patient's blood. Cary writes that he thinks the growing ovum acts as an antigen and stimulates the host to form antibodies but the host occasionally has a lowered immunity to the growth of the syncytium and unless the patient is fortified by something such as desiccated placenta, the vomiting occurs. Austin holds the same general idea but believes that up to the time the chorionic villi are developed into placenta, their syncytial cells secrete poison which is dumped into the mother's blood stream. Rubeska also gives credence to this theory.

Elaboration of the thory of anaphylaxis gave rise for a time to hopes that it might offer an explanation of toxemia during pregnancy, especially in connection with eclampsia. Further serologic studies seem to have discredited the idea, in spite of its having been supported by such men as Thies and Lockemann, Gräfenburg, Rosenau and Anderson, Lawrance and others. Obata has shown that the extract of normal placenta is as toxic as that of an eclamptic placenta and that no significant difference exists in the toxicity of serum from individuals of different groups. Furthermore, he has demonstrated that the neutralizing power of blood to the toxic property of placental extract is not increased during pregnancy, hence there is no evidence of an immunologic origin of a neutralizing power of the blood. Zweifel claims that there is no basis for the theory that toxemia—especially eclampsia—is the result of a hypersensitiveness on the part of the mother for fetal or placental proteins, since he has been unable to sensitize animals for homologous fetal and placental proteins.

IV. THE EFFECT OF HEPATIC, RENAL, AND OTHER METABOLIC DISTURBANCES

The metabolic viewpoint of this subject opens a tremendously broad and interesting field which is as yet far from completely explored. It links up closely with the gastrointestinal theory in the idea that the extra waste products of fetal metabolism thrown into the maternal blood stream cause an undue and unaccustomed strain on the mother's eliminative powers, thus producing a kind of autointoxication. This is not quite consistent, however, with the fact that the first evidences of toxemia are usually manifest early in pregnancy, after which there is a period during which the pregnant woman is fairly free from the likelihood of toxemia, followed by the interval of the later weeks when preeclamptic toxemia and eclampsia are prone to develop. The same fetal waste products are being thrown off into the maternal blood current in steady progression and with no remissions during the entire pregnancy.

Acidosis has been suggested by Zweifel as a cause of toxemia, but Van Slyke and Losee have demonstrated by a depletion of the alkaline reserve, that acidosis does not exist to any particular extent. It exists mildly even in normal pregnancy and is profound only in the last stages of toxemia. Otherwise, it never occurs to the same degree as in nephritis or diabetes and therefore may be considered merely as a symptom rather than a cause of toxemia.

Disturbances in hepatic and renal metabolism undoubtedly play an important rôle in toxemia. The recognition of hepatic lesions in fatal cases of toxemia has been established by Stone, by Ewing, and by Williams, but the cause of these lesions is still obscure. The fact that identical pathologic changes in the liver have been found in vomiting of pregnancy, chloroform, phloridzin, phosphorus, and arsenic poisoning, as well as in simple but complete starvation has been repeatedly emphasized.

Stone's theory of "suboxidation" based on his work in the "nitrogenous partition" of the urine was partially accepted by Ewing, but seems to have been disproved by the subsequent investigations of Van Slyke and Losee.

The work of Williams on the ammonia coefficient, especially from a prognostic standpoint in pernicious vomiting of pregnancy, has attracted wide-spread attention. Briefly his contention is, that the relation of ammonia nitrogen to the total nitrogen in the urine varies in normal pregnancy between 4 and 5 per cent, whereas in toxemic vomiting it rises to as much as from 20 to 50 per cent. Given a case of vomiting, therefore, he considered that a differentiation between neurotic and toxemic vomiting lay in the ammonia coefficient. Later his views underwent a slight modification in that he came to consider a low ammonia coefficient indicative of neurotic vomiting and therefore of negative value, whereas a high coefficient meant either a true toxemic vomiting which required immediate abortion, or that the starvation incident to prolonged vomiting of neurotic origin had produced the altered relation between the ammonia nitrogen and the total nitrogen. His procedure then was to undertake forced feeding whereupon the ammonia coefficient of the latter would fall, whereas that of the former would show no change for the better. Williams' work was sharply attacked by Underhill and Rand who considered the high ammonia coefficient merely an accompaniment of inanition and in no way connected with a toxemic process. Williams refutes their claims by such clinical methods as the presentation of a patient whose ammonia coefficient fell promptly after an abortion before she had been given any food. He still holds to the opinion that toxemic vomiting of pregnancy is either neurotic or toxic in origin and type.

Hepatic lesions are so constant in toxemia of pregnancy that liver involvement is indisputable. One important question which remains to be decided is whether or not a disturbance of liver function and metabolism is alone responsible, or if it be a combination of a specific and as yet unknown toxin elaborated by the fetal tissues acting in conjunction with an impaired liver. In such a review as this it is difficult not to intrude one's personal and possibly biased opinions. With this as a half-hearted apology it is desired to outline what seems to be a logical and consistent explanation of the rôle of the liver in the origin and progress of toxemia of pregnancy, at the same time admitting the point that the clinical and pathologic differences in the various toxemias of pregnancy intimate the elaboration of unknown and differing toxins which are able to seriously affect the patient only when the liver is already impaired.

The liver has several functions, of which two have a direct bearing on this subject. It is the carbohydrate storage organ of the body, maintaining a reserve supply of glycogen which can be drawn upon as needed in the general metabolism, and is also the great detoxicating organ of the body, being called upon to vigorously combat the effect of any poisons either ingested, or elaborated within the body. Direct starvation results in a drain upon the reserve glycogen stored in the liver, and likewise an unusual and prolonged demand for glycogen, to be consumed in the body metabolism, effects a similar glycogen depletion of the liver.

When the liver is not well stored with glycogen, it is far less able to perform its various functions, and its ability as a detoxicating organ is markedly impaired. This has been demonstrated by the experimental work of Roger, who tested the effect of various poisons on starving animals and found the lethal dose to be considerably smaller than for normal control animals. He also found that poisonous substances are less toxic if administered simultaneously with glucose. Davis, Hall and Whipple have found that yellow atrophy of the liver can be produced far more readily in experimental dogs which have been deprived of carbohydrates even though proteins have been allowed, and similarly that the ingestion of carbohydrates in various forms caused the central necrosis of the liver lobules in poisoned dogs to disappear much more rapidly than in control animals. They have thus been able to demonstrate a remarkable regenerative ability on the part of the liver.

Slemons has shown that the growing fetus makes a demand for carbohydrates far in excess of that of normal life, since the fetal tissues synthesize their protein from the material in the fetal blood, and that practically all of this nutritive diffusion from maternal to fetal blood streams takes place in the form of sugar. The mechanism by which a steady flow of glucose toward the fetus is maintained is explained by his finding that there is a higher mean glucose value on the maternal than on the fetal side. Lockhead and Cramer have shown that the fetus not only uses, but also stores, glycogen, the placenta acting in this capacity until the fetal liver can take up this function. Glinke and others have found that glycogen is especially abundant in fetal tissues, while McAllister has demonstrated that glycogen, present in the uterus and tubes independent of pregnancy, is most abundant at the time of childbirth, also being especially marked in the placenta.

Glycogen consumption during pregnancy translated into muscular energy would place a woman in the situation of running a nine-months long Marathon race usually without preliminary training. It is to be expected that her liver would become more or less depleted of its glycogen stores, unless constantly replenished by the proper kind of food, whereupon it promptly becomes less and less able to cope with any toxins in the system, be they merely metabolic or actually and specifically developed by the fetal tissues. With such disturbance in hepatic function by carbohydrate starvation, whether this be direct or indirect, and the establishment of nausea and vomiting, the food intake is lessened, so that a vicious circle is readily produced.

This "carbohydrate deficiency theory" as elaborated first by Duncan and Harding, and independently by Titus, Hoffmann and Givens, offers a simple explanation of certain peculiar facts pertaining to toxemia of pregnancy. It accounts for the occurrence of nausea and vomiting with such regularity in early pregnancy when the chorionic villi are especially abundant, since the chorionic tissue has been shown to be the glycogen demanding and storing portion of the fetus; it also accounts for the frequency of toxemia in hydatidiform mole and twin pregnancies where there is an unusual amount of chorionic tissue, so that the occurrence of pernicious vomiting and eclampsia in hydatidiform mole with no fetus present becomes the expected rather than the inexplicable thing; it explains the success to be obtained in vomiting of pregnancy by forced feeding and frequent meals; the reason why the restriction of such proteins as meat and eggs has been found empirically to be of value in toxemia is clarified on other grounds than a mere reduction in toxic waste products of protein metabolism; the similarity between the clinical symptoms and the pathologic lesions in the liver in starvation as compared to toxemia of early pregnancy is thus explained; on a purely physiologic basis the "carbohydrate deficiency" or "glycogen depletion" theory establishes fairly well the reason for individual resistance to the toxins which may be assumed to be present in every pregnancy, whether these be the "syncytiotoxin" of Weichardt, and Veit, or the "fibrin ferment" of Schmorl, and Dienst, or entirely unrelated to these theoretical toxins of pregnancy.

The disturbances in renal function seen so regularly in all profound toxemia of pregnancy may be merely incidental, precisely as in the case of any such toxemia as that of scarlet fever, pneumonia, bichloride of mercury poisoning, and so on. Even eclampsia occasionally is unaccompanied by nephritis, and Prutz concluded from a study of a large number of autopsies following death from eclampsia that it was unjustifiable to consider renal lesions as the anatomic substratum of eclampsia despite the frequency of their occurrence, assuming that they might well be secondary in the majority of cases.

In connection with the hepatic insufficiency idea there was a significant piece of work recently published by Mann of the Mayo Clinic. He, too, has demonstrated that the liver is able to regenerate rapidly even after surgical removal of as much as 70 per cent of its bulk. He has been able to remove the entire liver from dogs after having established a collateral circulation at a preliminary operation. The animals first develop muscular weakness, then fine muscular twitchings appear which increase in severity until definite convulsions occur, during one of which the animal dies. He concluded from his first work that there seems to be some change in metabolism whereby some intermediate toxic product is formed, or some necessary element for metabolism is lacking. In a further study, Mann and Magath found a progressive fall in blood-sugar after total extirpation of the liver and coincidently a decrease in glycogen content of the muscle. The first symptoms occur coordinately with this decrease in blood sugar, but if, during any stage after symptoms develop up to the point at which respirations have actually stopped, glucose is injected, the animal immediately and completely recovers. This process can be repeated many times before the animal finally dies with its blood sugar then not below normal. Transfusion of blood and saline were without effect, and no other substances than glucose, except maltose and galactose, produced this restoration.

Four main sources of possible trouble, as outlined above, have been carefully considered by innumerable investigators, and one after the other of these factors has been accused with neither conviction nor acquittal. Since each has been under suspicion it is by no means impossible that some combination of these various forces may be responsible for toxemia of early pregnancy.

The one tangible thing which stands out in all toxemia of pregnancy is that the liver is definitely involved, although it is not quite clear whether this involvement precedes or results from the toxemia. Knowing that liver lesions identical with those of vomiting of pregnancy may be produced by simple starvation, and that in early pregnancy a specific starvation results from the unusual demand for glycogen made by the fetus, it is logical to assume that this at least starts the trouble. Presently all the complexities of disturbed metabolism may be involved, and with the liver functions already disturbed and impaired, it requires very little imagination to complete the vicious circle.

The products of fetal metabolism which to an individual with an unimpaired liver would be harmless, may have a definitely toxic effect, although it is still possible that they would be without effect until combined with some such gastrointestinal disturbance as that following indiscretions in diet or a period of constipation. The interrelationship between the liver and the pancreas and spleen might play a rôle, while the thyroid and adrenals may even be involved.

Liver disturbance is, however, the constant factor in all this, and the way in which such disturbance may be instituted by the occurrence of a pregnancy can be outlined upon a rational physiologic basis, namely, the sudden and unaccustomed demand of the fetus for glycogen depletes the liver of its reserve sugar, whereupon its various metabolic functions are profoundly upset. What goes on thereafter is still a matter of conjecture.

BIBLIOGRAPHY

Albert: Arch. f. Gynäk., 1901, lxvi, 483. *Austin*: Med. Rec., 1914, xxx, 705. *Cary*: Surg., Gynec., and Obst., 1917, xxv, 206. *Cerecedo*: Siglo Med., 1913, lx, 546. *Davis and Whipple*: Paper I, Arch. Int. Med., 1919, xxiii, 612. *Davis and Whipple*: Paper II, ibid., p. 636. *Davis, Hall and Whipple*: Paper III, ibid., p. 689. *Davis and Whipple*: Paper IV, ibid., p. 711. *DeLee*: Year-Book of Obstetrics, 1920, p.

218. *Dienst*: Arch. f. Gynäk., 1910, xc, 536; ibid., 1912, xcvi, 43. *Dirmoser*: Wien. klin. Wchnschr., 1903, xvi, 405. *Duncan and Harding*: Canad. Med. Assn. Jour., 1918, vii, 1057. *Ewing*: Am. Jour. Obst., 1905, li, 145. *Foulkrod*: Amer. Jour. Med. Sci., 1905, cxxxvi, 541. *Glinke*: Biol. Ztschr., 1911, Moscow, ii, 1. *Gräfenburg*: Ztschr. f. Geburtsh. u. Gynäk., 1911, lxix, 270. *Hirst*: Jour. Am. Med. Assn., 1921, lxxvi, 772. *Lange*: Ztschr. f. Geburtsh. u. Gynäk., 1899, xl, 44. *Lawrance*: Paper read before Penn. State Med. Soc., Sept., 1921. *LeLornier*: Clinique Paris, 1913, viii, 631. *Lockhead and Cramer*: Proc. Roy. Soc., Series B, 1908, lxxx, 263. *Mann*: Amer. Jour. Med. Sc., 1921, clxi 37. *Mann and Magath*: Amer. Jour. Physiol., 1921, lv. *McAllister*: Jour. Obst. and Gynec., Brit. Emp., 1913, xxxiv. *McDonald*: Med. Rec., 1914, xii, 128. *Nicholson*: Med. and Surg. Jour., 1901, No. 6, p. 503. ibid., Trans. Obst. Soc., Edinburgh, March, 1902. ibid., Jour. Obst. and Gynec., Brit. Emp., 1902, v, 32. *Obata*: Jour. Immun., 1919, iv, 111. *Prutz*: Ztschr. f. Geburtsh u. Gynäk., 1892, xxii, 1. *Roger*: Thése de Paris, 1887. *Rosenau and Anderson*: Ref. Ztschr. f. Geburtsh u. Gynäk., 1911, lxviii, 27. *Rubeska*: Zentralbl. f. Gynäk., 1913, xxxvii, 307. *Schmorl*: Leipzig, 1893. ibid., Archiv. f. Gynäk., 1902, lxv, 504. *Slemons*: Am. Jour. Obst., 1919, lxxx, 194. *Stone*: Amer. Gynec., 1903, iii, 518. ibid., New York Med. Rec., 1905, xlviii, 295. *Talbot*: Jour. Am. Med. Assn., 1920, lxxiv, 756. *Thies*: Arch. f. Gynäk., 1910, xcii, 513. *Thies and Lockemann*: Biochem. Ztschr., 1910, xxv, 120. *Titus, Hoffmann, and Givens*: Jour. Am. Med. Assn., 1920, lxxiv, 777. *Tweedy*: Jour. Obst. and Gynec. of Brit. Emp., 1914, xxvi, 216. *Underhill and Rand*: Arch. Int. Med., 1910, v, 61. *Van Slyke and Losee*: Am. Jour. Med. Sc., 1917, cliii, 94. *Veit*: Wiesbaden, 1905, ibid., Monatschr. f. Geburtsh. u. Gynäk., 1913, v, 411. *Ward*: Surg. Gynec. and Obst., 1909, vii, 405. *Weichardt*: Arch. f. Gynäk., 1909, lxxxvii, 655. *Williams*: Obstetrics, D. Appleton and Co., N. Y., 1919, ed. 4, pp. 549-592. *Zweifel*: München med. Wchnschr., 1906, liii, p. 297. ibid., Ztschr. f. Immunitätsforsh., 1921, xxxi, 22. *Zulogoa*: Arch. Mens. d'Obst. et de Gynec., 1914, iii, 433.

Selected Abstracts

Physiology and Pathology of Menstruation

Morley: The Corpus Luteum of Menstruation and Pregnancy. New York Medical Journal, 1921, cxiii, 230.

This article is a review of a monograph published in 1851 by John C. Dalton, Jr., a work of considerable historical interest.

Dalton observed a series of eighteen carefully controlled cases at postmortem, eleven illustrating the corpus luteum of menstruation and seven that of pregnancy. He believed that ovulation and menstruation occurred synchronously though the precise time at which the rupture of the follicle occurred was not definitely ascertained. Shortly after the rupture of the follicle, the formation of the corpus luteum commences. He described its development in detail and mentioned also the fact that at the end of the third week from the close of menstruation it begins to retrogress.

The corpus luteum of pregnancy on the other hand arrives more slowly at its maximum of development and afterwards remains for a long time as a very noticeable tumor, instead of undergoing a process of rapid atrophy.

The corpus luteum of pregnancy retains a globular or only slightly flattened form and gives to the touch a sense of considerable resistance and solidity. Internally it has an appearance of advanced organization, which is wanting in the corpus luteum of menstruation. This gives the difference in the thickness of the convoluted wall of the two corpora lutea as a point in differential diagnosis. A more dusky and indefinite color is characteristic of the corpus luteum of pregnancy. If the period of pregnancy is at all advanced it is not found like the corpus luteum of menstruation in company with unruptured follicles in active process of development.   MARGARET SCHULZE.

G. Schickelé: Studies on Ovarian Function. Gynécologie et Obstétrique, 1921, iii, 171.

From observations made in 28 cases operated upon for various gynecologic conditions and amplified by reports of other authorities the writer draws the following conclusions: Ovulation may take place at any time from the beginning of one menstruation to another; the time of predilection would seem to be the week following menstruation, (17 in 36 authenticated cases); ovulation may take place during menstruation, but it more frequently takes place between the menstrual periods. As regards the relationship between the corpus luteum and menstruation, observations on 18 cases are tabulated, giving the time of the observation from the beginning and end of the last period, the type of menstrual rhythm, the condition of the corpus luteum and the condition of the uterine mucosa, and the following conclusions are drawn:

1. During the week preceding menstruation, the ovary often harbors a corpus luteum, but the corpus luteum will not always be found in the same phase of evolution. 2. One may find a corpus luteum at the height of its development in the week following menstruation. 3. During the week preceding menstruation the uterine mucosa often undergoes a change characterized by a hyperemia and a well marked glandular secretion. This change is not limited to the premenstrual period. One may find it during the week following menstruation. 4. Thus a corpus luteum in evolution will often be coincident with a uterine mucosa in a stage of change. This coincidence will occur more often during the week preceding than during the week following menstruation. In spite of the coincidence, the degree of development will not be markedly the same for the corpus luteum and the uterine mucosa.

Above all, the metamorphosis of the mucosa can take place without a corpus luteum, and a corpus luteum in a state of evolution may not force the uterine mucosa to metamorphose in its turn. Thus the corpus luteum and the uterine mucosa are reciprocally independent. 5. It is certain that menstruation may take place in spite of the absence of a corpus luteum.   R. T. LAVAKE.

Tschirdewahn: Ovulation, Corpus Luteum and Menstruation. Zeitschrift für Geburtshilfe und Gynaekologie, 1920, lxxxiii, 110.

The author states as his conclusions that in every healthy woman, one, or more rarely two follicles ripen periodically. Rupture of the follicle occurs from the 10th to the 26th day after menstruation, varying with the individual and also in the same individual. The ovum is received in the ampulla of the tube, there casts off its polar bodies and if it is not fertilized becomes disintegrated in 2-3 days. While the ovum is passing through the tube, the ruptured follicle is developing into a corpus luteum. Through action of the hormones, which have perhaps already been produced by the theca lutein cells, the uterine mucosa undergoes predecidual or premenstrual changes. After several days the fertilized ovum which has meanwhile been nourished by its deutoplasm arrives at the uterine mucosa, burrowing into it by the corrosive action of the outer trophoblastic layer. If this happens, the corpus luteum persists to exert a trophic influence on the uterus and its contents. If the ovum is not fertilized, the corpus luteum begins to retrogress. At the same time retrogressive changes occur in the predecidual mucosa and menstruation takes place. Ripening of new follicles, which has ceased while the whole blood supply was nourishing the corpus luteum, begins again and the process is repeated.

MARGARET SCHULZE.

Loeb: Effect of Undernourishment on Mammalian Ovary and the Sexual Cycle. Journal American Medical Association, 1921, lxxvii, 1646.

Loeb reviews the results of his work on this subject which has appeared in various publications.

He demonstrated by animal experiments that excision of the corpora lutea accelerated ovulation, while burning them did not do so, on account of the accompanying "tissue shock" to the rest of the ovarian tissue. This was evidenced by the slow growth of the follicles which had a tendency to become atretic when half developed. He next found this hypotypical condition in guinea pigs which had remained sterile for a long time and concluded that underdevelopment is one of the causes of sterility. Looking for a cause of these hypotypic ovaries, he found it possible to produce them artificially by undernourishment. He was able to demonstrate definite changes in the ovaries after six or seven days of underfeeding, but the results varied with the age and previous condition of the animals, as well as with the length and degree of underfeeding. The effect was most noticeable in the epithelial elements and in the partly developed follicles.

Further experiments led to the conclusion that the ovum is responsible for the growth of the follicle and, ultimately of the ovary itself. Other factors which produce underweight, such as thyroid feeding, were found to have the same effect on the ovaries. The uterus in such cases was found to be thin and inactive, however the structures representing the so-called interstitial glands in other species, were well developed.

R. E. WOBUS.

Steinach and Kammerer: The Relation of Climate to Puberty. Archiv fuer Entwicklungsmechanik, 1920, xlvi, 391.

It was found that by keeping young rats at relatively high temperature, evidence of puberty developed much earlier than in similar rats kept at ordinary room temperature. The higher the temperature, up to 35° C., the greater the development. Above this temperature, there was, if anything, a retardation. Primarily, the interstitial cells of testis and ovary were affected, which, in turn, caused enlargement of the seminal vesicles and prostate in the male and the uterus in the female.

This bears out observations on the development of puberty in man.

As we near the tropics, puberty appears increasingly early, while at, or near the equator, it is often retarded. Poor food and other deleterious factors may also retard puberty. Women in the far North menstruate sparingly, some Esquimaux only during summer. At high altitudes, puberty appears late. However, immigrants passing from one climate into another, frequently mature at the same age as if they had remained at home, even for several generations.

Another interesting observation on man, which was borne out by these experiments on rats, is the fact that, as we approach the tropics, the external sex characteristics, such as the distribution of hair, approach each other in the two sexes. R. E. WOBUS.

Wiltshire: Basal Metabolism in Menstruation. Lancet London, 1921, cci, 388.

The theory that the life processes of women undergo a periodic variation correlated with menstruation has been frequently suggested, and the effect of menstruation on the life processes of women studied in various ways.

The author undertook a series of experiments comparing the physiologic processes in the menstrual and intermenstrual periods. The points chosen for determination were: (1) the basal metabolic rate of normal women during menstruation and between menstrual periods; (2) the cost to the organism of a certain definite piece of work and (3) the rate of recovery from that work.

The observations were made on five subjects, the basal metabolism being determined each day during the menstrual periods and three or four times between these periods.

The results obtained showed that the basal metabolism was not appreciably affected by menstruation. The cost of work to the organism, and the rate of recovery from work were the same during the menstrual and inter-menstrual periods. The author concludes, that while more experiments must be done before any definite conclusions can be drawn, the processes appear to be identical during the menstrual and intermenstrual periods. NORMAN F. MILLER.

Clow: Menstruation during School Life. British Medical Journal, 1920, No. 3119, 511.

The author as medical inspector of a large girls' school had the opportunity of studying the menstrual function in 1200 healthy girls. The ages of these girls varied from 9 to 21 years. All of them were interviewed and examined once. The following information was secured: Regular menstruation occurred in 53.8 per cent; irregular menstruation in 46.1 per cent; no pain or discomfort in 73.0 per cent; discomfort or slight pain in 24.6 per cent; severe pain in 2.4 per cent; incapacitated 5.3 per cent; malaise 9.0 per cent; rest required during the period 23.0 per cent; baths taken during the period 23.4 per cent; games and usual exercise continued during the period 40.7 per cent; constipation during the period 9.0 per cent. The girls were advised to act normally during their periods, to bathe and exercise (except swimming) as they would do unless sick from some other cause. Of these girls 734 were seen more than once after having followed this advice and the following results were noted: Those having no disability rose from 67 per cent to 85 per cent; a reduction in those suffering from pain or malaise from 41 per cent to 17 per cent; that 6 per cent instead of 20 per cent lie down during the period; that there is an increase in the number taking baths and exercise and a decrease of those having constipation. Those suffering pain were greatly relieved by the use of the hot bath and taking exercise during the period. The general conclusions of the author are: (1) The majority of school girls are free from any menstrual disturbance; (2) If no unnatural restrictions are imposed, the proportion of girls free from any menstrual disturbance tends to increase; (3) girls in normal health should be encouraged to take baths and exercise during the menstrual period; (4) the amenorrhea to which school girls are subject is not caused by mental strain; (5) study *per se* is not a cause of dysmenorrhea, although if pursued to the exclusion of daily exercise it may become indirectly a contributory factor. F. L. ADAIR.

Rosenbloom: Influence of Menstruation on the Food Tolerance in Diabetes Mellitus. Journal American Medical Association, 1921, lxxvi, 1742.

Substantiating the claims of Naunyn and of Harrop and Mosenthal, Rosenbloom found the sugar tolerance markedly reduced during menstruation in two cases which he studied. R. E. WOBUS.

Schick: Menstrual Poison. Wiener klinische Wochenschrift, 1920, xxxiii, 395.

The author discovered accidentally that if his housemaid held flowers in her hand for several minutes, while she was menstruating, and then put them in water, the flowers withered more quickly than they did when she was not menstruating. He instituted experiments during four successive months using as controls women who were not menstruating and found that this same result was obtained each time, with the flowers held by the housemaid, while those held by the controls lasted a normal length of time; that the influence was most positive on the second, third, and fourth days of the flow; that sweat from the axilla seemed to contain the poison; that the blood corpuscles contained it and the blood serum did not; and that heating the menstrual blood up to 100° C. did not affect the result. A search of medical literature threw no light on the subject. A search of folk lore showed that the country people had traditions and ideas that menstruating women should not handle flowers or fruit; that florists laid off their workers during menstruation; that during menstruation women should not make bread, preserves, beer, wine, sauerkraut or butter because the various products spoiled. He calls the probable poison menotoxin and plans further experiments and considers its possible influence in the etiology of sterility, skin diseases, epilepsy and other diseases. FRANK A. PEMBERTON.

Stickel and Zoudek: The Menstrual Blood. Zeitschrift für Geburtshilfe und Gynaekologie, 1921, lxxxiii, 1.

The authors have made an exhaustive investigation of the morphologic and the physical properties of the menstrual blood, also a comparative study of the circulating blood of the menstruating woman. For a satisfactory study, the menstrual blood must be taken directly from the uterine cavity, as morphologic changes, especially sedimentation, take place on the way through the cervix. The blood must be thoroughly mixed before study as it has a tendency to deposit on shreds of mucous membrane.

The circulating blood shows no changes in morphologic constituents or in hemoglobin during menstruating except for a slight relative lymphocytosis.

The menstrual blood shows an oligocythemia, and a leucopenia; the white cells vary more than the red, the averages are 2,999,000 rbc and 3160 wbc. There is a relative lymphocytosis, 62 per cent with decreased polynuclears and no change in other types. Menstrual blood which has flowed through the cervix shows fewer lymphocytes.

The hemoglobin is regularly reduced but not proportional to the erythrocyte count. The color index is usually more than one. This is due to a partial hemolysis in the menstrual blood in the uterus. There are definite physical changes in specific gravity, osmotic pressure, etc.

There was no change in the fragility of the red cells either in menstrual or circulating blood. The hemolysis in menstrual blood is probably due to the action of a ferment produced by the uterine mucosa.

The coagulation time of the circulating blood is not changed during menstruation. Menstrual blood has lost its coagulability—showing no clots even after 24 hours. The coagulability is lost in the uterine mucosa. Blood obtained during menstruation by puncture of the cervix clots normally. MARGARET SCHULZE.

Graff and Novak: Regressive Gland Changes of the Endometrium in War Amenorrhea. Zeitschrift fuer Geburtshilfe und Gynaekologie, 1921, lxxxiii; 502.

The authors describe certain regressive gland changes in the endometrium in cases of so-called war amenorrhea, a condition which they regard as a nutritive disturbance secondary to the lack of protein in the war diet. These include changes in the shape, arrangement, and staining characteristics of the cells, which become pointed toward the base, lose their basement membrane, and are arranged almost circular to the gland axis, or may show a spiral onion-peel-like arrangement. The protoplasm becomes fibrillar, darkly eosin staining, the nuclei deep-staining homogeneous and of rod or comma-like form. The most marked changes of this type are found in the atrophic endometrium but they are also found in the resting stage and sometimes even in the mucosae which show definite cyclic phases. They are not dependent on the duration of the amenorrhea nor do they allow of conclusions concerning the prognosis. MARGARET SCHULZE.

Garling: On the Leucocytic Blood Picture during Menstruation. Deutsches Archiv fuer klinische Medizin, 1921, clxxv, 356.

The influence of menstruation on the endocrine system and the vegetative nerve apparatus has been much studied lately, but in view of the contradictory conclusions the writer undertook tests of the leucocytic picture in 37 normal and 9 diseased girls and women. The tests were made at the beginning of menstruation. The healthy persons were nearly all young women without stigmata of hyperexcitability of the vegetative nerve system; persons with accidental eosinophilia were also excluded. Of the 9 diseased persons, six showed eosinophilia even when not menstruating. The results of the tests were that there was no noticeable increase of the total number of leucocytes during menstruation. An increase in eosinophilia was seen in 15 out of the 37 healthy women, but in 14 there was a decrease. In the 9 pathologic tests, there was an increase of eosinophils in 4 cases and a decrease in 5. The lymphocytes increased in 17 of the 37 healthy women, and decreased in 11 cases. In the 9 diseased cases, there was an increase of lymphocytes 5 times. The mononucleates increased over 1 per cent in 11 out of the 37 healthy cases, and decreased over 1 per cent in 7 cases. In the 9 ill persons 5 showed increase up to 1.5 per cent, and 2 cases decreased up to 1 per cent.

AMERICAN INSTITUTE OF MEDICINE.

Novak and Graff: A Contribution to the Clinical and Pathological Anatomy of Amenorrhea. Zeitschrift fuer Geburtshilfe und Gynaekologie, 1921, lxxxiii, 289.

This report is based on the examination of curettings from 111 cases of amenorrhea in women from fifteen to thirty-nine years of age. Fifty-eight of the cases were the so-called "war amenorrhea," 16 cases presented marked grades of genital hyperplasia sufficient to account for the absence of menstruation, the others were distributed among cases of genital and extragenital tuberculosis, superinvolution, severe psychic trauma, extragenital hemorrhage, climatic change, etc. The authors found that even in the absence of menstrual bleeding, cyclic changes occur in the uterine mucosa which may be interpreted as the result of more or less complete ovulation. Three histologic types may be defined: Mucosae which represent a definite phase of the menstrual cycle; well-preserved mucosae without sign of proliferative change (resting endometrium) and finally mucosae which show well-marked atrophy. Transitional types may be seen, cyclic changes and signs of atrophy found in the same specimen. The severity of the change did not always depend upon the duration of the amenorrhea. The condition of the endometrium allows conclusions concerning the anatomical and functional condition of the ovaries which are of importance in making a prognosis. Curettage appears to favor the reestablishment of menstruation.   MARGARET SCHULZE.

Adler: Meno- and Metrorrhagia. Wiener klinische Wochenschrift, 1921, xxxiv, 378.

The author divides pathologic uterine bleeding into (1) Accidental and (2) Functional. The first group comprises bleeding due to erosions, polyps, carcinoma, etc. The second is concerned with the physiologic function of the genital organs as in (a) adolescence; (b) myoma, adnexal disease, retroversion, etc.; and (c) without gross pathology.

Hitschman and Adler have shown that endometritis and metritis do not cause bleeding. The author believes that the bleeding is controlled by the internal secretion of the follicles in the ovary. Salpingitis is not accompanied by bleeding until the ovaries are affected by the inflammation, which causes hyperemia and increased physiological activity. Examination of such ovaries shows many ripened follicles and no corpora lutea. On the other hand, if a corpus luteum is removed at an operation, menstrual-like bleeding appears in two or three days.

In addition to this the musculature of the uterus plays a part. The flabby uterus of the multipara and the weakly muscled uterus of the hypoplastic type, bleed longer than the normal nulliparous uterus.

Curettage is of little use as a treatment. The indications for it are (1) incomplete miscarriage; (2) question of malignancy and other diagnostic purposes; and (3) as a temporary means of stopping the flow. Curettage is useless as treatment for extrauterine pregnancy and myoma, and dangerous in salpingitis.

Medical treatment consists in the use of secacornin, ergotin and catorin, combined with climatic, balneologic and hygienic methods. Calcium preparations help sometimes. Lately organo-therapy by the use of hypophyseal, mammary, thyroid, pituitary, and especially corpus luteum preparations has found favor. Further, x-ray treatment is especially useful. Radium should not be used in the bleeding from benign causes because it is dangerous. The principal rule in treatment is to individualize each case.   FRANK A. PEMBERTON.

Phillips: The Treatment of Uterine Hemorrhage Not Associated with Pregnancy. British Medical Journal, Feb. 12, 1921, No. 3137, p. 224.

The author divides uterine bleeding into three groups, that occurring (1) at puberty, (2) during the childbearing years, (3) about the menopause. The first he considers as probably due to imperfect balance between the various internal secretions. This, he thinks, usually rights itself. The second is most commonly caused by the presence of fibroids. He thinks hysterectomy is indicated in almost every case associated with bleeding, either menstrual or intermenstrual. He also considers excessive bleeding as due to hypertrophy of the ovaries. He enumerates the following causes of hemorrhage at the menopause: (a) Cervical cancer (b) uterine fibrosis, (c) changes in endometrium which presumably cause uterine bleeding as the result of a deficiency in thrombokinase, (d) certain cases in which no abnormality can be found. These he considers to be due to some abnormality of the internal secretions.   F. L. ADAIR.

Herrmann: The Influence of Lipoids from Corpus Luteum and Placenta on Uterine Hemorrhages, the Menstrual Cycle and Menopause Symptoms. Monatsschrift für Geburtshilfe und Gynäkologie, 1921, liv, 152.

This investigator undertook a clinical experiment to determine the effect of a corpus luteum-placenta lipoid prepared by "Gesellschaft für chemische Industrie" in Basel.

The cases chosen were those with excessive bleeding due to an abnormality of ovarian function with or without an accompanying pelvic inflammatory condition.

Among 73 such patients he had good immediate results in 95 per cent and satisfactory permanent results in 74 per cent. The cases that responded best to the intramuscular injection of the preparation were those with menorrhagia or metrorrhagia; the presence of an inflammatory reaction in the pelvis apparently did not interfere with the regulatory action. Excessive bleeding in young girls at the time when the menstrual function was being established likewise responded extremely well. Hemorrhage at the menopause reacted promptly but the results were not lasting. EVERETT D. PLASS.

Forssner: The Results of Operative Treatment of Dysmenorrhea.
Uppsala Läkäreforeningens Forhandlingar, 1921, xxvi, 5.

No definite pathologic-anatomical change in the sexual organs of women is causing dysmenorrhea. There are, however, certain findings which usually go together with this symptom. For instance, myoma uteri and intrauterine polyps are very often accompanied by dysmenorrhea. In many patients with dysmenorrhea there is an aplasia of the sexual organs with retroflexio uteri, but in most of the cases no anatomical change can be found. The author started with the idea that dysmenorrhea was one of the symptoms of a nervous constitution, or in other words that it was one of the symptoms of a neurosis. This idea had to be given up. The actual cause of the pain is contractions of the uterus, but what the causes of these contractions are has never been determined. The pain is present before and during the first day of the menstruation and the author thinks that the most logical explanation is that hemorrhages take place in the mucous membrane of the uterus. A resulting tension seems to produce the painful contractions. When the tension in the mucous membrane, after some hours, has subsided, the irritation causing the contractions ceases.

It is his further experience that dysmenorrhea usually stops when a delivery has taken place. This harmonizes with the explanation mentioned above. After the delivery the uterine cavity never goes back to its former size. For this reason a hemorrhagic swelling of the endometrium will not cause the same degree of irritation as when the cavity is very small. Furthermore, the uterine musculature seems after delivery to be less able to go into convulsive contractions than before.

In the years 1910-1919 the author has had 153 cases of dysmenorrhea in nulliparae without any pathologic-anatomical findings. In 42.5 per cent of these cases an operation was advised, but never before psychic treatment had been tried. The patients were usually told that they did not suffer from any dangerous disease, that they must not pay any attention to the pain and go on with their usual work. If this treatment, after a longer period of time, did not seem to help, an operation was suggested. The operations were usually done in two steps; first, a dilation of the cervix. Hegar dilators No. 10-11 were introduced; then the uterine cavity packed with gauze for 48 hours. Second step: After removal of gauze, the cervix was again dilated up to Hegar No. 20, an abrasion done and the uterus repacked with gauze for another 48 hours.

Of the operated cases 46 per cent were completely cured, 34 per cent greatly benefited. They could perform their work which previously had been impossible for them. The pain still existed but they never had to go to bed. In the other 20 per cent the operation did not seem to have any effect. The author's patients have been followed for periods up to 10 years after the operation. KIRSTEN UTHEIM.

Item

AT a recent meeting of the Joint Committee of the American Gynecological Society and the American Child Hygiene Association, appointed to consider problems on Maternal Welfare, it was decided to give some publicity to the following report with the idea of eliciting constructive criticism. The personnel of the Committee is as follows: American Gynecological Society: Dr. Geo. W. Kosmak, New York; Dr. Fred Taussig, St. Louis; Dr. Fred L. Adair, Minneapolis. American Child Hygiene Association: Dr. J. Whitridge Williams, Baltimore; Dr. Anna E. Rude, Washington, D. C.; Dr. Merrill E. Champion, Boston. American Pediatric Society: Dr. Henry L. K. Shaw, Albany; Dr. Fritz Talbot, Boston; Dr. Walter Ramsay, St. Paul. The program has been tentatively accepted by the American Gynecological Society and the American Child Hygiene Association, but has not yet been presented to the American Pediatric Society for action.

It is suggested that communications be sent to Dr. Fred L. Adair, Chairman, 730 La Salle Building, Minneapolis, Minnesota. Any member of the above Committee, however, will welcome suggestions or inquiries regarding the above program.

The Committee considers its proper functions to be:

A. Elaboration of a complete scheme of maternal welfare as ideally developed, emphasizing the most important points for starting the development of such a plan with the idea of educating the public to the necessity of this work and to serve as a basis for governmental activity. The following skeleton plan is presented:

 I. Preservation of life and health of the mother.
  a. Decrease in the number of infections following abortion and childbirth.
  b. By providing better trained attendants.
  c. By educating the laity as to the proper preparation and necessity for proper supervision during pregnancy, etc.
  d. Inspection and control of institutions, etc., caring for maternity cases.
  e. Prevention and treatment of venereal disease in association with pregnancy.
  f. Control of toxemias.
 II. Increase in the number of fruitful pregnancies by
  a. Decrease in the amount of sterility.
   1. By diminution in the number of infections following abortion and childbirth.
   2. By diminution of venereal disease, especially gonorrhea.

b. Diminution in the number of abortions by
   1. Diminution in the number of spontaneous abortions by educating as to proper care when threatening symptoms develop.
   2. Diminution in the number of induced abortions.
      (a) self induced; (b) criminal operations; (c) therapeutic abortions.

N. B. (1) We recommend that hospitals require the written sanction of at least two reputable medical men before permission to perform an abortion is granted.
(2) We recognize the desirability of making abortions reportable to the health authorities.

c. Diminution of the number of premature births and deaths.
   1. Education and supervision.
   2. Provision for proper care of premature infants.
   3. Recognition and treatment of syphilis.
d. Diminution in the number of stillbirths.
   1. Improvement of statistics and methods of reporting stillbirths with causes.
   2. Education of laity and profession.
   3. Provision of better antepartum and intrapartum care.
   4. Better care of syphilitics.
e. Diminution in the number of neonatal deaths.
   1. Recognition of the importance of these deaths.
   2. Methods of prevention.
   3. Education of laity and profession.
   4. Provision of better antenatal, intrapartum and postpartum care.

N. B.—More careful scientific study of both stillbirths and neonatal deaths, together with causes of abortion, miscarriage and premature birth.

   III. Better facilities for the care of the unmarried mother for her own protection and that of her off-spring.
B. Definition of the relationship of this work to other health and welfare activities such as infant and child welfare; venereal disease campaign; antituberculosis; boards of health; Red Cross and nursing activities, as well as social agencies; certain eugenic problems.
C. To have some responsible agency of representatives and well qualified men to advise with the governmental agencies on the problems of maternal welfare. This may be enlarged to become a part of a sort of institute or academy of sciences which could well be an advisory body on matters pertaining to public health and welfare.
D. It is particularly important to work out problems of maternal and child welfare in cooperation with the pediatrists, by means of a joint committee representative of the leading national societies. We recommend that this joint committee on maternal welfare, work with one representing the American Pediatric Society to elaborate maternal and infant welfare programs.

Correspondence

Dec. 29, 1921.

Editor AMERICAN JOURNAL OF OBSTETRICS & GYNECOLOGY.
Sir:

I wish to bring to the attention of gynecologists and general surgeons, particularly the latter because of their radicalism and lack of general sound judgment where a gynecologic question is involved, the fact that we should be more conservative in our operative treatment of ectopic pregnancies. The great majority of operators are indiscriminately removing the tubes in these cases, even though they may leave the ovaries. I find that this is entirely unnecessary, no more necessary than it would be to remove the uterus for an incomplete abortion. This applies not only to the tubal abortions, complete and incomplete, but also to certain types of ruptured tubes where the bleeding can be easily stopped by a carefully applied suture of whipped over fine catgut. In some cases it is necessary to loop a suture around the pelvic side of the broad ligament, either above the ovary or sometimes below it. Tubes can easily be stripped of their contents through their fimbriated extremity or split open, doing a salpingotomy with removal of the contents and a closure.

Our object is or should be, primarily, a stopping of hemorrhage, if present, or the carrying out of such technic as will do away with the possibility of recurrence, and not mutilation.

This has undoubtedly been done by many. I cannot feel that there is any originality in the proposition, it is perfectly obvious and simple, but I wish to bring it to the attention of the profession generally.

Yours very truly,
ALBERT M. JUDD, M.D.

BROOKLYN, N. Y.

DR. E. GUSTAV ZINKE, of Cincinnati, Ohio, a member of the Advisory Editorial Board of the *American Journal of Obstetrics and Gynecology*, well known as a teacher and prominently identified with the organization and development of the American Association of Obstetricians, Gynecologists and Abdominal Surgeons, died at the age of seventy-six, on January 30, 1922.

The American Journal of Obstetrics and Gynecology

Original Communications

A CONTRIBUTION TO THE HISTOGENESIS OF OVARIAN TUMORS

BY SAMUEL H. GEIST, M.D., F.A.C.S., NEW YORK CITY

Associate Gynecologist, Associate in Surgical Pathology, Mount Sinai Hospital, N. Y.

THE question of the histogenesis of the epithelial tumors, both cystic and solid, arising in the ovary, has been the subject of much discussion. Virchow and Rokitansky ascribed them to the follicular epithelium or the Pflueger's cords, and Leopold a little later suggested the germinal epithelium as the site of origin. In the many descriptions and discussions that were published in subsequent years, various structures including the granulosa cells, rests of the wolffian body, ingrowths from the surface epithelium and the cylindrical or ciliated cell rests of Walthard, have been given prominence as possible sources from which these tumors may develop.

Recently Goodall has shown that all the parenchymatous structures in the ovary, namely, Pflueger's cords or tubules, the medullary cords, the rete ovarii, the follicle and its derivatives, are of germinal epithelial origin. Strictly speaking, then, one may trace to the germinal layer all epithelial ovarian tumors. By germinal epithelium Goodall means the epithelium covering the wolffian body which eventually gives rise to the genital gland, (ovary or testicle). However, it is still undetermined which differentiated cell of the germinal epithelium, i.e., Pflueger's cords, ray, rete, etc., gives rise to a specific group of tumors. As Goodall says, the various classifications of ovarian tumors have not as a rule been histogenetic but rather topical, clinical, or histologic.

In view of the wide variations in opinions any evidence that will at all tend to help in the classification of these common and clinically

---

NOTE: The Editor accepts no responsibility for the views and statements of authors as published in their "Original Communications."

important tumors and that may tend to indicate their origin is of sufficient value to make a record of it.

Through the courtesy of Dr. F. S. Mandelbaum, pathologist to Mt. Sinai Hospital, I obtained the material which furnishes the basis of this communication. The specimen consisted of a uterus and the adnexa. The patient had been operated upon by Dr. J. Brettauer, to whom I am indebted for the privilege of citing the clinical data.

The woman was fifty-two years of age and had complained of enlargement of the abdomen which had been noticed for several months. She had never been pregnant and since her twenty-ninth year had not menstruated. The physical examination of the patient showed an

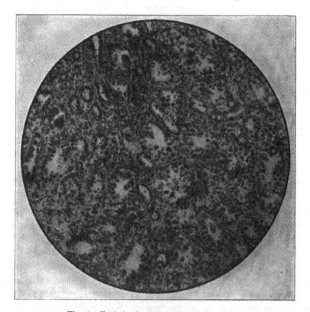

Fig. 1.—Typical adenocarcinoma of the ovary.

abdominal mass extending up to the umbilicus and apparently connected with the uterus. A laparotomy was done and a large ovarian tumor found. A complete hysterectomy was then performed.

On gross examination of the material it was seen that one ovary was the site of a rather large solid tumor, apparently a cellular neoplasm and histologically proving to be a typical adenocarcinoma (Fig. 1).

The tumor that I will describe was situated in the other ovary and because of the characteristic structure it seems possible to classify it histogenetically. The tumor was not of the type ordinarily seen in the ovary and could not be classified in any of the commonly accepted schemes. This ovary was somewhat enlarged but maintained its normal shape and consistency. On section it was polycystic and at one extremity (the pole opposite the ovarian ligament) presented a rather dense white appearance with minute cysts scattered in a rather cellular stroma resembling the ovarian stroma. This area was approximately 3 cm. in diameter.

Histologically the dense white portion was composed of epithelial masses in a connective matrix resembling stroma of unchanged ovarian type. These epithelial masses varied from a few cells to large agglomerated and branching strands (Fig. 2).

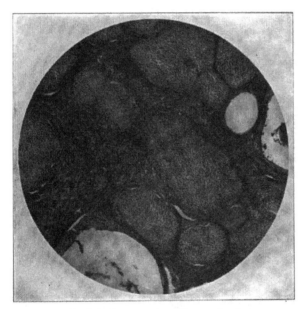

Fig. 2.—Epithelial cell groups and strands composing the tumor.

These cell groups were composed mainly of round or polygonal cells of rather large size with much protoplasm of a somewhat granular character and containing nuclei, rich in chromatin, small, round or oval in shape, and centrally situated. The cell masses, especially the larger ones, contained cysts of varying size. The epithelial lining of the cysts varied in thickness from one or two cells to ten or more. The cells that line the cysts resemble in the main the type seen in the solid cell masses, though in the larger cysts the lining epithelial elements were cuboidal and in some instances high cylindrical, approaching very closely the high cylindrical cells with pycnotic basal nuclei that line the loculi of the not uncommon pseudomucinous cysts of the ovary (Fig. 3). This appearance is rather important, as the histologic resemblance has a direct bearing on the interpretation of the possible origin of this type of cystic neoplasm. In most instances the cells adjacent to the cavities have a sharply defined membrane which seems to be formed by the fusion of the cell membrane forming the upper limit of this lining layer of cells.

In some of the cysts there can be seen a marked heaping up of the cells on one side while the other presents but one or two layers of cylindrical or cuboidal type. The impression is created that the cysts

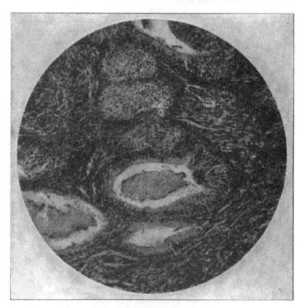

Fig. 3.—Acini lined by high cylindrical epithelium of the type seen in the pseudomucinous cyst adenoma.

may form eccentrically in the solid cell nests by liquefaction or degeneration of the cells and as these small cysts form they coalesce and give rise to the larger ones (Fig. 4). These cysts appear in their earlier stages as small spaces oval or round, containing a granular or fibrillar substance and often a large degenerated cell with a sharply defined limiting membrane but with very indefinite cell structure (Fig. 5). Occasionally instead of these cells in the cyst lumen there is found a round homogeneous or granular mass which stains deeply with eosin and has been interpreted by some observers as a degenerating ovum. Careful study of all the structures found in these cysts has failed to reveal at any time the characteristics that would make it possible to definitely identify these elements as true ova. They are in all probability secretion masses, disintegrating cells, or products of their degeneration.

This process of cyst formation or cavity formation resembles the pseudo-oögenetic process described by Goodall and in a personal communication from him after study of my slides he states, "In many of the circular cell masses there is a strong tendency to the formation of a pseudo-oögenetic process." The attempts at oögenesis can be studied from the agglomeration of a few cells into a giant cell, the

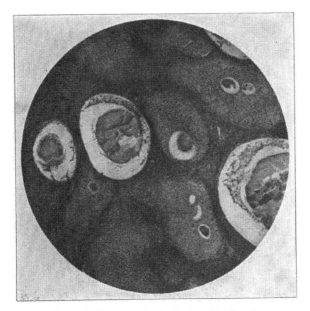

Fig. 4.—Cavities of varying size in the solid cell nests.

fusion of these and later slow destruction leaving only a circular or oval cavity filled with detritus. In many of these cell masses there are as many as eight oögenetic attempts.

The cell masses both large and small are separated from the ovarian stroma by a definite connective tissue layer, resembling the theca externa, which limiting membrane runs at right angles to the stroma proper, just as the true theca surrounds the normal follicles.

It seems that the tumor starts with the small cell proliferation and gradually as these grow, the connective tissue capsule surrounding the collections is absorbed or breaks down (Fig. 6) and so two or more cell masses fuse to form the large bizarre shaped complexes with multiple cysts of varying size. These cysts in turn coalesce until there is formed a single cyst of fair size. The process can easily be visualized as one that continues in this manner until we have the formation of a large multicystic tumor lined by cuboidal, columnar, or cylindrical cells. It has been suggested that in this manner ovarian cysts are formed, either the simple type lined by columnar epithelium or the more complicated pseudomucinous variety.

Both Pfannenstiel and Voigt have described tumors similar to the one above and suggested them as possible stages in the development of pseudomucinous cysts. On the other hand Brenner does not believe

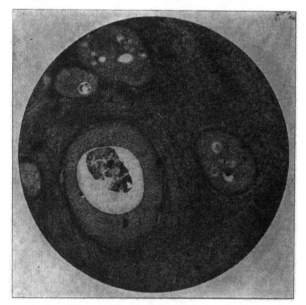

Fig. 5.—Cysts containing detritus and degenerating cells.

that these tumors form any but microcysts. In view of the fact that the tumor that I have described presented cysts lined by epithelium of the type found in the typical pseudomucinous tumors and in view of the probable method of development as we suggested it seems rational to suppose that the viewpoint of Pfannenstiel, Voigt and myself is possible.

There are no normal follicles to be seen in the tumor proper or even atretic ones. In the rest of the ovary while there were the scars of previous corpora lutea, there were no follicles seen in any stage of development. This of course in view of the age of the patient and her history of amenorrhea was to be expected. The cells in the compact masses resemble morphologically the cells of the granulosa cells of the follicles. We have an agglomeration composed of varying layers of cells oval or polyhedral with a deeply staining oval nucleus centrally placed, the basal layers having a somewhat radical appearance (Fig. 7). The masses may remain solid with a definite limiting connective tissue capsule a structure resembling a true theca, closely simulating a follicle without an ovum. On the other hand with the development of a cavity we have a picture that mimics the true ovarian follicle. From this stage there are the variations that compose the tumor.

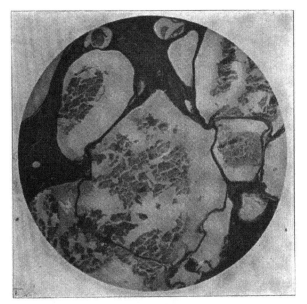

Fig. 6.—Cysts of varying size showing the thinning of the septa and gradual formation of larger cysts.

The question as to the histogenesis of this tumor is the point of interest. What type of cells in the ovary can give rise to a tumor that so closely mimics the follicles and also possesses the potentiality of reproducing so varied a picture and so divergent structures?

We know from the work of Goodall that there are found in the ovary structures whose origin can be traced to the original germinal cell layer of the fetus and that these structures located in the medullary cords or rete have the potentiality of developing follicle-like structures and of reproducing all the characteristics of the true follicle, even to the extent of imitating the oögenetic processes. In a personal communication from Goodall he stated ''the growth can be seen in any of the following stages, simple glandular growth, racemose glands with tall columnar cells in a single layer, gland acini with many layered cuboidal cells, solid masses of circular cells with much protoplasm, resembling an endothelioma or perithelioma and other circular masses of granulosa-like cells. This leads us to the presumption that can give rise to so many variations in growth, it is a cell of great potentiality and primitive characters, that is a cell from the parenchyma of the ovary.''

The tumor under discussion does not present the characteristics of

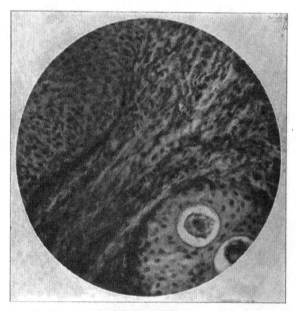

Fig. 7.—Edge of two cell nests, one showing small cavity with degenerating cell, the other showing polyhedral cells with radial arrangement resembling the granulosa layer of a follicle.

a malignant tumor. There is no tendency to invade the rest of the ovary, there are no mitotic figures to be seen, the individual cells are well-developed, normal-appearing structures with no abnormalities in the nuclei, and the entire structure of the growth is orderly. However, I agree with Goodall that a tumor with so many variations must arise from cells with primitive characteristics. This would preclude the possibility of origin from any of the mature cells of the ovary or follicle such as the granulosa cells of the primordial follicles as in these elements the potentiality is limited. Pflueger's cords might be considered as a possibility except that these structures rarely persist for so long a time in the ovary and furthermore the cells composing them give rise to one structure only, the follicle. It would seem that the cell rests from the original germinal epithelium that one finds in the medullary rays or rete as described by Goodall are the only possible source of a tumor with such wide variations as we have described. Further it would seem that these developmental anomalies may be the source of origin of the other forms of cystic ovarian tumors.

To recapitulate: In the ovaries of a woman fifty-two years of age were found on the one side a typical adenocarcinoma and on the other a process involving the greater portion of a somewhat enlarged ovary that also resembled a new growth. It is composed of masses of cells varying in number either isolated or in large branching strands. The cells in these solid masses resemble those of the granulosa layer of the follicle. In these masses are found cysts of varying sizes lined by cells of a cuboidal, columnar or the high cylindrical type as seen in the pseudomucinous type of ovarian cyst. Often in these cysts are found oval granular bodies which on superficial examination might be taken for degenerated ova but which are undoubtedly degenerated tumor cells or secretion masses. The origin of this process is the point of interest. It seems to be independent of the tumor of the other side, first as it bears no histologic resemblance to it, and second as it has none of the distinguishing criteria of a malignant tumor. The stroma resembles that of the unchanged ovary and is a predominant part of the process. The stroma and cells always maintain a definite relationship and at no point is there a proliferative or invasive tendency or an inflammatory infiltration. Mitoses were not found.

The cells composing the tumor resemble in their appearance and arrangement the granulosa cells and the general structure of the growth in parts suggests the developing follicle with many variations. Because of this morphologic appearance, the arrangement of the tumor and the wide variation in its structure, it is suggested that a cell of great potentiality must play the rôle of origin. Such a cell type we find in the embryologic rests that have been described by Goodall.

In addition the development of cysts which form by degeneration of the larger cell masses and grow by coalescence suggests this as one method of development of the microcysts and later of the larger cysts that occur in the ovary. Furthermore the cells lining these cysts are often cuboidal and occasionally high cylindrical mucin containing elements and can be traced by direct observation from the large cell masses of granulosa-like cells. This leads us to the presumption that some of the so-called simple cysts, follicular cysts and even the more complex pseudomucinous cysts may be the products of these same embryonal remains.

The nomenclature employed for the classification of this type of tumor is still indefinite, as each writer has selected a name that has fitted his theory of origin or the fancied resemblance to some structure of the ovary. At the present time there are tumors similar to the one above described that have been termed adenoma of the graafian follicle, folliculoma malignum, carcinoma folliculoides, oöphoroma folliculare, and folliculoma. Von Werdt described a group of tumors in which are included several somewhat similar to the above-mentioned type and has called them granulosa cell tumors. Several of the names can be discarded, such as adenoma of the graafian follicle, folliculoma malignum and carcinoma folliculoides as the tumor is neither a malignant tumor nor an adenoma. Personally I believe that the best way to classify these tumors is not to give them a name but to group them as tumors arising from persistent embryonal structures.

I wish to thank Dr. F. S. Mandlebaum, director of the laboratory, for the excellent microphotographs.

REFERENCES

Von Kahlden: Zentralbl. f. Allg. Path., vi, Part 7. *Gottschalk*: Arch. f. Gynäk., 1899, lix. *Schroeder*: Arch. f. Gynäk., 1901, lxiv. *Voigt*: Arch. f. Gynäk., 1903, lxx. *Liepmann*: Ztschr. f. Geburtsh. u. Gynäk., 1904, lii. *Von Werdt*: Beiträg. z. path. Anat., 1904, lix. *Brenner*: Frankf. Ztschr. f. Path., 1907, i. *Pfannenstiel*: Veit's Handbuch der Gynäk., 1898, iii. *Walthard*: Ztsch. f. Geburtsh. u. Gynäk., 1903, xlix. *Goodall*: Surg., Gynec. and Obst., 1920, xxx.

300 CENTRAL PARK WEST.

THE ACTION OF EMETINE HYDROCHLORIDE UPON THE UTERUS*

By PAUL MARTIN, M.D., (BRUSSELS), BOSTON, MASS.

From the Pharmacological Laboratory of Yale University School of Medicine.

IN Central Africa a few years ago I treated a white woman, in the sixth month of pregnancy, suffering from a dysenteriform enteritis (without amebae in the stools). Not responding to ordinary treatments she was given for three consecutive days one hypodermic injection of one grain of emetine hydrochloride. The drug had no action upon the enteritis and on the morning following the last injection, my patient went into labor and aborted the same evening. This suggested to me to test the action of emetine upon the uterus.

Since the work of Vedder[1] and of Rogers,[2] emetine has been the object of many experimental and clinical studies among which the following relate especially to the action of this drug upon the smooth muscle of the uterus.

Maurel,[3] who published the first experimental work on emetine, apparently performed no experiment upon the uterus. He, however, made the following suggestions after observing that smooth muscle is more sensitive to the action of emetine than any other tissue of the body: "By its action upon the smooth muscle of the uterus it must be able to control hemorrhage and perhaps to facilitate labor. But it must be able, too, in large doses, to cause abortion."

Nielson[4] states as a result of tests upon the pregnant and the nonpregnant guinea pig's uterus "it may be said that emetine apparently does not influence the tonic contractions, while it does seem to increase slightly the number and the volume of the rhythmic contractions."

Pellini and Wallace[5] experimented also with the isolated uterus of the guinea pig; they found on adding emetine to the fluid no change in uterine movement except a slight increase in tone.

In the present investigation we studied:

(1) The action of emetine hydrochloride upon the pregnant and the nonpregnant isolated uterus of the rat, dog, and rabbit.

(2) The action of emetine upon the pregnant and nonpregnant uterus of living animals (dogs, rabbits).

(3) We tried to produce abortion in rats by injecting emetine hypodermically.

---

*The expenses of this research were defrayed from a grant from the Therapeutic Research Committee of the Council on Pharmacy and Chemistry of the American Medical Association.

1. EXPERIMENTS WITH THE ISOLATED UTERUS

Our method was similar to that used by Dale[6]: A 100 c.c. beaker filled with Locke's solution was immersed in a larger vessel containing water kept at a constant temperature of 39° C., affording in the beaker a constant temperature of 37.5° C.

A constant flow of oxygen was kept bubbling through the Locke's solution by means of a glass tubing reaching the bottom of the beaker.

One end of the uterine muscle strip was fastened to the glass tubing in the bottom of the beaker, the other end being connected with a lever. Although the organ was prepared immediately after excision, a delay of about a half hour usually ensued before relaxation to a constant level occurred and regular rhythmic contractions were established.

The drug was added after a period of about ten or fifteen minutes of regular contractions.

The concentrations used were: 1/100,000; 1/20,000; 1/10,000. Emetine hydrochloride (Lily) was used in these experiments.

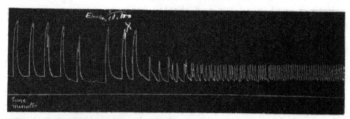

Fig. 1.—Isolated uterus of rat (nonpregnant). Time is recorded in minutes. Emetine (1/10,000) produced a decrease in the amplitude of contractions and an increase in the rate; the time being unchanged.

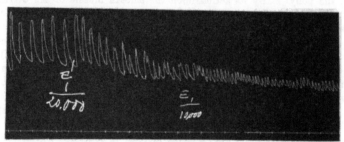

Fig. 2.—Excised uterus of rat (early pregnancy.) Shows the same as Fig. 1, plus a definite fall in the tone.

(A) *Experiments Upon the Nonpregnant Rat Uterus.*—The amplitude of contractions was found strikingly diminished, the rate much increased, and the tone unchanged. (Fig. 1 was selected from eight similar experiments to illustrate these points.)

(B) *Experiments upon the Pregnant Rat Uterus.*—The effects of emetine were found similar but there was also some decrease of the tone. (See Fig. 2, one of five experiments.)

(C) *Experiments upon the Rat Uterus During Involution.*—The

MARTIN: ACTION OF EMETINE HYDROCHLORIDE 243

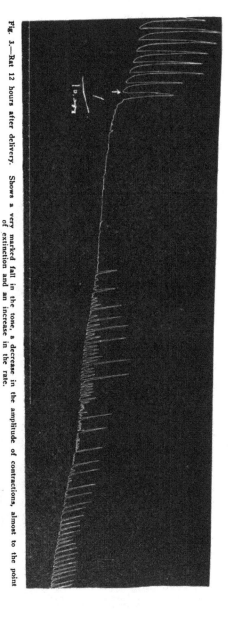

Fig. 3.—Rat 12 hours after delivery. Shows a very marked fall in the tone, a decrease in the amplitude of contractions, almost to the point of extinction and an increase in the rate.

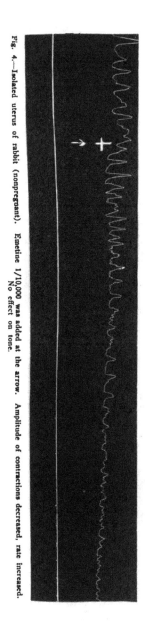

Fig. 4.—Isolated uterus of rabbit (nonpregnant). Emetine 1/10,000 was added at the arrow. Amplitude of contractions decreased, rate increased. No effect on tone.

uterus became completely paralyzed by emetine and the tone considerably decreased. However, this was not permanent as, after fifteen minutes the contractions were resumed with accelerated rate but diminished amplitude. (See Fig. 3, one of four experiments.)

The results are summarized in Table I in which + indicates increase; (–) decrease; and 0, no effect.

TABLE I
EXPERIMENTS UPON THE EXCISED UTERUS OF RATS

STATE OF UTERUS	AMPLITUDE	RATE	TONE
Nonpregnant	(–)	+	0
Pregnant	(–)	+	(–)
In involution	(–)	+	(–)

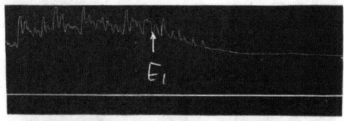

Fig. 5.—Isolated uterus of rabbit (pregnant). Decrease of tone and amplitude of contractions. (Emetine 1/10,000 added at the arrow.)

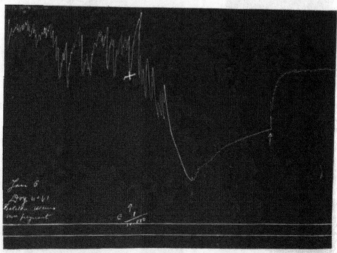

Fig. 6—Nonpregnant isolated dog uterus. Emetine 1/10,000 was added at the first arrow. Marked fall in tone, decrease in the amplitude of contractions and increase in the rate. (There was a little friction in the middle part of the tracing which was relieved at the second arrow.)

Emetine in a concentration of $1/100,000$ does not markedly affect the uterus. At $1/20,000$ the effect of emetine is well marked; at $1/10,000$ the effects were always very striking.

Some Tests with Quinine.—The fact that in tropical practice one very frequently prescribes emetine for patients who are accustomed to take preventive doses of quinine brought forward the question whether the effects of emetine added to those of quinine were not able to cause a special reaction upon the uterus. A few experiments upon the isolated uterus of rats revealed:

(1) That quinine given alone ($1/50,000$) failed to produce any effect upon the uterus.

(2) That introduction of emetine subsequent to that of quinine ($1/50,000$) has the same effect as when it is introduced alone.

(3) That emetine introduced at the same time as quinine ($1/50,000$) has the same effect as when it is added alone.

(D) *Experiments upon the Isolated Uterus of Rabbits.*—Emetine exhibited approximately the same effect in rabbits as in rats. (See Fig. 4 (nonpregnant rabbit) and 5 (pregnant rabbit) taken from groups of respectively three and two similar records.)

(E) *Experiments upon the Isolated Uterus of Dogs.*—Results similar to the above were given with the nonpregnant dog uterus except for a depression of tone by emetine exceeding that noted in pregnant rats and rabbits. (See Fig. 6, one of four experiments.)

2. EXPERIMENTS UPON LIVING ANIMALS

Dogs and rabbits were used.

Technic.—In the first experiments a finger cot was introduced into the vagina and to record muscular activity connected with a Marly's tambour. This method had the advantage that it could be used, at least in rabbits, without an anesthetic and without sacrificing the animal. But it was soon found unsatisfactory because intestinal peristalsis and vesical contractions were sometimes recorded at the same time.

The method finally chosen was that described by Barbour.[7] This requires anesthesia. The dogs were given 5 mg. morphine sulphate per kilo hypodermically, followed one-half hour later by 0.15 gm. of chloretone per kilo administered by means of a stomach tube. This gave a satisfactory anesthesia which lasted about five or six hours. However, the anesthesia being very light, it has sometimes been necessary to give a small quantity of ether when starting the laparotomy.

The rabbits were anesthetized with 1 gram of paraldehyde (by stomach tube). The uterus exhibits an apparently normal rhythmic activity under these anesthetics but the possibility of their exerting some influence upon the action of other drugs cannot be overlooked.

After anesthesia was obtained, usually a half hour after the chloretone was given an abdominal incision was made in the median line directly above the pubis for a distance of about 8 cm. The contents of the bladder were expressed. Then the two horns of the uterus were cut between two ligatures, near the ovaries. The broad ligaments were then dissected gently in order to liberate the uterus without injuring the blood vessels. A glass cylinder of about 10x2.5 cm. was inserted in the wound and the abdominal wall sewed around it.

The uterus was connected with a lever by means of a thread which passed through the cylinder. Warm albolene was poured into the abdominal cavity until it filled the cylinder.

The carotid blood pressure was recorded; emetine was injected through a cannula inserted into the femoral vein.

A. *Rabbits.*—With nonpregnant rabbits the result obtained was opposite to that recorded with the excised uterus. Emetine (2 mg. per kilo) gave an increase in the uterine tone and did not seem to influence the amplitude and the rate of contractions. (See Fig. 7, one of four experiments.) No experiments were performed on pregnant rabbits.

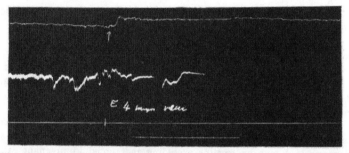

Fig. 7.—Nonpregnant rabbit, 1700 grams (intact uterus). Four mgs. of emetine were injected at the arrow. The injection was followed by an increase in the tone of the uterus.

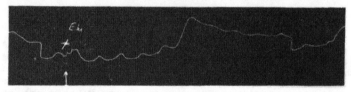

Fig. 8.—Nonpregnant uterus of dog *in situ*. Shows the rise in tone caused by an intravenous injection of emetine (1 mg. per kilo).

B. *Dogs.*—(1) Nonpregnant Uterus. The only change obtained was an increase of the tone. There was no marked change in the amplitude and the rate of contractions. (See Fig. 8, one of six similar records.)

(2) Pregnant Uterus. Here also an increase of tone was seen in each of the three cases tested. The amplitude also usually became slightly increased, the rate remaining approximately the same.

3. INJECTIONS IN UNOPERATED PREGNANT RATS

Hypodermic injections of fairly large doses of emetine were given to pregnant rats with the intention of determining whether abortion could be provoked. "Timed pregnant rats" supplied by the Wistar Institute were used. In one series each animal was given a single dose of 2 mg. of emetine hydrochloride. In another series two 1 mg. doses were injected in each rat on two successive days.

The results are tabulated as follows:

TABLE II
FIRST SERIES. (SINGLE 2 MG. DOSE OF EMETINE)

RAT NO.	STAGE OF PREGNANCY	WEIGHT	DATE OF INJECTION	RESULTS
1	14 days	210	1- 6-21	Died on 1-8-21. Vaginal hemorrhage. Uterus removed several hours after death showed microscopically an aborted fetus.
2	18 days	240	1-22-21	No effect. Delivered at term of pregnancy. (22d day.)
3	14 days	200	1-23-21	No effect. Delivered at term of pregnancy. (22d day.)

SECOND SERIES. (TWO 1 MG. DOSES OF EMETINE ON SUCCESSIVE DAYS)

RAT NO.	STAGE OF PREGNANCY	WEIGHT GM.	FIRST INJECTION	SECOND INJECTION	RESULTS
1	16	...	1- 8-21	1- 9-21	No effect. Delivered at term.
2	18	220	1-22-21	1-23-21	" " " " "
3	19	240	1-23-21	1-24-21	" " " " "

Thus the attempts to induce abortion with nearly lethal doses failed except in the one case which ended fatally. Here the uterus was not removed until five hours after death so that the histopathology may have been due to some postmortem uterine change. Furthermore, since this occurred on the fourteenth day of pregnancy it is most probable that if the emetine was responsible for the abortion similar results would have occurred in the other rats, which were in a more advanced stage of pregnancy.

DISCUSSION

The most important finding in this work was that the action of emetine upon the uterus differed *in vitro* and *in vivo*.

The failure of the uterus *in vivo* to relax after emetine can be accounted for by the probability that by the time the organ was reached by the drug an effective concentration (such as $1/20{,}000$) was not available. Furthermore the presence of the serum colloids is known to detract from the action of some drugs on smooth muscle.[8]

To account for the positive finding of an increase in tone it becomes necessary to seek an explanation by which some tissue or organ of the body exerts an intermediary action. My first idea was that emetine might act by an influence upon the secretion of a ductless gland. With regard to the ovary Athias[9] claims that the uterus of a castrated female guinea pig does not exhibit any contractions *in vitro*.

I performed experiments upon three ovariectomized dogs but emetine produced an increase of the tone of the uterus in these cases as in other animals. (See Fig. 9.)

Another explanation might be found in a possible indirect influence by the adrenal secretion, but two adrenalectomy experiments gave no positive results.

The rise in uterine tone seen *in vivo* is always accompanied by the

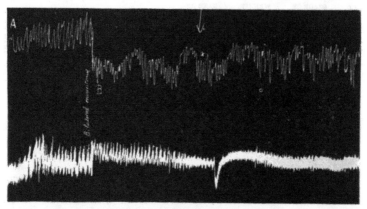

Fig. 9.

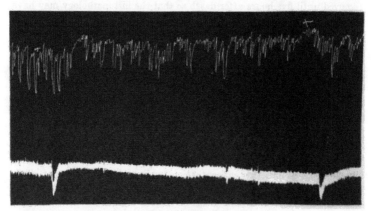

Fig. 9. (Continued)

Fig. 9.—Dog (intact uterus). The first part (*A*) of the tracing shows the normal activity of the uterus. The second part (*B*) shows the uterine movements after bilateral ovariectomy has been performed. Emetine (1 mg. per kilo) was injected at the crosses. There is a slight increase in tone after each injection.

secondary blood pressure rise so that it may be due to stimulation of the medulla, analogous to the emetic action of emetine. Another plausible hypothesis is that emetine may act by stimulating some (non-peripheral) part of the sympathetic system. The nerve physiology of the uterus is not, however, clearly enough defined to allow of further speculation on the matter.

CONCLUSIONS

1. *In vitro* emetine lessens the activity of pregnant and nonpregnant uterus (dogs, rats, rabbits). It causes a decrease in tone and amplitude although increasing the rate of contractions.

2. *In vivo* emetine causes an increase in the tone of the uterus both pregnant and nonpregnant (dogs and rabbits).

3. Emetine probably does not act as an abortifacient in rats.

4. Emetine might be tested with caution in the treatment of metrorrhagia and menorrhagia owing to the fact that it increases the tone of the uterus *in vivo*.

Professor H. G. Barbour, in whose laboratory this work was performed, gave many valuable suggestions and advice and had the kindness to revise the manuscript. We beg him to accept our best thanks.

REFERENCES

(1) Jour. of Tropical Med., 1911, xiv, 149-162. (2) Brit. Med. Jour., 1912, 1, 1424. (3) Arch. de méd. expér. et d'anat. path., 1914, xxvi, 225-250. (4) Am. Jour. Clin. Med., 1915, xxii, 227-235. (5) Am. Jour. Med. Sc., 1916, clii, 325-336. (6) Jour. Pharm. and Exper. Therap., 1912, iv, 75-95. (7) Jour. of Pharm. and Exper. Therap., 1915, vii, 547. (See also Jackson's Experimental Pharmacology, pp. 363-364, Fig. 306.) (8) *Storm Van Leeuwen*: On the Influence of Colloids on the Action of Noncolloidal Drugs, Jour. Pharm. and Exper. Therap., 1921, xvii, 1-20. (9) Jour. de physiol. et de path. gén., Paris, 1920, xviii, 731-743.

PETER BENT BRIGHAM HOSPITAL.

CARCINOMA UTERI*

By Charles L. Bonifield, M.D., Cincinnati, Ohio

CANCER is still the most dreaded of all diseases. Cancer of the uterus is one of the most frequent and at the same time one of the most fatal and most disagreeable manifestations of this disease. Its treatment still leaves much to be desired. We have two other papers on the program on this subject, one dealing with its treatment by radium, and the other with the extending of the radical operation for its surgical removal. I will simply speak of a few points, with which I have been impressed as a result of my own medical experience, and the observation of the work of others.

The cause of cancer has not yet been determined, but there are two factors in its etiology that have impressed every observing clinician, as being very important. The first is the age of the patient at the time cancer occurs, and the second is chronic irritation. The period at which cancer of the uterus is most prone to occur begins about forty, and ends about fifty-five. Many cases are seen in earlier life, many later, but this is the real cancer age. It cannot be emphasized too strongly or too frequently that the patient should be brought to that period of her life in the best possible condition, physically, particularly as regards her uterus. Therefore, all lacerations of the cervix that produce any irritation at all should be repaired, and if a chronic endometritis exists, it should be cured before this period arrives.

The next point I wish to emphasize is that for a number of years we have been trying to preach to the laity the danger of cancer, and in this way to get to operate and treat cancer in its earliest stages, but that our efforts have not produced the results which we hoped. To my mind there is some objection to carrying on the propaganda as it has been carried on in the past. Something like a year ago, we had "Cancer Day," in Ohio, and a number of Protestant pulpits in Cincinnati were filled with speakers on cancer. I know of at least one instance where a woman fainted, and had to be carried out after hearing a discussion on this subject by one of the speakers, and many more were so frightened that the talks did them no good. I maintain that to arouse hysteria in regard to these things is folly, and does not bring results.

The thing I wish to suggest instead of this, is that every woman who has borne children, and therefore has the strongest predisposition

---

*Read at the Thirty-Fourth Annual Meeting of the American Association of Obstetricians, Gynecologists, and Abdominal Surgeons, St. Louis, Mo., September 20-22, 1921.

or the strongest predisposing cause that we know of, when she reaches the age of thirty-five or forty should go to her family physician and be examined to see if any symptoms of cancer are manifesting themselves. It is necessary for us to go to our dentists every six months in order to save our teeth, and so it certainly seems worth while for the woman to subject herself to this little inconvenience and expense for the purpose of saving her life.

It has been my experience, and I believe that of most of us, that 75 per cent of the cases of cancer that come into the office are already so far advanced that the hope of permanent and complete cure has already gone by.

The next point I wish to speak of is the treatment. I think this might be divided into four methods; cautery, x-ray, radium and surgery. The cautery is one of the oldest treatments and has given good results, but it is not applicable to all the cases and has not become very popular. The same may be said of the Percy treatment by heat. The x-ray I believe is capable of further development, and I have great hopes that some time it will be a more powerful remedial agent than any we have at present. I understand that in Germany they are making tubes that will make it more potent, but at present it does not, in my opinion, answer the purpose as well as other methods.

In some places, the most popular and to some people the most attractive treatment is radium, but the very expense of this treatment will for many years to come, prevent its applicability to the vast majority of cases of cancer of the uterus, but this to me is not a very depressing fact because I still believe that the thorough removal of cancer by the surgeon is the best treatment that has yet been devised. Just what the procedure shall be must depend upon the judgment of the surgeon into whose hands a given patient falls. When we first operated for cancer, the vaginal hysterectomy was done, and by and by the operation was extended and extended as we became more radical, and of late years, we have been preaching and practicing that the radical operation should be limited to those cases in which we feel very sure that we are able to remove the disease in its entirety. I concurred in that belief for many years, but my observations in recent years have convinced me that I was mistaken. Up to that time when a case came to me, that I regarded as inoperable for thorough cure, I was satisfied to curette away the tissue as far as possible and then cauterize with the actual cautery, following that with applications of formaldehyde. I relieved these patients somewhat and prolonged their life, but all the time these patients knew that the disease was still there. The psychologic effect was bad and death followed, preceded by those dreadful complications such as vesicovaginal and rectovaginal fistula. In operating I occasionally made mistakes. I thought when I examined a patient, I would be able to do a complete hysterectomy, but when I opened the abdomen, I found I could not get quite all the disease. Observation has convinced me that my mistake was a fortunate one for the patient, for she lived longer than the others, and when she died, she passed away with less discomfort.

Such cases have now become sufficiently numerous to convince me that my former teaching and practice was a mistake, that wherever it is at all practical to do a hysterectomy, it should be done. These are the points that I particularly wish to emphasize, but I also wish to say: The advocates of radium claim that if they do not cure the patients, they relieve the pain, and they die happily. It has been my fortune or misfortune, to see a number of cases dying after treatment by radium, and one of them, I think, died the most miserable death of any patient with cancer of the uterus that has been under my care.

409 BROADWAY. (*For discussion, see p.* 312.)

SOME PHASES IN THE EVOLUTION OF THE DIAGNOSIS AND TREATMENT OF CANCER OF THE CERVIX[*]

By ROLAND E. SKEEL, M.D., F.A.C.S., LOS ANGELES, CAL.

ONE who peruses the literature of the preceding century in a search for data on cancer of the cervix, is likely to be the victim of conflicting emotions when his labor is completed. He will be deeply impressed by the magnificent advance which the profession has made in its knowledge of pathology, the prevention of infection, and improvement in operative technic; and as profoundly depressed by the absence of corresponding improvement in the ultimate mortality rate of the disease.

It was my intention in planning this paper to consider the diagnosis and treatment of cancer of the cervix in four principal epochs of the last one hundred years; first, the preanesthetic; second, from the discovery of anesthesia until the time of general adoption of antiseptic methods; third, from the preceding until the publications of Wertheim's panhysterectomy; and fourth, from the latter to the present, a time when it is felt that a new era is dawning, one which is likely to persist until the discovery of the ultimate cause of cancer leads to the development of a positive cure.

Somewhat to my surprise there appeared to be no significant change either in methods of operation or the results obtained following the

[*]Read at the Thirty-Fourth Annual Meeting of the American Association of Obstetricians, Gynecologists, and Abdominal Surgeons, St. Louis, Mo., September 20-22, 1921.

general introduction of anesthesia; and operations for cervical cancer were denounced, thereafter, in almost the identical language used before, excepting that the term painful occurred less frequently. So the plan of study was changed to make the first era extend to the time when aseptic and antiseptic principles were universally adopted, i.e., the 1880-1890 decade, the second from 1890 to 1907; the third from 1907 to 1921.

Diagnosis and treatment are considered together since, at least, some of the improved results of modern treatment can be conclusively traced to earlier and more accurate diagnosis as well as more effectual treatment. It also seems logical to begin our study with the opening of the last century; for while there had been casual mention of operative procedures for the relief of cancer of the cervix for many years, the first systematic attempt at amputation of the cervix seems to have been made by Osiander in 1802, at vaginal hysterectomy by Sauter in 1822, and Langenbeck's first abdominal hysterectomy was performed in 1825.

At this time the diagnosis of cancer was accomplished by clinical methods only; and while the microscope was occasionally employed for the study of pathology, there was no definite demonstration of the difference between the minute anatomy of cancer and other new growths. The microscopic differential diagnosis of early cancer was unknown.

As late as 1857 Churchill[1] wrote: "As our microscopic knowledge increases we may arrive at some definite distinctive mark by which to recognize the disease," while ten years earlier J. Hughes Bennet[2] read a paper on "The more exact diagnosis of cancer by the use of the microscope," in which he said: "we are only on the threshold of inquiry. What may we expect when surgeons are more extensively assured of the diagnosis?" At this same period, 1850 and thereabouts, Rokitansky and Virchow definitely established cellular pathology and the pathology of cancer. Paget's *Surgical Pathology*, published in 1865, gives the minute anatomy of cancer practically as we know it today; while the method of transmission and metastasis to other areas is erroneously attributed to the blood stream.

During the latter part of the preantiseptic era other lesions which had not been considered to be true cancers, especially that condition known as cancroid, were gradually recognized as being of a genuinely cancerous nature. The earliest and most thoroughgoing emphasis upon the epithelial character of the cancer cell and the diagnostic importance of its minute anatomy by any English writer of renown, was made by Lawson Tait[3] in 1879.

It is interesting to note that long before Emmet's discovery of laceration of the cervix, the prevalence of cancer of the cervix in women who had borne many children and those having had many difficult labors, was not only known, but given almost universal recognition, and this explanation for the greater frequency of cervical cancer in Europe than in America is mentioned by more than one writer of the period.

As regards prognosis and treatment, it is also interesting to note the same occasional recovery after the use of some simple or bizarre remedy, and the same discrepancy of opinion as to whether any case actually made a permanent recovery that we find at present; the pessimistic note gradually diminishing towards the end of the era.

Dewees[4] in 1847, says that "Our duty in the treatment of uterine cancer is to mitigate suffering which we cannot remove." Tait, *ibid,* in 1879, said of cancer of the cervix that it is "the most painful and terrible disease from which mankind suffers, because nothing can be done for its cure" and that he "has never had a cure."

Emmet[5] in 1884 said: "When at the time of operation no doubt existed as to the character of the malady it always returned."

Other writers mention an occasional cure running over a two year period, an inadequate time as we understand it today; but this mention of what we would consider uncertain cures, grows more and more frequent as operative procedures became more common and less dangerous.

During this period, also, we see a gradually increasing effort at more radical extirpation; a wave of enthusiasm for each procedure being succeeded by revulsion of feeling as improved results failed to materialize in the hands of any one aside from its sponsor.

It is difficult to avoid undue and untimely philosophizing when considering the methods of treatment in use and "there is nothing new under the sun" occurs to one's mind over and over again. Thus early writers contended that low diet and local and general venesection prolonged life. In 1842 Montgomery[6] quite accurately described as an early type of cancer, what we now regard as laceration with cervicitis and hypertrophy, which, he said, should be treated by local blood letting and the application of nitrate of silver. Douches of chloride of lime solution were recognized as efficient deodorizers in advanced cases with fetor.

Byrne,[7] in 1871, reported a case in which he was unable to apply his galvanocautery loop and in which a cautery knife was used instead; while Courty[8] in 1882 advocated amputation with a peculiar shaped cautery knife made by Colin of Paris, the vagina being protected during its application by a box wood speculum.

Noeggerath[9] in the discussion of Byrne's paper fifty years ago, announced his conviction that radiating heat destroyed cancer cells beyond the point of application and thus prevented recurrence.

From the time of Osiander's demonstration, amputation of the cervix, as a definitive method of treatment for cancer, easily maintained its supremacy throughout the preantiseptic era. Performed at first with knife, scissors or écraseur, the operation was greatly improved by the introduction of various types of galvanocautery loops and knives.

Marked palliation of symptoms and, occasionally, a permanent cure, can be said to have been the result of amputations until the time of Byrne who, first with the galvanocautery loop and later with cautery knives and dome-shaped irons, established a record which surpassed anything previously known. As early as 1871, he was enabled to report several cases without recurrence after from six to nine years.

Vaginal hysterectomy began also to have its advocates; but vaginal hysterectomy was endowed with a peculiar fatality for many years after its introduction, especially if performed with the uterus *in situ*, while the death rate was low if the uterus was prolapsed or inverted. Indeed, these two conditions were considered to be the indications *par excellence* for the operation. Until 1830, there were but ten authentic cases of removal of the uterus, per vaginam, and the operation was called the most serious and painful in surgery. The editor of the *Medico-Chirurgical Review* remarks at this time, "We consider the extirpation of the uterus, not previously protruded or inverted, one of the most cruel and unfeasible operations that ever was projected or executed by the head or hand of man."

Thus the dangers were so great that, in 1856, but 25 vaginal hysterectomies had been performed, with 22 operative deaths and three recurrences. In 1863, Sir James Y. Simpson[10] said that "excision of the uterus is an unthinkable procedure at present;" and, in 1882, Courty wrote that "extirpation of the entire uterus and supravaginal cervix were common enough at one time to afford material upon which to base a serious opinion as to their advisability. Only the infravaginal cervix should be amputated and with this some cures result."

The decade 1880 to 1890, was marked by a renaissance of vaginal hysterectomy following the lead of numerous German surgeons abroad and Fenger in America.

This same decade saw a decline in abdominal panhysterectomy which had been taken up by a number of European surgeons of note, following Freund's[11] report, 1878, of ten operations with but five deaths. Despite this mortality, some operations continued to be performed; but vaginal hysterectomy was, at this time, so much safer that the surgical profession continued to lean towards it despite the high percentage of recurrence.

During this decade and, indeed, until his death, Byrne continued, as pointed out by Werder, to be as one crying in the wilderness, and at the time of his death he had nearly 400 cases to his credit without an operative death and with a 19 per cent permanent recovery rate.

It is assumed that all of us are more or less familiar with the situation as it existed from the beginning of the antiseptic era until the complete development of the Wertheim operation and the publication of his studies[12] in this country in 1907, from which may be said to date the general, although by no means universal, adoption of this method of operating for cancer of the cervix.

In this era vaginal hysterectomy continued to lead other operative procedures, and the mortality was continuously lowered; but, at the same time, the safety of all abdominal operations was almost unbelievably increased through the practice of surgical asepsis. Ovariotomy, salpingectomy and hysteromyomectomy, heretofore approached with great apprehension, became so safe that recovery was anticipated as a matter of course. In view of this it is not strange that the improved results from more extensive operation and glandular excision in cancer of the breast, called the attention of several operators to the possibilities inherent in a more radical extirpation of the periuterine structures and pelvic lymph glands, so that Mackenrodt, Rumpf, Ries and Clark, in 1894 and 1895, independently evolved methods which differed somewhat in detail but not in principle. In 1898, Werder[13] published his method of total removal of the uterus with a large portion of the vagina, and in the same year Wertheim began the study which eventuated in the operation bearing his name.

The complete development of the Wertheim operation seems to have been brought about by serial studies of the iliac glands together with a knowledge of the high ratio of local recurrence after vaginal hysterectomy. Wertheim's appearance in this country, with the publication of his statistics to date, was but the culmination of a series of events which gave the Wertheim operation its widespread vogue.

In his Chicago address, Wertheim reported 345 operations (about 50 per cent of all the cases applying for treatment). Especial attention is directed to his assertion that his early mortality was 18 per cent following a 2 to 2½ hour operation, while he was able, later to reduce this to 8 per cent for the same operation if its performance did not require more than an hour.

From 1907 to the present may be considered the Wertheim era, although Schauta continued to contend valiantly for his extended vaginal method during the early years of the epoch.

In order to obtain a correct perspective of recent developments, the introduction of statistics becomes necessary despite their known unreliability.

Fortunately modern methods of microscopic diagnosis remove one element of uncertainty in that, practically, all cases reported as cancer of the cervix are that and not something else, so that the greatest element of uncertainty does not pertain so much to the percentage of cures as to the stage which had been attained when the cure resulted, the percentage of operability reported running all the way from

Clark's estimate of only 10 per cent, applying to the University of Pennsylvania Clinic, up to Graves'[14] latest figures of 64 per cent. Obviously the difference between these figures represents a difference in the material seen by each and, probably, also a different viewpoint as to what does and what does not render a case inoperable.

One may consider operation worth while even though permanent cure is improbable, while another may be taking a very broad view of the community and sociologic aspect of an operation, which, although an improvement on what has preceded it, still has so disastrous a general mortality and recurrence rate, as to frighten prospective good operative risks, thus leading them to delay examination and treatment until they, in turn, become poor operative risks; the whole constituting what might be termed a sociosurgical vicious circle. Of the writers consulted, Clark alone seems to emphasize this broad humanitarian viewpoint. Moreover the value of statistics depends upon the relation between the constant and the variable factors: When the known constant factors remain the same, multiplication of numbers tends to average the variables and leads to increasing accuracy, so that case reports running into the thousands mean something rather definite, while a few may mean much or nothing.

A comparison of results as between vaginal and abdominal hysterectomy for cancer during the past ten years would be unfair to vaginal hysterectomy, since most surgeons now choose the latter in obese patients or those obviously unable to bear the shock and hemorrhage of the abdominal operation, the bad risks, while a comparison of the two in 1900, let us say, would be unfair to abdominal hysterectomy which then was in a state of earlier evolution than the vaginal operation. A comparison of the results when each operation may have been said to be at its acme, however, is not unfair; and, counting the available statistics, gives the following results for vaginal hysterectomy: Operability 37 per cent, operative mortality 4.5 per cent; five year cures 28 per cent; absolute cures, per one hundred applying for treatment, 12.5 per cent.

Applying the same method to the Wertheim operation, Janeway[15] completed the following figures. Of 5027 cases 35 per cent were operable, operative mortality 18 per cent. Five year cures 35 per cent; absolute cures, per hundred applying for treatment, 12 per cent.

A comparison of these two sets of statistics is interesting. Operability rate is nearly the same, the absolute cures are almost identical. The superiority of five year cures from the Wertheim operation, being figured on survivors of the operation, is offset completely by the greater number that succumb to this operation as compared to vaginal hysterectomy.

Some smaller but later sets of statistics serve somewhat to dissipate the gloom produced by a comtemplation of figures which appear to show that we have not succeeded in advancing very far even with the aid of what may be termed a super-major operation.

Thus Lincoln Davis[16] gives, in 64 cases, an operable rate of 42 per cent; mortality rate, 11 per cent; five year cures, 42 per cent; absolute cures, 8 out of 64, again 12.5 per cent. Graves[14] reports 64 per cent operable out of 189 cases or 119 operated upon with a 5 per cent mortality rate; and Cobb, in his last 30 cases, had the same mortality rate with an average of absolute curability of 18.5 per cent. Weiss[18] in 1918, reporting on the Werder operation, gave 25 per cent operability, 6 per cent mortality, 45 per cent five year cures, making 11 per cent absolute cures. Faure[19] says he has treated 71 by abdominal hysterectomy, 50 per cent free from recurrence; but adds that of "early cases 88 per cent survive, of late, 27 per cent."

In contemplating the subject and reading the available literature two things stand out with great distinctness. First, the mortality rate goes down with increasing experience. Thus many writers refer to their last thirty, or fifty, or one hundred cases when stating the possibilities inherent in the Wertheim operation. Second, the operative recovery rate and freedom from recurrence are enormously increased by early diagnosis and early operation. Of the importance of the latter all of us are aware and it is not my intention to go into this phase of the subject on this occasion.

Though the data do not justify so high an operability rate, so low a general mortality rate, nor so high an absolute curability rate, let us observe, in liberal round numbers, what has happened at the expiration of five years to 100 women with cancer of the cervix, if 50 per cent were operable; there was only a 10 per cent mortality rate, and 20 per cent of absolute cures. Out of 100, twenty are now well; fifty inoperables have gone on and died, all presumably having had a Percy cautery. curette and cautery, or some other form of local treatment; five of the fifty operated upon died at once, and the remaining twenty-five died from a recurrence. Of the fifty who underwent a tremendously severe painful operation, thirty were dead within five years. Were the operation less serious, less heroic, and less frequently complicated by postoperative sequelae, such a showing might be justifiable; but with the reverse true, it, in my opinion, lacks justifiability when performed upon the present indications of operability.

The Present Era.—Cobb[17] says: "It is absolutely certain that radium and cautery cannot cure cancer of the cervix." Between this and the opinion of ardent radiotherapists, there is room for a wide difference of opinion, opinion which must be based upon impressions rather than large arrays of statistics, since radium has been used extensively and intelligently for too short a period to permit the completion of conclusive statistics.

Allowing for the exaggeration which attends every new method, the legitimate and illegitimate enthusiasm attaching to any new operative painless treatment, utilizing so mysterious a force as radium, there still remains the fact that radium has been used in a sufficient number of inoperable hopeless cases with results so startling as to make us pause; and, on reflection, question whether bloody means ever are justifiable in cancer of the cervix, and if so, when?[20]

That Cobb's statement is extreme,[21] and that radium does sometimes cure cancer of the cervix, can be proved by a limited number of cases in the records of many surgeons and radiotherapists. Personally, I have one with no recurrence after seven years following cautery amputation and radium; but it is the apparent cure of a considerable number of inoperable cases extending over two, three, four, and five years that makes it impossible to rule radium out of the field. Thus Burnam reports 30 patients without recurrence out of 200 treated by radium more than five years ago, and these were either borderline or inoperable cases. If only we knew whether late recurrence was rendered more likely after radium than after the knife, we would have some definite data for comparison; but of this we are not certain. We can at least conceive that living carcinoma cells may be imprisoned in the mass of connective tissue, left after the use of radium, to again become active many years later. That postoperative sequelae do occur after radium treatment, is well known; that an occasional death may result from overradiation in an advanced case may be granted; but there is no perceptible mortality rate in cases which are operable when measured by our present standards.

From a careful personal observation and checking up of my own results, and taking into consideration all the concomitant circumstances, I have been gradually driven to certain conclusions but, before putting them before this body, I felt it wise to obtain the opinions, pro and con, of a few distinguished authorities with much greater experience than my own, who are not members of the Association and, therefore, would not be present to give their personal views in the discussion.

Accordingly, letters were sent to W. J. Mayo, Reuben Peterson, John G. Clark, and Howard C. Taylor, asking them to criticize, favorably or unfavorably, the thesis that "Only such cases of cancer of the cervix should be submitted to the Wertheim operation, as are discovered so early in the course of the disease as to require the microscope for a positive diagnosis." At the time these letters were written the papers of Clark and Keene,[22] Schmitz,[23] and Duncan[24] had not been published. If they had been available, Clark's opinion could have been obtained by quotation from his paper rather than by personal solicitation; and Schmitz's statement would have been presented earlier in the present discussion since it so accurately corresponds with my own experience. This paragraph of Schmitz is as follows: "In my experience, almost all the patients that survived an operation for carcinoma for the customary five year limit had been either subjected to a panhysterectomy on account of unexpected microscopic findings or the recurrence and persistence of the underlying pathologic process after minor surgical procedures instituted for the correction of apparently benign disease," whereas I had endeavored to put the matter concisely by stating that in those who survived, the discovery of malignancy had been accidental.

Concisely stated, cancer of the cervix was practically hopeless until the introduction of the galvanocautery amputation by Byrne. Unfortunately this was not widely adopted and the results obtained by vaginal hysterectomy, when that operation was fully developed, were probably superior to cautery amputation alone. Certainly it was more extensively used so that many more cures resulted.

Panhysterectomy, by the Wertheim method, has in general no higher rate of absolute cure than the vaginal operation; but in the hands of the most expert it is, probably, superior to vaginal hysterectomy. All of the major operative procedures, performed upon the ordinary indications of operability, leave so large a proportion untreated, have so high a mortality rate, and such a large number of recurrences, as to have a profoundly bad effect upon what may be termed the community surgical morale; and, therefore, I wish to present the following theses for discussion, all but the first being offered in the hope of standardizing our procedures, as well as in the belief that more cures will be effected than at present.

CONCLUSIONS

1. Any expectation of an increased number of cures of cancer of the cervix by surgical methods must be based upon earlier diagnosis.

2. Panhysterectomy should be reserved for cases in which a positive diagnosis can be made with the microscope only.

3. The parametrium being free so far as digital examination can determine, but the case far enough advanced to be diagnosed, clinically, a high cautery amputation of the cervix, followed by radium treatment, offers the greatest hope of cure.

4. The advanced, surgically hopeless case should be treated by radium rather than with the knife, curette and cautery, chemical caustics, or Percy cauterization, unless profound toxemia or serious infection contraindicates local interference of any kind.

The replies to my letter were as follows:

"In reply to your letter of July ninth, asking my opinion as to the position you are about to take on the question of the diagnosis and treatment of cancer of the cervix, I will say that I am afraid that I cannot agree with you.

"I have nothing against the use of radium, although I have no personal experience with it. However, you must remember that comparatively few men have enough radium to carry out such treatment. Cancer of the cervix is widespread and should be seen and treated by many surgeons. The greatest good will result, in my opinion, where cases of cancer of the cervix are seen early by the surgeon and subjected to radical surgical treatment. The poor results of the radical operation came from unfamiliarity with the technic and subjecting too far advanced cases to the knife. However, many cases which can be diagnosticated as cancer of the cervix by inspection and palpation can be cured by the radical operation. This does not mean that every case should not be checked up by the microscope. But the criterion of surgical treatment for carcinoma of the cervix diagnosticated by the microscope *only* in my opinion is not broad enough.

"Have you seen Graves' last article? His work, that of Cobb, and possibly my own show what can be accomplished by the radical operation. It only remains for surgeons to strive to have the patients come to them early and to operate only upon these early cases.—*Reuben Peterson.*"

"Relative to your question as to when to apply the radical operation in cancer of the cervix, I would say that I have almost reached the point where I believe radium is the best treatment for all cases regardless of the extent of the lesion. During the last year we have operated upon very few cases; so few, indeed, as to make our statistics almost negligible. I cannot help but feel, therefore, that when we consider the remarkably good results in inoperable cases which follow radiation, the very early case ought to respond infinitely better. I do not feel, however, that I have quite reached the point yet where I am able to take the stand squarely in favor of radiation alone; but I have so nearly come to this point, I very seldom do a radical operation.—*John G. Clark.*"

"I have your letter of July 9 in regard to the use of radical (Ries, Clark, Wertheim) hysterectomy for cancer of the cervix. The Wertheim type of operation has today only a very small field of usefulness. Personally, I have not done one in three years. Radium is taking the place of the extensive operation for the cure of carcinoma of the cervix with the exception of very early cases and it is possible that it will soon be the method of choice in all cases, either alone or combined with operation. For carcinoma of the body of the uterus, total hysterectomy is the operation of choice.—*W. J. Mayo.*"

"I do not go so far as your letter would indicate in the use of radium instead of operation for carcinoma of the cervix uteri. There is no question that all of us have changed our ideas with regard to the cases that are operable, but personally I would prefer operation in a case in which carcinoma is limited to the cervix with no involvement of the vaginal walls or the bases of the broad ligaments.

"It is my custom if the growth seems limited to the cervix to first make an application of radium (100 milligrams for twenty-four hours) and then to wait for two weeks. At the end of that time I do such hysterectomy as the case seems to indicate. If the patient is in good condition and is a good operable risk I would do a radical abdominal operation. If the patient is not in good condition I would be satisfied with a less extensive hysterectomy.

"The only theoretical objections to this plan are the risk of the operation and the theoretical possibility of liberating some live cancer cells by the operation which have been encysted by the action of the radium. I consider that the risk of the operation is a very small one. Selecting only favorable cases the mortality from the radical abdominal operation is small. The risk of cancer cells which have become encysted ultimately causing trouble seems to me to be considerable. For these reasons I still consider that there is a definite group of cases that should be operated upon and that this group is more extensive than your letter would indicate. There is another group of cases on which I operate though I appreciate that I may be wrong in doing so. I refer to the class of cases that are inoperable when first seen on account of extension to the vaginal walls or to the bases of the broad ligaments but which become operable, that is, any induration extending outside of the uterus is removed, by the application of radium. On these cases, assuming that they are favorable operable risks, I still do a hysterectomy. I have in mind one case in which the growth had extended upward into the fundus of the uterus to such an extent that it was well away from reach of radium and in my judgment beyond doubt carcinomatous tissue was removed by the operation that would not have been cured by radium alone.

"I appreciate that many of our best men have largely given up operations in these cases and are relying entirely on radium. I think only time can decide which course is the better to follow. That great benefit is derived from the use of radium is beyond question but I have not given up operation for cancer of the cervix uteri.
—*Howard Canning Taylor.*"

REFERENCES

(1) *Churchill*: Diseases of Women, 1857. (2) Am. Jour. Med. Sc., Feb. 3, 1847. (3) *Tait, Lawson*: Diseases of Women, 1879. (4) *Dewees, W. P.*: Treatise on Diseases of Females, 1847. (5) *Emmet*: Principles and Practice of Gynaecology, 1884. (6) Am. Jour. Med. Sc., July, 1842, iv. (7) Tr. of Am. Gynec. Soc., 1877. (8) *Courty*: Practical Treatise on Diseases of Uterus, Ovaries and Fallopian Tubes, 1882. (9) *Noeggerath*: Tr. Am. Gynec. Soc., 1877. (10) *Simpson, Sir James Y.*: Clinical Lectures on Diseases of Women, 1863. (11) *Freund*: Centralbl. für Gynäk., 1878, pp. 497-503. (12) Surg., Gynec. & Obst., Jan., 1907. (13) Am. Jour. Obst., 1898, xxxvii. (14) Surg., Gynec. & Obst., June, 1921. (15) Surg., Gynec. & Obst., Sept., 1919. (16) *Davis, Lincoln:* Surgical Clinics of North America, June, 1921. (17) Jour. Am. Med. Assn., Jan. 3, 1920. (18) Am. Jour. Obst., Dec., 1918. (19) Jour. Am. Med. Assn., Feb. 12, 1921. (20) *Percy, J. T.*: Jour. Am. Med. Assn., Mar. 19, 1912. (21) Bull. Johns Hopkins Hosp., Dec., 1913. (22) Jour. Am. Med. Assn., Aug. 20, 1921. (23) Jour. Am. Med. Assn., Aug. 20, 1921. (24) Jour. Am. Med. Assn., Aug. 20, 1921.

TITLE INSURANCE BUILDING.

(*For discussion, see p. 312.*)

VALUABLE METHODS USED TO EXTEND OPERABILITY IN ADVANCED CANCER OF THE CERVIX*

BY G. VAN AMBER BROWN, M.D., DETROIT, MICH.

THE history of cancer is as old as that of medicine. Up to the present its cause is unknown with the mortality alarmingly on the increase, so that, today, one out of every eight individuals dies of this malady, and one wonders whether we are not facing the danger of extermination of the race by its ravages. The mortality is about equally divided between men and women, there being eleven men to every thirteen women. It is most interesting to note that, in the past twenty years, the mortality of tuberculosis has decreased 30 per cent, while that of cancer has increased 30 per cent. The death rate, in this country, shows that, in the last five years, while radium and x-rays are being actively exploited as the treatment *par excellence* for cancer, the annual increase in mortality is from 2 to .3 per cent. Such a mortality exists in New York City where x-rays and radium are, probably, used more than in any other medical center; and in this same city in the last year, the death rate of cancer far exceeds the death rate of tuberculosis. Carcinoma of the cervix constitutes about one-third of the cases of malignancy occurring in women. Statistics from the American Society for the Control of Cancer show that in the year 1918 there was, in the United States, a mortality of 11,965 from uterine cancer. Reports from the various clinics throughout this country show that in the cases of carcinoma uteri presenting for treatment, from 60 to 90 per cent were inoperable when first seen.

It is not my intention, at this time, to discuss the etiology or symptomatology of this malady. I wish only to speak of two methods which greatly extend the operability in advanced cancer of the uterus: (1) the "Starvation Ligature," (2) radiotherapy. It is not known who first employed the starvation ligature; but ligation of vessels for control of hemorrhage is mentioned in the writing of Celsus (30 B.C. to 50 A.D.), and of Galen (131-211 A.D.). The ligation of arteries is said to have been practiced at least 1800 years before Harvey discovered the circulation of the blood (1616-1619). With the discovery of the circulation and the development of knowledge concerning a part played by the blood in the nourishment of normal as well as abnormal tissue, the method of ligating arteries increased in scope. It then came to be applied not only for the control of hemorrhage, but for the

---
*Read at the Thirty-Fourth Annual Meeting of the American Association of Obstetricians, Gynecologists, and Abdominal Surgeons, St. Louis, Mo., September 20-22, 1921.

purpose of causing atrophy of organs or other parts of the body, and to lessen the nutrition of inoperable new growths, thus checking their further development and often causing their disappearance.

The last named use of the ligature has given rise to the term starvation ligature. It has been said that Johann Muys, in 1626, recommended the starvation method by means of arterial ligature. However, the discoverer of the circulation of the blood is credited with originating this method, which procedure he used in 1651, when he is said to have treated successfully a case of elephantiasis of the scrotum and testicle by ligating the spermatic artery. It is recorded that, in 1707, Lange employed it in the treatment of goiter. A hundred years elapsed before the method was again employed when, in 1809, Travers employed it in a tumor of the orbit. Since then its field of usefulness has been gradually extended, so that the procedure has been applied to the tongue, thyroid gland, spleen, buttocks, prostate, testes, ovaries, uterus and other parts of the body. Neither in the earlier days of its use, nor in later times, has the method received the attention it merits.

During the latter part of the last century Dr. John A. Wyeth of New York, reported 789 cases of ligature of the common carotid, of which 95 were for malignant tumors of the orbit, and 91 cases of the external carotid alone were tied to relieve, or cure, so-called malignant growths. He also analyzed 18 cases of ligation of the internal carotid. He gives no statistics upon starvation ligature as applied to the internal carotid alone, and from his other cases nothing reliable can be deduced as to the practicability of this operation; though this procedure was used about the same time by many others, both in this country and in Europe, it was not until the appearance of an essay by Samuel D. Gross, "The Treatment of Certain Malignant Growths by Excision of the External Carotid," by Robt. H. M. Dawbarn, that the starvation ligature became the modified "starvation treatment," which is now an established procedure in the treatment of advanced cancer of the mouth, the face, and of the uterus. In cancer of the cervix, Fritsch was the first to use tying of the uterine arteries. In 1888, Baumgarten was the first to use it in inoperable cancer of the uterus. Howard A. Kelly, in 1893, was the first to ligate the internal iliac, which was done in an emergency on account of a violent hemorrhage that occurred during the operation. Afterwards it was used by him as a method of choice, as was also done by Pozzi and many others. Later, Bainbridge from a seven years' experience, reported in 1915, 48 cases of ligation of the internal iliac, mediosacral, and ovarian arteries, for malignant disease of the uterus. In two of his cases he ligated the common iliac with satisfactory results. In another case both common iliacs were ligated.

We will now turn from the starvation ligature to a consideration of radiotherapy and then to the use of the two jointly. In 1792, George Adams, mathematical instrument maker to His Majesty, and optician to his Royal Highness, the Prince of Wales, reproached the medical profession for lack of tenacity of purpose in its use of electricity, at the same time, forecasting the history of electrotherapy as applied to cancer at the present time. Adams declared that electricity had considerable scope for action in surgery, in tumors, particularly of the glandular type. In glancing over the literature of the electrotherapeutic treatment of cancer, the prophetic insight of this observer is borne out one hundred and thirty years later. What applies to electrotherapy is equally true of its concomitant, radiotherapy. Radiotherapy includes radium, x-rays, and the radiant energy of heat.

The x-rays, discovered by Roentgen in 1895, were first employed in the treatment of malignant disease. The history of the use of the x-rays from then until now again verifies the prophecy of Adams. In 1913 Sir Malcolm Morris in the preface of the first treatise on radiumtherapy (Wickham) expressed an opinion parallel to that voiced by Adams in 1792, with the result that, today, the use of radium has verified this prophecy. Radium and x-ray have a selective action, producing masses of bundles and bands of scar tissue which may delay the advance of the growth; but they make late subsequent operation difficult and often ineffective. Heat prevents progress of the cancer and does not interfere so seriously with late secondary operative procedures.

Five hundred years ago Guy de Cheulic, though he used the knife in cutting out cancer at an early stage, recommended and used in growths, particularly of the fungus type, the actual cautery. The electrocautery introduced by Middledorpf, crude as it was, was considered by many surgeons as preferable to destructive chemical agents in the treatment of uterine cancers. This method was later adopted by John Byrne, of Brooklyn, who (1892) gave his first paper in the use of the galvanocautery in cancer of the cervix. This he used in doing vaginal hysterectomy and high amputation of the cervix. The method, later improved upon by him, came to be known as the Byrne method.

In recent years, J. F. Percy developed a technic for the use of moderate heat in treatment of advanced cancer of the cervix. As he calls attention to the point that by his procedure there is in no sense a burning or cauterization of the parts, for this, according to Percy, only defeats the effort to get a maximum penetration of heat. To quote Percy: "Experimental work has shown that a low degree of heat has a much greater penetrating power in a mass of cancer than has a high degree. High degrees of heat carbonize the tissues, inhibiting penetration. Low degrees of heat coagulate the tissues, encouraging heat dissemination. High degrees of heat, with a resulting carbon-core, prevent drainage in the cancer mass. This prevents in a certain number of cases the absorption of an excessive quantity of broken down cancer cells, which are dangerous to the life of the patient. When the temperature in the heating iron is the right degree for the greatest penetration, its shank can be wrapped with cotton and remain there for forty minutes or more. The color or texture of the cotton will not be altered in any way by this degree of temperature, and this merely emphasizes the fact that a burning temperature is not used.''

W. J. Mayo calls attention to the point that, for a certain distance, cancer cells are killed and that at a greater distance they are sickened or sterilized by this method, that is, they have lost their ability to reproduce and, before the recovery of the latter is the most favorable time for the radical operation hysterectomy.

Percy states that his work is based on laboratory experiments, which show that the cancer cells cannot be successfully transplanted after an exposure of 45° C. for ten minutes, while normal tissue cells can stand a temperature of from 55° to 60° C. without being devitalized. Doyen, a number of years before Percy, experimented to determine the thermal death point of cells and came to the same conclusions. Doyen also showed that cell destruction is the result of tissue coagulation, and, that it is possible to coagulate tissues to a depth of five to eight centimeters in from one to two minutes by diathermy.

The normal cell has three periods of existence; growth, function, regeneration for purposes of growth. During the period of function, reproduction is most active. The malignant cell has no period of function; its entire reproductive activity is thrown into the first stage, and only embryonic cell growth is produced. The normal functioning cell, as a part of the community life, is protected by the entire organism of which it is a part. The nervous system, the blood supply, and the lymphatics are all a part of this mechanism. The malignant cell has no such protection, hence it is five times more vulnerable than the normal cell and is treated by nature as a foreign body. Malignancy is the property of the cell; the stroma is not a part of the neoplasia, but is a measure of nature's defense. Therefore, since the malignant cell is five times more vulnerable than the normal cell, it is not hard to see that, by cutting down the blood supply by ligature and still further lessening it by sealing the smaller vessels with heat and, also, through the heat produce increase of connective tissue which further protects against the ingress of the malignant cells, we may by this method completely destroy them, still leaving enough blood to the parts to nourish the normal cell.

Then, too, if not supplemented by the starvation ligature, radiotherapy often fails in the destruction of the malignant cells when their nests are in or near the blood vessels from which they draw sufficient nourishment to withstand its effect.

As regards the value of combining the heat with the starvation ligature method, it has been extensively tried out in this country, and though opinions vary considerably, the most reliable evidence is in its favor. The most complete report on the use of the method has been made by Smith, who records 100 cases treated at the Mayo Clinic. Of these it was possible later to perform a radical extirpation of the uterus in 26 cases; the time chosen for the hysterectomy being about four weeks after the heat treatment. In 19 of the 26 cases operated on, no carcinoma was found in the specimen removed at the final operation. Smith's results compare favorably with, if they do not surpass, the best reports from the use of radium in the same class of cases.

I wish here to supplement this report by giving briefly results obtained in a series of eight cases.

1. CASE NO. 3568, housewife, age thirty-five, weight 150 pounds, multipara, metrorrhagia for two months, constant bleeding, many large clots. Tissues bleed freely upon careful examination. Cauliflower growth of cervix. Operation, August 6, 1921. Ligation of both internal iliacs and ovarians. Heat applied. Recovery uneventful. Left hospital end of third week. Cervix is normal in appearance except that the canal is larger than normal and the surrounding mucous membrane pale.

2. CASE NO. 1479, housewife, age forty-six. Had 11 children; no instrumental deliveries; no previous operations; menopause two and a half years ago. Present complaint: For six weeks has been bleeding almost constantly, never profuse. Diagnosis carcinoma of cervix not confirmed by laboratory. Operation: March 30, 1921, Percy heat applied for one hour. Patient left hospital the fourth day. Has since been in good health.

3. Mrs. L. B., housewife, age forty-seven, mother of four children; normal deliveries; laceration of perineum and cervix with first. Chief complaint: Bleeding from vagina; pain in pelvis, back and legs. Physical examination negative, except cervix. Three excavating ulcers, the largest about the diameter of a dime. Bleed upon touch. Feb. 3, 1921, radical hysterectomy was attempted but patient became profoundly shocked at the time the broad ligaments had been cut from the uterus. We hurriedly withdrew from the abdomen without completing the hysterectomy. Her immediate recovery was prompt. The patient refused further operative measures, but on Feb. 19, 1921, she returned. Under anesthesia a treatment of Percy heat was given. Following this, bleeding and pelvic pain ceased. Her condition locally was improved. The patient was, the third day, up and about. She gained in weight and color and was doing her own work until one month later, contrary to her physician's advice upon her own initiative, she had radium treatment. Within 8 hours after this pain became intense, accompanied by backache and bloating of abdomen and she has never been free from pain since, refusing all other surgical and mechanical intervention. (14 hours radiation, with 50 mg. radium.) There is now an extension to bladder, rectum, and sacral lymph nodes.

4. Mrs. D. S., age forty-five years, weight 220 pounds, present illness began in 1917, chief complaint was leucorrhea and increased flow at menstrual periods. Was advised to have operation at that time, but refused, and was not seen again until October, 1919, at which time she was confined to bed too weak to stand from loss of blood. She was white as parchment. Examination negative, except vagina revealed an old laceration of perineum. The vagina was filled with blood clots. The cervix

was large and hard around the vaginal attachment. The os was crater like and the tissue broke down when examined and precipitated a fresh hemorrhage. Diagnosis: Carcinoma of the cervix, confirmed by microscopic examination. Heat and ligation of both iliacs and ovarians October 19, 1919. Results: Two weeks after operation condition changed from fungating mass as large as an orange to what resembled a normal uterus two days after a four months' miscarriage. The patient, however, being a very fleshy woman, with deep abdominal fat, and very anemic, her R. B. C. less than a million and a half, developed, evidently from her lowered resistance, a fat necrosis with infection about the abdominal incision resulting in general sepsis, and death at the end of a month.

5. Mrs. D., age forty-eight, weight 160 pounds, has had no miscarriages. Three normal births, youngest child twenty years old. Present illness: Menopause was regarded as normal until the middle of May, 1920, when bleeding became so profuse as to be alarming. Examination revealed old laceration of perineum. The cervix was hard and the os was filled with fungating material which broke down and bled freely when examined. Diagnosis: Carcinoma of cervix uteri. Pathologist's report of curetted specimen dated May 26, 1920, was, that condition was not malignant. August 28, 1920, the same pathologist was taken to her home and allowed to examine patient and take specimen for examination which he reported to be actively malignant. Operation was advised to which patient consented, but afterwards changed her mind and was not seen until March 10, 1921, at which time her condition was the same as before, only that disease was much more advanced. The cervix, at this time, filling the whole vagina and broke down when examined, bled freely. Operation: Ligation of both internal iliacs and both ovarian arteries plus heat, March 16, 1920. Results: Two weeks after cervix looked smaller and only anterior border looked unhealthy. Heat again applied April 4, 1921. Sept. 15, 1921, the uterus feels and appears like a normal senile uterus. The patient is perfectly well and is doing her own housework.

6. CASE No. 235, Mrs. M. S., age forty-two, weight 155 pounds. Mother died of cancer of uterus; father died of cancer of liver. Personal history: Had abdominal operation, February, 1913, when left ovary and both tubes were removed, and a Gillian suspension done. Since then she has been well. Present complaint: Backache, slight bloody vaginal discharge and irregular menstrual periods. Friday, Feb. 4, 1921, on account of a chill, physician was called. A slight pinkish discharge has been present for some days. Also has abdominal pain and backache with sensation of fullness in bladder. Vaginal examination revealed a large very nodular mass filling upper portion of vagina with an area of induration extending toward the anterior vaginal wall, with a uterus that was somewhat, but not freely, movable. Diagnosis: Advanced carcinoma of the cervix uteri. Laboratory report, medullary mixed cell, basal and squamous, carcinoma of the cervix uteri. Operation: Feb. 9, 1921, Percy heat was used coupled with ligation of both internal iliacs plus crushing and ligation of upper portion of each broad ligament. The adhesions resulting from the previous operation were so extensive that a hysterectomy would be mechanically impossible. This patient made a nice recovery, leaving the hospital four weeks later. Since then she has had a series of x-ray treatments attacking the pelvis anteriorly, posteriorly, and laterally. From each of these treatments she always had a marked radiation sickness lasting for days. She has had one radium treatment which also was followed by a severe sickness for several days. No such reaction followed the use of the heat treatment. This woman was examined in my office within the past week. She says that she is well except that she has not fully regained her strength. She looks well; the cervix is normal, except that the contour is changed as is also the upper portion of the vagina.

7. CASE No. 632C. House wife, age twenty-eight, weight 165 pounds, nullipara, denies ever being pregnant, has never been ill. Cause for consultation: First noticed bleeding five years ago. It is accompanied by pain. At first noticed a spot of blood on clothing, occasionally, three or four times a month. Some discharge before her periods; this has gradually been getting worse. About a month ago she took a great deal of exercise, walking, climbing hills, and bathing daily. This seemed to make her bleeding worse. Has worn napkins daily for the past month. For the last two months she has had a yellowish discharge mixed with the blood, and of foul odor; probably pus. Vaginal examination reveals a fungus mass bleeding readily. Diagnosis: Advanced carcinoma of uterine cervix. Diagnosis by pathologist, from curettings: Medullary, basal celled type of carcinoma of the cervix uteri, actively growing. Consultation: Diagnosis concurred in and advice of consultant to abstain from operation as case is hopeless. Operation, August 16, 1920. Percy heat, coupled with ligation of both iliacs and both ovaries. Patient left hospital during third week after an uneventful recovery. Though no bleeding ever occurred after this operation, there was a small area about the cervical canal which was slow in clearing up. One radium treatment promptly disposed of this. I saw her in my office one week ago today. She is perfectly well. Now weighs 190 pounds, having gained 25 pounds since the operation. The cervix is healthy and she menstruates normally and regularly three days in each month.

8. CASE No. 305. Housewife, age thirty-eight, has five children, last baby eight months old. Present illness: For over a year patient had noticed a slight bleeding between periods. Flowed twice while carrying last child. This occurred about the fifth or sixth month. Flow regular since birth of last child, except that during the last three weeks some clots passed. No pain or other disturbance associated with the bleeding. Patient otherwise well. Vaginal examination reveals a large round, hard, bleeding mass growing from the cervix and extending well out into the anterior and posterior vaginal walls. Vaginal examination, under anesthesia, showed further that the rectum is infiltrated with the growth, as is also the perimetrium. Infiltration is so extensive that the whole is as if it were set in masonry. Diagnosis: Advanced carcinoma of the cervix uteri. Prognosis: Case deemed hopeless. Pathologist's report, Jan. 22, 1920; early active, rapidly growing, medullary, squamous celled carcinoma of the cervix uteri. Since no other form of treatment seemed to offer any hope whatever, we decided to resort to the heat and ligature method. Operation, Feb. 18, 1920. Bilateral salpingo-oophorectomy, ligation of both internal iliacs, Percy heat. Just below the bifurcation of the iliacs was an enlarged and broken down lymphatic gland which was removed. Pathologist's microscopic diagnosis: Passive congestion and early atrophy of the fallopian tubes, cystic degeneration of the ovaries, and far advanced rapidly growing carcinoma in the extrinsic tissues. Recovery from operation was rapid and without incident. May 3rd, ten weeks later, examination shows that the indurated area is much lessened. The uterus is freely movable, general condition of patient good. No hemorrhage in six weeks. June 7, heat applied for forty minutes without anesthesia. Aug. 3, examination in the office shows no induration about the vagina or cervix, that the contour of the cervix is good. The tissues are smooth and gliding, the uterus small, the fundus forward and in a good position. The parts are normal in color except some slight thin scarring of tissue in the vault of the vagina. The woman looks well, has a ruddy complexion, has gained in weight, and states that she feels as well as when she was sixteen. Clinically, she is apparently cured. August 24, three weeks later, the condition is the same; at this time, by sharp dissection, a portion of the cervix was removed for microscopic study. This was followed, immediately, by another application of the Percy heat which was used

for two hours. Pathologist's report: From this tissue which seemed to be normal, microscopic examination shows that there are still some growing cancer cells. Two weeks later it was deemed opportune to do the radical operation, which was done Sept. 11. Preceding the operation, cystoscopy was done and the bladder was found normal in appearance. In the abdomen we encountered broad extensive adhesions, binding the bladder and sigmoid to the uterus, these were freed with much difficulty. The uterus was small, the walls of the blood vessels appeared much thickened and the lumen materially narrowed. It was noticeable that the uterus and broad ligaments were quite anemic. There was one lymphatic gland the size of a small almond taken from the left side near the cervix and between the folds of the broad ligament. A hysterectomy was done, going well out into the broad ligaments, including the upper portion of the vagina, using for dissection the cautery knife. Pathologist's report: Microscopic examination (partial). The specimen is labeled—uterus. Most of the areas appear to be distinctly contracting. This is less noticeable, however, in the smaller cell nests. All of the neoplastic tissue presents the general cell picture of degeneration in addition to being quite markedly swollen and blurred. The neoplastic tissue appears to have undergone more degenerative change than the supporting tissue. Histologically, there remains an open question as to whether all other cancer cells are devitalized. Diagnosis: Caloric and atrophic change in carcinomatous and uterine tissue following ligation of blood vessels and repeated cautery treatments. Later this patient was given a series of x-ray treatments. Each treatment was followed by a radiation sickness; other than this she has remained well. I received a letter from her husband within the last few days expressing to me their gratitude.

Of the eight patients every one has shown improvement locally. One died of sepsis. One in which ligation was not done, but heat used after uncompleted operation, improved locally and in her general condition, until later, when radium was employed. This was immediately followed by extension of the growth. One, the last, operated, has cleared up locally and is improved generally. Seven of the patients (87.5 per cent) are living, two (25 per cent) are improved, five (62½ per cent) are clinically cured. If no permanent cure has been effected, the relief from symptoms and prolongation of life, has made this work worth while. The purposes of this method are:—
(1) To control hemorrhage which is sufficient to cause a constant drain on the patient's vitality or is so severe or frequent as to warrent fear of a fatal return at any time. (2) To facilitate the discharge of pus and necrotic tissue, also diminish the absorption of poisonous products. (3) To control the progress of the disease thereby lessening pain and suffering. (4) To render a later total extirpation possible. (5) That suffering may be lessened and life prolonged in many cases when all other methods have failed. (6) That in many apparently hopeless cases life may be saved and a clinical cure effected. Having observed these eight cases with as much precision as I am capable, coupled with a perusal of recent literature on the subject, I am prompted to offer the following as points that should be emphasized.

(1) The use of the starvation ligature mechanically accomplishes

instantly in the blood supply what a study of a microscopic specimen of carcinoma shows nature is endeavoring to accomplish. (2) The vessels should be tied at two points with either kangaroo tendon or heavy catgut ligature, as finer catgut may cut the vessel wall and precipitate a hemorrhage. Between the ties the arteries are crushed to a ribbon. Absorbable suture is used to avoid, as far as possible, the irritation factor that will, undoubtedly, arise from the use of the nonabsorbable material. (3) In applying the heat the temperature is kept at 122°-140°F. and the abdomen should always be opened so that the heating iron can be properly guided from the vagina through the cervix to the fundus. By so doing, not only is the iron properly adjusted, but the gloved hand of an assistant placed over the fundus is an aid in determining the amount of heat to be used, and the danger of injury to the bladder, rectum and ureter, with the formation of fistula, may be avoided and sealing of the smaller blood vessels and lymphatics accomplished. (4) Should one not care to depend upon the heat and starvation ligature, and extirpation of the uterus is to follow, it should be done as a thermocauterectomy between the second and fourth week before the sickened cells have recuperated, and before the deposit of scar tissue is sufficient to interfere seriously with operative procedures. (5) With no other method can the fixed pelvic structures be loosened and mobilized as by the heat and ligature. (6) Adequate x-ray and radium treatments cause a decided radiation sickness from which the patient does not fully recover for from one to six weeks, rendering a hysterectomy hazardous. Hence, in this respect the heat has advantage over the x-ray or radium. (7) (a) After surgical procedures have been completed, x-ray or radium, or both, may be employed to advantage as was done in three of my cases; (b) if hysterectomy is not to be done and the growth is well within the cervix, radium alone is indicated; (c) if involvement is broad x-ray, combined with radium, is used; (d) if hysterectomy had been done, then later x-ray is used if doubt exists as to whether all cancer bearing tissues have been removed or if there is a recurrence. (8) (a) Postoperatively to pursue a set course, without variations, is hazardous. As far as postoperative cure is concerned, we should individualize the carcinoma of the cervix. (b) Along with the details above mentioned, attention should be given to diet, fresh air, and other measures that will raise the general resistance of the individual. (c) Inattention to details will lead, as it too often does, to failure of cure and bring unjust criticism upon the method. (9) In advanced carcinoma of the cervix, heat and starvation ligature are methods that should precede a contemplated panhysterectomy. While x-rays and radium are useful postoperative adjuvants, they should never be used as preoperative measures.

REFERENCES

Bainbridge: The Cancer Problem, 1915. *Garrison*: History of Medicine, 1914. *McLean*: Surg., Gynec. and Obst., April, 1915, pp. 457-461. *Bernheim*: Surgery of the Vascular System, 1913. *Bulkley*: Medical Record, March 12, 1921. *Percy, J. F.*: Trans. Am. Assn. Obst. and Gynec., 1917, p. 97. *Graves*: Text Book Gynecology, 1918. *Balfour*: Mayo Clinics, 1916. *Saltzstein*: Modern Medicine, Oct., 1920. *Balfour*: Surg., Gynec. and Obst., 1916, xxii, 74-79. *Mayo, W. J.*: Surg., Gynec. and Obst., 1920, xxx, 1. *Balfour*: Lancet, 1915, xxxv, 347-350. *Duncan*: Jour. Am. Med. Assn., Aug. 20, 1921. *Bailey*: Am. Jour. Obst., Sept., 1919, p. 300. *Clark*: Ann. Surg., June, 1920, p. 688. *Schmitz*: Ibid. *Clark and Keene*: Ibid. *Stone*: Surg., Gynec. and Obst., June, 1921. *Graves*: Ibid. *Burrows*: Annual Reports of the Manchester Radium Institute, 1919.

(*For discussion, see p. 312.*)

THE CONTROL OF THE MORTALITY OF ABDOMINAL OPERATIONS FOR CANCER*

By George W. Crile, M.D., F.A.C.S, Cleveland, O.

ON THIS occasion I wish to report the methods and management of operations upon that group of patients who constitute a large portion of the group of handicapped cases whose successful treatment taxes to the utmost the resources of the surgeon, namely, abdominal operations for cancer.

The two outstanding principles which we shall describe were developed as the result of experience in the war. These two principles may be briefly formulated as follows: I. Protection of the patient in advance of the emergency. II. Control of infection (a) by the separation of contaminated surfaces from each other; and (b) by prevention of the pooling of wound secretion.

I. *Protection of the Patient in Advance of the Emergency.*—To achieve this end all the restorative measures that would be employed after it is recognized that the patient's life is threatened are employed *in advance of the probability* of the advent of danger. That is, when an operation, the mortality of which according to general statistical reports is from 10 to 25 per cent, is to be performed upon a patient, the patient is given the benefit of all the restorative and protective measures *before the positive indication* for their use has developed. In other words, we utilize the principle of prevention in surgery, as the principle of prevention is employed in medicine.

We shall never know in how many of the cases in which we have applied preventive measures those measures would have been required; just as no one can say how many of the individuals inoculated against smallpox or typhoid would have developed either of those diseases without that protection. In either case the value of the preventive measure

---

*Read at the Thirty-Fourth Annual Meeting of the American Association of Obstetricians, Gynecologists, and Abdominal Surgeons, St. Louis, Mo., September 20-22, 1921.

must be judged by the effect upon the gross mortality as established by mass statistics.

Thus, as we might say, we do not treat the patient but the probability. One may, at first, feel that a disadvantage to this plan appears in the fact that if all our protective and restorative measures are employed in advance of the emergency, there will be nothing left to be done for the patient should he "go bad." The answer is, that the emergency will rarely develop; and, as shown by our experience at least, the mortality rate of operations upon bad risk cases will be markedly reduced.

The specific application of this principle in bad risk cases requiring resection of the stomach or resection of the intestine consists in (a) *the establishment of water equilibrium;* (b) *maintenance of a failing circulation;* (c) *psychic and physical rest;* (d) *completely anociated operation;* (e) *the application of heat.*

(a) *The establishment of water equilibrium* is secured before and after operation by subcutaneous infusions of novocaine $\frac{1}{32}$ per cent in normal saline (Bartlett). (b) If the *circulation* is feeble and in the presence of *anemia* a transfusion of blood is made before operation. This is repeated before, during, or after operation according to the requirements in the individual case. (c) *Psychic and physical rest* are promoted to the utmost degree possible before and after operation; morphine being given if it is required to assure the maintenance of the state of negativity. (d) *The performance of an anociated operation* means that in these cases the utmost precaution must be exercised to avoid further impairment of the internal respiration. Lipoid solvent anesthetics and complete surgical anesthesia therefore are contraindicated. The operation is performed under nitrous oxid analgesia and local anesthesia. (e) The internal respiration is promoted by heat and is markedly impaired by chilling of the viscera. During the operation therefore the exposure of the viscera is reduced to the minimum and, after the operation, heat is applied to the whole abdomen in the form of moist hot packs.

II. *The Control of Infection.*—It was long ago recognized in civilian practice, but was dramatically demonstrated during the war, that contamination may be prevented from going on to infection by preventing the contact of one raw contaminated surface with another raw contaminated surface, and by preventing the pooling of wound secretion. The control of infection is further promoted by the protective and restorative measures already described; for the greater the resources of the patient, the better the local defense.

The application of these principles in resection of the large intestine is accomplished as follows: The operation is divided into two stages. In the first stage by means of a colostomy or by visceral anastomosis, the fecal stream is diverted from the field of resection, so that there will be no danger of fecal leakage at the point of resection anastomosis. There is no doubt that in many cases it may be safe to perform the entire operation at one seance; but, on the other hand, if too great a chance is taken in an operation, it may be regretted, but the opportunity to save the patient cannot be returned.

After the preliminary operation every effort is made to increase the resistance of the patient. In attaining this end, the application of the general principles of restoration and the length of the interval before the resection is performed are varied according to the needs of the individual case. Generally, however, about a week elapses after the preliminary operation at which the operability of the case has been ascertained and the fecal stream diverted from the field of resection. At the end of this period the patient is a much safer risk.

At the end of the resection, the technic of which is now so well standardized, a single layer, or at most two layers, of iodoform gauze are interposed between the contaminated raw surface areas. This is removed in from four to six days and the wound dealt with either by a similar redressing or by the intermittent use of Dakin's solution.

The restorative measures already described are used. If restoration lags, blood transfusion is given and even repeated several times. The dietetic and hygienic regimen employed in the treatment of tuberculosis aids the convalescence.

The protective value of these measures is strikingly illustrated by the fact that in my last 66 operations for cancer of the rectum and large intestines there has been but one death; while the mortality rate in operations on the stomach and the intestines has fallen to 2.6 per cent, the operability has been extended until no case is refused for operation unless anatomically inoperable; and the postoperative morbidity has been progressively diminished.

CLEVELAND CLINIC.   (*For discussion, see* p. 312.)

THE NEW TREND IN GYNECOLOGICAL THERAPY*

BY GEORGE GELLHORN, M.D., F.A.C.S., ST. LOUIS, MO.

IT was the name of this organization that decided my choice of a subject. The very name suggests that close relationship of the sister sciences of gynecology and obstetrics from which, practically, all the progress of the last decades has sprung. This intimate kinship, this physiologic union of the two branches of medicine has repeatedly been assailed of late years and in several seats of learning it has actually been disrupted. In some of these instances, the sincere though mistaken idea may have prevailed that gynecology was nothing but a surgical specialty, while in others, personal and, therefore, all the more regrettable, motives seem to have been at work.

Be that as it may, it is a curious irony of fate that just at the moment when the general surgeons claim the gynecologic field as their own, gynecology has entered into a new phase of development where efforts are being made to replace surgical methods of treatment largely by nonsurgical means. It will be an easy and, I hope, an interesting matter to substantiate this statement by a brief survey of the situation.

Let us begin with cancer of the cervix—a surgical disease in the truest sense of the word. I will not again go over the ground that has been so well covered in today's discussions, nor will I present the statistics prepared for my own paper. These have been published elsewhere.[1] In a deadly disease like cancer every single case which is permanently cured is a decided gain and a triumph of our surgical endeavors; thus the operative cures of approximately 25 per cent might well be a source of satisfaction to us. But when we contrast this figure with the number of all patients afflicted with cancer, our achievements dwindle in importance.

For practical purposes the proposition amounts to this: Of 400 women who seek our aid for the relief of cancer of the cervix, barely 100 are actually and radically operated upon.[2] The other 300 are hopeless cases; their doom is sealed even though we may inflict some sort of superfluous surgery upon them. Of the 100, on whom the radical abdominal operation is performed, about one-fourth die of the operation, about one-half die from recurrences, and about one-fourth are alive and well after five years. A material change in this sum total is hardly to be expected because the technic of the operation seems to have reached the zenith of perfection.

And now comes radiotherapy as an earnest competitor of the

---
*Read by invitation at the Thirty-fourth Annual Meeting of the American Association of Obstetricians, Gynecologists, and Abdominal Surgeons, St. Louis, Mo., September 20-22, 1921.

surgical treatment in cervical cancer. To be sure, radiotherapy is still on probation. The first five-year period of observation has passed only recently and the percentage of radium cures is still a point or two below that of the surgical cures. But if we look upon these statistics in their true light, they will assume a new significance. The radium results reflect, to a large extent, the infancy of the new method which is just about to emerge from the crude empiricism of its initial stages. Better results, therefore, are bound to come in the future. Even now, one authority[3] at least has already obtained results with radium that are in every way identical with those derived from surgery. Then, too, the cases treated with radium are on the whole more unfavorable than those subjected to operation. And to offset the slight difference in final results, there is a primary mortality from radium of 3 per cent as compared with the 20 or 25 per cent after operation.

If men of vast experience and superior technical skill, like Doederlein and Bumm,[4] eliminate surgery altogether in the treatment of uterine cancer and rely exclusively on radiotherapy, we should pause to think. As long as the subject is still a matter of discussion, the advocates of operation are, of course, justified in adhering to surgery; but the fact stands out in clear relief that surgery is no longer the only mode of attack and, unless all signs fail, the future of the treatment of uterine cancer belongs to radiotherapy,—at least until a biological method of treatment will have been discovered.

Personally, I had arrived at a formula which, until recently, seemed highly satisfactory to me.[1] Inoperable and borderline cases were treated exclusively by a combination of radium and x-rays. Early cases were operated upon by the radical abdominal method and received a preoperative treatment with radium and a postoperative treatment with x-rays. But I confess that my former confidence has deserted me, and at present my efforts are confined strictly to radiotherapy.

Another field of gynecology in which the therapy has, until recently, been exclusively surgical, is that of fibroids. As we look back upon the brilliant development of the operations for fibroids and consider the steadily decreasing mortality and the benefits reaped by our patients, we can well understand that the feeling became established in the profession that the question of the best treatment was definitely and satisfactorily settled.

The first reports on the effect of x-rays upon fibroids came as a complete surprise and met, in many quarters, with considerable incredulity; but extensive confirmation came in a very short time, and today it may be accepted as a fact that x-rays and radium check the hemorrhages in about 98 per cent and reduce the size of the tumors in from 70 to 80 per cent of the cases. Further improvement may be expected from a more careful selection of the cases, the use of more powerful x-ray apparatus, and, perhaps, also from a judicious combination of radium and x-rays. At any rate, the surgical method of treatment, hitherto supreme, has now found a very strong rival in radiotherapy which can point to a mortality of 0 as against an average mortality of 3 to 5 per cent or even more, after surgical procedures.

Radiotherapy, however, cannot supplant surgery altogether. There are still enough cases of fibroids left in which an operation alone is indicated; but it is a significant fact that it is just the case with a poor surgical risk, the exsanguinated or the very fat woman, the patient with kidney or heart complications, that is particularly suited to, and benefited by, the new treatment. This is not the place to go into details as to indications and contraindications or a comparison of the complications following the two methods. The reader is referred to two previous publications.[5,6] Suffice it to say that, approximately, only 30 per cent of the cases need operation while the overwhelming majority can be cured by nonsurgical means. Doederlein applied x-rays in 222 cases of fibroids and used the knife in 91 others in the same period of time. Kelly used radium in 210 cases and operated on 45.

The treatment of chronic inflammations in the pelvis, particularly those of gonorrheal origin, forms one of the most changing and interesting chapters of gynecologic therapy. We have all witnessed and participated in these changes. It did not take long to realize that the so-called conservative treatment, that is, rest in bed, douches, tampons, and the like, only served to hasten the transition from the subacute to the chronic stage, and that an operation was required to bring about a cure. The surgical treatment itself underwent a long and varied evolution within the memory of most of us. At first satisfied with removing only the affected tube, we soon learned that the apparently healthy tube of the other side quite regularly developed into a pyosalpinx and demanded a second operation. Then, the persistence of the inflammation in the interstitial portions of the tubes required deep excisions of the uterine horns. And yet, the patients continued to complain of symptoms that arose from the uterus and did not cease until that organ was eliminated. To reduce this dreary train of operations, Beuttner, of Switzerland, devised an operation which was sponsored by Polak, in this country, and revived by Bell, in England, and consisted of the removal of both adnexa and a part of the uterus. Other operators believed that an ascending gonorrhea in the female was, in a way, an incurable disease and, following the lead of Schauta and Landau, extirpated the entire uterus with both adnexa. Whatever method was adopted, it ultimately mutilated and unsexed the patient; and, as the disease occurs only in the reproductive age and is found more often in persons young in years, even the most successful outcome of our operations could not possibly fill us with wholehearted satisfaction. It was just this state of mind that induced many of us to attempt more conserving operations, such as injecting the tubes with some antiseptic fluid, splitting and draining them, etc., but you all know that these measures ended in signal failures.

More recently, however, a determined effort is being made to attack gonorrhea of the internal genitals by nonoperative means. Two novel methods have thus far been proposed. The first of these originated with Van de Velde,[7] of Holland, who started from the familiar observation that the approaching menstruation exerts an untoward influence upon an acute salpingo-oophoritis. The inflammatory process, which above all else requires rest and protection, is stirred up by the cyclic changes in the ovaries and the resulting phenomena in the pelvic organs. In these cases, Van de Velde applied radium and x-rays alone or combined and claims to have produced a "temporary" castration. The ovarian function was suppressed for from several months to one and one-half years; there was no exacerbation of the inflammation but fever and other symptoms subsided, and complete cure could be brought about by a simple absorbent therapy. Similarly good results were obtained in cases of chronic recurrent adnexal inflammation.

The second method is the adoption of foreign protein therapy in gynecology of which the vaccine therapy was an early though inefficient forerunner. By the introduction of foreign proteins, the protoplasm of the cells is stimulated to greater activity and the afflicted organs are, thereby, enabled to restore themselves to normal conditions. This, at least, is the theoretical explanation of the astounding results observed after the intramuscular or intravenous injections of milk or casein. A very recent article by Zill[8] includes a report of 90 cases of large adnexal tumors treated in this manner for several weeks. Of these 90 cases, 59 were cured completely, that is, the palpatory findings were perfectly normal; 27 were improved, in that there was still a slight thickening of the adnexa, but the subjective well being of the patients was unimpaired; and only in four instances there was no improvement.

A very similar rationale underlies the treatment of ascending gonorrhea by means of injections of turpentine. This substance deposited in the subfascial tissues, produces a reaction which sets free homologous proteins, and these, in turn, are apt to activate the protoplasm of the cells of the inflamed structures. A diminution, and even disappearance, of the adnexal tumors has been claimed in a large percentage of the cases thus treated.[9, 10] It is not surprising that a number of authors[11] have failed to observe such satisfactory results, for all these efforts of treating an ascending gonorrhea are still in an experimental stage; but they are highly promising and indicative of the present nonoperative trend in gynecologic therapy. Their final success would confer a blessing upon our patients whom we can *cure* by operation only at the expense of their genital function.

The abuse of the curette has been a much discussed evil, and the attempts at restricting this favorite instrument to its legitimate use in abortion, polyps, and, for diagnostic purposes, in cancer, have been numerous. We have now advanced far enough into a better appreciation of the pathologic physiology of the female genital organs to know that dysmenorrhea and sterility very rarely require curettage. The profuse hemorrhages of adolescence, once the indication for repeated curettages, are now explained by endocrine disturbances and treated accordingly. As we learn to recognize a syphilitic metrorrhagia, we shall have no need for surgical treatment in cases of this kind. Uterine discharges of any kind used to call, automatically as it were, for the curette while today this instrument would be the very last thing an up-to-date gynecologist would consider in the treatment of this most common of all symptoms.

Another illustration. About a year ago I demonstrated before the St. Louis Medical Society the amazing effect of radium upon condylomata acuminata, and since then two papers have appeared reporting the same results with x-rays.[12] All along the line then, we see, today, a tendency to replace surgical means by nonoperative means in the treatment of gynecologic affections.

But the factor that promises to do more than any other towards reducing the need for surgical intervention, is the product, the very child of that much maligned and wantonly disturbed union of obstetrics and gynecology—*preventive obstetrics*. It mattered little to the midwife of whatever sex, whether or not the cervix was torn in delivery as long as the bleeding was not excessive. It was the gynecologist with obstetric training and obstetric practice who realized the relations of cervical lacerations to subinvolution and its sequels, and their possible bearing upon cancer, and who insisted upon the necessary care in applying forceps. Neither did the midwife pay much attention to the position of the uterus four or six weeks after confinement; and again, it was the gynecologist who recognized that more than 75 per cent of all displacements occur after labor, and that these may be prevented by the proper hygiene of the puerperium or cured by the temporary use of pessaries.

I trust that nothing that has been said in these pages, will be misinterpreted as a disparagement of surgery, its brilliant progress, or its marvelous results. Any such thought would ill befit one who himself is a gynecologic surgeon. But I take it that our ultimate object is the *cure* of the patient, not the *specific method* by which we arrive at our goal, and it seems to me that, as far as our present attitude goes, this ultimate object is attainable in a large percentage of the cases by nonoperative means.

It is, therefore, not illogical to suggest, at this time, a revision of our previous therapeutic conceptions and to point to the necessity of a recasting of our fundamentals of treatment. It may, then, be seen that gynecology is, after all, not an exclusively surgical specialty, that with all the tremendous importance and value of surgical treatment, it is neither the only nor even the most important means at our disposal.

When a business house takes over another business concern, an inventory is made prior to the transfer. You may say that such stock should have been taken *before* gynecology was bound over to surgery. Precisely; but since the transaction seems to have taken place without such a procedure, it might be well to provide an inventory *post festum*, so as to have it on hand in the future if a readjustment should be under discussion. It may be that gynecology will revert from the security of present nonoperative gains to former surgical methods; but this is highly improbable because the present status of affairs indicates, to my mind, a *higher* phase of development. It may also be that gynecology in its present form and with a growing leaning towards nonoperative lines, will not appear as attractive to surgery as it has seemed in the past, so that the realignment of gynecology and obstetrics will meet with less opposition.

BIBLIOGRAPHY

(1) *Gellhorn:* Jour. of Radiology, 1921, ii, 23. (2) *Taylor:* Tr. Am. Gynec. Soc., 1912, xxxvii, 314. (3) *Kehrer:* Tr. German Gynec. Soc., 1920. (4) *Doederlein and Kroenig:* Operative Gynäkologie, ed. 4, 1921, p. 574. (5) *Gellhorn:* AM. JOUR. OF OBST. AND GYNEC., 1921, i, 767. (6) *Gellhorn:* Jour. Missouri State Med. Assn., 1921, xviii, 220. (7) *Van de Velde:* Zentralbl. f. Gynäk., 1920, xliv, 994. (8) *Züll:* München. med. Wchnschr, 1921, lxviii, 803. (9) *Friedrich:* Zentralbl. f. Gynäk., 1921, xlv, 353. (10) *Sonnenfeld:* ibid., 686. (11) *Kronenberg:* ibid., 257. (12) *Stein:* Wien. klin. Wchnschr., 1921, xxxiv, 315.

METROPOLITAN BUILDING. (*For discussion, see* p. 316.)

THE HYPERTROPHIC-ULCERATIVE FORM OF CHRONIC VULVITIS. (ELEPHANTIASIS, ESTHIOMENE, SYPHILOMA)*

BY FRED. J. TAUSSIG, M.D., F.A.C.S., ST. LOUIS, MO.

A FREQUENT source of confusion in medical literature lies in the attempt to call by one name conditions that are really manifold in their etiology and clinical appearance. A good illustration of this is to be found in the peculiar chronic infectious enlargement of the vulva to which the terms elephantiasis, pseudoelephantiasis, esthiomene, rodent ulcer, lupus, granuloma, and syphiloma of the vulva, have been applied. Perhaps the term that is most nearly justified is that suggested by Stein, "syphiloma," for syphilis is doubtless the most frequent etiologic factor in the formation of these hypertrophic ulcerating growths. Granuloma fails to express the hypertrophic character of many of these cases. Lupus is identified with tuberculosis, which is only rarely present. Esthiomene and *rodent ulcer* would apply more to the ulcerating cases and elephantiasis, though most generally adopted, has the least to recommend it, because of the confusion with filarial lymph stasis and the absence of any consideration of the chronic infectious character of the condition.

I would prefer to get along, as far as possible, without any hard and fast term but rather to group this condition as the *hypertrophic ulcerative form of chronic vulvitis.* Under this general head, the cases due to syphilis, to tuberculosis, to the "climatobacterium granulomatis," to filariasis, and to other sources of infection can be separately considered. Any attempt, however, to individualize these cases will meet with difficulties, for symptomatically, anatomically and even histologically, they are often so much alike that their etiology cannot be determined.

As I see it, we should not be concerned so much with the particular microorganism, that may be present in any one case, as with the special anatomic, physiologic, racial, and social factors that lead to the production of this characteristic lesion. Beside the infecting agent or agents there are, I believe, five factors that can be held responsible: (1) A racial predisposition to fibrous hypertrophy. (2) The manner of lymphatic distribution in the vulva. (3) The looseness of the vulvar skin predisposing to edema. (4) Lack of cleanliness from secretions and excretions in this region. (5) Repeated excoriations from coitus with resulting chronic wound infection.

---
*Read by invitation at the Thirty-fourth Annual Meeting of the American Association of Obstetricians, Gynecologists, and Abdominal Surgeons, St. Louis, Mo., September 20-22, 1921.

(1) When we consider that the negro makes up but one-tenth of the population of this country, it is striking that, practically, all these cases of vulvar hypertrophy in American literature are found among colored women. Stein's two cases, Gallagher's four cases and the 13 cases considered in the present report were all negresses. In fact I can recall having seen but one such case in a white woman, a prostitute, in whom, moreover, an admixture of negro blood was suspected. Even the filarial form of elephantiasis of the vulva has been noted primarily in the colored races. In European literature the condition has been found almost exclusively among prostitutes. That this tendency to fibrous hypertrophies of the vulva among colored women has some relationship to the similar tendency to keloids and uterine fibroids in

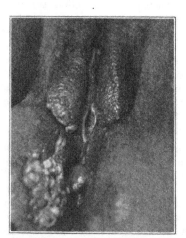 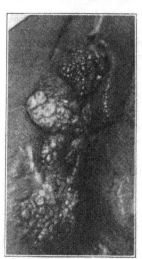

Fig. 1.—(Case 11) Combination of ulcerative and nodular form of chronic hypertrophic vulvitis. On the left side we see beginning hypertrophy with extensive ulceration. The right hand picture was taken 2½ years later and shows the continued ulceration with marked hypertrophy of clitoris and right labia.

this race, seems more probable. There can be no question as to the pronounced racial predisposition to this condition existing among the negroes. I have seen neglected syphilitic ulcerations in white women, even prostitutes, produce only slight thickening or edema of the labia, while in the negress there usually developed a considerable pendulous tumor.

(2) The anatomic distribution of the lymph channels of the vulva predispose to lymph stasis. In filarial infections, the occurrence of a lymphatic enlargement in the inguinal and femoral region not only blocks the flow to the leg, but also to the labia on the same side, Koch has reported cases following removal of the inguinal glands.

The two most pronounced hypertrophies in my series occurred in women who had had a chronic infection of the inguinal and femoral lymph glands preceding the development of the mass in the inguinolabial fold on the same side. Lymph stasis of some degree, whether in the groin or in the vulvar tissue itself, must be considered as a *sine qua non* in the production of these enlargements.

(3) The looseness of the vulvar skin makes possible the formation of chronic edematous deposits with resulting fibrosis and enlargement of these parts. Together with the eyelids and the back of the hands, the vulva is one of the first points at which a tendency to edema will be manifested. The edema of pregnancy is often localized in the vulva.

(4) Uncleanliness is an important etiologic factor. In no instance is this disease found among women of the better classes. Persons with neglected syphilis and gross lesions about the external genitals may develop a slight thickening of the tissues; but, if they are clean about

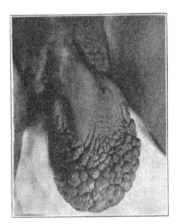

Fig. 2.—(Case 13) The nodular type involving clitoris and left labium minus in a patient who had been confined two days previously. The tumor hung between the thighs and was very edematous. No ulceration whatsoever in this case.

their person, they do not develop these extreme hypertrophic ulcerations. Often a syphilitic rectovaginal fistula, together with a gonorrhea, makes it almost impossible to keep the parts clean. On the other hand, once the condition has developed, the best care and hospital nursing trying to keep the parts clean, will not materially influence the size of the mass or the extent of the ulcerations.

(5) The disease is found solely during the period of greatest sexual activity, and it is certain that the repeated traumatisms of coitus, especially in prostitutes, has much to do with the production of hypertrophy. The frequent occurrence of tertiary syphilitic ulceration about the vestibular ring results in repeated injuries with resulting wound

infection following coitus. The poor nutrition of these parts produced by the lymph stasis and obliterating endarteritis make wound healing slow; so that, in most instances, these ulcers do not heal entirely and must be excised.

As to the nature of the infecting agent in this disease there is, as has already been stated, much difference of opinion. Syphilis is found in 80 to 90 per cent of the patients; but there is some difference of opinion as to whether the lesion is to be classified as a tertiary gummatous deposit or as a postsyphilitic process. Many of these cases have a negative Wassermann with positive evidence of a previous syphilis. One or two of my cases, that have been under observation a long time, had a positive Wassermann in the first year of ulceration and then, later, when the hypertrophy became more pronounced, developed a negative Wassermann. Even after therapeutic excitation, the test remained negative. Such cases were, usually, totally uninfluenced by treatment; so that I feel we cannot properly class them as syphilitic lesions, but rather as chronic ulcerations on the basis of syphilitic scar tissue.

While textbooks on gynecology have, in the past emphasized filariasis as a factor, it is apparently rather rare, not nearly as frequent as the filarial elephantiasis of the scrotum in men and limited to certain tropical areas. In only a small portion of those in whom the diagnosis of filarial elephantiasis vulvae is made are the filaria actually found circulating in the blood. Some believe it to be purely a postfilarial condition.

Dermatologists have made special studies of a form of vulvar hypertrophy found in Porto Rico, British Guiana, and tropical regions, in which the development of ulcers is more pronounced than in filarial infections. They have found a peculiar germ called the "climatobacterium granulomatis" in all of these lesions. Most authors feel certain that this disease is not syphilis. The slow advance, superficial character, and the vascularity of the lesions, tend to differentiate it from gumma. Goodman's recent reports in the Archives of Dermatology emphasize the contagious character of these lesions and its occurrence, primarily, in prostitutes.

Tuberculosis of the vulva has been found in some few cases associated with these hypertrophic tumors and, in one of my series, the absence of any syphilis, the presence of giant cells in the ulceration, and the positive signs of an active tubercular lesion in the chest, make the suspicion of a tubercular factor in the production of the lesion very strong.

Gonorrhea is, probably, never a primary factor, but will often greatly increase vulvar irritation and so, secondarily, aids in the growth of the vulvar enlargements. In the presence of a profuse leucorrhea the tendency to the papillonodular form of hypertrophy is more pronounced.

In two instances of my series tissue was removed and specially stained for Ducrey's chancroid bacillus, but with negative results. A suppurating bubo will, however, predispose to lymph blocking and so, in the presence of syphilis, may lead to more pronounced enlargements.

In general we may distinguish three types of cases according to location: (1) An inguinal-labial type involving, usually, only one side, and leaving the clitoris unaffected. (2) A clitoral type involving

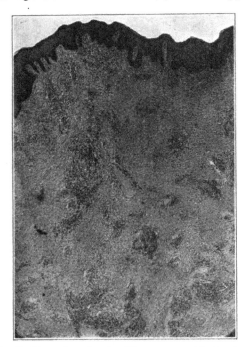

Fig. 3.—(Case 6) Microscopic section of nodular mass removed by operation. Everywhere are areas of lymphocytic infiltration. The epithelium shows increased keratin but less papillary extensions with the connective tissue than ordinarily is formed. No superficial ulcers present at time of operation.

the clitoris and, usually, also both labia minora; but not the labia majora. (3) A diffuse type in which the hypertrophy is more general, involving the entire vulva more or less.

A further grouping of these cases is also possible according to the prevailing type of pathologic lesion. We can have: (1) A *hypertrophic* form, in which large pendulous tumors are found, usually with but slight ulcerations. · (2) An *ulcerative* form, in which the ulcerating granuloma makes up the bulk of the enlargement. (3) A *papillary* form, in which the tumor surface is covered with small nodular or papillary excrescences. Often there is a combination of two or more of these forms.

Symptoms are usually insignificant in this disease. This may, in part, be due to the low state of intelligence and lowered pain sense in these individuals. Some discomfort from the weight of the pendulous mass, interference with walking, and urinary and rectal irritability may be noted. If the mass becomes more acutely inflamed, for some cause or other, there may be pain. Dyspareunia is often the

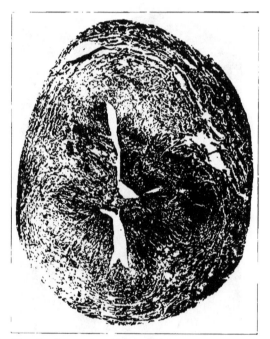

Fig. 4.—(Case 6). Cross section of blood vessel formed in tumor mass showing obliterative endarteritis.

main reason for their seeking medical advice. When we think of the severe pain some women experience from small burns or chancroidal sores about the vestibulum, it is amazing that these extensive ulcerations produce so little discomfort. Very meagre, and often contradictory statements as to the duration and course of the disease, are given by these dull-witted individuals.

From a diagnostic standpoint this condition is of interest because of its confusion with carcinoma. In the latter, however, we have a circumscribed lesion that is brittle, bleeds easily, and is practically never found in the negress before the menopause. The differentiation from fibroid tumors of the vulva is usually easy, since fibroids are circumscribed, have a smooth skin surface, and present no evidence of ulceration.

A word must be added regarding the treatment of these cases. Antisyphilitic treatment, even the most persistent and vigorous, will not cure these cases and will only rarely and temporarily affect the size of the tumor mass. It is well, however, that such treatment be employed to promote prompt healing after surgical intervention. The record in the seven cases that underwent operation in my series, shows the uniformly satisfactory results of vulvectomy in these cases, provided only, that the incision be wide enough to include all indurated and ulcerated tissue. It is better to make this incision with the cautery, though in some of the cases here recorded such a plan was

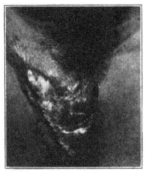

Fig. 5.—(Case 10). Inguinolabial type showing extensive ulceration as well as hypertrophy associated with suppurative adenitis.

not adopted. One case, that was followed for eight years after vulvectomy, remained perfectly well except for a rectal stricture that required further dilatation.

In conclusion I append a brief record of the 13 cases included in the present study. It will be noted that four of these patients were seen in the services of my colleagues, Drs. Gellhorn, Crossen and Otto Schwarz, and thanks are due for permission to include them in the present analysis of the question.

CASE REPORTS

CASE 1.—Ophelia T., twenty-seven years, colored, two children, one stillborn and one living, came to Washington University Hospital in 1907 complaining of partial incontinence of feces and the formation of a lump in the genital region that had grown to the size of a lemon during her last pregnancy one year previously. Examination showed a rectovaginal fistula, a stricture of the rectum, ulcerations about the fourchette and urethra, and a nodular enlargement occupying the region of the clitoris and both labia minora. Antiluetic treatment produced but slight improvement. Vulvectomy and repair of rectovaginal fistula, followed by further treatment, gave good results. She was delivered of a full-term normal child in 1912. When seen last, in 1915, there was no recurrence of the vulvar condition, although the rectal stricture and gummatous deposits in the rectum still required treatment. Microscopically, the organs removed, showed typical sclerosis and chronic infection.

CASE 2.—Mattie L., twenty-five years, colored, never pregnant, entered St. Louis Skin and Cancer Hospital, May 14, 1910, with a swelling of the vulva that had persisted for one year associated with ulceration over the perineum. It had been diagnosed as rectal cancer. Examination showed rectum uninvolved. Both labia and clitoris enlarged to size of a man's fist. Urethra normal. Antiluetic treatment caused no change in the mass; hence, on May 31, 1910, excision of mass. A latent tuberculosis of the lungs was also diagnosed and, after the operation, a pleuritic exudate developed, but this was gradually absorbed. No tubercle bacilli found in the mass removed, but numerous giant and epithelioid cells were found. There was also marked proliferation of the papillae of the vulvar skin and infiltration with lymphocytes and plasma cells.

CASE 3.—Mamie F., thirty-one years, colored, entered Barnes Hospital Dec. 16, 1914, with old luetic scars over body, no pregnancies, history of rectal abscesses three years ago, and for the last year a vulvar enlargement. No bleeding or discharge. Mass occupying left labium majus eight inches long and four inches wide with small base. Ulceration over perineum. No mention of urethral or rectal lesion. Wassermann positive. The vulvar skin was thick, wrinkled and cracked. Very slight tenderness. Refused treatment.

CASE 4.—Mattie J., thirty-seven, colored, entered Barnard Skin and Cancer Hospital August 22, 1919, five pregnancies, two miscarriages, luetic eruption at 23 years. Bubo in left groin one year ago. Since then vulvar swelling. Examination shows entire vulva seat of ulcerations serpiginous with raised border. Left labia edematous and enlarged. Rectum negative. Wassermann negative. Ducrey's bacillus not found. Tissue removed for microscopic study showed only chronic granulation. Refused treatment.

CASE 5.—Nettie T., twenty-five, colored, no pregnancies, entered Barnes Hospital Jan. 13, 1919, with history of labial swelling for past three years. Treated for lues in skin clinic during 1917. Tumor became painful two weeks ago. Temp. 99., no leucocytes. Labia minora and clitoris forming a mass 10x5x4 cm. Ulcer beneath it. Vulvectomy, by Dr. O. Schwarz, with good final result.

CASE 6.—Johanna O., thirty-four, colored, entered Barnes Hospital January, 1920, gave history of pruritus and swelling in left labia, the size of an egg, four years previously. In two years it was the size of a grape-fruit, and for the past year had grown to the size of a man's head. Antiluetic treatment and amenorrhea for past year. Pain and discomfort on walking during month before entering hospital. Examination showed a suppurating sinus in left inguinal region above Poupart's ligament. An indurated mass, 20x18x8 cms. in size, involving groin and left labia. Right labia also somewhat enlarged. An ulcer the size of a half dollar on top of the mass. Large whitish scars from former ulcerations. Urethra not involved. Papillary projections over vulva and perineum. Vulvectomy Jan. 15, 1920, by Dr. H. S. Crossen. Wassermann negative before and after operation. Histologically it is noteworthy that the entire mass showed evidence of chronic inflammation, plasma cells, lymphocytes, and sclerosis of connective tissue in the absence of any active ulcerations.

CASE 7.—Nona M., thirty, colored, entered Barnard Skin and Cancer Hospital May 14, 1919, one child, ulcers and vulvar enlargement of moderate extent that began one year ago. Pain on defecation. Examination showed considerable general hypertrophy with many rectal tags. Stricture of the rectum. Vigorous antiluetic treatment. Six salvarsans and many deep injections up to July 8, 1919, produced no visible improvement. Vulvectomy refused.

CASE 8.—Rose J., twenty-four, colored, entered Barnard Skin and Cancer Hospital October 11, 1917, one miscarriage. History of lues for previous year. Clitoris enlarged to size of a thumb with ulcer beneath it extending up to urethra. Attempt at autoinoculation from ulcer to test for chancroid gave a negative result. Wassermann negative. Returned two years later, Sept. 15, 1919, with condition only slightly worse. Antiluetic treatment produced no change. On Nov. 8, 1919, vulvectomy. Mass removed included both labia as well as clitoris, somewhat pendulous, hard, nodular, with many ulcerations. It was three inches long and one and three quarter inches in diameter.

CASE 9.—Bessie K., twenty-six, colored, entered Barnard Skin and Cancer Hospital Feb. 11, 1920, four pregnancies, no living children, had a vulvar lump and ulcer for two years. Pronounced leucorrhea. Some dribbling of urine. Wassermann positive. Both labia involved in a mass the size of a fist with numerous ulcerations. Antiluetic treatment produced very slight change. Refused operation.

CASE 10.—Irene J., thirty, colored, entered Barnard Skin and Cancer Hospital Dec. 22, 1919, two pregnancies, one miscarriage, gonorrhea at 21. Present trouble began one year ago with pimple in right groin that was opened with a needle, but mass rapidly grew larger until it hung between thighs and interferred with walking. Wassermann positive. Entire right half of vulva involved in a hard mass with areas of ulcerations extending up to the right groin. Preliminary antiluetic treatment; then, on Feb. 19, 1920, operative removal of mass by Dr. G. Gellhorn. This mass was 26x16x5½ cms. and weighed 620 grams. Good operative result. Referred to skin department for further antiluetic treatment.

CASE 11.—Dora W., forty-two, colored, came to Skin and Cancer Hospital May 24, 1919, no pregnancies, history of rectal abscesses for five years and for two years an ulcer and warty growths on vulva. Small rectovaginal fistula. Wassermann positive. Radium in form of plaque over site of perineal ulcer applied tentatively by Dr. G. Gellhorn. No improvement following. Intermittent antiluetic treatment. Returned two and one-half years later with considerable increase in vulvar swelling, especially in region of the clitoris as seen by the two photographs. (Fig. 1.) On Sept. 15, 1921, vulvectomy and excision of perirectal ulceration.

CASE 12.—Emma P., twenty-two, colored, entered City Hospital No. 2, August, 1921, no pregnancies, very dull witted, stated that she had noticed a hard swelling of her genitals for about one year with a sore in that region. Examination showed a pendulous mass consisting of labia minora and clitoris with ulcerations around the urethra the mass being about the size of two fists. Wassermann negative, but spirochæte found in dark-field of ulcer. Refused operation and left hospital without treatment.

CASE 13.—Lillie M., twenty-nine, colored, entered City Hospital No. 2, September 17, 1921, in labor. She was delivered by version by Dr. L. Dorsett. This was her fifth living child. She stated that the tumor mass, hanging from the vulva, had been present for 11 years. During each pregnancy the mass became much larger and after delivery again returned to its former size. She had been operated for rectal fistula and abscess. Examination eight hours after delivery showed a soft pendulous mass the size of a child's head springing from the left labium minus. (Fig. 2.) Scars from old ulcerations visible on the inner aspect. No active ulceration. Urethra normal. The mass showed marked nodular papillary surface. Within 24 hours the edema had decreased and the mass was visibly smaller.

4506 MARYLAND AVENUE.   (*For discussion, see p. 320.*)

ATRESIA AND STRICTURE OF THE VAGINA*

By James E. King, M.D., F.A.C.S., Buffalo, N. Y.

ATRESIA and stricture of the vagina are problems that not infrequently confront the gynecologist. They lay claim to his attention not because they of themselves are a source of suffering, but because they prevent the woman so affected from fulfilling her mission as a wife and mother. There is a voluminous literature on various phases of the subject. Most writers have confined their discussion to congenital absence of the vagina and the operative procedure for rectifying it. A review of the literature seems also to indicate that certain of the acquired forms have been regarded and described as congenital.

Atresias of the vagina may be divided into the congenital and acquired forms. Of the congenital atresias, imperforate hymen is the most frequent type. Absence of the vagina, strictly speaking, is not an atresia, inasmuch as in such cases a vagina never existed, but for convenience it may be placed under this heading. Finally transverse septa may also be found as a congenital anomaly. These defects are rarely discovered until puberty, when presence of the menstrual molimen with absence of flow, prompts an examination.

Congenital absence of the vagina is a rare anomaly and it is almost invariably associated with either a very rudimentary uterus or its complete absence. Indeed, cases that show an apparent absence of the vagina but in which there is found a well developed cervix and uterus, should be studied carefully, as it is very probable that they belong to the acquired rather than to the congenital type. Congenital types present no etiologic problem and they are interesting mainly from the viewpoint of their surgical treatment. It is not the purpose of this paper to enter into the discussion of these forms.

The acquired types of atresia are much more interesting. It is convenient to classify them in three groups, based upon the time of life when they occur; namely, those cases that develop during infancy and childhood, those that develop during the childbearing period, and those that develop after the menopause. This classification finds justification not only by reason of the different clinical aspects presented by each of the three groups, but more especially because of the distinct etiology found to cause the atresia during each of these three periods. Considering the etiologic factors in the three groups of our classification, we find the atresias produced during infancy and childhood to

---
*Read at the Thirty-fourth Annual Meeting of the American Association of Obstetricians, Gynecologists, and Abdominal Surgeons, St. Louis, Mo., September 20-22, 1921.

be due to trauma and vaginal infections. During the reproductive period they result from injuries and infections of labor, and very rarely to other vaginal infections, while after the menopause almost the sole cause is an atrophic vaginitis with a superimposed infection. Although the atresias produced during the childbearing period and after the menopause are interesting and worthy of discussion, only those atresias that develop during infancy and childhood will be discussed.

Atresias due to trauma during childhood present no question as to their etiology. The history of an injury, and the evidence of malformation and scar tissue about the vulva, clearly determine the causal factor. On the other hand, in the cases of atresia resulting from infantile vaginal infections, it is often impossible to obtain a history of the vaginal discharge and it may thus be difficult to establish the real cause of an atresia discovered in adult life.

Undoubtedly by far the most common cause of an atresia developing during childhood is infantile vaginitis. The bacterial cause of vaginitis in childhood is generally conceded. Grouped broadly, these infantile vaginal infections may be classified under two headings; those due to the gonococcus, and those due to other bacteria. With regard to the miscellaneous infections there seem to be many views, having but little foundation in scientific observation, that have found their way into many text books unquestioned. Most text books, for example, give first place to the exanthemata as a cause of vaginitis in children. The writer has never seen vaginitis associated with or following any of the exanthemata. Such cases he believes to be rare, and if they do occur, to be of short duration. However, children exhausted by any severe or long illness, or those suffering from malnutrition, are not infrequently subjects of vulvitis when cleanliness is not maintained. The possibility of a severe streptococcus ulcerative infection, or of a true diphtheritic infection of the vagina, is conceded. In such instances the great severity of the constitutional symptoms dominates the picture. A chronic purulent discharge in young children that bacteriologically shows no gonococci is not infrequently considered to be due primarily to a mixed infection. As a matter of fact, this mixed infection finds its origin in a gonorrhea and the persistence of the discharge is due to the pathology caused by, and remaining after the disappearance of, the gonococcus itself.

That the gonococcus causes a very large majority of vaginal discharges in children must be generally admitted. A committee representing the American Pediatric Society attempted by means of a questionnaire sent to hospitals and physicians, to obtain information on which might be based some definite data on this important subject. The result emphasized the fact that there existed among a considerable proportion of those approached, a failure to appreciate the real seriousness and importance of gonorrhea in childhood, and it made it clear that there still remains much to be done in placing squarely before the general profession the real truth concerning vaginitis in children.

A discussion of the atresia due to gonorrhea in childhood necessarily comprehends a consideration of certain features of gonorrheal vaginitis. It is well established that gonorrhea of the vagina is a disease of infancy and early childhood. The stratified epithelium of the glandless membrane of the adult successfully resists attacks of the gonococcus, while the more delicate vaginal tube of the child offers a field easily infected by, and difficult to rid of, these germs. The epidemics in institutions are now well understood to be due to contact infections, through the media of a large variety of agents. A discussion of the various means by which the gonococcus may find entrance to the vagina of a child is not pertinent to this paper.

Of the clinical manifestations following infection it may be said that as in adults, they vary in different individuals. Certain cases present but a moderate discharge, that attracts little attention and soon subsides. In other children the vaginal discharge may persist for months. To understand the variation in the clinical course in these little patients, one has only to keep in mind the fact that the gonococcus is a pyogenic organism that causes ulceration, and that in any gonorrheal inflammation mixed infection is the rule. The clinical manifestation of a gonorrheal vaginitis in the period just following the infection, often proclaims the severity of the process, and makes easily understood some of the sequelae which are seen later in life. Other things being equal, the amount of discharge and its persistence will depend upon the extent of ulceration. A discharge will continue until the ulcerated vaginal areas have been replaced by healed scar tissue, or until apposing granulating surfaces become united, and the obliteration of those surfaces is thus accomplished. It is doubtless just as true in gonorrheal vaginitis in children, as it is in urethritis in the male, that the less marked lesions may heal, leaving no trace. In every case, however, in which ulceration and mixed infection are pronounced, sequelae are certain to result. It is obviously quite impossible to estimate with any degree of accuracy the percentage of permanent structural changes that follow vaginitis in children. Probably, however, it is not high, inasmuch as some men of large experience have never encountered a case. That these changes do not occur more frequently is rather surprising, when one considers the delicate vaginal membrane of the child, and the indifference and difficulties encountered in the treatment of these infections.

The structural changes found in the adult vagina as a result of gonorrhea in early childhood, may be divided in two groups: a narrowing of the vagina due to scar tissue involving to a greater or lesser degree its circumference, and a more extensive condition, consisting of partial or complete obliteration of the vagina, brought about by the fusion of vaginal surfaces. It is seldom that either of these types is discovered until the woman marries. The first type may be found during a vaginal examination prompted by other conditions, or the stricture may interfere with normal married life to an extent that will lead to the discovery of its presence.

In cases belonging to the first group a wide variation in the extent of scar tissue is found but usually it is not sufficient to produce trouble. The examining finger comes in contact with a cord-like process felt in the vaginal wall. The lateral walls are the most frequent location. In view of the fact that such conditions do not interfere with normal processes, they possess but little clinical interest. The writer has met with a number of such conditions that were presumably the result of gonorrhea, but in only one could a definite history of a vaginal discharge in childhood be obtained.

In the cases belonging to the second group, the obliteration of the vagina naturally prompts an examination after marriage. In this group the vaginal defect is marked and the vagina is found almost completely closed, with the exception of the lower one, or one and a half inches. The vagina is represented by a pouch an inch or two in depth. Somewhere along the line which marks the fusion of the vaginal walls, is located the opening connecting with the uterus. This external opening may be extremely small and difficult to locate, and when found may admit only the smallest probe. Beyond this point the fusion of the vaginal walls will vary in extent. The fornices of the vagina in some instances may not be involved, while in others the vaginal walls may closely encompass, and be adherent to, the cervix.

The union that takes place between the vaginal walls is very firm. In the cases described, and in those seen by the writer, there has always been the small pouch representing the vagina just inside the vulva. This rather constant lower limitation to the vaginal adhesions may possibly be explained by the fact that the lower end of a child's vagina is gaping. If the labia be separated, and if the opening of the hymen be not too small, one may easily see the portion of the vagina just above the hymen as a cavity. At puberty the development of the levator muscles and the vaginal constrictors bring the lower part of the vaginal tube closely in contact. The fact of the imperfect vulval closure in the child may possibly explain why the bath tub commonly acts as the medium of infection in some of the institutional epidemics of vaginitis. The water of the bath finds ready entrance to the vagina, and if germ laden, infection is accomplished.

The writer's experience with acquired vaginal atresia as a result of infantile vaginitis, is confined to three cases.

The first was a young woman of nineteen who began menstruating at sixteen. With each period she experienced much pain, and the flow came very slowly. The feeling complained of was that of pressure in the vagina. Increasing discomfort with each month's flow, prompted an examination. It was found that the vagina was closed an inch and a half from the hymen by the firm union of the vaginal walls. No attempt was made at this time to find the opening along the line of union. Later, under anesthesia, a small opening was found that admitted only a probe. The union of the vaginal walls was dissected for about one half inch. Above this was the vaginal cavity where an adhesion of much lesser extent was found and corrected. Following this procedure menstruation occurred without pain. A year later the young lady married, and although no examination was permitted, her married life was reported normal. The discomfort at menstruation in this patient was due to the small opening not permitting a sufficiently rapid discharge of the menstrual fluid. During the time when the discharge from the uterus became greater than could be drained by the fistula through the atresia, the accumulation produced pain and pressure. Based upon the best of circumstantial evidence the cause of this atresia was an infantile gonorrhea. The mother stated that when the girl was four years old a persistent vaginal discharge required treatment for nearly a year. The mother herself gave a distinct history of pelvic inflammation, following which she had had years of pelvic symptoms, and finally she was operated upon by the writer for a chronic gonorrheal pelvic pathology.

The other two cases of atresia may be briefly cited. A Russian Jewess, twenty-six years old, four months after marriage consulted the writer because intercourse was impossible. Examination showed the vagina to be represented by a shallow pouch. The opening connecting with the uterus could not be found. The patient was requested to return during her menstruation, at which time it was possible to locate the lower opening of an apparently tortuous channel. At operation extensive vaginal adhesions were found to almost completely obliterate the vaginal tube. Following this attempt to open the vagina, although there was much improvement, in two months a second operation was undertaken, followed by vaginal dilatation. Shortly after the second operation pregnancy occurred. The labor was terminated by a difficult forceps delivery in the hands of a competent obstetrician. The baby died. Examination three months after this labor showed considerable scar tissue in the vagina, but a lumen that admitted two fingers comfortably. Pregnancy again took place and at term the woman was delivered by abdominal section with happy results. No history could be obtained here of any discharge during childhood. The patient could not, however, give any information concerning her early childhood in Russia, and there was none of her family who could supply such information. While in this case all direct evidence of infantile gonorrhea was wanting, the atresia was in the writer's opinion undoubtedly due to such a cause.

The third case was a young woman of twenty-three, married three months, referred because intercourse was impossible. Examination showed that the vagina was closed an inch and a half beyond the introitus. At operation, after dividing the lower union, a small vaginal cavity was encountered, and above this the vaginal walls were found closely adherent about the entire cervix and united in front of it, in such a manner that it was with considerable difficulty that the os was finally located and the cervix freed by a careful dissection. Very shortly after the patient left the hospital she became pregnant. At the seventh month of pregnancy examination showed the cervix free of adhesions. The obstetrician in whose hands this patient was placed deemed it wisest to deliver by abdominal section. This patient was able to secure the information that in early childhood she had had a profuse discharge that persisted for many months. Although positive evidence proving the source of this discharge to be a gonorrhea is wanting, our knowledge today of such conditions justifies an assumption that the gonococcus was the exciting germ.

If we grant that all such cases of atresia and stricture are due to a gonorrheal vaginitis that existed in childhood, it presents a strong argument for more prompt and active treatment of these discharges.

The operative technic for the relief of atresia of the vagina must depend naturally upon the needs of each individual case. There are a few general principles that can be applied, however. In atresia due to the union of vaginal surfaces, the dissection should be most carefully done, and when possible it should be accomplished by the finger. The sharp knife, unless great care is used, will penetrate into the deeper layers of the membrane, thus favoring the development of a scar in the deeper structures. A denuded vaginal surface in contact with a similar denuded area, will result in their union. If, therefore, after separating an area of vaginal union, it is possible to do on one wall a plastic procedure that brings an area of normal epithelium opposed to the denuded area of the opposite side, the denuded area will in due course be covered by a modified epithelium, such as is seen in the scar of the lacerated perineum. Where this cannot be done, the surfaces separated must be kept apart by frequent packing with iodoform gauze heavily impregnated with vaseline.

The atresia due to stricture seems to present greater difficulties than the atresia due to vaginal adhesions. As a rule the scar of these strictures is deep and its base broad. Before proceeding with the operation itself the strictures should be most thoroughly stretched with dilators and finger, until sufficient dilatation is obtained to permit one to determine the limits of the scar. Good dilatation also affords greater room for any plastic work. Plastic procedures are difficult. If the scar be not too wide, a resection of a part of the circumference of the stricture should be done, substituting for the resected portion, a union of membrane drawn from above and below the scar. This procedure was helpful in one of the writer's cases. Whatever operative plan is adopted, the vagina should be systematically dilated as soon as possible following the operation. In two of the writer's cases pregnancy took place within four months after operation. It would seem that the vaginal congestion accompanying pregnancy renders contractions of scar less prompt.

The question as to how such patients are to be delivered must of course be decided in each case by the condition of the vagina. If a delivery through the natural passages can be terminated with safety to mother and child, there can be no question as to the advantage derived from the dilatation. It would seem that such cases might also present a valid indication for the induction of premature labor. If however, considerable resistance is offered to the progress of the head, the chances that a premature infant will survive the labor are rather remote. For the safety of the child abdominal cesarean section undoubtedly is the best procedure.

1248 MAIN STREET. *(For discussion, see p. 320.)*

NITROUS OXIDE AND OXYGEN CONTINUOUS ANALGESIA AND ANESTHESIA WITH REBREATHING, IN OBSTETRICS. TECHNIC OF ADMINISTRATION AND SUMMARY OF RESULTS*

By A. E. Rives, Ph.G., M.D., East St. Louis, Ill.

THE WORLD-WIDE propaganda on painless childbirth and twilight sleep formed a nucleus for a greater future for motherhood than was anticipated. That the world is growing weaker and wiser is clearly demonstrated in obstetrics, childbirth becoming a more difficult problem in each generation, with the expectant mother well versed through the press and magazines of the advancement of the scientific methods of relief to be had by merely demanding them. We no longer believe that labor pains do not hurt and the old maxim of letting nature take its course in the sense in which it has always been applied in obstetrics, is a thing of the past. The demand for better obstetrics and safer analgesia and anesthesia must be respected. Today nitrous oxide is accepted as the safest analgesia and anesthetic for this purpose.

My personal experience with nitrous oxide and oxygen in obstetrics has been limited to private practice and dates from March 4, 1917. During this period I have kept complete records of each individual case, including the number of child in order of birth, urinary findings during pregnancy if abnormal, pituitrin if any, amount used and time given, time of beginning and termination of administration of the analgesia, ether used if any, amount of nitrous oxide used, calculations being on the basis of one hundred gallons for every two and one-half hours of continuous administration, lacerations if any, instrumental, difficult or abnormal labors, postpartum hemorrhage if any, condition of child, patient's version of entire procedure relative to amount of pain experienced, presence or absence of exhaustion following delivery, comparative flow of milk and results other than normal between date of delivery and date of last call.

There are a number of factors necessary to insure success in this work as with any other. The most important are, first, that the physician be a trained obstetrician; second, he must be thoroughly familiar with the technic of the administration of nitrous oxide and oxygen and must be able to differentiate between the stage of mild and deep analgesia and anesthesia, and must be able to interpret every sign and

---
*Read at the joint meeting of the Midwestern Association of Anesthetists and the National Anesthesia Research Society, at Kansas City, Mo., October 24-26, 1921.

symptom with the patient as his guide, and an apparatus that will deliver known quantities of the gases and capable of changing proportions in any quantity quickly. Third and equally important, the intelligence and the physical and mental attitude of the patient. I insist upon an early engagement, a specimen of urine every ten days previous to the sixth month, and weekly thereafter, and the usual physical examination and suggestions.

During this antepartum period the doctor and patient become acquainted, confidence is established, and the nature of the analgesia is explained with much stress laid upon the importance of cooperation before and during delivery. This greatly helps to overcome the fright and lack of confidence resulting from the usual neighborhood advice.

One of the greatest advantages of nitrous oxide in obstetrics is that it can be given at the home as well as the hospital. Personally, I prefer the delivery at home whenever possible. The expense is lessened, with less fear and more contentment, with home comforts and surroundings. The sanctity of the joys of the birth are not interrupted by the embarrassment caused by the presence of strangers and strange surroundings.

By insisting upon being notified when the first symptoms of labor make their appearance, preliminaries are early arranged. My equipment consists of a fiber case, made especially for me, which carries one tank of oxygen and two tanks of nitrous oxide, a Gwathmey portable outfit, an obstetrical bag with complete equipment, and a nurse.

No preliminary narcosis is used except in a case of rigid os. Early in the first stage of labor, when the os has softened and dilated one and one-half to two inches in diameter, and sometimes less, I begin the analgesia, after again reassuring the patient of her safety and comfort, explaining the necessity of cooperation and describing the symptoms and sensations she is going to experience.

The position of the patient is prone, on the right side of the bed, the patient being properly sterilized and draped. The right hand is inserted in a sterile glove; and with my left hand I manipulate the machine, which has a long rubber tubing with the breathing bag and Gwathmey face piece at the other end. My nurse is trained in fitting the face piece on the face to exclude all outside air, and manipulating the rebreathing valve and the face control. Before beginning, the face control is closed until the bag is about one-half to two-thirds filled with the mixture of approximately 95 per cent of nitrous oxide and 5 per cent of oxygen. We begin with this mixture and continue until a stage of analgesia is reached with whatever changes are necessary in the mixture. Within from two to four minutes the patient is completely anesthetized, in which condition she is allowed to remain for from five to ten minutes. This is done for two reasons, first to establish a blood saturation of the gases which, when once established, renders the patient more acutely susceptible to any necessary changes of the mixture from time to time as labor progresses. The other reason is that in 90 per cent of all the cases under the effect of the nitrous oxide and oxygen, more so than any other anesthetic I have ever used, the os rapidly dilates, so that usually in from two to fifteen minutes, the first stage of labor terminates. At this time, the sac is ruptured and if indicated, a hypodermic of 5 ℳ of pituitrin is given and the progress of labor is painlessly hastened. In place of the contractions and expulsive power being lessened and at longer intervals, as is sometimes the case with chloroform and ether, and always with scopolamin-morphine narcosis, they are more than doubled or trebled, the second stage being complete usually in from one-fourth to one-sixth the time of labor under any other circumstances, except instrumental or surgical.

In a short time the mixture required for the individual is found and is seldom changed until just before the termination of the second stage, when analgesia is deepened to nearly or complete anesthesia. The usual precautions are taken to prevent lacerations and at this time, I have sterile gloves on both my hands and the gases are not changed until the termination of this stage, when my nurse or myself, closes the nitrous oxide valve and opens wide the oxygen, allowing the mother to inhale pure oxygen for one to two minutes. The cord is then cut, and the mask is removed from the face of the patient.

During the entire procedure there is partial rebreathing, the bag being kept from one-half to two-thirds full, as near as possible. In nervous or excitable patients, a few breaths of air are given from time to time, when needed, as indicated by rapid, deep breathing, a tendency to excitement or cyanosis. Cyanosis is avoided throughout and semiconsciousness is maintained, likewise the ability of the patient to respond quickly to suggestions at all times.

The immediate family is allowed to be present, but they are requested to remain quiet, as the patient is instructed that I will be the only one to prompt her and that she should respond quickly each time. The result is that she bears down or remains quiet at my command.

The placenta is delivered under analgesia, as are repairs of the perineum made if any laceration.

The type of the individual must govern the depths of the analgesia and her susceptibility and acceptibility, physiologically and mentally, must be recognized and respected. The hysterical primipara is difficult to handle where the analgesia is begun before she has had enough hard pains to make her appreciate the difference. I have found, as yet, no contraindications for nitrous oxide in obstetrics when properly administered.

Rebreathing plays an important part in anesthesia and analgesia in major and minor surgery as well as obstetrics, a fact that has been denounced in no mild terms until a few years ago, on account of numerous postoperative and postpartum, disagreeable and dangerous symptoms that resulted from lack of knowledge of its application, effect and control. By close observation, the amount of rebreathing suited to the individual is soon discovered and the result is a smoother maintenance, more comfort to the patient, and economy of the gases. There is less tendency to shock, less depression and a lessened postpartum exhaustion.

During my first year I conducted my cases with interrupted analgesia, the patient taking three or four deep breaths of a 95 per cent-5 per cent mixture, just before the onset of each pain, holding the last one and bearing down as long as possible. The disagreeable feature of this was that I had failures because I was unable, in some cases, to "beat the pain." Unless the analgesia is established before the height of the contraction, the effect is lost. I observed in the hospitals while giving gas-oxygen anesthetics for major and minor surgical procedures that a great many cases could be carried from one-half to two and three hours on a light anesthesia or deep analgesia by continuous administration with partial rebreathing, and it occurred to me that this method should be applicable in obstetrics. It has proved successful in 94 per cent of my obstetrical cases in the last three and one-half years.

The total number of deliveries during this four and one-half years were 238, of which 121 were primiparae and 117 multiparae; of the babies, 132 were boys and 106 were girls; 218 cases delivered at home and 20 cases in hospitals. Ages of the primiparæ were from 16 to 39 years with average of 22.8 years. The following table contains further details of interest.

	PRIMIPARAE	MULTIPARAE
Total average time of delivery	1 hour, 13.4 min.	31.2 min.
First year, with interrupted administration, average time	1 hour, 47.3 min.	40 min.
Second year, with continuous administration, average time	1 hour, 15.1 min.	39.1 min.
Third year, continuous administration, average time	1 hour, 19 min.	29 min.
Last one and one-half years	1 hour, 6.6 min.	26.4 min.
Abnormal presentations—face	4	1
2 of primiparae delivered instrumentally, and 2 by version: multip. normal.		
Abnormal presentations—breech	7	3
Instrumental to perineum	7	2
Instrumental complete	4	
Instrumental, high application	3	
Rigid cervix	3	
No relief from pain		11
Ether at delivery		39
Over 10 days in bed		5

One phlebitis developed fifth day, right leg, recovery complete in four weeks
One 12 days, 3rd degree laceration, face presentation, 12½ lb. child, rupture of sac 4 days previous to delivery, instrumental.
Two—pyosalpinx, with temperature 104°, with chills, 36 and 38 hours after delivery. Recovery at 5 and 8 weeks.
One hemorrhage during and after delivery from laceration, recovery 2 weeks.
Postpartum hemorrhage — None
Stillbirths — 2
Macerated fetus, premature, 6½ and 7 mo. — 2
Atrophy of cord — 1
Full term that died within 10 days; One, congenital hemophilia, 7 hours. One, anancephalus, 2 hours.
Full term that received oxygen after birth. All lived. — 6

Types of pathological conditions existing in the mothers were pulmonary tuberculosis, hemiplegia, asthma, cardiac lesions, nephritis, diabetis, high blood pressure.

SUMMARY

I find less cyanosis in the babies but have been unable to get a record of the difference of loss of weight. Absence of postpartum hemorrhage, less surgical shock, less postpartum exhaustion, noticeable by the patients themselves where one or more deliveries have been made previously, with and without other anesthetics. No maternal deaths, greatly lessened first and second stage and more comfort to the mother and a greater satisfaction to the patient and family. Saving of time for the obstetrician.

MURPHY BUILDING.

INDICATIONS AND CONTRAINDICATIONS FOR THE USE OF PITUITARY EXTRACT IN OBSTETRICS*

BY ROLAND S. CRON, M.D., ANN ARBOR, MICHIGAN

From the Department of Obstetrics and Gynecology, University of Michigan.

IN THE Department of Obstetrics and Gynecology at the University Hospital pituitary extract has been used since the year 1911 without any very serious accidents directly attributable to the drug. It has been administered for the induction of labor, during labor, and also during the puerperium. In 1914 Seeley analyzed forty cases from the clinic and, although much has since been learned, the conclusions which he reached are for the most part still accepted as correct. In 150 additional cases an attempt has been made to elaborate on and extend the use of this drug.

The preparation used during the majority of our experiments is "pituitrin" manufactured by Parke, Davis & Company, of Detroit. Occasionally it has been necessary to substitute "pituitol," a Hollister-

---
*Abstract read before the Section on Gynecology and Obstetrics, Michigan State Medical Society Annual Meeting, May 24-26, 1921, Bay City, Michigan.

Wilson laboratory preparation. The action of the two preparations in so far as our observations have advanced has been identical. One cubic centimeter of this solution is equivalent to 0.1 grams of the fresh gland. Surgical "pituitrin" also marketed by Parke, Davis & Company has been used but its potency is approximately twice that of the obstetrical preparation and therefore when used not more than one-half the customary dose has been administered.

The dosage has varied according to the indication for its use from 3 minims to 1 c.c. Our maximum fractional dosage has never been more than 3 c.c. in twenty-four hours. Watson in a recent paper has advocated much greater dosage, having administered in cases of induction of labor as much as 8 to 10½ c.c. in ½ c.c. doses at intervals of one-half hour, while Bandler has given 12 to 14 c.c. in twenty-four hours without disastrous results.

The extract should be injected intramuscularly, either directly into the skeletal or into the uterine muscle. For the usual obstetrical case satisfactory results are obtained by injection into the gluteal or deltoid muscles. In cesarean section and postpartum hemorrhage it may be given directly into the uterine muscle.

INDUCTION OF LABOR

Our results in cases of induction of labor have been more successful than those reported by Seeley, Mundell and Bandler but not as successful as those of Watson, Stein and Wilson. They compare quite favorably with those reported by Adair. Forty-five individual cases ranging from the eighth month of pregnancy to three weeks' postmaturity were subjected to induction of labor. Thirty-one, or 69 per cent, responded to one of the methods mentioned below. Of these 31 cases in 26, or 65 per cent, labor was brought on by means of a combination of castor oil, quinine, and pituitrin. Five were induced by the insertion of a Voorhees bag and repeated small doses of pituitrin. Fourteen, or 35 per cent, did not respond sufficiently to the combination of castor oil, quinine, and pituitrin to bring on labor.

The method which in our hands proved most successful was the administration by mouth of one to two ounces of oleum rinci, followed two hours later by ten grains of quinine sulphate. The quinine was repeated and at the time of the last doses of quinine five minims of pituitrin were injected intramuscularly followed two hours later by a second and sometimes a third dose of pituitary extract. Not more than three injections of this extract were administered during a single attempt at induction. The object of the combination of these drugs is to secure a maximum oxytocic action on the uterus. The castor oil besides congesting the pelvis has a direct irritant action on the uterine musculature. The quinine acts as a continuous oxytocic, while the pituitrin has a rhythmical stimulating action of relatively short duration. Therefore it is most important to administer repeatedly the pituitrin in order to secure a completion of the onset of labor. Many patients apparently go into labor but the uterine contractions do not continue long enough to secure sufficient cervical dilatation and separation of the ovum unless the drug is repeated two to three times.

There were sixty-nine attempts made to induce labor by means of the aforementioned drugs. A few attempts, namely ten, were made with only castor oil and quinine, about an equal number with pituitrin alone. The results as far as successful inductions are concerned cannot be compared with the combination of the three drugs. It is quite evident that in some individual cases repeated attempts were made to bring on labor. As many as six courses at intervals of three to six days have been given to a single case. It is very interesting to note the increasing success with this method as the gravida reaches maturity and postmaturity. At eight months two attempts were unsuccessful; at eight and one-half months one attempt was unsuccessful; at nine and one-fourth months one attempt was successful while four were unsuccessful; at nine and one-half months two were successful while nine were unsuccessful; at nine and three-fourths months one was successful and six unsuccessful. At ten months nineteen were successful while six were unsuccessful; at ten and one-fourth months one was unsuccessful; at ten and one-half months five were successful and at eleven months one was successful. Judging from these results it is quite apparent that the irritability of the uterus and its response to oxytocic drugs increases as term is approached. Pauliot and others have reached the same conclusion. Furthermore it can be concluded that for bringing on therapeutic abortion or premature labor, pituitary extract alone or in combination with other drugs is practically useless.

Resort to the Voorhees bag for induction of labor had to be made in two cases of polyhydramnion. Both pregnancies had gone beyond term and although as many as six attempts with castor oil, quinine, and pituitrin had been made, all were unsuccessful. Undoubtedly the uterine musculature had been so stretched and thinned that it could not be stimulated by medicinal irritants. Following the introduction of the Voorhees bag one can administer small doses of pituitrin and thereby shorten the onset of labor pains from six to ten hours.

This drug is also a great help in differentiating false from true labor pains. A few minims of the drug will augment true pains so that there is no further doubt about the status of the uterine irritability. In cases of premature rupture of the membranes during the latter months of pregnancy or at term, small doses of pituitrin will influence the uterus in the same way as after bagging. Many cases of intrapartum infection due to long exposure have undoubtedly been prevented in this way.

FIRST STAGE OF LABOR

Our experience with pituitary extract during the first stage of labor has been very limited. Except for those rare cases of primary uterine inertia its use during this stage is most dangerous. There were six labors complicated by primary inertia. Five of them responded to small doses of the extract but the sixth one was not benefited. In two of the cases the pains became continuous and the uterine contractions so severe that the fetal circulation was considerably embarrassed. It became necesary to complete the labor in both cases by internal podalic version under deep anesthesia. A third case was similarly affected. The uterus went into a state of tetany and the labor was terminated by manual dilatation of the cervix and forceps extraction. The baby of this last case suffered from asphyxia pallida and was resuscitated with great difficulty.

Primary uterine inertia can and should be recognized before labor. The uterus is atonic and flabby and indifferent to stimulation; the blood pressure is generally low and the calcium index is subnormal. Bell advises that such a state be treated by the oral administration of calcium salts and the dried extract of the posterior lobe (gr. v, t.i.d.) or the whole pituitary gland (gr. xx, t.i.d.). He has seen women with bad obstetric histories in regard to primary uterine inertia, go through easy and rapid labors after the treatment described.

There may be another indication for the use of pituitrin during the first stage of labor, namely in cases of marginal or partial placenta previa with incomplete dilatation of the cervical os and rupture of the membranes. A small dose of the extract in some cases may be sufficient to force the presenting part down into the pelvis and against the placenta. The head then acts as a very efficient tampon.

SECOND STAGE OF LABOR

"It is probable, other conditions being suitable, that the use of pituitrin in secondary uterine inertia, a very common condition, far exceeds all other applications of the effect of this preparation on the uterus." That is Bell's opinion of the extract when used as an adjunct during the second stage. Bandler speaks even more favorably of the preparation. He claims that by the administration of the drug he has excluded the use of forceps except in sudden emergencies and that he has not used them at all in private practice for over two years. Mosher's expression fits in with our opinion of the value of this drug much better than either of the previous two. His dictum, namely, "To a mother who has had the test of labor with an inability to deliver a head already on the perineum, it is a boon. To a primipara in the first stage of labor it is a menace" can be universally adopted by those practicing obstetrics.

It has been suggested to the writer, after having observed Doctor Irving W. Potter "iron out" a perineum for selective version and extraction that his technic can be applied to the vulval outlet of primiparae. After completion of the first stage of labor and with the patient fully anesthetized the perineum can be completely dilated with the aid of green soap. Then the patient can be kept in the obstetrical degree of anesthesia and the labor completed by the administration of 0.5 c.c. of pituitrin. This procedure has been carried out in a limited number of cases but cannot as yet be recommended for adoption.

Bell has advocated the combining of pituitrin with scopolamine pantopon anesthesia (twilight sleep) for shortening the period of labor. In our hands twilight sleep has not been a success but in those cases with which we have had experience the oxytocic is of value in completing the prolonged labor. Stein's results in combining nitrous oxide and pituitrin have been excellent. We are inclined to concur with him in regard to this technic.

Any practitioner who has used pituitary extract in either the first or second stage of labor must have at some time in his career found it necessary, because of an abnormal fetal heart, to complete a delivery with forceps. Frequently the infant is in a state of livid or pallid asphyxia. Occasionally it is stillborn and sometimes it does not show symptoms until later in life. The pituitrin circulating in the maternal blood causes rapid, recurrent and more forceful uterine contractions, shutting off the placental circulation and also directly compressing the fetus. Kerley, Holt, Heard, Norris and Chapin and Pisek have called our attention to the late effects of pituitary extract on infants. They have found in many of their cases at autopsy meningeal and cerebral hemorrhages which in the living child lead to paralysis, epilepsy and idiocy. In view of these findings and the frequent disastrous effects to the mother should we not as medical men be most conservative in the use of this popular drug?

THIRD STAGE OF LABOR

Bell mentions that Strassman and others observed that when pituitary extract was administered during the first stage of labor, the third stage was much shortened. Advantage has been taken of this suggestion and one cubic centimeter has been injected deep intramuscularly immediately following the birth of the infant.

Our results in the first 135 consecutive cases have been so uniform and offer such brilliant hopes for the future that we feel justified in reporting them at the present time. The amount of blood lost during delivery, the length of the third stage of labor, the method of expression, and the mechanism of separation of the placenta and frequency of postpartum hemorrhage have been recorded and analyzed.

The loss of blood was accurately measured by placing a flat douche pan under the patient as soon as the second stage was completed. The hemorrhage occurring before the separation of the placenta, at the time of separation and that after separation was used in the estimation. The loss varied from three cubic centimeters to 840 cubic centimeters for the normal cases, the average being 255 cubic centimeters. Seven cases were excluded from this estimate; six had adherent placentae due to a syphilitic chorionitis and prematurity. The actual loss of blood in these six cases was 270 cubic centimeters, 360 cubic centimeters, 600 cubic centimeters, 840 cubic centimeters, 1050 cubic centimeters and 1800 cubic centimeters. The seventh case was complicated by a marginal placenta previa and a loss of 2010 cubic centimeters of blood.

The length of the third stage of labor in the normal cases varied from one to thirty-two minutes, the average being 12.1 minutes. Five of the seven cases mentioned above were excluded because of adherent placentae. These placentae remained *in utero* forty-three minutes, one hour and eighteen minutes, two hours and thirty-three minutes, two hours and fifty minutes and twenty-one hours and thirty minutes.

The separation of the placentae in 69 per cent of the cases was by the Schultze mechanism, the fetal surface appearing first. This method of separation is acknowledged as the most favorable and accompanied by the least amount of bleeding. The remaining 31 per cent except two placentae which were manually removed, separated by the Duncan mechanism.

The delivery of the placenta was completed in 94 per cent of the cases by modified Credé expression. The remaining 6 per cent were cared for as follows: four cases of adherent placentae, two by true Credé and two by manual removal, two by the Michael Reese method of expression and one came away spontaneously.

The height of the fundus of the uterus above the symphysis pubis one hour after delivery averaged 15.9 cm. for full term pregnancies.

When these results are compared with controls and also with the textbook picture of the third stage of labor, it will be found that the third stage of labor has been materially influenced by the pituitrin. The loss of blood was reduced from 330 c.c. in the controls and 300 to 500 c.c. (Williams) to 255 c.c. in our pituitrin cases. The third stage was shortened from thirty-five minutes in the controls and twenty to thirty minutes (De Lee and Williams) to twelve and one-tenth minutes. The methods of separation and expression were kept in the same ratio one to another as those of the controls as well as those of the textbooks. The frequency of adherent placentae and complications might appear unusually high, but it must be remembered that approximately 20 per cent of our pregnancies are complicated by lues.

We have not observed any cases of hour-glass contractions. It is possible but not probable that in partially adherent placentae especially in premature labors this complication may occur. We believe, however, that the intermittent retraction and contraction of the uterus would have a tendency to free such placentae.

POSTPARTUM HEMORRHAGE

Pituitary extract as an etiologic factor in the causation of postpartum hemorrhage was not in our hands an important one. When the drug brings on tetanic contractions of the uterus followed by atony then, of course, it can be blamed for the condition. Fortunately, because pituitrin is only rarely used during the first and second stages, this has never been our experience.

For the treatment of postpartum hemorrhage the usual method of intramuscular injection of 1 c.c. of the solution was used. De Lee suggests in such cases that the drug be injected directly through the abdominal wall into the uterine muscle. Naturally the hemostatic effect is much more rapid. Its action on the uterine muscle is not of as long duration as ergot preparations but the length of time necessary for it to circulate in the arterial system to stimulate the uterus to contract is three to five minutes, while intramuscular injections of ergot take some fifteen to twenty minutes.

CESAREAN SECTION

Formerly pituitrin was administered by the usual method of intramuscular injection at the time of, or immediately after, the removal of the placenta. More recently operators have infiltrated the uterine incision with 1 or 2 c.c. of the extract. When used in this manner the closure of the uterine wound is greatly facilitated. An excellent procedure recommended by many operators is to supplement the action of pituitrin by injecting intramuscularly at the beginning of the operation one of the sterile preparations of ergot. Then one secures besides the immediate effect of the pituitrin the lasting and tetanic action of the ergot. During the postoperative period of cesarean section cases repeated small doses of either the obstetrical or surgical preparation of pituitary extract may be used most efficaciously.

CONCLUSIONS

1. At maturity labor can be induced in about 65 per cent of the cases by oral administration of castor oil, quinine and repeated small intramuscular injections of pituitary extract.

2. For the treatment of primary inertia the extract should be used most cautiously and only in very small doses.

3. Judiciously pituitary extract can be used to great advantage in the cases of secondary inertia.

4. The third stage of labor can be most favorably influenced by the intramuscular injection of 1 c.c. of the extract.

5. Pituitary extract should be included in the obstetrician's armamentarium for combating postpartum hemorrhage.

6. The extract facilitates the closure of the uterine wound in cases of cesarean section.

REFERENCES

Adair, F. L.: Interstate Med. Jour., 1916, xxiii, 1111. *Bandler, S. W.*: Am. Jour. Obst., 1916, lxxiii, 77. *Bandler, S. W.*: Am. Jour. Surg., 1916, xxx, 121. *Bell, W. B.*: Brit. Med. Jour., 1909, ii, 1609-1613. *Bell, W. B.*: The Pituitary, Monograph, New York, 1919, Wm. Wood & Company, pp. 319-320. *Chapin and Pisek*: Diseases of Children, 1915, Wm. Wood & Company, p. 8. *De Lee, J. B.*: Principles and Practice of Obstetrics, 1916, W. B. Saunders Co., pp. 581, 318. *Heard, A. C.*: Texas State Jour. Med., 1916, xii, 265. *Holt*: Diseases of Infancy and Childhood, 1919, p. 104. Appleton. *Kerley*: Practice of Pediatrics, 1914, W. B. Saunders Co., p. 495. *Mosher, G. C.*: Surg., Gynec. and Obst., 1916, xxii, 108. *Mundell, J. J.*: Am. Jour. Obst., 1916, lxxiii, 306. *Mundell, J. J.*: Jour. Am. Med. Assn., 1917, lxviii, 1601. *Norris, R.*: Am. Jour. Obst., xxi, 471. *Pauliot, L.*: Rev. mens. de gynec., d'obst. et de pediat., 1919, xiv, 27-40. *Potter, I. W.*: Am. Jour. Obst. and Gynec., 1921, 1, 560. *Seeley, W. F.*: Jour. Mich. State Med. Soc., July, 1914. *Stein, A.*: Am. Jour. Obst., 1919, lxxx, 470. Also: Zentralbl. f. Gynäk., 1920, xliv, 1152. *Strassman, P.*: Zentralbl. f. Gynäk., 1912, xxxvi, 438. *Watson, B. P.*: Canad. Med. Jour., 1913, iii, 729. *Watson, B. P.*: Am. Jour. Obst. and Gynec., 1920, i, 70. *Williams, J. W.*: Obstetrics, 1919, D. Appleton & Co., pp. 250, 315. *Wilson, H. C.*: Med. Jour. Australia, 1918, i, 171.

REPORT OF A CASE OF B. WELCHII BLOOD STREAM INFECTION OF UTERINE ORIGIN*

By HARVEY BURLESON MATTHEWS, M.D., F.A.C.S., BROOKLYN, N. Y.

(From the Department of Obstetrics and Gynecology of the Long Island College Hospital)

MRS. B. H., age twenty-three, para ii., was admitted to Long Island College Hospital (No. 3605) by ambulance on August 2, 1921. She was acutely ill, and stated that three days previously, believing she was two months' pregnant, she inserted a slippery elm stick into the uterus for the purpose of producing an abortion. Almost immediately she began to bleed and passed numerous clots. The bleeding continued that night but ceased on the following day. Twenty-four hours later, believing that the ovum had not been passed, she took a mustard foot bath after which she began to flow, vomited, had a severe chill, followed by a headache but was not particularly feverish. The following day, that is forty-eight hours after the uterine bleeding first began, she was very feverish and weak and for the first time called a physician who made a diagnosis of an inevitable abortion and recommended hospital treatment. This she accepted and entered the hospital, as stated above, at 11:00 A. M., Aug. 2, 1921.

Past and menstrual histories, negative. Obstetrical history: One child, two years old, normal delivery and puerperium.

---
*Presented at a meeting of the New York Obstetrical Society, November 8, 1921.

Physical examination on admission showed a young adult female, acutely ill, skin dry and flushed, conjunctiva and skin deeply jaundiced, lips and skin dry and a marked fetor from the mouth. There was definite cyanosis of the lips and finger tips with an associated coldness of all extremities. Temperature 104, pulse 120 regular, fair quality, respiration 34. Head, eyes, ears, nose negative. Teeth in poor condition, many fillings, slight gingival infection. Tongue dry and covered with a thick white fur. Tonsils and pharynx, lungs and breasts negative. Heart muscular tonus fair, moderate venous pulsations in the neck veins. Pulse 120 fair quality. Abdomen moderately distended and tympanitic throughout, no masses palpable, no abnormal rigidity, marked tenderness in both lower quadrants, particularly on the right side.

Pelvic Examination.—Multiparous introitus, fair pelvic floor with relaxed levators, some relaxation of the anterior vaginal wall. Cervix bilaterally lacerated, soft, open, admits one finger, points in the axis of the vagina and is quite sensitive on motion. Uterus the size of a two months' pregnancy, soft, boggy, and retroverted to the first degree, movable and very sensitive. There was moderate tender infiltration in the left broad ligament. Exudate is more extensive and more sensitive in the right fornix but is still confined to the pelvis. Adnexa not palpable. The entire pelvis is extremely tender and painful on manipulation.

Diagnosis.—Septicemia following septic abortion and old laceration of the cervix and pelvic floor.

Laboratory Findings.—Red cells 3,000,000; white cells 51,200; polys 89; small lymphocytes 11 per cent; hemoglobin 60 per cent; blood pressure, 100/68.

Treatment.—Hypodermoclysis 750 c.c. was given immediately and blood for blood culture taken at this time. The Fowler position, ice cap to lower abdomen, low enema followed by Harris drip of 5 per cent glucose in 2 per cent bicarbonate of soda solution. Digalen minims 20 every four hours, alternating with camphor in oil 30 minims and enough morphia to quiet the patient.

Follow Up Notes.—Aug. 2, 1921, 6:00 P.M. Patient irrational, had two chills since admission. Temperature remains 104.2°, pulse 120 but of good quality. Cyanosis of the fingers and lower portion of the forearm more marked. 8:00 P.M. Patient delirious, very restless and noisy. Cyanosis of extremities more marked. Temperature 105°, pulse 140, irregular, weak, respirations 40 and shallow.

Aug. 3, 1921, 9:00 A.M. Patient having chills about every half hour, almost constantly shaking. Pulse 130, bad quality. Respiration 50 and shallow. 6:30 P. M. Patient semicomatose for last few hours. Had to be restrained on several occasions. Had repeated chills about every twenty minutes, very cyanotic. Respirations irregular and shallow. Definite rigidity of neck, pulse 140, weak, thready and imperceptible at times. Crepitation felt in both inguinal regions, more marked on right side. 7:30 P.M. Pronounced dead 37 hours after admission and 109 hours after passing the elm stick into the uterus.

Autopsy Findings (by Dr. A. Murray).—Body well nourished, rigor mortis present, no marks of violence. Body jaundiced throughout, crepitates and enormously swollen. Both lungs showed intense congestion with a possible septic pneumonia. Pericardial sac contained two ounces of bloody fluid, gas bubbles are seen in the epicardium and throughout the myocardium. Heart normal in size, all valves normal, myocardium very soft. Spleen is firm, congested, and about normal size. Both kidneys contain gas bubbles throughout but otherwise apparently normal. Adrenals normal. Stomach pancreas, intestines, and gall bladder all apparently normal. Liver weighs 1447 grams and is filled with gas bubbles. Uterus very soft and contains the remains of placenta. Gas bubbles over the surface of the uterus and broad ligaments. All organs showed marked autolysis.

Microscopic Findings.—Spleen, intense congestion and a few gas holes. Pancreas showed areas of necrosis. Liver riddled with "gas holes" throughout and stained sections show many B. Welchii about "gas holes." Considerable fatty infiltration and autolysis. Kidneys advanced necrosis. Lungs edematous and congested.

Cause of Death.—Bacillus aerogenes capsulatus infection.

Blood Culture Reports.—Aug. 2, 1921, on admission, specimen of blood sterile. Aug. 3, Blood culture showed numerous B. Welchii. Aug. 4, Smear of; 1. Heart blood large number of capsulated gram-positive rods. 2. Peritoneal fluid large numbers of capsulated gram-positive rods. 3. Pus from uterus, gram-positive and gram-negative rods and streptococci.

Cultures of heart blood showed enormous numbers of B. Welchii in pure culture. Peritoneal fluid enormous numbers of B. Welchii in pure culture. Pus from uterus showed numerous B. Welchii, B. proteus, and staphylococci.

COMMENTS

Since Professor Wm. H. Welch of Johns Hopkins first described the B. aerogenes capsulatus in 1891 surgeons have reported innumerable cases of "gas gangrene" both in civil and military practice. During the World War many thousands of cases of infections by "the gas-producing group of microorganisms" occurred and the literature from 1917 to 1920 is literally full of dissertations upon this very interesting and usually fatal infection. Perhaps no other surgical subject usurped as much attention along the front line hospitals as did the management of these infections and due to this fact we undoubtedly know far more today than we would have otherwise known. Regarding the puerperal and postabortal infections by this microorganism we know comparatively little except in so far as our surgical confreres have informed us. Only a very few completely detailed cases with bacteriologic and pathologic reports have been made. Curiously enough Professor Welch reported in 1891, the first case of puerperal sepsis caused by the B. aerogenes capsulatus. Since this time Dobbin, P. Ernst, Graham, Stewart and Baldwin of Columbus, Ohio, Krönig and Menge, E. L. Hunt, have studied and reported a few cases of puerperal and postabortal infections that were either caused by B. aerogenes capsulatus or in which it played an important rôle. Herbert V. Williams found the bacillus complicating a case of suppurative pyelitis. At autopsy the body presented all the characteristics of B. Welchii infection.

The symptoms are those of a profound toxemia, e.g., high temperature, rapid pulse, and respiration, chills, sweats, dryness of the mucous membranes and skin, cyanosis and acidosis. There have been many and varied explanations of how death is caused by the B. Welchii but perhaps Bull and Pritchett are correct in their assumption that death is produced by a specific bacterial toxin and not by a blood stream invasion of the microorganism or by an acid intoxication (butyric, succinic). It is generally believed that when the organism is found in the blood stream, and there are very few case reports where blood cultures were positive, circulatory failure has begun and since the blood stream is at this time poorly oxygenated or even in certain parts or the body devoid of oxygen, the B. Welchii begin to multiply very rapidly and within from four to forty-eight hours death ensues. Following death their growth is extremely rapid and within a few hours unless the body is kept on ice it is swollen to twice its normal size or even larger. There is marked crepitation and upon opening the ab-

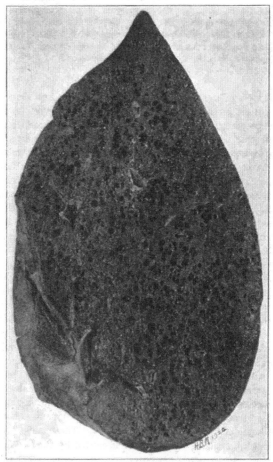

Fig. 1.—Photograph of gross section of liver from case of B. Welchii infection, showing surface riddled with "gas-holes",—the so-called "foamy liver."

dominal or other cavities there is escape of gas. The gas burns with a blue flame and is composed largely of hydrogen with some CO_2 and a small percentage of nitrogen (Hunt).

Treatment.—The management of puerperal and postabortal infections by B. aerogenes capsulatus is expectant. If the diagnosis is made early enough, cleansing of the uterine and vaginal cavities of all clots, dead tissue and other debris that is known to grow these microorganisms is indicated. I could find no report where hysterectomy or other operative procedure in such cases had been done and indeed it would seem a useless procedure. Simultaneous with the diagnosis,

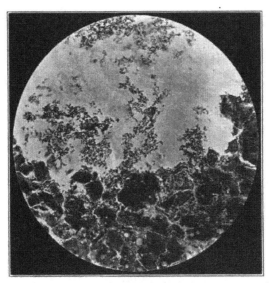

Fig. 2.—Microscopic section of liver tissue showing B. Welchii infection. Section shows edge of a "gas-hole" with bacilli in between liver cells and lying loose in "gas-hole."

the specific antitoxin as recommended by Bull and Pritchett or Henry and Lucy or any standardized antiserum should be administered forthwith. Transfusion may offer something but as yet there is no data to prove or disprove the efficacy of this procedure.

BIBLIOGRAPHY

(1) *McFarland*: Pathogenic Bacteria and Protozoa, Philadelphia, 1919, W. B. Saunders Co., ed. 9. (2) *Park and Williams*: Pathogenic Micro-organisms, Philadelphia, 1920, Lea and Febiger, ed. 7. (3) *Esty, J. E.*: Jour. Bacteriol., 1920, v, 375. (4) *Bloodgood*: Surg., Gynec. and Obst., 1916, xxiii, 182. (5) *Bull and Pritchett*: Jour. Exper. Med., 1917, xxvi, 119. (6) *Bull and Pritchett*: Ibid., p. 867. (7) *Graham, Steward, and Baldwin, J. F.*: Columbus Med. Jour., 1894, xii, 55. (8) *Adams, D. S.*: Boston Med. and Surg. Jour., January to June, 1920, clxxxii, 373. (9) *Hunt, E. L.*: Ibid., p. 385. (10) *Welch, W. H.*: Bull. Johns Hopkins Hosp., 1900, ii, 185. (11) *Welch, W. H.*: Boston Med. and Surg. Jour., July to December, 1900, cxliii, 73. (12) *Welch and Nuttal*: Bull. Johns Hopkins Hosp., 1892, iii, 81. (13) *Welch and Flexner*: Jour. Exper. Med., 1896, i, p. 5. (14) *Dobbin, G. W.*: Am. Jour. Obst., 1898, xxxviii, 185. (15) *Williams, H. V.*: Bull. Johns Hopkins Hosp., 1896-1897, vii-viii, 66. (16) *Henry and Lucy*: Proc. Roy. Soc., London, 1919, xci, 513.

643 ST. MARKS AVENUE.

Society Transactions

AMERICAN ASSOCIATION OF OBSTETRICIANS, GYNECOLOGISTS, AND ABDOMINAL SURGEONS. THIRTY-FOURTH ANNUAL MEETING HELD AT ST. LOUIS, MO., SEPTEMBER 20, 21, AND 22, 1921

(*Continued from the February issue.*)

Dr. Charles L. Bonifield, of Cincinnati, Ohio, read a paper entitled **Carcinoma Uteri.** (For original article see page 250.)

Dr. Roland E. Skeel, of Los Angeles, Cal., presented a paper entitled **Some Phases in the Evolution of the Diagnosis and Treatment of Cancer of the Cervix.** (For original article see page 252.)

Dr. G. Van Amber Brown, of Detroit, Mich., read a paper entitled **Valuable Methods Used to Extend Operability in Advanced Cancer of the Cervix.** (For original article see page 263.)

Dr. George W. Crile, Cleveland, Ohio, read a paper entitled **The Control of the Mortality of Abdominal Operations for Cancer.** (For original article see page 272.)

DISCUSSION OF THE PAPERS OF DRS. BONIFIELD, SKEEL, BROWN AND CRILE.

DR. GEORGE GELLHORN, St. Louis, Missouri, (by invitation).—I rise chiefly to applaud the paper of Dr. Skeel. Hardly ever have I heard or read as excellent an exposé of the whole subject. I would like to make just one comment. In one of his conclusions Dr. Skeel suggests that in borderline, or inoperable cases of cancer of the cervix, the use of the thermocautery should precede the radium application. On the strength of a rather extensive experience gained at the Barnard Free Skin and Cancer Hospital in this city, I venture to say that by doing so one would deprive himself of a very valuable filter. No filter that we can devise in any way takes the place of the filter supplied by Nature, and by thrusting radium needles into the diseased tissues themselves, the latter will act as a very efficient filter.

On the other hand, if the tumor be removed by curet or cautery, there are very thin walls left between the cavity and the adjoining organs, and it was due to that practice that we had a number of fistulae in former years when we did just what Dr. Skeel advocates. Now that we eliminate all kinds of preliminary surgery, such fistulae have not occurred and the palliative result of radium has been even better than before.

DR. WILLIAM SEAMAN BAINBRIDGE, New York City.—The consensus of opinion today is that we have more careful dosage and deeper effects of x-ray, with more refined technic; radium is emphasized as a more important agent with better technic and larger dosage. The German school is divided into two very hostile camps; the first advocating that the x-rays should replace all surgery in cancer of the uterus and that, very soon, radium will be forgotten; and the second insisting that the combined method is the only worth while one, using the x-rays externally and radium internally. Sittenfield says that surgical work on uterine cancer is practically ended and that in ten years it will be superseded by the x-rays and radium. Others of our colleagues say there is nothing in these two agents to be hoped for. Hadley remarks that surgery should be employed as heretofore, but with finer technic, and that x-rays and radium should be tried as aids to the surgeon.

Such papers as Crile's, and others, that we have heard today make us realize the difference between surgery and surgery. As the application and dosage of radium and the x-rays are being perfected, it is for the surgeon to prevent cancer by early surgery, while groping for its cause. It is important to eliminate scars and other contributory factors, and the duty of the surgeon is to dwell more upon the prevention than the cure of the disease.

Pinch, the head of the London Radium Institute, is an advocate of radium and the x-rays, and says that "surgery still holds its place, but radium, a pocket x-ray as it may be called, and the x-rays are on trial but seem to warrant the belief of their being great additions in the treatment of cancer of the uterus. However, the extreme views expressed by German observers, and recently by some Americans, are unfortunate, for the facts do not justify their conclusions and only bring discredit upon the whole problem before us. Remember that radium and x-ray may cause harm as well as good. Let us give them a fair trial. Let us not forget, while testing these things, that surgery is our mainstay."

The question of tying off the larger blood vessels has been discussed. In 1908, and again in 1911, I published papers advocating the starvation ligature and lymphatic-block operation, and in 1913 read another paper on the same subject before this Society. Why have we been so slow in taking up this procedure? Why not ligate and block even though radium and the x-rays are to be used? To ligate both internal iliacs, both ovarians, and the sacralis media, controls the blood supply to the pelvic organs, checks the local nutrition, and stops the rapid spread of the disease. I have cases living today, many years after operation, who are apparently perfectly well. Of course, most of the cases died, but they had been given relief from pain and hemorrhage for a time.

At Guy's Hospital they are doing the starvation ligature and lymphatic-block operation in many cases. Recently, I have seen uterine cases treated by starvation ligature by Brown of Detroit, who has had some admirable results.

Referring to Dr. Bonifield's paper, in connection with age, it is well to remember that it is not the number of years we live, but the age of the tissues as a whole and not the passing of the years which is the important factor in disease.

DR. JAMES E. DAVIS, DETROIT, MICHIGAN.—The body resistance may be divided into two types, general and local. The local is involved in the general. All of the speakers have referred to both types of resistance. I wish to call attention to the picture that one sees in the histopathology of these tissues. There is an acquired fibrosis, a change in the blood vessels, and lymph vessels; also a small round cell infiltration. There is some question as to just how valuable the small round cell infiltration is as a measure of resistance, but to my mind it is one of the most positive and reliable evidences of resistance. All of these conditions obtain in cases that are not treated, if the body is able to acquire the ideal of resistance. You may produce all these conditions by the use of slow heat, or radium, or the x-ray, making a replica picture of natural tissue resistance. The same picture is also produced if you deprive the tissues of their blood supply.

I cannot see why there should be many points of difference in regard to the treatment. It is only the problem of application of the treatment to the tissues involved—getting the penetration to the exact area involved in the cancer.

I want to speak briefly in regard to one of Dr. Brown's cases. It was my privilege to study carefully the tissue from one of the cases he has reported. It was interesting to find the occlusion of the blood vessels in all of the tissues involved, and also the cellular change. In many cells there was distention of the cell envelop, in other cells extrusion of the protoplasm, while in some the protoplasm was completely demobilized. In places it was impossible to tell whether the cells were virile, without considering the difficult chemistry of the cell. It was interesting to note the depth of penetration and the change in the cell where the penetration was less deep than in other places. Hence the problem can be summed up in terms of resistance, and the application of the remedy to the most remote parts of the cancer growth.

DR. MILES F. PORTER, FORT WAYNE, INDIANA.—I do not know whether Dr. Bonifield's published paper will contain the statement I understood him to make regarding the possible danger of the publication of facts to the public concerning cancer or not. If it does I think it would be a great mistake for this Association to even seem to support the idea that the public should not know the things that we know regarding the early manifestations of cancer. We lose in the United States about 100,000 people every year from this disease. The increase of cancer has been great until the last year or two, when it has stopped, and it is the opinion of those who know that the reduction, together with the increase in the percentage of cures, that those two favorable changes are due to the fact that the public is coming to understand something more about cancer and presenting themselves to the doctor in time to be cured. I think it would be a great mistake for this Association to even seem to put any drag upon the movement which seeks to get these men and women to the doctor in time to be cured. If we can save 50 per cent of these people we can afford to haul out now and then a few fainting, neurotic patients—male or female.

DR. SKEEL (closing on his part).—It might be thought from some things that have entered the discussion that I had become a radiotherapist. This is not the case, however, as I remain a surgeon although I hope the day will not arrive when I shall be only an operator, and cannot use or advise the use of radium or the x-ray if they offer more hope for the patient than operation, just as I hope the day will not come that I can't listen to Dr. Crile's advocacy of physiological principles in surgery and follow such of them as appeal to my judgment. Also I trust the day will never come when I shall not think of the welfare of the patient as the primary consideration in determining what form of treatment shall be used.

I quite agree with Dr. Noble that radium is an unknown quantity, but such it will remain unless we study it sufficiently to determine its value. Instead of spending time in discussing this phase of the matter at length, however, I prefer to read these letters, since they are of greater value in elucidating the matter than anything I could say, the reading of which was prohibited by the time limitations set upon papers before the Association.

I do wish to insist, however, that we were discussing cancer of the cervix and nothing else.

All of us know the difficulties and dangers encountered in doing a radical extirpation for cancer of the cervix by any method, as well as the high mortality and recurrence rate; and for this reason one phase of the matter was emphasized, that which might be called its sociosurgical aspect, the ultimate effect upon society of unsuccessful operative procedures. For this reason, if for no other, we should in all cases, but the very earliest, abandon an operation which shows so low a final re-

recovery rate and continue our search in other directions until such time as a more satisfactory and successful operation is devised for those plainly diagnosable by clinical methods.

DR. BROWN (closing on his part).—Recently I had a letter from William Mayo in reply to a letter I wrote him regarding their experience with the Percy cautery heat. His reply was that results had been entirely satisfactory in their hands, but as it was more cumbersome than radium, they were employing the latter oftener now only because of its convenience.

I wish to give you some opinions from men like Stone, Clark, Schmitz, Graves and others, to tell the other side. William S. Stone of New York (Surg., Gynec. and Obstet., June, 1921) from observations in over four hundred cases says: "On account of lymph node involvement in certain cases of cancer of the cervix, radium cannot entirely supplant operation in all such early lesions. A strong plea is made to avoid treatment of primary cases that are too far advanced." He further states that the chief error in the use of radium seems to be an overdosage, with the subsequent disastrous results to the neighboring tissues.

Bailey, in a recent article, deals with 336 cases. He says that practically all cases that have a complete radiation of the local lesion and the lymphatics and other involved tissues, pass through a period of improvement, disappearance of ulceration, lessening or disappearance of discharge, gain in weight, and improvement of health are secured in all but the advanced conditions. After a longer or shorter time of well being, many of the cases have further development of cancerous tissue behind the vault of the vagina.

Burrows (Annual Reports of the Manchester Radium Institute) states that among 363 cases of carcinoma of the cervix of the uterus that were treated by radium, most of them were inoperable, 10 per cent showed a complete disappearance of symptoms and signs, but at least one-half of them recurred in twelve months.

Clark and Keene (Jour. A.M.A., August 20, 1921), in a list of 313 cases treated with radium, state that in eleven cases, which were advanced when treatment was given, the patients are dead. Also that irradiation is dangerous immediately before or soon after operation, or when employed in fresh operative fields.

Schmitz, reporting 163 consecutive cases (Jour. A.M.A., August 20, 1921) says: "Radiation treatment always causes a decided radiation sickness. During this period the patient could not be safely subjected to the additional trauma of a capital surgical procedure. The operation must be postponed for from three to six weeks, during which time the patient will have recovered from the radiation toxemia. If the operation is performed within a few days after radiation the patient succumbs to sepsis and shock with an alarming frequency. Should the operation be postponed to a later period the same danger is still present on account of necrosis of tissue in the cervical canal, which cannot be avoided. These factors and the intense connective tissue formation in the parametrium, which renders hemostasis difficult, therefore do not let it appear advisable to resort to preoperative radiation."

W. P. Graves (Surg., Gynec. and Obst., June, 1921) speaking from his own experience, states: "It may be said that we have not—so far as we know—cured with radium a single case of inoperable cancer of the cervix." And further, in view of his unfavorable experience with radium, and his favorable operative results, of which he gives statistics, he does not feel justified in substituting radium for radical surgery in cases favorable for operation.

John G. Clark (Annals of Surgery, June, 1920) after five years' experience with radium, states that he considers it an adjunct to surgery and that in the certainly operable cases they still advocate a radical operation followed by postoperative radiation. As yet they claim no cures from radium.

Since a permanent cure for uterine cancer by radium has not yet been proved, it seems to me that Dr. Skeel must find himself in the same position that Victor Hugo once found himself when he said, "I stand for a thing which does not exist!" If, however, radium has no other use, as one of our number declared to me this morning, it is an excellent refuge for a coward.

DR. CRILE (closing).—I have nothing to say in behalf of my paper, but I wish to express my great appreciation of the brilliant presentations of my two good friends, Dr. Skeel and Dr. Brown. I am sure before this question is finally settled you will hear many other papers on the same subject.

DR. GEORGE GELLHORN, St. Louis, Mo., read a paper entitled **The New Trend in Gynecological Therapy.** (For original article see page 275.)

DISCUSSION

DR. JOHN O. POLAK, BROOKLYN, NEW YORK.—Personally, I am of the belief that the subjects of obstetrics and gynecology should be combined. My reasons for that are, first, a large amount of our gynecology is the result of our obstetrics. Were it not for the lacerations of the cervix and the incidence of infection, we would not have cervicitis and parametritis. Were it not for the trauma to the anterior vaginal wall by prolonged labor, or administered in the course of delivery, prolapses and displacements would not occur.

Dr. Gellhorn has called attention to the value of radium in myomata of the uterus. I cannot let that pass without a word of warning, namely the danger from using radium in myomata where there is parametrial inflammation, as radium apparently, notwithstanding the observations recently made in Holland, particularly where there is streptococcic infection or the results of streptococcic infection, has the property of lighting up that infection.

His remarks concerning gonorrhea I do not think can be too enthusiastically endorsed. Personally, I feel that all the operations we have done have lost to these women the privilege of ovulation and menstruation. We feel that ovulation without menstruation is very unsatisfactory, that ovulation without menstruation is not cured by all the surgical means we have at hand. Consequently, I have adopted much the same method the doctor has suggested, particularly in gonorrhea, namely to let these women alone and insist on rest at the menstruation period. I shall put into effect his other suggestion as soon as I can try it out. I do know that many patients with definite gonorrheal salpingitis have, eventually, become pregnant and borne children, while the women I have operated never have.

DR. STEPHEN E. TRACY, PHILADELPHIA, PENN.—It is evident that the treatment of carcinoma of the cervix uteri is still under consideration. It is undoubtedly true that in a certain type of simple, uncomplicated fibromyomas radiotherapy will give satisfactory results, but we must not overlook the fact that 30 per cent of these patients, as they come to the surgeon, have either a degeneration in the tumor or a malignancy of the pelvic organs; an additional 40 per cent have closely associated abdominopelvic lesions. This leaves only 30 per cent of simple, uncomplicated cases. It is generally agreed that, in patients under the age of forty years, the treatment should be conservative surgery—myomectomy. In patients past the age of forty years, only 16 to 18 per cent have simple, uncomplicated tumors. By surgery we not only get rid of the tumor, but at the same time remove the associated pathological lesions, and cure the patient of all symptoms in from 96 to 98 per cent of the cases. Pfahler claims 75 per cent of cures by x-ray treatment. He treats only cases referred to him by gynecologists or surgeons, and, therefore, has simple, uncomplicated cases and I know his results are excellent. As only 18 per cent of cases are uncomplicated, he would cure only 13.5 per cent of the patients as the surgeon sees them. Kelly claims 45 per cent of cures by radium, which is even less favorable than Pfahler's results. The question of what cases should be treated by radiotherapy depends on the diagnosis, and no one can determine with any degree of certainty whether he is dealing with a simple or complicated case.

The radiotherapists say but little about complications. Kelly acknowledges that 8 per cent of his cases subsequently require surgical treatment. Ward reported a case treated by radium in which a loop of bowel adherent to the uterus became necrotic, resulting in a peritonitis and death. The difficulty in diagnosis explains the complications of the radiotherapists. I trust Dr. Gellhorn will tell us, in closing, of his complications.

I endorse what Dr. Polak said about conservative treatment of inflammatory disease of the appendages. Some of these cases will recover and later on bear children; while those subjected to operation seldom do.

DR. HUGO O. PANTZER, INDIANAPOLIS, INDIANA.—Dr. Gellhorn in his clear, eloquent, and rather convincing paper has mentioned that radium is still on probation. I wish to cite a case, recently deceased, of inoperable cancer which had been treated with radium. The patient, cured of the cancer, died within one year with occlusion of both ureters as a result of the fibrosis brought on by the radium. Control, i.e., safe limitation of the radium effect, must be yet achieved.

Regarding the use of radium or x-ray in fibroid tumors of the uterus, we should individualize carefully before applying the remedy which entails sterility. I will cite a given case. Miss H., forty-three years old, came to me suffering from protracted and excessive menstrual flow due to multiple fibroids of the uterus, owing to which the organ extended to the umbilicus, and an associated toxemia, due to chronic suppurative tonsillitis and intestinal (ileocecal torsion) stasis. A swarthy skin and spare body, she looked pitiably ''minus.'' To associate with her the hope of future marriage and motherhood was audacious, indeed! But here was a phase of her history, which induced me to make effort to effect a *restitutio ad integrum*. She was the oldest of seven children, when her father, a wage-earner, had died and had left his family practically destitute. With fine spirit she jumped into the arena; during the day she worked away from home and at night assisted her mother in the manifold duties of caring for her six brothers and sisters. This she had kept up through the long years, uncomplainingly, zealously, and happily, but at the cost of her own health and prospects of life. After due attention was given to her general and throat condition, I surgically removed eight fibroid tumors from her uterus, taking pains to carefully resuture; and, also, cut extensive ileocecal membranes, which were distorting and unfitting for function these anatomical parts. It will suffice to say here, she made a fine recovery, put on the color and spirit of youth again; and, in turn, attracted a fine discriminating man who made her his wife. The culmination of it all: they have a fine boy, two years old now, born unaided *per via naturalis*, and the three constitute a volume of happiness, which, were it to fall out would make this world of ours perceptibly less happy.

DR. GORDON K. DICKINSON, JERSEY CITY, N. J.—I am sure the time is coming when surgeons will rely, more and more, on rest and depend more on physiological means. One of the most distressing things is the operating that is being done, not by true surgeons, but by operators, not men who are going around from school to school to see what they can see and how poor their work may be. For us to stand up for physiological methods and for time in the treatment of cases speaks well.

DR. FRED J. TAUSSIG, St. Louis, Missouri, (by invitation).—I think that one of the good features that will come as the result of the nonoperative trend in gynecology is that women will not hesitate so long before they come to the gynecologist. In the past, how often have we all heard, "Yes, Doctor, I did not come right away because I thought it would be a matter of operation if I was referred to a specialist, and so I put off coming." This fear that nothing but operation will be suggested has deterred many people from coming. Particularly in the case of fibroids I believe we have in radium a treatment for the early stages which will lead to the prevention of these enormous tumors which have come to us in the past.

I do not think we can stress too much the importance of research study in our specialty. The moment you separate obstetrics from its sister branch gynecology you are going to cripple the amount of research study to a very great degree.

As to the indications for treatment, Dr. Gellhorn and I are almost in accord, particularly with regard to the use of radium. My personal feeling is still, however, that in early cervical cancer we should employ operative measures, in association with radium to be sure, but primarily an operative procedure. With the research and educational work that is going on each year, we are getting more and more of the early cases. I believe surgery still has an important place in cervical cancer.

DR. G. VAN AMBER BROWN, Detroit, Michigan.—The essayist has called attention to the desirability of getting temporarily rid of the menstrual flow in certain pathological conditions. On the other hand, it is often our aim and desire to preserve the menstrual function. I would like to call your attention to a case which brings out the advantage of using ligation and heat rather than radium. The case is one of a young woman, aged twenty eight, a nullipara with advanced carcinoma of the cervix. She was not willing to have her uterus removed, and refused to have anything done that would interfere with her menstrual flow; so we promised not to interfere with that. Had we resorted to radium we know we would have checked the menstrual flow for some months and, possibly, permanently. By doing the ligation and using the heat she made a mighty good immediate recovery with, apparently, a cure. The operation was performed a year ago last August, she has remained perfectly well, has gained twenty pounds in weight, and has not missed a single menstrual period, three days out of every twenty-eight, which is natural to her.

DR. CHARLES E. RUTH, Des Moines, Iowa.—I had become so thoroughly satisfied with my results in hysterectomy, that I had no hesitancy in recommending any case of fibroid of sufficient size and producing symptoms, to operation. In one case, six years ago, in which a fibroid of large size was becoming a serious matter, I recommended operation which was promptly and emphatically declined. I then turned the patient over, with what advice I felt competent to give, to our roentgenologist who gave her two treatments of heavy cross-fire x-rays, with the result that a careful examination after four years showed the patient practically well with only the slightest vestige of fibroid still recognizable.

The next case of striking possibilities along the same line, came a few months later. This was a patient with a fibroid and the symptom of bleeding had existed for a sufficient length of time and was of sufficient severity to have practically exsanguinated the patient. Her hemoglobin was only 18 per cent. I did not feel justified in attempting a hysterectomy. She was twice transfused in the interim between menstrual periods, and then received x-ray treatment in the same manner as the other case in the hope that we could get a stay of execution sufficient to permit of a hysterectomy with greater safety. This patient also received two treatments and now, after two years, she has had no hysterectomy and is well.

DR. ROLAND E. SKEEL, LOS ANGELES, CAL.—I desire to offer a word of appreciation. On my way here I stopped at Salt Lake City to read a paper on the limitations imposed upon gynecologic surgery by our present day knowledge of radium therapy. In this I called attention to the fact, that so far as we know definitely at present, there are three gynecological disorders in which we should stay our hands in operating; first, carcinoma of the cervix; second, small fibromata without complications but causing hemorrhage, and third, that condition variously known as hemorrhagic endometritis, fibrosis uteri, and subinvolution, all of course with bleeding as the predominant symptom. I shall be glad to be convinced that there is some way of handling gonorrheal salpingitis, other than by surgery, if that method does not stop ovulation.

By surgical methods one waits until the infection has ceased, then amputates the tubes, and does not remove the ovaries. The recurrent infections, which occur because ovulation and menstruation continue, are, in my opinion, due to persistent cervical infection and, if a high cervix amputation is performed at the same time, I believe we can allow menstruation and ovulation to continue without difficulty. I am afraid of radium in the presence of infection, but I sincerely hope Dr Gellhorn is right, for the further away from surgery we get in cases that can be treated otherwise, the further we remove ourselves from the men who operate indiscriminately.

DR. MILES F. PORTER, FORT WAYNE, INDIANA.—My impression is that real surgeons stopped years ago operating for gonorrheal or any other kind of salpingitis. Real surgeons have not been operating for gonorrheal salpingitis for years and it is wrong to condemn surgery for operations that real surgeons have not, in my estimation, been doing. To operate for gonorrheal salpingitis and to operate for the results of it are two different things entirely, and, if we want to get at the correct solution of this question, we have to stop and figure out exactly where "we are at" and what we mean.

I do not think it is correct to say that one out of every four cases, operated for cancer of the cervix, dies. That is not correct. We will never get anywhere, and stay there, unless we start from a correct premise. One out of every four cases operated for carcinoma of the uterus does not die in the hands of men whose work we look up to. On the other hand, there are multiplied thousands of women throughout the United States, who are bearing children today, who have been operated by good men for the results of gonorrheal salpingitis; and there are other thousands who have been operated for fibroids and are now bearing children.

DR. GELLHORN (closing the discussion).—Dr. Tracy will find the desired information in two previous publications which are referred to in my manuscript. In answer to Dr. Porter's question. I have quoted from H. C. Taylor, of New York. This author has computed a mortality of 25 per cent after the radical operation, and this method is the only one under discussion.

May I interpret your silence as your assent to my first point that gynecology and obstetrics should never and nowhere have been divorced, and that, after the mismating of gynecology and surgery has been annulled, the divorced parties should be remarried?

My second point was the growth of nonoperative tendencies in gynecology. After a man has worked a lifetime along surgical lines, it seems hard to have to abandon the altar one has helped to erect and to worship new gods. But it is always thus that the better has to give way to the best, and time will show whether or not the claims of the nonoperative methods are of enduring value.

DR. FRED J. TAUSSIG, St. Louis, Mo., read a paper entitled **The Hypertrophic-Ulcerative Form of Chronic Vulvitis**. (For original article see page 281.)

DISCUSSION

DR. JAMES E. DAVIS, DETROIT, MICHIGAN.—I have had one case which belonged to the diffuse hypertrophic type and the labia and clitoris were involved. The patient was a colored woman and there was a very large number of clearly defined tubercles and giant cells throughout the entire growth.

DR. GORDON K. DICKINSON, JERSEY CITY, N. J.—I would like to ask what relation this lesion has to esthiomene.

DR. TAUSSIG, (closing).—Esthiomene is only another name for this lesion. I believe that the sooner we get a simple name for things the better it will be. This particular type of chronic vulvitis with hypertrophy should be grouped as a part of the chronic affections of the vulva. Of course, in hospital records I suppose it is difficult to avoid the use of special terms.

DR. JAMES E. KING, of Buffalo, N. Y., read a paper on **Strictures and Atresias of the Vagina**. (For original article see page 290.)

DISCUSSION

DR. CHARLES W. MOOTS, TOLEDO, OHIO.—I desire to present the two following cases of congenital atresia of the vagina.

CASE 1: Patient, age twenty-three, rather short and stout with a very short neck. Family history negative except that the patient and a younger sister were both psychoneurotic. She was referred to me by an internist, not because she was sick but because she had been sent to him owing to the fact that she had never menstruated. I found no evidence of endocrine disbalance, the usual growth of hair was present in the axillae and in the pubic region, the vulva and clitoris were perfectly normal. There was present a thin, red streak about two inches long where the introitus should have been. On careful rectal examination I found absence of the uterus, ovary, and tube on the left side; but a small mass, probably an ovary, on the right side. She had never had any violent love affairs, she had no desire to marry, she was happy in her work, and apparently had no sexual feeling. I advised no treatment whatever in this case, except that she return to the village where she was teaching and try to absorb herself in her work.

CASE 2: Patient thirty years of age, married and the mother of two children. She was not brought on account of illness, but because her family physician had found a peculiar condition of the vagina, which was double, the tracts being of about equal size, the septum in about the midline, and deflected to the right side of the cervix, ending in a blind pouch. The doctor said this septum stretched easily on delivery, there was no difficulty whatsoever, and he simply wished to know what to do about it. In this case I also advised no treatment.

DR. FRED J. TAUSSIG, ST. LOUIS, MISSOURI.—I think it is well that Dr. King has emphasized the significance of gonorrhea in children and its seriousness. Having had occasion to be in charge of a clinic for the study of such cases, and having followed them for a long period of time, I am in doubt as to the responsibility of this form of vaginitis as a cause of atresia. Nagel and Veit claimed that atresia of the vagina was due to an acquired vulvovaginitis in children. That statement has been passed down from year to year and has been accepted by many but I defy anybody to show me proof that vulvovaginitis produces atresia of the vagina. If so, why do we not find strictures of the vagina more frequently? Gonorrhea in children is very common, but Dr. King was able to find only one case of stricture. Why do we not find any intermediate steps in the production of the atresia? If it produces a complete obliteration we should find stricture frequently. We do find it occasionally, I grant you that, but we should find many cases. The development of the hymen shows that there is a tendency for the obliteration of that portion of the tract, and I believe we must accept the theory that these so-called atresias are congenital and are only noticed later in life, because only upon the onset of menstruation do they give symptoms.

DR. IRVING W. POTTER, BUFFALO. N. Y.—I have no cases of atresia to report, probably because most women are pregnant when they come to me. I had the pleasure of delivering both of the patients the doctor mentions. The first by cesarean section, because she had lost her first baby. The second case I delivered without the knowledge of Doctor King. She was seen by him at the seventh month and he thought she could be delivered. I thought she could not be, so I sectioned her with equally good results.

DR. CHARLES E. RUTH, DES MOINES, IOWA.—I wish to speak of two cases, one congenital. Both of these patients were school teachers. One was pregnant and sought to terminate this by the introduction of several 7½ grain tablets of bichloride of mercury into the vagina, with the result that she had mercury poisoning that came near terminating her life. She lost the fetus and she also lost the entire vagina, because it was obliterated absolutely from cervix to vulva, with the exception of a drainage tract too small to permit the passage of even a small probe. After she had suppression of the menstrual flow, her physician persisted until he got a probe in, making an opening which permitted a menstrual flow. This had so contracted when I saw her that it could not be followed by a probe. She insisted on the construction of a vagina but the attempt to reconstruct a vagina from the labia has not, to the present time, been entirely successful.

The other patient consulted me because she did not menstruate. She was normal in development and sexual feeling, masturbated and found great difficulty in controlling that tendency. I could find no sign of a vagina, uterus, and ovaries except that, on the right side, there seemed to be a little thickening or cordlike structure extending from what should have been the top of the vagina. So I presume she had a vestige of an ovary on that side which accounted for her sexual tendencies.

DR. HUGO O. PANTZER, INDIANAPOLIS, INDIANA.—Forty years ago, as a dispensary interne, I had such a case. When first seen by me the patient had been in labor for forty-eight hours with a breech presentation, making little headway against an almost obliterated vagina, owing to scarring by nitrate of silver, which had been used on venereal warts. The dead fetus was finally delivered by embryotomy.

DR. KING, (closing).—As Dr. Taussig has said, it is very difficult to determine with absolute certainty the cause of such atresias as I have described. In every case, unless there is a clear history and record of examination during the presence of discharge, there will always be a question as to the bacterial factor where atresia is discovered later in life. Where atresias are due to streptococcus or diphtheritic infection in childhood there would be a clear history indicating the severe constitutional reaction associated with such infections.

As to the frequency of these atresias we might also ask why strictures of the male urethra do not occur more commonly. It is doubtless true that the vaginal mucous membrane of the child is more resistant to the ulcerative process than the urethra. This subject has been presented with the purpose of bringing to your attention this sequela of vaginal discharge in children to the end that it may prompt a more careful study of such cases.

NEW YORK ACADEMY OF MEDICINE. SECTION ON OBSTETRICS AND GYNECOLOGY. STATED MEETING, OCTOBER 25, 1921

DR. HAROLD BAILEY IN THE CHAIR

DR. STAFFORD McLEAN reported a case of **Sarcoma of Uterus in Infant.**

He stated that carcinoma of the uterus was extremely rare in infancy and childhood and only twelve cases were reported in the literature. Primary sarcoma of the vagina, however, was not so unusual. The case he reported came under observation in April, 1920, and was followed for sixty-nine days. The baby exhibited pallor and a bloody discharge had been noticed on the diaper for the past two months. The birth weight of the infant was eight pounds; she was born at full term; delivery normal. The baby was fed on milk powder and sugar. The stools had occasionally contained mucus, and blood was noticed two months before. The child had four or five stools daily. The appearance of the infant was that of a well nourished, well developed child. The head was normal, there being no cranial tabes. The heart, lungs and abdomen were absolutely normal. There was no enlargement of the lymph nodes. There was bleeding from the vulva. The blood count showed 2,800,000 red cells and 14,800 white cells. A specimen of the uterine growth was submitted to Dr. Wollstein who reported that it was a sarcoma. There was much infiltration into the surrounding tissues. Radium treatment was given, 100 millicuries for three hours. There was no oozing after the first treatment. Three radium treatments were given, the third being a month after the first. Six weeks from the day of admission the mass was well down in the abdomen and the size of an adult uterus. The child suffered from anorexia, showed extreme pallor, became rapidly weaker and finally died. The autopsy findings confirmed the original diagnosis.

DISCUSSION

DR. HAROLD BAILEY.—One frequently hears of sarcoma of the kidney in young children, but it is extremely rare to hear of sarcoma of the uterus. A feature of particular interest brought out by Dr. McLean was that one child with sarcoma of the uterus had been cured by operation.

The case reported was seen by Dr. Studdiford, Dr. Downes and myself, and we all felt that it was an inoperable condition. Only one finger could with difficulty be inserted into the vagina. By rectal palpation a considerable mass could be felt which extended beyond the outline of the vagina and uterus. Autopsy showed an abscess cavity opening into the vagina and filled with sarcomatous tissue. Treatment with radium was hopeless though we have had some remarkable results in large polyhedral cell growths and in large round cell tumors. As a matter of fact we had one woman with a surcoma, proved by operation, where the tumor extended into the broad ligament who was treated only by raying with massive doses on the surface and through the vagina. Six months later she was again operated upon in another clinic. The pelvis was found normal. When she learned this she wanted to bring suit against the original surgeon on the ground that he had performed an unnecessary operation. In radiating this case we used a small silver applicator but could only get a short distance into the vagina, and with the finger in the rectum we determined the location of the capsule. There seemed to be some immediate results. In view of the fact that we were unable to determine what was the proper skin dose, we used ¼ the adult dosage of radium from the outside of the abdomen. However, we apparently hit the correct dosage because there was an erythema. At autopsy a small opening into the culdesac was found, and it is possible that the silver wire punctured the wall of the vagina.

Dr. McLean's case is exceedingly interesting inasmuch as it is one of only about a dozen similar cases recorded in the literature. The autopsy findings suggest that possibly the case might have been treated more successfully from the surgical standpoint as the growth was found to be localized entirely around the vagina and cervix.

Dr. HARBECK HALSTEAD read a paper entitled, **Pyelitis During Pregnancy.**

This study was based on 24 cases of pyelitis during or immediately following pregnancy, occurring at the Sloane Hospital for Women, from July 1, 1919, to July 1, 1921. The incidence of pyelitis in this period at Sloane Hospital was about 0.7 per cent. The inciting organism was in nearly all cases the bacillus coli communis, mostly alone, but occasionally associated with the streptococcus or staphylococcus. In one case an unidentified organism closely allied to the bacillus coli occurred in pure culture. The most important contributory cause of infection seemed to be an interference with the free outflow of urine from the ureter. Further contributory causes were constipation, bad teeth, infected tonsils, or other focal infections.

There were two types of onset common in this series. First, a slow onset with gradually increasing symptoms. The second, an acute onset with a chill, fever, rapid pulse, and severe pain in one or both costovertebral angles. The slow onset was more common. The more marked general symptoms were: malaise; chills; fever; sweating; increased pulse rate; vomiting; headache; rapid loss of weight. The local symptoms included pain in one or both kidney regions; frequent and painful urination; occasionally, a dull ache in the bladder region; cloudy urine with a foul odor or hematuria. In some patients, there were periods with chills, fever, and other marked symptoms, followed by periods when the patient was entirely or nearly free from symptoms.

The following is the procedure now followed at Sloane Hospital in treating these cases: During the acute symptoms, absolute rest in bed. Raising the head of the bed, and in pregnant patients, if strong enough, the knee-chest posture twice a day for a few minutes. Force fluids. Rapid alkalinization of the urine with large doses of alkalies, usually using sodium bicarbonate, a dram every two hours, with one-half dram of sodium or potassium citrate. As soon as the urine becomes markedly alkaline, the amount of the alkalies is decreased by lengthening the time between doses. This treatment often relieves the symptoms, brings down the temperature and clears the urine of pus; but in none of these cases has it rendered the urine sterile.

After the urine has been alkaline from one to two weeks, depending on the symptoms, all the alkalies are stopped, even in the colon irrigations, and hexamethylenamin and sodium benzoate are given, ten grains of each every three or four hours. This is kept up for two weeks, if the patient is improving, and if she shows no signs of bladder or kidney irritation from the hexamethylenamin. Periods of alkalies and of hexamethylenamin and sodium benzoate are kept up alternately until the patient is well and the urine sterile.

If the patient is not much improved, very soon after the urine becomes alkaline, a cystoscopy should be done and the kidney pelves washed with an antiseptic, 20 per cent or thirty per cent solargentum or argyrol is usually used. This treatment is repeated from one to three times a week and is kept up until three negative cultures are obtained. As there is nearly always an associated cystitis, the bladder is washed several times before each cystoscopy with boric acid solution, and after the cystoscopy argyrol or solargentum is instilled, to remain in for ten minutes and then to be passed by the patient.

The above treatment has proved satisfactory in the early months of pregnancy and postpartum, but in the later months it has been unsatisfactory, as have all other methods, with the exception of the induction of labor.

If, despite all treatment, the patient grows progressively worse, especially if her pulse rate progressively increases, induction of labor or abortion should be considered. The treatment of these cases should not be stopped as soon as the temperature and pulse are normal and the patient symptomless. It should be kept up until the urine cultures are sterile.

DISCUSSION

DR. HENRY DAWSON FURNISS.—I do not believe that pyelitis is limited to pregnancy or that the pyelitis of pregnancy has peculiarities differentiating it from pyelitis at other times. I think the percentage of 0.7 which Dr. Halsted reports is far less than we have had on the gynecological service at the Post-Graduate Hospital. There is never a year when there are not quite a number of cases that develop pyelitis after operation. When after operation there is a rise in temperature with no exudate, no wound infection and no respiratory trouble, one should be on the lookout for renal involvement. At times the symptoms may be very slight. There may be just slight pain or discomfort in the back and you will find the patient with her hand under her back. This pain may be elicited by tapping the patient on the back or by deep palpation. This pain usually lasts only two or three days. Dr. Halsted spoke of the way in which the kidney became involved. I believe the majority of infections are through the blood stream, but a few show all the evidence of having ascended along the course of the ureter. There will be a slight temperature and pain which gradually goes up along the course of the ureter. It is a question whether the infection ascends along the ureter by the way of the lymphatics or is a surface infection of the mucosa. I believe, however, that as a rule infection is by way of the blood stream; the infection is first in the parenchyma and localizes later in the kidney pelvis. If lavage of the pelvis is instituted during the first few days the results are not very satisfactory because the infection is still localized in the kidney substance. I do not believe the infection is cleared up so much by the antiseptic property of the drugs as by the active hyperemia that is set up.

Dr. Halsted speaks of hematuria and of ecchymotic areas limited to the trigone. It has been my experience that the trigone is no more involved than the rest of the bladder, but if one does a cystoscopy during pregnancy, the bladder walls are so collapsed by the pressure of the enlarged uterus that one does not see the entire bladder wall so easily as in the nonpregnant state. One will find ecchymotic areas all over the bladder wall, which makes one think the infection an embolic process. In one case of pyelitis in which there was hematuria for one or two days I found on cystoscopy that there were as many as fifty ecchymotic areas scattered over the bladder. I believe most of these infections come through the intestinal tract. Kidd claims that bacteria are often carried in the blood stream of every individual, and it is only when there is lowered resistance as from exposure to cold, wet, or from excessive fatigue, that the organism is unequal to combating the infection.

In the pregnant woman there is greater hydronephrosis than in the nonpregnant, though even in the nonpregnant one finds a moderate dilatation of the pelvis and ureter. In treating a pyelitis the pelvis of the kidneys should be well emptied before introducing the medicament, as such drainage allows the pelves and ureter an opportunity to contract and regain tone. In pyelitis there is a marked swelling of the mucosa and the good effects of drugs are undoubtedly due to their shrinking the mucosa.

Dr. Halsted spoke of nephrectomy. I do not think we are so radical in regard to nephrectomy as formerly. Often in pyelitis both kidneys are more or less involved, and we feel that conservatism is safer than taking out one kidney and leaving a slightly damaged kidney. It is not a question of the patient standing the operation of nephrectomy, but of getting well with a remaining kidney as badly diseased as the one removed. There are undoubtedly instances of the fulminating type in which nephrectomy is life saving.

DR. A. J. RONGY.—I disagree with Dr. Halsted in several particulars. To my mind the etiology of the pyelitis of pregnancy in a very large number of patients can be traced to a latent pyelitis which either complicated or followed the infectious and contagious diseases of infancy and childbirth. Particularly is this true of patients who have had scarlet fever in a severe form. These patients do well when their system is not unduly strained, but when pregnancy occurs every secreting organ in the body is overtaxed so the latent pyelitis which existed for a great number of years very often assumes an acute aspect and all the symptoms that are associated with it.

Pregnancy very often leads to a mechanical impediment in the flow of the urine through the ureters and in that way will cause disturbance in the pelvis of the kidney. I do not see how washing out of the pelvis of the kidney two or three times a week can benefit the patient, for the involvement of the tissues is very much beyond where the irrigating fluid can reach it. Catheterization of the ureters should be used for diagnostic purposes only. Patients who suffer from pyelitis complicating pregnancy should be kept in a sitting posture as much as possible, for in that way the weight of the pregnant uterus is prevented from pressing upon the ureters at a point where they enter the pelvis.

Operative interference is very seldom indicated in this class of patients. If, however, the patient does not seem to improve, as indicated by constant rise of pulse and temperature, labor should be induced.

DR. WILLIAM H. WELLINGTON KNIPE.—I think the incidence of pyelitis reported at the Sloane Hospital is too low for the reason that they have not reported pyelitis unless a cystoscopic examination had been made. At the Gouverneur Hospital pyelitis is so common that we do not think anything of it. At the Gouverneur Hospital I feel confident that the incidence of pyelitis is five times 0.7 per cent. Our treatment differs a little from that at Sloane. We believe in posture and we give urotropin, not in 10 grain doses, which we think inadequate, but in 60 grain doses daily and enough acid sodium phosphate to make the urine completely acid. With this treatment we have had no occasion to employ lavage of the kidney. We have had cases in which we have used ordinary stock vaccines, and the patients have responded to the treatment. I think we should be conservative in the treatment of these cases. The temperature may keep up for a week or ten days but I have never seen a case that required operative interference.

DR. HERMAN LORBER.—Dr. Halsted said the differential diagnosis of pyelitis was quite easy. I know of a patient seven months' pregnant, who had pain and rigidity in the lower right quadrant and ran a temperature of 103°. The doctor who attended her assured me the urine showed no pus cells. She was taken to the hospital and the blood count showed a high differential count. An operation for appendicitis was performed and perfectly normal appendix removed. A catheterized specimen of urine later showed pus cells. The woman was delivered two months later and made an uneventful recovery. I think it well to call attention to the fact that pyelitis may cause symptoms very similar to those of appendicitis.

DR. HARVEY B. MATTHEWS.—I have had two cases similar to the one just reported in which the symptoms were those of appendicitis, though fortunately the patients were not operated upon. The diagnosis of appendicitis in one case was made by two surgeons and two general practitioners and in the other by two surgeons only. In a third case the diagnosis of pyelitis in a woman six months' pregnant was made just as she was being prepared to be taken to the hospital for an operation for appendicitis. In one of the first two cases mentioned operation was advised, but was delayed. In a short time both patients recovered.

DR. WILLIAM HEALY.—I have been especially interested in listening to the discussion on the treatment of pyelitis because some years ago I heard Dr. Furniss say that practically all cases of pyelitis should be treated by lavage of the kidney pelvis. My experience up to that time had been so uniformly favorable by simple medical treatment without cystoscopy or lavage that I was very firmly opposed to his point of view. But in the last two years I have had three cases that did not respond to the most approved methods of medical treatment in the effort to relieve the pyelitis and relief was only obtained by catheterization and lavage of the kidney pelvis. Then they were so promptly relieved that I am quite convinced that some cases have to have that done in order to be cured.

DR. BAILEY.—I wish to bring out a point merely for reiteration. Of course we have all for years adopted the conservative method of treating pyelitis. As Dr. Healy has said there are very few of these cases in which the kidney pelvis has to be emptied by catheterization. The whole question is what happens to the woman later on; does she develop pyelonephritis or is she cured? Merely because she has no fever does not mean that the pyogenic bacteria have been entirely eliminated. Many may continue to have pyogenic bacteria who feel comfortable and well.

Another important point is the administration of drugs. I question the advisability of giving these drugs for three or four weeks,—hexamethylenamine for two weeks and alkalies for two weeks. I do not see how the stomach can tolerate this treatment for such a length of time, especially when acid sodium phosphate is combined with urotropin.

DR. W. E. CALDWELL.—The small number of really serious cases of pyelitis which have occurred in this series is surprising. It was my impression that a much larger proportion of women during pregnancy would show infection of the pelvis of the kidney. Seven-tenths of one per cent does not seem much higher than the percentage of cases occurring among women not pregnant.

Considering how frequently pyelitis is found among children, I expected that Dr. Halsted would find a past history of pyelitis in a large number of cases,—probably a history of chronic nose and throat infection or acute contagious diseases. However, the majority of patients were clinic cases and it is possible that the histories are inaccurate on this point, but it seems that very few were found who gave a history of previous pyelitis attacks.

I have been impressed in private practice with the frequency of pyelitis in women with faulty development,—the enteroptosis type, who frequently have distorted fascias causing anteflexion of the uterus and distortion of the ureters and who frequently gave a history of dysmenorrhea before pregancy and marked vomiting in the first three months of pregnancy. It does not seem possible that the weight of the uterus alone will cause an obstruction in the ureter.

I have been desirous for statistics on pyelitis cases from clinics where frequent routine rectal examinations are made throughout labor. If the infection of the kidney pelvis occurs through the lymphatics from the rectum, we would expect a larger incident of pyelitis among cases where unskilled rectal examinations are made.

Unfortunately, Dr. Halsted has not had the cooperation of a good dentist and consequently focal infections in the mouth have not always been checked up with cultures to see whether the same bacteria are found as in the urine culture. Apparently the colon bacillus is frequently found in infections of the mouth.

In the treatment of these cases Dr. Halsted has not become overenthusiastic about any one form of treatment. He has used all the recognized forms of treatment and has individualized his cases. Apparently the infection can be cleared up more quickly with local applications and the establishment of drainage than by purely medical means. It is seldom that a premature labor or abortion becomes necessary in these cases. His "follow-up" on the pyelitis cases is the most valuable part of his work, in my opinion, as it shows how long these infections persist and the necessity of active treatment for a long period of time.

Dr. Harvey B. Matthews read a paper entitled **Pregnancy after Nephrectomy.**

As is well known, after nephrectomy, for any cause, there is a compensatory hypertrophy of the remaining kidney so that the urinary function is not decreased for any length of time after operation, and frequently this hypertrophy has taken place before the diseased kidney has been removed. Physiologists tell us that the total amount of renal tissue possessed by normal individuals is three to four times what is actually needed to meet the ordinary demands of the organism. While chemical and microscopical examination following nephrectomy usually reveals complete return of renal function in some instances, this is not always the case. In a goodly number of nephrectomized individuals albumin is present in the urine many years after nephrectomy. In about 25 per cent of cases of nephrectomy for unilateral renal tuberculosis there is an abnormal condition of the remaining kidney, as is shown by albumin in the urine, irritable bladder, etc. For years there has been the feeling that pregnancy is greatly to be feared in a woman who has had a nephrectomy. In view of these facts the writer has made a study of 200 cases from the literature in which pregnancy occurred following nephrectomy; 37 cases collected in Greater New York, and four cases coming under his personal observation. Before analyzing this series of cases it may be noted that there are two classes of cases in which nephrectomy is performed. In one it is done for pyonephrosis, pyelonephrosis, benign tumor or cyst; in the other for unilateral renal tuberculosis or malignant disease. In the former group the remaining kidney is much more likely to be competent and remain so than in the latter.

In the 200 nephrectomized patients collected from the literature there were 215 pregnancies, in 10 of which there were complications, and two died. In the 37 cases in Greater New York there were 43 pregnancies; five of these pregnancies were complicated by severe toxemia. In the writer's four cases nephrectomy was performed three times for unilateral tuberculosis and one for pyonephrosis; all of these patients had albumin in the urine ranging from 1 to 4 plus. These four nephrectomized women had seven pregnancies and seven living children, with no serious complications. Blood chemistry observations in three of these women, as compared with three nonpregnant women with only one kidney showed the urine to be normal. Taking these cases all together there was a total of 265 pregnancies with 250 normal labors and two deaths; and 15 labors in which there were complications. From a study of these cases it would seem that pregnancy in the nephrectomized woman is little more hazardous than in normal women, provided the remaining kidney is functionating properly. Albumin occurs in a certain proportion of these cases, usually in the latter months of pregnancy but if treated properly clears up just as in the normal case with two kidneys. In 60 per cent of the cases studied there was albumin from 1 to 4 plus during the latter weeks of pregnancy. Some of the nephrectomized women had albuminuria all thorugh pregnancy. There is little to be said regarding the conduct of labor in nephrectomized patients. They stand morphine and anesthesia well. Chloroform, of course should never be used for reasons needing no elucidation. Chloral hydrate and veronal are badly borne by these patients. Lactation is not interferred with in nephrectomized women, but if the nephrectomy has been done for unilateral tuberculosis or the kidney, lactation should be prohibited. Marriage after nephrectomy is permissible if the remaining kidney has functioned normally for one year or more. If there are symptoms of renal insufficiency in the remaining kidney after marriage, pregnancy should not be allowed to take place and contraceptive methods should be employed. If nephrectomy has been performed for unilateral tuberculosis of the kidney, pregnancy may be permitted provided the remaining kidney has functioned normally for three years or more. If nephrectomy has been performed for a malignant tumor, pregnancy must never be permitted. Finally there is need of a full study of nephrectomized women with well worked up reports of urinary findings and blood chemistry on every case of pregnancy after nephrectomy.

DISCUSSION

DR. A. J. RONGY.—I can very well recollect the first patient who came to engage me for her confinement and who told me that one of her kidneys was removed some three or four years previously. I really was reluctant to accept her. Evidently I was not familiar with the literature on the subject. However, in looking up the literature I quickly discovered that there was really no great cause for alarm, which practically coincides with what Dr. Matthews said tonight. I had three cases of pregnancy and labor in patients with only one kidney. In two the kidney was removed for benign tumors and in one for tuberculosis. One of these patients had a great deal of albumin during the early months which gradually diminished until she reached the ninth month, when it reappeared in large quantities. At one time when the urine contained no albumin she passed as much as 120 oz. of urine in twenty-four hours. I recall a patient telling me that she had had seven children after one of her kidneys had been removed. On the whole it seems to me that these patients stand labor and pregnancy very well.

DR. ALFRED M. HELLMAN.—I have a case of pregnancy following nephrectomy for tuberculous kidney. The right kidney was removed eight years ago. She is married five years and has a child three and a half years old. She is now in the fourth month of her second pregnancy and has no complications in any way related to the nephrectomy. She had a slight uterine hemorrhage during the second month. She has had no albumin in the urine, and her systolic blood pressure has ranged from 95 to 110.

DR. BAILEY.—One case reported by Dr. Matthews is very interesting. When there is an elevation of the nonprotein nitrogen and high uric acid in the blood it is almost certain that the woman has a badly damaged kidney. One can estimate the years of life on the basis of such findings. In cases where the total nonprotein nitrogen goes above 100 the patient has a very short time to live.

Department of Reviews and Abstracts

CONDUCTED BY HUGO EHRENFEST, M.D., ASSOCIATE EDITOR

Selected Abstracts

Carcinoma

Ochsner: Cancer Infection. Annals of Surgery, 1921, lxxiii, 294.

People who eat largely of raw vegetables fertilized with human excreta, as the Japanese and Chinese, are very prone to stomach cancer, while the Hindus, who boil all food and water, are practically free from cancer of the digestive organs. In northern Europe, where human excreta are largely used as fertilizer, stomach cancer is much more prevalent than in Russia, Australia and America. The Japanese, who are very cleanly, seldom have skin cancer, which is relatively frequent among the less fastidious Hindus. These figures do not change when these people live together in other countries, e.g. the Philippines.

These and similar data incline Ochsner to the infectious theory of cancer. He holds that such factors as chronic irritation only prepare the soil for the infection. R. E. WOBUS.

Nuzum: An Organism Associated with a Transplantable Carcinoma of the White Mouse. Surgery, Gynecology and Obstetrics, 1921, xxxiii, 167.

Nuzum found a minute, filtrable, gram-positive coccus in the Crocker mouse carcinoma No. 11. It occurred with considerable regularity in all the growths examined. He was enabled to obtain a pure culture of the coccus and found that by injecting this culture subcutaneously, he was able to produce tumors which were practically identical with the original growths, but usually disappeared after a while. These new growths, however, were transplantable, the transplants developing typical carcinomata in 80 per cent of the animals experimented upon. R. E. WOBUS.

Evans: Malignant Myomata and Related Tumors of the Uterus. Surgery, Gynecology and Obstetrics, 1920, xxx, 225.

In the hope of determining the criterion of malignancy, Evans examined a series of 4000 myomata removed at the Mayo clinic. Among these there were 72 cases classed as malignant. These he divides into three groups; (1) those showing from 2200 to 12000 mitotic figures per c.mm.; (2) those having from 200 to 800 per c.mm.; and (3) those showing only an occasional figure or none at all. In this connection it is remarkable that there were none containing between 800 and 2200 mitotic figures.

The number of giant cells varied considerably, but, on the whole the more malignant growths showed the greater number. However they did not occur in any exact ratio to the mitotic figures. Hyperchromatic nuclei, and nuclei elongated and showing direct cell division, occurred frequently, the latter especially in the less malignant forms without mitotic figures.

All recurrences were in Group 1. There were 13 in this group and 11 had recurrences at from one to 18 months after removal. The other two patients were living 4 and 7 months respectively, after operation, too short a time to be classed as cured. The average age of the patients in this group was 50 years, while the average of those in all three groups was 40½ years.

Metastases were not located in any distant organ in any case. Where they did occur, they were found in the pelvis or abdomen.

Evans tentatively classifies tumors of Group 1 as definitely malignant; those of Group 2 as transitional; and those of Group 3 as premalignant or having malignant tendencies. He does not believe that these tumors are *a priori* malignant, but that there is a gradual transition from fibroids with very active cell division to the malignant tumor classed as sarcoma. He finds the only dependable feature to be the abundance of mytotic figures in the very malignant cases. Other important features are: (1) The large size of the great mass of tumor cells in a given case and a marked inequality of their size; (2) the relative decrease in the amount of fibrous stroma; (3) the growth among the tumor cells of blood vessels with very thin walls or walls entirely wanting and (4) the relative increase in the size of the nucleus of the tumor cells as compared to the mass of the cytoplasm of the cell body.

R. E. WOBUS.

Berreitter: The Question of the Frequency of Malignancy in Myomata. Zentralblatt für Gynäkologie, 1921, xlv, 1592.

Since the development of conservative methods of treatment of uterine myoma, the question of the frequency of malignancy in these tumors has increased in practical interest and importance, particularly as a diagnosis is in the majority of cases clinically impossible.

Berreitter gives tables from the literature, showing various percentages of malignancy, running from nil (in 1000 cases) reported by Pfannensteil to 10 per cent as reported by Warnekros. In 1905 Mackenrodt suggested from 6 to 7 per cent as a probable figure, but never before had 10 per cent been suggested, and Berreitter undertook to examine a large mass of pathologic material with a view to discovering the actual figures.

In his 716 cases 6 malignant tumors were found, each of which is described at considerable length. In each instance the tumor showed the presence of numerous giant cells. This finding has not been characteristic of other reported cases. The histologic findings on which a diagnosis of malignancy was made in other instances is questioned, notably in the cases reported by Warnekros, 5 of which Berreitter believes to have been benign. He concludes that malignant tumors are *very infrequently* associated with myomas, and that 0.5 per cent is about a true average of incidence; perhaps even this figure is a little too high. Frequently, indeed almost always, in the true malignant type numerous irregular giant cells are present, and on this a diagnosis may be made. They were present in all of the six cases described by Berreitter. H. M. LITTLE.

Engelkens: Primary Cancer of the Vagina. Nederlandsch Tijdschrift voor Geneeskunde, 1922, i, 27.

Quoted statistics show that primary carcinoma of the vagina constitutes from .26 to 1.5 per cent of all cancers of the female genitalia. The etiology is quite obscure. Carcinoma cells have been found in the ulcers caused by pessaries, but in view of the many women who wear pessaries and the scarcity of carcinoma of the vagina, such a sequence is quite exceptional. The most common form consists of one or more discrete nodules, but there exists a diffuse infiltrating variety which Schlundt found 20 times in a total of 184 cases. While operation, on the whole, has been futile, due in part to the rich network of lymphatics around the vagina, there are authentic cases recorded which were free from recurrence after a period of five years.

Engelkens reviews the various operative measures advocated, especially by the German gynecologists. Though often heroic, they have, on the whole, been quite disappointing, and he feels that the hope of cure lies in radiation, or a combination of rays and surgery, but that it is still too early to judge ultimate results.

He reports two cases, the one, apparently, being caused by lysol. An unmarried woman, being pregnant, went to an abortionist who injected pure lysol into the uterus. The patient experienced acute pain for several days and had continuous bleeding for ten months, when she presented herself at the clinic. At that time, the entire vagina consisted of a diffuse infiltrating carcinoma. R. E. WOBUS.

Zweifel: The Significance of Early Symptoms in the Management of Cancer of the Uterus. Zentralblatt für Gynäkologie, 1921, xlv, 1126.

The nonoperative treatment of cancer of the uterus has undoubtedly two great advantages in the absence of a primary mortality and in its painlessness—matters of great import for the laity. The deciding point, however, is the question of absolute cure.

Statistics must be concerned with (1) primary mortality; (2) apparent cure after at least five years; (3) the frequency of operability; (4) absolute cure.

The greatest importance must be placed on whether patients come sufficiently early for treatment. Statistics will have to be altered in future and be arranged to show whether the cases were operable, border-line cases, or entirely inoperable; whether deaths are the results of the operation, or due to intercurrent disease; finally, the frequency of recurrence, and deaths from recurrence.

Zweifel still holds that operation is the best means for the cure of cancer, provided cases may be definitely classed as operable. Inasmuch as primary operative mortality has reached the lowest possible figure, any improvement from the standpoint of operation must depend on early diagnosis—a matter for the general practitioner, but chiefly for the patient herself. That improvement is possible, cannot be doubted.

Zweifel notes especially the importance of the early symptoms, which he believes are not sufficiently considered, e.g., bleeding after cohabitation; bleeding after gentle manipulations during examination; nodules other than follicular cysts on the cervix. In all these, snipping for microscopical examination will help when in doubt. Further symptoms are pruritus vulvae and an irritating discharge, even without the appearance of blood. The public must be educated by means of pamphlets, etc.

Of the greatest importance is the recognition that cancer is a disease of irregular discharge, and in the early stage *without pain*. No physician fulfils his duty by prescribing in such cases without local examination. Cancer may develop absolutely without symptoms before there is an onset of irregular bleeding, and an attempt should be made to overcome the instinctive disinclination of the patient against examination when menstruation or other vaginal bleeding is present (for which the physician is as much to blame as the patient), and, particularly, to spread the belief that any bleeding in the climacteric years should automatically bring the patient to the physician.

H. M. LITTLE.

Winter: Increasing Inoperability of Uterine Cancer and Its Remedy.
Zentralblatt für Gynäkologie, 1921, xlv, 1733.

The inoperability of uterine cancer has increased markedly in Germany since the beginning of the war. This has been due in large part to neglect. Winter has analyzed these neglected cases and found the fault to lie in 74.5 per cent with the patients themselves; in 21.5 per cent with physicians, and in 3.4 per cent with the midwives.

Winter has much to do with the campaign in Germany (commenced in 1904) for the early reporting of cases of carcinoma, and believes that the increasing number of cases of neglect is not directly attributable to war conditions, inasmuch as he gives at length the reasons for delay in bringing patients for treatment. The only hope for improvement is a return to the system of propaganda used before the war, which for a time showed such marked results: wide diffusion of the knowledge of the early symptoms of carcinoma (bleeding after cohabitation; bleeding in the menopause; bleeding with urination or defecation; and bleeding absolutely independent of the ovarian function).

Winter does not agree with Zweifel that pruritus may be an early symptom, but does agree that obstinate discharge may be a sign. With any of the symptoms, positive findings on palpation or inspection indicate a further and more careful examination. Excision and curetting for diagnosis must be more frequently undertaken by the general practitioner.

Statistics on operability are essential, if there is to be improvement. Radiation has given enormous aid to the healing of cancer, and at the moment the primary results of operation are better than ever, thanks to the development of technic. On the other hand, the ravages of carcinoma are as bad as ever. Therefore it is imperative, in order to make any advance, that treatment be undertaken at the earliest possible moment.

H. M. LITTLE.

Highsmith: The Importance of Early Diagnosis of Uterine Cancer. Southern Medicine and Surgery, 1921, x, 521.

The importance of early diagnosis lies in the fact that if the disease is diagnosed in time all patients are curable, while if not diagnosed in time, all must die. W. K. FOSTER.

Frankl: Early Diagnosis of Carcinoma of the Uterus. Dublin Journal of Medical Science, 1921, iv S., No. 21, p. 491.

After a compilation of the cases of carcinoma of the uterus in Schauta's Clinic at Vienna, Frankl states that early cases showed an increasing proportion from 1909 to 1913; while during the years of the war, the incidence of early carcinoma materially diminished; but is once more, in 1920 and 1921, on the increase—showing that by reason of the economic stress of the war, patients neglected to consult physicians in regard to suspicious symptoms. But circumstances have improved in this regard with the change in economic life. The early cases are those in which the cancer can only be demonstrated microscopically, or those in which the tumor was present without invading surrounding structures. Obviously, the diagnosis depends upon test excision or curettage in all specific cases. The article details the pathologic diagnosis of beginning malignancy. A. N. CREADICK.

Warthin and Noland: The Differential Diagnosis of Chancre and Carcinoma of the Cervix. The American Journal of Syphilis, 1921, v, 553.

Agreeing with Gellhorn and Ehrenfest, Warthin holds that the primary cervical chancre offers no truly characteristic and pathognostic features clinically, and that the diagnosis and a differentiation from carcinoma can be made only through its characteristic histological picture. The finding of Spirochetae pallidae in a smear is not conclusive, as a syphilitic woman may have carcinoma of the cervix and it is known that the spirochetes occur in the cervical secretions of syphilitic women. Finding them, however, in the tissues of the characteristic lesions offers valuable confirmatory evidence.

A case is reported substantiating these facts. In a married woman, aged 42, examination revealed a cauliflower growth covering the entire cervix, containing an ulcer which was covered by a grey membrane, the growth bleeding readily on examination. Since the Wassermann test was negative and the appearance of the growth seemed typical for a cervical carcinoma, a panhysterectomy was done in a private hospital. After leaving the hospital, the patient developed secondaries and brought suit against the hospital for $100,000, on the ground that she had contracted syphilis in the hospital from the needle used in drawing the blood for examination. Her husband brought suit for a like amount, since he had meanwhile also developed evidence of syphilis. The growth was sent to the University of Michigan, where Warthin found it to be a typical chancre of about four to six weeks' duration. He also demonstrated the spirochetes in the tissues. Upon this evidence the suit was lost.

The article contains some exceedingly good photomicrographs, showing in detail the characteristic picture of such a lesion. According to Warthin, the tissue changes due to primary syphilis are more typical in the cervix than in any other tissue. R. E. WOBUS.

Fink: Early Diagnosis of Chorionepithelioma After the Birth of Viable Children. Zeitschrift für Geburtshilfe und Gynäkologie, 1920, lxxxiii, 63.

The author believes that chorionepithelioma develops in all cases in the early months of pregnancy while Langhan's layer and the syncitium are both present. The tumor usually leads to abortion and hence the great majority of cases are reported following abortion or hydatiform moles. Occasionally, however, pregnancy may continue to near term, though the labor is usually somewhat premature. There is frequently atonic bleeding immediately postpartum with acute or chronic hemorrhages in the puerperium and subinvolution of the uterus. Any tissue removed from cases giving such a history should be examined most carefully microscopically with this point in view. The author reports such a case in a twenty-one-year old primipara who had had a severe attack of influenza in the second half of pregnancy. The labor was 3 to 4 weeks premature, severe bleeding followed the spontaneous separation of the placenta. Lochia still bloody and uterus subinvoluted on the eleventh day postpartum. Severe hemorrhage on 18th day with removal on 20th day of polypoid growth from uterus, histologically suspicious of chorionepithelioma. Cessation of bleeding until 40th day when she had another severe hemorrhage. Renewed examination of tissue confirmed diagnosis and the uterus with left adnexa was removed by vaginal hysterectomy on the 43rd day. MARGARET SCHULZE.

Geist: The Diagnosis and Treatment of Chorio-Epithelioma. Surgery, Gynecology and Obstetrics, 1921, xxxii, 426.

While adhering to the classification of Marchand, Geist prefers to term typical chorioepithelioma as choriocarcinoma and the atypical form as syncytioma. Between these, there are numerous transition stages and, in addition, there is a form presenting an exaggerated reaction to pregnancy without definite tumor formation, which he terms syncytial hyperplasia.

The diagnosis from curetted or expelled material is extremely difficult except in the clear-cut cases of the two groups. In the transitional types prognosis is doubtful. A positive diagnosis of syncytioma would call for conservatism, yet, the clinical course might still necessitate hysterectomy. In choriocarcinoma and the transitional types, abdominal hysterectomy is indicated and offers a fair prognosis even in the malignant type. R. E. WOBUS.

Smiley: Prophylaxis in Carcinoma of the Cervix. New York Medical Journal, 1921, cxiv, 384.

According to Bland's statistics, one woman of every eight dies of cancer; one-third of all cancers in women are of uterine origin; 85-90 per cent of uterine carcinoma are cervical in type. Cervical carcinomas are found almost exclusively (97 per cent) in women who have borne children or who have been subjected to some form of cervical traumatism with incidental infection. Chronic endocervicitis is, therefore, definitely a precursor of cervical cancer, and as such should be subjected to surgical treatment, which alone is curative. Low amputation and trachelorrhaphy are not curative. High amputation is frequently followed by serious functional disturbances. The Sturmdorf tracheloplastic operation, on the other hand, removes the entire diseased area, yet leaves the cervical musculature intact. The author has used this operation for eight years in a large number of cases with entire satisfaction. He regards it as an efficient prophylactic of cervical cancer and believes that there is no contraindication to its use during the childbearing age. MARGARET SCHULZE.

Cullen: Early Squamous-Cell Carcinoma of the Cervix. Surgery, Gynecology and Obstetrics, 1921, xxxiii, 137.

This case represents the earliest carcinoma which has come to the attention of Cullen. An unmarried woman of 46 presented herself on account of uterine bleeding. Curettage showed a glandular hyperplasia of the endometrium with a small area of carcinoma. The curettage was repeated in order to make the diagnosis positive, the second specimen showing typical carcinoma. A complete hysterectomy was done. The uterus contained a submucous fibroid which, together with the hyperplasia, accounted for the bleeding. At the internal os was found a small, wartlike projection, this being the only remaining evidence of the carcinoma. R. E. WOBUS.

Schweitzer: Attempts to Decrease the Mortality of Operation for Uterine Carcinoma. Archiv für Gynäkologie, 1921, cxiv, 213.

The Rumpf-Riess-Wertheim operation for carcinoma of the uterus has increased the proportion of curable cases; but the primary mortality from peritonitis, extraperitoneal sepsis, and pyelonephritis has remained high. It is not possible entirely to abolish peritonitis, because in some cases the infection is in the parametria or the lymphatics; but infection of the peritoneum by the unsterilizable vaginal surface of the carcinoma has been obviated by Zweifel, who after wide extirpation of the diseased pelvic organs, frees the uterus from all but its cuff of vagina. Three sutures are put into the posterior border of the bladder wall, left long, and the free ends put into the uterine wall. The uterus is then pushed down into the pelvis and the peritoneum closed over it. The abdomen is closed. The uterus is easily removed by cutting around the vaginal cuff, and the latter is attached to the bladder with the sutures that were pulled down with the uterus. The wound space above the vagina is filled for 10 days by loosely packed iodoform gauze. The bladder thus has an attachment for efficient contraction and the patient can void, while it is also protected from extension of infection from the vaginal wound.

Within 10 years the Leipzig clinic has employed this method in 322 cases of carcinoma of the uterus, of which 41 involved the body and 281 the cervix. There were 16 deaths, a primary mortality of 4.96 per cent, peritonitis claiming 0.93 per cent.

Among the 281 cases of carcinoma of the cervix, there were 15 primary deaths (5.8 per cent), peritonitis claiming 1.06 per cent and pyelitis 0.4 per cent (one death, in a case with extensive involvement and suppuration of the bladder); compared with 362 cases of the unmodified Wertheim operation with a primary mortality of 14 per cent, peritonitis 5.8 per cent and pyelitis 1.7 per cent. The Zweifel operation is seldom accompanied by injuries to the neighboring structures (7.5 per cent, while Wertheim himself reports 16 per cent and other operators up to 37 per cent). Peritoneal shock does not occur and ⅔ of the cases in the series studied made an afebrile recovery.

The operation is not suitable for all cases, especially not when the vagina is small and senile. In about 4 per cent of the cases the difficulty of pelvic hemostasis prevented the modification being used. In about 3 per cent of cases the peritoneal cavity was already invaded by the infected carcinoma and in such cases nothing is to be gained by the Zweifel operation over the Wertheim.

The objections that vaginal hemostasis is difficult and that the operation takes longer, are not valid. The vaginal artery and the communications with the hemorrhoidal vessels may be ligated before the abdomen is closed, and if nothing is left but the vaginal wall to be cut from below there is no hemorrhage. The intraabdominal part of the operation is actually shortened, and the vaginal part can be done after the anesthetic is stopped. RAMSAY SPILLMAN.

Bonney: The Radical Abdominal Operation for Carcinoma of the Cervix. British Medical Journal, 1921, No. 3183, p. 1103.

Bonney gives a report of 100 cases with an operative mortality of 20, death from recurrence 33, death from other diseases 3, not traced 4, well after five years 40. The author uses spinal anesthesia in conjunction with general anesthesia. Vaginal sterilization with "violet green" has reduced the number of cases of postoperative infections. Without vaginal drainage the patients do better. Operation will endure until some other method of therapy will cure more than 35 per cent of the patients. Radium on the whole has been disappointing.
F. L. ADAIR.

Cunéo and Picot: The Technic of Vaginal Hysterectomy for Carcinoma of the Cervix. Journal de Chirurgie, 1921, xviii, 193.

In an extensive article containing 11 excellent illustrations the authors describe minutely the technic which they employ in vaginal hysterectomy for carcinoma of the cervix. They favor this method above the abdominal route because they find that, especially in adipose individuals, it is an easier and faster operation while at the same time it permits a wider excision of the vaginal cuff. They find also that it does not necessitate the use of such an exaggerated Trendelenburg position, which fact tends toward better respiration, smoother anesthesia and less postoperative shock.

They favor the use of spinal anesthesia aided, where necessary, by small amounts of ether or narcotics. The position used is that of an exaggerated lithotomy with the patient's head lowered slightly and the table of sufficient height to allow the operator to stand.

The main incision is similar to the "Perineal Laparotomy" of Zuckerkandl, and passes from one ischium to the other in a convex line falling two centimeters below the posterior fourchette. From this point they divide the operation into four main steps. The first is that of separation of the bladder and rectum from the vagina. The next is that of ligation of the various arterial pedicles. At this point the authors call especial attention to the fact that the anatomic relation of the bladder, ureters and uterine arteries is greatly altered by the traction downward on the freed vagina and cervix and the upward pressure on the bladder which is being applied at this time. The arterial pedicles having been ligated and sectioned, the next step, comprising the ligation and section of the various uterine ligaments, is undertaken. Here again they call attention to the rich lymphatic supply of the uterosacral ligaments and plead for as wide an excision of these tissues as possible. The final step is that of closure.

When the malignant process has extended further than was first thought and has invaded the bladder or rectum, and injury is done to these organs by the attempted removal of the cancer, Cunéo and Picot claim that such injury may usually be repaired with a satisfactory result.

The postoperative treatment is simple and consists of frequent catheterization, induced paralysis of the intestines for five to six days, and tampons in the vagina to help hold the vault in place. The tampons should be changed every two days. They find that complete healing usually occurs in from 20 to 25 days.

In the hands of these operators the immediate mortality has compared most favorably with that of the abdominal route, while the ultimate results have been even more satisfactory.   T. W. ADAMS.

Adler: The Treatment of Cancer of the Uterus. Wiener klinische Wochenschrift, 1921, xxxiv, 312.

Of 52 cases of inoperable cancer of the cervix treated with radium in 1913 and 1914, thirteen (25 per cent) are still free from recurrence. Of six operable cases treated during the same time only one is free.

The technic of radium treatment is uncertain because there is no definite dosage on account of the impossibility of defining the extent of the disease. Each case is an experiment. If too strong a dose is given severe burning and fistulae may result, if too weak a dose is applied, the growth may be stimulated.

There is a primary mortality with radium treatment, Bumm and Von Schäfern having reported deaths from sepsis following treatment. A large percentage of patients do not return for further treatment, some because they are symptomatically relieved for the time being; some because the severe reaction and pain makes them fearful of another treatment.

The operative treatment has probably reached its highest possibilities. The vaginal operation has a lower primary mortality than the abdominal, being in the last ten years in the Schauta clinic only 3.5 per cent. The five-year cures in the Schauta clinic amount to 22 per cent, in the Weibel (Wertheim) clinic 20 to 25 per cent. The vaginal operation may be used in elderly women, especially under local anesthesia, and when the abdominal route is contraindicated.

The object now must be to combine radiotherapy, x-ray and operation to get better results. Since 1913, 29 cases have had prophylactic radium treatment four weeks after operation, usually 50 mg. in the vagina for from 10 to 12 hours. Five to six years after operation 58.8 per cent of these were free from recurrence. Of those not having the treatment only 42 per cent were cured.

Eight cases operated on 3 and 4 years ago had 30 to 35 mg. of radium placed in the parametrium on each side at the time of operation for 5 to 8 hours. Of these six (75 per cent) are still living. (The author does not make any statement as to recurrences in these six cases.)

In the last year he has combined operation with radium as above, and intensive x-ray treatment for from 8 to 14 days after operation.

Summary—Every operable case should be operated on, the method, vaginal or abdominal, depending on the custom of the surgeon; the operation should be followed by radium and x-ray treatment.

FRANK A. PEMBERTON.

Seitz: Carcinoma Treatment and Dosage. Muenchener medizinische Wochenschrift, 1921, lxix, 1107.

The author very generally considers chemical and physical irritation in their etiologic relationship to carcinoma. Roentgen rays belong to the latter class and may cause carcinoma, aggravate an existing neoplasm, or kill a malignant growth. The author has studied the effect of the rays with the object of determining the various dosages which will produce these different results and reached the following conclusions: (1) The irritating dose is 35 to 40 per cent of the unit skin dose; (2) The destructive dose is 100 to 110 per cent of the unit skin dose; (3) Between these extremes the dose leads to neither irritation nor to destruction, unless it be repeated, and then it becomes destructive.

S. B. SOLHAUG.

Schmitz: The Treatment of Cancer of the Uterus. Journal American Medical Association, 1921, lxxvii, 608.

Schmitz urges the correction of all pathologic lesions of the cervix and uterus as a prophylactic measure. In operable cases, he urges abdominal panhysterectomy, but limits operability to those cases where the growth is distinctly limited to the uterus. He considers postoperative radiation as useless. His standard dose for inoperable cases is 50 milligrams applied for 30 hours. This he supplements with x-ray treatment. Of 7 operated cases 5 are alive after periods of from one to five years. Of his radiated cases, 161 in all, 27 or 16.8 per cent are alive after the same period of time; this includes also the cases of recurrence, of which only one out of a total of 46 is alive. R. E. WOBUS.

Frankl: X-ray and Radium Treatment in Gynecology. Dublin Journal of Medical Science, 1921, iv S., No. 21, p. 500.

The author calls attention to the fact that statistics from the clinics of Wertheim and Schauta, where radical surgery for malignancy originated, is a good field for comparison in interpreting the results arrived at by combined x-ray and radium therapy. Admittedly, surgery and the physical methods of treatment have their limitations. In gynecology the treatment is essentially a deep treatment, and for this a powerful dosage is necessary, symmetrically applied over large areas, guaranteeing deep penetration; he advises 100-110 per cent of the erythema dose of x-ray, cross-fired through three to five avenues of entry on the abdomen, three to four routes from the back, and one or two from the perineum. At the same time 50 mg. of radium element are inserted in the cervix and allowed to remain from 12 to 24 hours. The author demonstrates the action on carcinoma cells removed on different days and from different distances, following radiation. This treatment has shown a small percentage of cures of otherwise inoperable cases, and a decided benefit in preventing recurrence following operation. It is much more readily applicable to cancers of the cervix than it is to cancers of the uterine body, is serviceable in milder dosage for menorrhagic metropathia, and is of use in myomata when the patients are near the menopause with intramural tumors which are not degenerated. A. N. CREADICK.

Boggs: The Treatment of Carcinoma of the Cervix and Uterus by Radium: Supplemented by Deep Roentgen Therapy. New York Medical Journal, 1921, cxiv, 381.

Results in radiotherapy of uterine carcinoma cannot as yet be definitely formulated. Progress is hindered by the practice of superficial and inadequate radiation so widespread among persons in possession of small amounts of the drug. The Wertheim operation with its high operative mortality shows only a very low percentage of five-year cures. Proper radium treatment locally, supplemented by sufficient cross-firing from radium packs from the x-ray from outside as an anteoperative procedure would cure many more cases. The best results are obtained by the cooperation of a well trained surgeon and a well trained radiologist. Remarkable palliative results are obtained by the use of radium in inoperable cases. The author employs 3000 mg. hours in the vagina, using 1½ mm. brass and sufficient gauze and rubber to make 15 mm. filtration. Three tubes are employed, one directed toward the cervix, one toward each broad ligament. Where it is possible to insert radium in the cervical canal, an additional 3000 mg. hours is given in this way. The local radium treatment should be supplemented by deep Roentgen therapy, for which the author details the technic. MARGARET SCHULZE.

Graves: Present Status of the Treatment of Operable Cancer of the Cervix. Surgery, Gynecology and Obstetrics, 1921, xxxii, 504.

Graves is not ready to discard the operative treatment of cervical cancer. He feels that, while better results are being obtained from radium, the results from operation are also improving. This he ascribes not only to improvement of technic, both in the application of radium and of operation, but also to the fact that patients appear earlier for treatment. He sums up the situation very aptly in the following words: "Cancer of the cervix uteri, notwithstanding the ghastly consequences of which it is capable, is nevertheless peculiarly amenable to curative treatment in the early stages. Whether the ultimate treatment of curable cases shall continue to be surgical or whether surgery shall yield to radiation, the general outlook is encouraging."
R. E. WOBUS.

Shaw: The Present Position of the Treatment of Carcinoma of the Cervix. British Medical Journal, 1921, No. 3183, p. 1101.

The author discusses the present status of therapy from the standpoint of the Wertheim hysterectomy and the use of radium. The author gives his own operability percentage as 26.8. The mortality in 89 cases was 19.1 per cent. Of 59 cases operated over one year, 12 died from the operation; 21 died of recurrence; 26 (or 55.3 per cent) are alive and well. He uses radium only in inoperable cases, but has done the Wertheim operation, after the use of radium, in 10 cases and found increased technical difficulty. He now operates about one week after the application of radium.

Duncan: Uterine Cancer. Journal American Medical Association, 1921, lxxvii, 604.

Duncan has treated a total of 236 cases of uterine cancer with radium. Of these, 96 or 40.6 per cent are clinically well after from one year to four years. Of recurrences treated, 22 per cent are well after a period of from one to four years. He advocates the use of radium in all cases of uterine carcinoma, but emphasizes that proper dosage and technic are of utmost importance. He usually employs 200 millicuries with a total dosage of 4000 to 6000 millicurie hours. R. E. Wobus.

Burrows: The Treatment of Advanced Carcinoma of the Cervix of the Uterus by Radium. British Medical Journal, 1921, No. 3170, p. 525.

All cases were inoperable. The author analyzed 100 cases treated from 1916 to 1918. Six are still well after 3 to 3½ years; 5 were well 12 months after treatment. These 5 have not been traced since. Seven were well 3 to 6 months after treatment, also not traced since. Six were rendered operable, and operation was performed. Thirty-two were made comfortable and were able to work for 6 months to 2 years. Twenty-six were not improved, and 16 cases were not followed. The author uses a dosage of at least 120 millicuries for 24 hours.

F. L. Adair.

Drueck: Excision of Cancerous Rectum through Vaginal Section. New York Medical Journal, 1921, cxiii, 21.

Drueck recommends the vaginal route for the perineal removal of carcinoma of the rectum. Section of the posterior vaginal wall and perineum provides ample working space, there is little traumatism and hemorrhage and consequently little shock. The operation is practical only when the tumor is movable and is situated in the lower half of the rectum. If it is as high as the rectosigmoid junction, then the combined abdominal and vaginal operation should be employed. He gives a detailed description of the technic. Margaret Schulze.

Book Reviews

Pneumoperitoneal Roentgen Ray Diagnosis (A Monograph with Atlas). By Dr. ARTHUR STEIN, M.D., F.A.C.S., Associate Gynecologist, Harlem Hospital and Lenox Hill Hospital, New York City, and Dr. WILLIAM H. STEWART, M.D., F.A.C.P. Roentgenologist, Harlem Hospital and Lenox Hill Hospital, New York City. The Southworth Company, Troy, New York. 1921.

The authors describe in detail the method employed by them of inflating the peritoneal cavity with oxygen in order to make the contents of the abdomen capable of transillumination with the x-ray. The procedure was first introduced into this country by them in June, 1919. Practically 17 years had elapsed since Kelling of Dresden first demonstrated the value of inflating the abdominal cavity with air. This author, however, had in mind the visualization of the viscera by means of the endoscope introduced through a small abdominal incision. Jacobaeus later, 1910 and 1911, practiced this new method of laparoscopy and reported his results in 100 cases. The outstanding feature was the absence of any infection as a result of the diagnostic method.

Roentgenologic procedures were adapted to the method of abdominal inflation by Weber in 1912 and by Lorey in the same year. Weber's roentgenograms showed that the following viscera and areas may be rendered visible by means of gas inflation of the abdomen. (1) The liver and spleen as a whole including the region of the gall bladder. (2) Coils of large and small intestine without bismuth filling. (3) The pyloric portion of the stomach. (4) The walls of the stomach and large intestine with gas contents. (5) The bladder filled with urine. (6) Parts of the mesentery. (7) The subphrenic space, not readily accessible to diagnosis. (8) Many intraabdominal tumors. These conclusions were based upon experiments on animals and on fresh cadavers of adults and children. Lorey was the first to demonstrate the diagnostic value of peritoneal inflation and his findings were published in 1912.

Rautenberg in 1914 introduced air into the abdominal cavity in a case of disease of the liver complicated with ascites for the purpose of obtaining more distinct contours of both liver and spleen. About the same time Meyer-Betz recommended withdrawing the ascitic fluid and replacing it very slowly by oxygen injected by means of an ordinary insufflation apparatus such as is used for the application of therapeutic pneumothorax. In 1918 Goetze published very remarkable roentgenographic data obtained by means of the new method and concerning nearly all the abdominal viscera. Other observers were Decker, Kirscher and Allessandrini, who reported on the valuable data arrived at through the employment of the new procedure of induced pneumoperitoneum and roentgen examination. Meantime French investigators reported favorable results; while in this country Alvarez, impressed with "the beautiful plates taken with this method by Drs. Stein and Stewart," recommended the use of carbon dioxide gas (CO_2) because of its rapid absorption (one-half hour as compared to 24 to 100 hours for the oxygen). A. F. Tyler reported his findings in the study of 36 cases and stated that the method proved of great value in making a positive diagnosis of adhesions, early uterine enlargement gastric tumors and gallstones. He points out that the entire kidney, ovaries and tubes can be visualized by these means.

The indication for gas inflation of the abdomen in connection with roentgenology is chiefly in those cases where the clinician is baffled. (1) It is singularly valuable in demonstrating intraabdominal adhesions especially those between the viscera and the abdominal walls. (2) To diagnose cases of early peritoneal tuberculosis and (3) adhesions or the contents of herniated abdominal coverings; (4) diseases of the liver such as cysts, gummas and metastatic tumors are best diagnosticated by this method. (5) Affection of the gall bladder and bile ducts especially gallstones; (6) spleenic disease; (7) renal disease. (8) It was especially useful in locating extraperitoneal tumors and in distinguishing whether a projectile is above, within or below the diaphragm and (9) whether a tumor is intraabdominal or intrathoracic when it is situated near the diaphragm. (10) The presence or absence of subdiaphragmatic tumors, abscesses and adhesions and finally, (11) lesions in the pelvis.

The contraindications to the method are chiefly in elderly persons, notably men who have used alcohol in excess, and those suffering from valvular disease and other circulatory diseases. Acute abdominal conditions such as acute appendicitis or peritonitis naturally prohibit the employment of abdominal inflation.

The danger of infection is theoretical because in none of the 150 cases of the authors' experience has this been noted. Puncture of the intestine has been reported as occurring in two cases. In neither of these was any ill effect observed. About one-third of the authors' cases complained of pain in the shoulders, especially the right, following distention of the abdominal cavity with gas. This has largely been remedied by avoiding full distention, by deflating the patient after the roentgen examination, (when oxygen has been used) and by using a gas which is rapidly absorbed, such as carbon dioxide. Superficial emphysema can easily be avoided if one follows exactly the rule stated in reference to introducing the needle into the abdominal cavity before the gas is turned on. Puncturing the epigastric arteries is best avoided by introducing the needle in the median line (linea alba) about two fingers below the umbilicus where there is no artery to be encountered; this technic would also avoid the danger of gas entering these vessels.

The absence of danger from the method is further borne out by the actual therapeutic use of oxygen in certain abdominal conditions. A brief note upon inflation of other body cavities concludes the monograph. Of special interest here is the mention of Stewart and Luckett's case of traumatic fracture of the skull where the ventricles were distended with air following the fracture as demonstrated by the roentgenograph. This experience was utilized by Dandy in outlining roentgenographically the cerebral ventricles by injecting air into the cavities of the brain.

The authors describe the inflation technic and the roentgen ray technic with very illuminating photographs.

The Atlas consists of 34 plates which represent the principal lesions in a beautiful and graphic manner. Explanatory notes are given on pages opposite to the plates in English, French and Spanish. These plates are original photographs and not halftones as ordinarily employed. Naturally this feature makes the price of the book considerably higher than can be met by many to whom the book would be useful. It is to be hoped that this change may be made so as to reach a greater number of roentgenologists and others interested in general diagnosis.

The authors deserve great credit for bringing this valuable method to the attention of the profession; for their personal contributions in the matter of indicated uses and technical improvements, and finally for presenting the method in that clear, concise and compact form in the present volume. As the authors have aptly said, "a great future can be confidently predicted for this interesting method of examination, which during the short period of its existence has already passed through several phases, with constant enrichment of its diagnostic value or extension of its clinical applicability."

The transuterine insufflation test for tubal patency, while not directly resulting from the authors' publication, was nevertheless made possible by them because the induction of a pneumoperitoneum which in itself is harmless, was the very thing needed to complete the work on tubal patency. It had been possible to demonstrate tubal occlusion by injecting collargol, thorium and bromide solutions into the uterus and then employing roentgenography. To demonstrate patency of the fallopian tubes this method had not proved so satisfactory. With oxygen or CO_2 gas as a medium and the production of a pneumoperitoneum tubal patency is at once demonstrated. Likewise in the event of failure to produce a pneumoperitoneum by injecting the gas into the uterus, tubal occlusion may at the same time be diagnosed. Other features and details of this diagnostic test, such as pressure control, soon developed. The reviewer is glad of the opportunity to record here the fact that his work on tubal patency and tubal occlusion begun by him in 1913 was finally made possible in 1919 when his attention was called to the demonstration given by Dr. Stein and Dr. Stewart of the method of pneumoperitoneum induced by oxygen for general abdominal diagnosis.

I. C. RUBIN.

The Problem of Abortion from the Medical and Legal Standpoints.—By FRANZ KISCH, M.D., Urban and Schwarzenberg, Vienna, 1921.

This is a well-written treatise of 110 pages, containing numerous references and intended to defend the practice of abortion from various points of view. On page 6 the author says: "It is the duty of the State to guarantee safety and protection to its citizens and to secure the physical and moral well-being of all who are willing to work. Above all, it is the duty of the State to so manage, that a sufficient quantity of food is provided, that in return for work every one may be assured of a sufficiency to satisfy all needs in this direction. If the State is unable to guarantee this, the natural consequence will be, that procreation must be considerably reduced. The amount of available food and procreation . . . . stand in direct proportion." The communistic idea that the State must supply food to all who are willing to work, is a Utopian dream which it is not our purpose to discuss here. Referring to the statement, that the amount of available food and procreation stand in direct proportion to each other, one can only say that the facts are against the author. It is common knowledge that the very poor are blessed with large families, while the rich usually boast of but few children.

In the chapter dealing with the indications for the production of abortion and the induction of premature labor, the author seems to go a little beyond the generally accepted medical opinion. He counsels the interruption of pregnancy, if the consent of the patient has been obtained, in the following cases: Organic heart disease, namely valvular lesion, even if perfect compensation exists, pulmonary tuberculosis, nephritis, diabetes, goitre, cirrhosis of the liver, tetany, lupus, extensive varicose veins of the vulva or legs, chronic appendicitis, hernia, abdominal tumors and in absolute pelvic contraction if the patient desires it.

It would take much more space than is allotted to us to take up each one of these indications for criticism. One can hardly refrain, however, from pointing out the very broad indication for abortion when extensive varicosities on the legs is one of them. This is an incident in the majority of pregnancies and if at the behest of all women who have them and desired relief, the pregnancy were terminated, we might become very busy abortionists indeed.

S. D. JACOBSON.

Die Prophylaxe und Therapie der Enteroptose.—By PROFESSOR LUDWIG KNAPP, Prag. Urban & Schwarzenberg, Berlin, 1921.

This is a scholarly and well-written treatise characterized by excellent diction and good literary style. In the chapter on Prophylaxis of Enteroptosis the author points out that inherited weakness of tissues plays an important part in the later development of ptoses. He emphasizes the importance of breast milk in infant feeding and quotes Esser that it is especially harmful to subject milk to prolonged boiling. In this way the constituents of milk are injured and its value as a plastic food diminished. He protests against physical overexertion and mental strain in children and declares that co-education is particularly harmful if girls compete with boys in school. He believes that gymnastics and outdoor sports especially in the winter are beneficial and that swimming is to be highly recommended because the positions assumed counteract the tendency to ptosis.

The author lays stress on the importance of care during menstruation and particularly during the weeks following childbirth, so as to secure proper involution of the genitals and a return to normal of the tension of the abdominal and pelvic musculature. He sounds a note of warning against intensive courses of reduction for obesity especially after the menopause and quotes Menge as saying that nervous collapse and heart failure are to be feared in such cases. In the chapter on therapy the author takes a decided stand against operative interference. He extols the use of mechanical support, massage, general tonic treatment, and in thin, nervous individuals a prolonged rest cure combined with forced feeding.

S. D. JACOBSON.

Item

The Forty-Seventh Annual Meeting of the American Gynecological Society will be held at the Hotel Washington, Washington, D. C., on May 1, 2, and 3, 1922.

The American Journal of Obstetrics and Gynecology

Original Communications

NORMAL VARIATIONS IN TYPE OF THE FEMALE PELVIS
AND THEIR OBSTETRICAL SIGNIFICANCE

BY JOHN T. WILLIAMS, M.D., F.A.C.S., BOSTON, MASS.

IN 1543, less than four hundred years ago, Andreas Vesalius gave the first correct anatomical description of the normal pelvis. Eighteen years later his pupil, Arantius, first recognized the existence of contracted pelves. Two hundred and thirty more years elapsed before Baudelocque, in 1789, invented the pelvimeter and put the study of the pelvis in the living woman upon a scientific basis. Scientific obstetrics may be said to date from this invention, although the study advanced so slowly that it was not until 1861, seventy-two years later, that Litzman published the first classification of pelves based upon form as well as size. It is not remarkable, therefore, that, since the recognition of gross abnormalities developed so slowly, the study of variations in the normal pelvis should have received little attention. Ethnologists have long been familiar with variations in the form of the pelvis in different races, but since from an obstetrical standpoint we are concerned mainly with women of the white race, I shall not refer further to such racial differences.

The rarity of deformed pelves in white American women has been remarked by a number of observers. Reynolds[1] found only 1.34 per cent of contracted pelves in 2,227 women, but as he measured the pelvis in those cases only in which dystocia occurred, we must regard his figures as too low. Flint[2] found 8.46 per cent of contracted pelves in 10,233 women delivered by the New York Lying-in Hospital. Williams[3] found, in Baltimore, 8.49 per cent of contracted pelves among 2,178 white women. Among the 300 primiparous women upon whom

---

NOTE: The Editor accepts no responsibility for the views and statements of authors as published in their "Original Communications."

the study of this paper is based I found 27 in whom I felt the measurements were small enough and the disproportion between the pelvis and fetus great enough to demand cesarean section for mechanical reasons alone. In the majority of these the pelvis was perfectly normal in shape but of small size.

The normal female pelvis, as described in all textbooks of anatomy or obstetrics, presents the following characteristics: the bones are lighter and thinner than in the male. The flare of the ilia is greater resulting in broader hips. The superior strait is elliptical and wider in all its diameters than is the case in the male. The pelvic outlet is wide in the female and the descending rami of the os pubis form an arch rather than an angle. According to Dieulafé[4] the arch in the female intercepts an arc of from 70 to 100 degrees, while in the male the rami form an angle of always less than 70 degrees. The outlet is therefore wider in all its diameters in the female than in the male. The sacrosciatic notch is also wider in the female. The obturator foramen is more triangular in the female and more oval in the male. Quain[5] gives the following average measurements from a number of full sized male and female pelves:

	MALE	FEMALE
Intercristal diameter	28.6 cm.	31.9 cm.
Interspinous diameter	24.1 "	25.0 "
External conjugate	18.4 "	18.0 "
Transverse of outlet	8.8 "	12.1 "
Anteroposterior of outlet	8.5 "	10.8 "

J. Whitridge Williams[6] gives the following internal measurements:

	MALE	FEMALE
Superior Strait.		
Anteroposterior	10.5 cm.	11.0 cm.
Transverse	12.5 "	13.5 "
Oblique	12.0 "	12.75 "
Inferior Strait.		
Anteroposterior	9.5 "	11.5 "
Transverse	8.0 "	11.0 "

With the development of the study of the pelvic outlet by Williams, Thoms and others, the great frequency of pelves with small outlet measurements became recognized. Thoms[7] found that 5.3 per cent of 4000 consecutive patients at the Johns Hopkins Hospital had contractions of the pelvic outlet. Williamson,[8] in New York, found outlet contraction in 7.7 per cent of 1,579 cases at the Manhattan Maternity Hospital. These figures include only those cases in which the transverse diameter of the outlet was 8 cm. or under. If all cases where the diameters of the outlet were less than those given by Quain or Williams had been included the percentages would have been considerably higher.

Two explanations have been advanced for the occurrence of outlet contractions in women. J. Whitridge Williams[9] believes the majority of them to be due to assimilation of the fifth lumbar vertebra with the sacrum. This results in a higher articulation of the ilium with the spinal column which causes the ischia to converge. He was able to confirm this mechanism in a number of patients by palpating six sacral vertebræ. On the other hand, this explanation does not hold good for all cases. I have had several cases of outlet contraction x-rayed in which the sacrum showed definitely only five segments.

Berry Hart[10] explains the incidence of contractions of the pelvic outlet by what he describes as inversion of certain parts of the female pelvis to the male type. He differentiates two forms of inversion, an iliosacral and an ischiopubic type. In the iliosacral form the ilium and sacrum invert to the male type resulting in contraction at the superior strait. In the ischiopubic inversion the outlet is contracted; the pubic arch is angular, and the ischia close together as in the male pelvis. Hart's views are based upon the examination of one autopsy and seven museum specimens.

Impressed in the course of routine antepartum examinations by the large number of contracted outlets found in women with broad hips and large external measurements, I found after a time that I could predict almost with certainty that when the external measurements exceeded 30 cm. in the intercristal, and 20 cm. in the anteroposterior, the transverse diameter of the outlet would be more or less contracted and the pubic arch angular. On the other hand, in women with measurements which did not exceed 20 cm., 25 cm., and 28 cm. for the external conjugate, the interspinous and intercristal diameters, respectively, I could with equal certainty predict a wide arch and an ample transverse diameter of the outlet. These observations led me to believe that there are two distinct types of female pelvis both of which must be regarded as normal. Further study has revealed other characteristics of both types which I shall enumerate.

The more common type corresponds rather closely with the ordinary textbook description of the normal female pelvis. The external measurements are normal or often slightly below normal. An external conjugate of 18 cm. or 19 cm. is not uncommon and from the usual course of labor in these pelves must be regarded as within normal limits. The intercristal is almost never over 28 or 29 cm. The pubic arch is wide and the transverse diameter of the outlet ample. The bones are thin and internal examination gives a sense of roominess. The os pubis is vertical or nearly so, and its vertical diameter is short. The general development of the patient is in keeping with the form of the pelvis. The entire skeleton is lighter than in the other type. This type of pelvis is more commonly found in slender women, although it may be found in obese subjects. The perineum is usually elastic and not particularly thick or muscular. For purposes of designation, I shall call this the feminine type of pelvis.

The other, which is also the less common type of pelvis is, as I have indicated, characterized by broad external measurements and a narrow outlet. The external conjugate varies from 21 cm. to 23 cm., the interspinous from 26 cm. to 28 cm., and the intercristal diameter from 30 cm. to 32 cm. The pubic arch is narrow and the ischia close together. The bones are usually thicker and heavier than in the first type of pelvis. This is especially noticeable in the os pubis, which is considerably increased in height, and is horizontal rather than vertical so that its anterior surface is directed downward instead of forward. This is due in part to an increased pelvic inclination. The

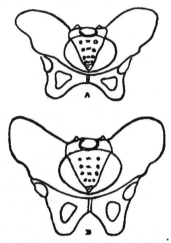

Fig. 1.—Feminine type above. Muscular type below. Purposely exaggerated to show differences. Note the wider pubic arch and lighter bones in the first type and the narrower outlet but wider hips in the second.

skeleton is heavier than in the type of pelvis first described. The patients are either large and muscular, usually obese, but with distinctly feminine type of figure, or short and thick set with heavy figures. The perineum is thick and muscular. I shall call this the muscular or heavy type of pelvis. Although difficult to measure or even estimate in the living woman, I believe the superior strait to be normal or increased in area in this type.

These two types are as a rule readily distinguished upon examination, although some modifications of each will be met with and an occasional case which is hard to classify. A pelvis of the feminine type in which the measurements are very small constitutes a justominor pelvis. A pelvis of the muscular type in which the outlet contraction is particularly marked is usually described as a funnel pelvis. These two are very naturally the most common forms of contracted pelvis in this country.

EFFECT OF TYPE OF PELVIS UPON THE COURSE OF LABOR

This study has been based upon three hundred consecutive primiparae attended in private practice, although confirmed by observations upon multiparae and patients at the Boston City Hospital obstetric ward. I have restricted my figures to primiparae for three reasons. First: because it is only in the first labor that the effect of type of pelvis can be accurately estimated. Second: to prevent the same patient appearing in the statistics more than once. Third: to exclude an undue proportion of cases referred because of difficulty in a previous labor. These primiparae were with few exceptions delivered in private hospitals around Boston between Jan. 1, 1918, and April 30, 1921. I have selected private cases only because I have been able to give them more detailed study than the hospital cases and in all instances to follow them through from beginning to end.

Proportion of Types.—The first or feminine type made up 221 cases or 73.6 per cent; and the second or muscular type 79, or 26.4 per cent.

Rupture of Membranes.—Rupture of the membranes before labor or at the onset of labor occurred in 18.3 per cent of the feminine type, and 38.4 per cent of the muscular type of pelvis. (Cesarean section was performed before onset of labor or rupture of membranes in eight patients of the first type and in one patient of the second type.)

Presentation and Position.—The accompanying table gives the number and percentage of the various presentations occurring in each type of pelvis.

PRESENTATION AND POSITION	FEMININE NUMBER	PER CENT	MUSCULAR NUMBER	PER CENT
O.L.A.	140	63.3	40	50.6
O.D.P.	50	22.6	25	31.6
O.D.A.	10	4.5	6	7.6
O.L.P.	9	4.0	5	6.3
Brow	1	0.4	1	1.2
Face	1	0.4	0	0
Breech	10	4.5	2	2.4

These figures show that in the muscular type of pelvis there is a decided increase in the proportion of the two posterior positions of the occiput, but a smaller number of abnormal presentations (brow, face, breech). This I attribute to the larger superior strait. To the same cause and the larger number of posterior positions of the occiput must be attributed the much larger percentage of premature rupture of the membranes, which is the most striking effect of the muscular type of pelvis upon labor. In the feminine type the head as a rule engages before labor and molds early. It also passes the plane of greatest resistance, which in this type is the superior strait, before the pains have spent themselves and the patient become exhausted. In the muscular type the pelvis narrows toward the outlet and the resistance increases as the head descends. In the muscular type the perineum and the muscles and fasciae of the pelvis are stronger and offer greater resistance, and it is my belief that the cervix is more apt to be rigid.

Difficult Labors.—There were among the three hundred primiparae, three stillbirths due to difficult delivery, all in instances of the muscular type of pelvis, all associated with premature rupture of the membranes. In all of these patients because of the duration of the rupture of the membranes, cesarean section seemed contraindicated. Cesarean section was performed 33 times. In the feminine type of pelvis the measurements seemed sufficiently small to justify cesarean section as an elective operation in 11 patients. In six it was done after failure of the test of labor to bring the head into the pelvis. In six more it was done for nonpelvic reasons: placenta previa centralis, threatened eclampsia, multiple fibroids or elderly primiparity. Among the muscular type of pelvis the outlet was so small in three cases that elective cesarean section was performed. In seven more cesarean was performed after failure of the test of labor.

Reducing the above figures to percentages: in the feminine type elective cesarean section was performed for justominor pelvis in 4.9 per cent and after failure of the test of labor in 2.7 per cent, a total of 7.6 per cent for this type requiring cesarean section. As would be expected because of the greater difficulty in estimating disproportion in advance of labor in the muscular type of pelvis, elective cesarean section was performed in only 3.8 per cent but cesarean section after failure of the test of labor was done in 8.8 per cent bringing the total requiring abdominal delivery to 12.6 per cent, without counting the three stillbirths in which cesarean would have been performed had there been no contraindications. Therefore it will be seen that, excluding cesarean section performed for other than pelvic reasons, the muscular type of pelvis is considerably the more unfavorable of the two. This is still further borne out by the greater number of posterior positions of the occiput and the enormous percentage of premature rupture of the membranes.

Furthermore in the muscular pelvis, as has been stated, the resistance to the presenting part increases as the fetus descends, making interference more difficult, whereas in the feminine type the greatest difficulty is over once the head has passed through the superior strait, and low interference is relatively easy.

CONCLUSIONS

1. There are two distinct and easily recognizable types of normal female pelvis, which for purposes of designation may be called the "feminine" and the "muscular" types.

2. The first or "feminine type" presents external measurements closely approximating the 20, 25, 28 cm. of the textbooks with thin bones and a wide outlet.

3. The second or "muscular type" is characterized by large external measurements, but a narrow outlet and an angular pubic arch. The bones are as a rule heavier. The os pubis is thicker and more horizontal, and the pelvic inclination increased. The muscles and fasciae are firmer than in the first type.

4. Although both of these types must be considered as normal, the "feminine type" is much the more favorable for labor. In the "muscular type" premature rupture of the membranes occurs in nearly 40 per cent and posterior positions of the occiput are more common. In spite of the larger external measurements, cesarean section was necessary in a greater percentage of pelves of the muscular type. Both the normal mechanism of labor and operative interference are unfavorably affected by the horizontal os pubis and the greater pelvic inclination in this type.

REFERENCES

(1) Trans. Amer. Gynec. Soc., 1890, xv, 367. (2) Report Soc. Lying-in Hosp., N. Y., 1897, p. 258. (3) *Williams*: Obstetrics, 1920, p. 739. (4) Quoted by Quain: Anatomy, iv, pt. 1, p. 177. (5) *Quain*: Anatomy, iv, 1, pp. 176-178. (6) *Williams*: Obstetrics, 1920, p. 15. (7) Amer. Jour. Obst., 1915, lxxii, 121. (8) Amer. Jour. Obst., 1918, lxxviii, 528. (9) Amer. Jour. Obst., 1918, lxxvii, 714. (10) Edinburgh Med. Jour., 1917, xix, 82.

483 BEACON STREET.

EXOPHTHALMIC GOITER AND PREGNANCY

By Israel Bram, M.D., Philadelphia, Pa.

THE clinical implications arising from a combination of exophthalmic goiter or Graves' disease and pregnancy in the same individual are noteworthy. The problem is important and often difficult, for upon its solution depends the life both of the patient and offspring. During the past decade the author has seen a considerable number of subjects of Graves' disease in whom pregnancy was a factor and believes that the topic permits of the several subdivisions briefly discussed in this paper.

ENGAGEMENT AND GRAVES' DISEASE

The state of "engagement" is commonly replete with moments of emotionalism in which the sexual instinct plays an important part.

In all females with Graves' disease, the sexual instinct and emotions must be suspected as partially or wholly an etiologic factor until the contrary can be reasonably proved. In each patient a careful sexual history should be obtained and all possible sexual factors taken into proper account. The nature of the probable underlying predisposition should also be ascertained if possible.

The unengaged girl must be considered apart from the girl already engaged. Her sexual thoughts and possible habits must receive the necessary attention of the clinical attendant and should be tactfully corrected. This task is a delicate one, often difficult and at times apparently impossible. It may be inadvisable for such a person to become engaged until such time as the Graves' disease is sufficiently improved to render her relatively safe for marriage to a compatible mate. Such a union should be preceded by a minimal engagement period.

On the other hand, the already engaged girl with Graves' disease is often an individual in whom engaged life plays an important etiologic rôle. Since the continuation of the engagement is usually detrimental, it must be discontinued by an immediate estrangement or by immediate marriage. If the young man involved appears temperamentally and sexually compatible, it is prudent to advise immediate marriage, with admonitions regarding the practical side of the married state, in accordance with prevailing indications. Marriage is especially commendable if the patient's condition indicates the existence of an active recuperative power, and if her fiancé has the physical and mental virtues qualifying him not only as a devoted husband but also as a sensible assistant to the medical attendant. Under such favorable conditions, marriage is usually followed by rapid improvement and ultimate recovery, often within a few months. This applies to the average, especially the early subject of the disease; but there are glaring exceptions to the above. In a patient whose vital

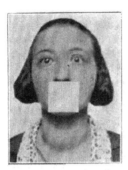

Fig. 1.—Exophthalmic goiter of one year's duration in a nonpregnant patient married thirteen months.

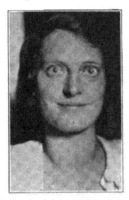

Fig. 2.—Exophthalmic goiter, the onset of which occurred three years ago following a narrow escape during an accident. Patient is married one year and is in the fifth month of pregnancy.

organs are too far degenerated to withstand a prospective pregnancy, it is preferable to face the danger of a broken engagement rather than the peril of marriage.

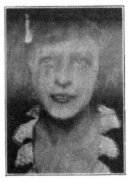

Fig. 3.—Exophthalmic goiter of six months' duration in a patient married one year. Syndrome appeared shortly after a miscarriage and curettement. Weight of patient 107 pounds; beginning exophthalmos and swelling of thyroid gland; heart rate 140; moderate gastrointestinal irritability and psychic disturbance.

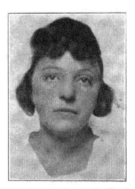

Fig. 4.—Same patient as in Fig. 3, after six months' nonsurgical treatment. Weight, 143 pounds; complete subjective and objective recovery.

FECUNDITY IN A SUBJECT OF GRAVES' DISEASE

In both sexes, in the presence of Graves' disease sterility is common, but not the rule. In the male who had not been sterile prior to the onset of the syndrome, I have observed an increased fecundity. Indeed, the sexual activity of the patient is at times increased to such a degree that it constitutes an important problem in treatment. Priapism may require especial therapeutic attention. The patient's moral sense may become all but eliminated, and gratification may be sought away from his own household. Sexual excitability increases the endocrine dysfunction, especially that of the thyroid; the latter seems in turn to increase the sexual excitability,—thus there is added another vicious circle to those already characterizing this affection.

In the female suffering with Graves' disease, though the libido may be normal or acute, there frequently occurs a degree of vaginismus and a dread of coitus. Often this status bears an etiologic relationship to Graves' disease. Here, also, the vicious circle obtains: ungratified desire leads to an aggravation of the syndrome of Graves' disease; the aggravated syndrome in turn leads to increased libido. In consequence of diminished frequency of coitus and because of the probable coexisting menstrual disturbances and ovarian hypofunction in these patients, there may be sterility in some instances and lessened fecundity in others, especially during the active stage of the disease. Many patients become pregnant, however, and when this occurs, other problems present themselves.

PREGNANCY AND GRAVES' DISEASE

Here, too, in an important percentage of cases pregnancy seems to have been the exciting cause of the affection. Omitting this phase of the question, I would state in general that pregnancy helps rather than hinders improvement where Graves' disease already exists. Especially is this true if the disease has not led to marked degeneration of the vital organs, and if the patient is under the care of a well equipped internist who understands the management of these subjects. A moderate aggravation of the syndrome, especially the thyroid swelling, may occur in pregnancy, to disappear shortly after delivery. On the other hand, the occurrence of pregnancy in a markedly advanced case of the disease is usually detrimental, as the vital organs are unable to cope with the increased demands made upon them. Sooner or later Nature either expels the uterine contents, or, if this does not occur, the physical condition may require a therapeutic abortion.

MISCARRIAGE IN GRAVES' DISEASE

It has been taught in some quarters that in this disease not only is sterility the rule, but that when pregnancy occurs, miscarriage is apt to result within the first few months. In my experience, sterility and miscarriage occur in the minority of these women. All things equal, the patient who miscarries is worse off than she who is delivered at term. The reasons are (1) *mental*, i.e., on the one hand, the unhappiness re-

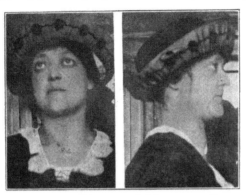

Figs. 5 and 6.—Five years ago, this patient applied for treatment of a very severe type of exophthalmic goiter of four years' duration, the onset of which occurred shortly after engagement to be married. After six months of nonsurgical treatment, patient was so improved as to render marriage safe. In the above pictures taken shortly after marriage, though all other symptoms have been eliminated, there is a still prevailing thyroid swelling and some exophthalmos, due to anatomic changes incident to the chronicity of the affection.

sulting from the loss of the fetus, especially if this be the first pregnancy, and on the other, the happiness and contentment of motherhood; and (2) *physical*, i.e., the disturbance of the endocrines, especially the

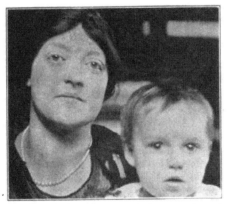

Fig. 7.—Same patient with normal child. There was a postpartum hemorrhage for which the obstetrician was prepared, and patient made an uneventful recovery. She feels better than ever in her life. There is a peculiar redundancy of skin over site of former thyroid swelling.

sexual organs and the thyroid during abortion, and the tendency toward adjustment or rectification of the internal secretions and the nervous system following normal delivery at term. I find that subjects of Graves' disease who have recently miscarried are comparatively more difficult to manage than those patients who have recently become mothers. The latter respond promptly to the treatment of the individualizing internist, if favorable personal and environmental cooperation prevails.

PARTURITION IN GRAVES' DISEASE

Parturition in a subject of Graves' disease is fraught with at least two problems. The first is that of straining with each pain. Bearing down not only adds to the undue strain of an overworked heart, but also increases the size and vascularity of the thyroid gland. In addition, the accompanying pain is a kind of shock which had preferably be avoided. I advise the obstetrician to employ his art in such manner as would obviate the necessity for bearing down, and suggest the use of a few whiffs of chloroform and whatever other measures may be deemed advisable at the time. The second problem is that of postpartum hemorrhage. The coagulation time of the blood in a subject of Graves' disease is delayed, in some instances to such an extent that the patient should be managed with the same degree of caution as is directed toward a subject of hemophilia. I suggest the use of prophylactic injections of "thromboplastin" or similar preparations during labor. It is essential also to be in readiness for packing the uterus after delivery of the placenta. Postpartum injections of pituitrin are harmless and frequently useful in this connection.

EFFECT OF THE MOTHER'S GRAVES' DISEASE ON THE INFANT

Theoretically, a child born of a mother with Graves' disease would be either predisposed to or afflicted with an endocrinopathy. In view of the fact that the average subject of Graves' disease presents a history in one or more members of the family of this disease, Raynaud's disease, angioneurotic edema, hay fever, bronchial asthma, hysteria, neurasthenia, and other affections involving the neuroendocrine system, it would seem that the offspring of such patients would be prone to these affections. However, my observation of a goodly number of these youngsters, some of whom are attending school, proves them to be enjoying the average good health, and a few are exceptionally robust. What puberty and adolescence have in store for them is to be seen; attempts at prophylaxis in these persons should be seriously considered.

There is one peculiar phenomenon which is noteworthy in this relation. Occasionally, *an infant born of a mother suffering with this affection may present congenital goiter with or without evidences of hypothyroidism or of cretinism.* Several observers have called attention to this occurrence, and I have seen three instances of this sort in the past few years. This should give the surgeon much food for thought, as it presents one of the most striking arguments against thyroidectomy in this affection. It seems strongly to indicate that the body requires all the thyroid substance which the thyroid gland can manufacture in order that toxins originating elsewhere in the body may be combated, and that the thyroid swelling in Graves' disease is a defensive reaction on the part of Nature in its efforts toward recovery.

EFFECT OF LACTATION ON THE COURSE OF GRAVES' DISEASE

Lactation is decidedly harmful to a subject of Graves' disease. The patient is already suffering with a high plus basal metabolism and further to drain the body of nutriment by lactation makes for greater loss in weight and aggravation of the disease. Lactation must be discouraged after the first week or two, and the baby should be fed by a wet nurse or placed on an artificial mixture as soon as possible. I have often seen a very miserable patient improve with surprising

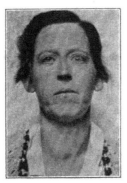

Fig. 8.—Exophthalmic goiter with unilatral exophthalmos; onset during pregnancy. Patient was nursing her six weeks' old baby when treatment was instituted. Heart rate 120.

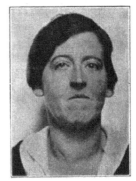

Fig. 9.—Same patient as Fig. 8 two months later, following cessation of lactation and institution of nonsurgical therapeutic measures. Eyes nearly normal, thyroid smaller, pulse is normal, and there is a gain of 20 pounds in weight. Patient is still under treatment and is rapidly approaching complete recovery.

rapidity very soon after breast feeding was discontinued. Moreover, the infant in taking the milk of such a mother, is receiving food contaminated with the toxins of Graves' disease. It is evident then, that such infants do far better away from the mother's breast.

REPEATED PREGNANCIES IN SUBJECTS OF GRAVES' DISEASE

Sufferers from Graves' disease as a rule do not become multiparae during the course of the affection, for reasons already implied above. When repeated pregnancies do occur, there is a tendency on the part of the thyroid toward hyposecretion. Such patients are especially prone to present a combination of hypo- and hyperthyroidism simultaneously, with a predominance of the former. Also, among such patients an occasional "burned out" thyroid is observed, in which the patient, evidently tending toward spontaneous recovery, is seen to overlap this point and soon takes on the clinical picture of a varying degree of myxedema. It is well for both endocrinologist and obstetrician to advise against repeated pregnancies in these patients. With regard to contraceptives, it must be borne in mind that considerable thought should be given the matter before final advice is offered the patient, lest great harm result from improper measures. This is a vital matter, and if carefully studied in advance will be of assistance in the ultimate restoration of our patient to health and happiness.

In conclusion, we must emphasize the fact that since no two cases of Graves' disease are alike, there is no standard management applicable to all patients of the type indicated in this discourse. Individualization must guide our course. The hereditary trends of the patient, her age, temperament, social stratum, financial resources, peculiarities and idiosyncrasies, the probable pathogenesis of the affection as well as its duration and severity,—all these must be taken into serious account and properly evaluated when the problem of pregnancy with its antecedents and sequences becomes a factor during the course of Graves' disease.

1431 SPRUCE STREET.

OBSERVATIONS ON THE DISTRIBUTION AND FUNCTION OF THE UTERINE CILIATED EPITHELIUM IN THE PIG, WITH REFERENCE TO CERTAIN CLINICAL HYPOTHESES

BY FRANKLIN F. SNYDER, B.S., AND GEORGE W. CORNER, M.D., BALTIMORE, MD.

From the Anatomical Laboratory of Johns Hopkins Medical School.

THE ciliated epithelium along the path of the ovum has long been a subject of interest as a possible factor in determining the movements and ultimate resting place of the ovum, and also because it has been believed to take part in the periodic changes of this pathway, such as those occurring during menstruation and estrus. The evidence has rested upon observations on the human and practically all the laboratory animals.

According to Mandl (1911) and Hoehne (1908), in the human uterus the cilia diminish in number before menstruation, vanish entirely during that period, and gradually reappear afterwards. In material from the human, examined *in vivo*, Mandl found no cilia during menstruation or on the second, third, and fourth days thereafter. He saw cilia again on the seventh day after menstruation and from 1 to 8 days preceding the next flow. Other evidence in agreement with this supposed absence of cilia during menstruation has been offered by F. Christ (1892), Bayer (1906), and Hitschmann and Adler (1908), while on the contrary Wendeler (1895), Moericke (1882), and Geist (1913) record finding cilia during menstruation.

Hitschmann and Adler (1908) in examining fixed material found cilia only sparsely or not at all in the uterine mucosa, though in the late interval and pre-menstrual periods frayed-out surfaces on some of the epithelial cells were described as resembling epithelium from which cilia had broken away. At the same time these cells had the appearance of secretory epithelium (Drüsenzellen). It is further stated that "in the pre-menstrual period, during which the ovum probably reaches the uterus, the cilia disappear at the onset or perhaps coincidently with the secretion. Thus it would appear that the further transport of the ovum is impeded and implantation favored."

Other evidence of secretory activity coincident with the loss of cilia rests (according to Mandl) upon Schaffer's observations in animals. In sections of the isthmus at times the latter found only glandular epithelium, at other times ciliated cells, and hence inferred the transformation of the latter into the former. In the human, Hoehne states that in pregnancy, disappearance of cilia from the cervix becomes evident, especially as the cervical canal becomes filled with secretory masses. And finally Mandl (1911), pointing out that during menstruation (at which time he found no cilia) a serous secretion is mingled with the hemorrhagic discharge, concludes that in the uterus secretory epithelium periodically develops where before it was ciliated, and vice versa.

With such possible variations in the activity of the ciliated epithelium in mind, explanation of various pathologic conditions has been attempted by several authors. In placenta previa, the abnormal site of implantation has been regarded by Hoehne (1911) as the result of an abnormal extensive ciliation which increases the strength of the ciliary current so as to sweep the ovum farther along toward the cervix than normally. That the influence of cilia in the transportation of the ovum may be a factor also, even before fertilization, was suggested by R. Jolly (1911), who stated that the closer to the uterine end of the tube the fertilization occurs, the farther along toward the cervix will the fertilized ovum be carried before it becomes developed sufficiently to be capable of implantation. Likewise, sterility may result from abnormal ciliation, as the ovum finds no resting place for implantation (Hoehne, 1911). In some recent observations regarding tubal pregnancy this author (1917) concludes that insufficiency of ciliation, either through inflammatory or developmental disturbances, is a factor among the mechanical obstructions by which he would account for implantation at an abnormal site.

In chronic hyperplastic conditions of the uterine mucosa, Hoehne (1911) has found that "the extent of the ciliated epithelium and the strength of the current is increased in proportion to the hyperplasia * * * and that cilia are present even during menstruation." Such observations included cases of profuse and long continued menses, myoma uteri, excessive bleeding after absorption, and pre-climacteric menorrhagia.

Among the lower animals, particularly swine, the presence of cilia in the uterus has been both affirmed and denied by various authors. Lott (1872), Storch (1892), Ellenberger and Gunther (1908), found cilia present, while Schmalz (1911), Keller (1909), and Beiling (1906) deny the presence of cilia on the surface epithelium, and Beiling doubts their occurrence even in the uterine glands. Mandl (1911) holds that there is a transitory ciliation. Having observed 39 animals, including 24 dogs, he states that the animal uterus is covered by a secretory cylindrical epithelium, which at times, though indeed but briefly, changes into a ciliated epithelium. It may be noted that this brief phase of ciliation in the lower animals stands in sharp contrast to the longer phase described by him in the human, since he believes that the mature human uterus is covered by ciliated epithelium during the greater part of its cycle and that the period when cilia are absent coincides with menstruation.

During estrus, both a diminution and an increase in cilia have been described, dependent upon the site. Stegu (1912) saw fewer cilia on the surface epithelium in the sow's uterus during heat, and just before and just after it, than at other times in the cycle. An increase in ciliation between the ovary and the ostium of the tube at the time of estrus, as a result of transformation of the squamous epithelium of the peritoneum to a ciliated cylindrical type, has been described by Morau (1892) in the sow, dog, cat and mouse.

PERSONAL OBSERVATIONS

In evaluating the data and hypotheses which have been reviewed, it may be pointed out that they have not always been based upon the fullest possible knowledge of the normal uterine cycles of the animals studied, or upon the full range of available technical methods. A satisfactory idea of the functions and possible pathologic relations of the uterine cilia must take into consideration the periodic alternations of structure and function in the reproductive tract; especially must the state of the cilia be correlated with the time of passage of the ovum. This of course is not yet possible in the human species, in which, moreover, many of the observations as to the presence of cilia have extended no further than sections of fixed material. Among the lower animals, while observation has been practically as extensive as the number of domesticated species permits, in no case has investigation of any one species been complete.

The following pages outline an attempt to carry out a complete study of the uterine ciliation in one species, throughout the cycle. For this purpose the domestic sow was chosen, on account of the abundance of material available, and also because of the fact that recent work on the reproductive cycle of this species makes it possible to select from the uteri obtained at the abattoir a series which shall be representative of all stages of the cycle, and to study these in the light of accurate knowledge of the time of ovulation and the wandering of the ova and embryos in this species.

The choice of material representative of the successive stages in the 21-day cycle of the sow was made, upon the basis of previous acquaintance with the events of the cycle, by inspection of the ovaries and by search of the fallopian tubes and uteri for ova, and was confirmed by microscopic study of sections of the corpora lutea and the uterine mucosa. The necessary data have been given in a monograph by one of the present authors (Corner, 1921 a) and need only brief mention here.

Thus, during the three days following ovulation there are freshly ruptured follicles (i.e., early corpora lutea) in the ovaries, and the ova may be recovered from the fallopian tubes. About the fourth day the ova pass into the uterus, whence they may be recovered by washing out the uterine canal. By the seventh day the corpora lutea are solid, and have reached a diameter of 9 mm. The microscopic picture is now that of full maturity. About the seventh or eighth day the ova disappear by degeneration within the uterine cavity, and thus the second week is characterized by the presence of fully matured corpora lutea in conjunction with the absence of ova from the tube and uterus. About the end of the second week the corpora lutea suddenly degenerate, as indicated by a beginning diminution in their size, by an increase in the firmness of their texture, and by a change of color from the flesh color of maturity to a yellowish tone. The microscope reveals degeneration of the granulosa lutein cells. During the latter part of the third week the new crop of Graafian follicles begins to exceed the resting stage of 4 to 5 mm. diameter, until finally they reach the mature diameter of 8 to 10 mm. Their rupture at the end of the third week marks the beginning of a new cycle. Figure 1 presents a graphic representation of the reproductive cycle as just described.

By the aid of these criteria, and by comparison with the characteristic cyclic histologic changes of the uterine mucosa, as illustrated in the above-mentioned monograph, it is possible to assign a given specimen of the internal genitalia of a sow to its correct place in the cycle, within a few days, and thus to collect any desired series of stages directly from abattoir material. The following list enumerates the specimens upon which our present observations are based:

First to 3rd day of pregnancy cycle, 4 specimens; 4th to 7th day, 5; 8th to 10th day, 4; 10th to 15th day, 3; 15th to 20th day, 2. Blastocysts in uterus, 1; embryos of 17-18 days, 2.

As soon as the specimens arrived at the laboratory, usually within an hour after killing, bits of the mucosa were snipped off and flattened down under a cover-slip, as Nylander had done in Leydig's laboratory in 1852 when he first discovered active cilia in the uterus of the pig. In such preparations from the tubes and uterus, cilia were always seen actively beating even under low powers of the microscope. Neither a

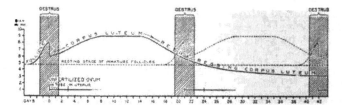

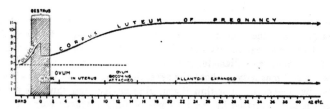

Fig. 1.—Diagram showing in graphic form the relations between estrus, ovulation, the development of the corpus luteum, and the progress of the ova in the sow.*
Above: events of the average cycle of 21 days in the nonpregnant sow.
Below: events of the first weeks of pregnancy.

warm chamber nor nutrient media were found necessary, for at ordinary room temperature, even without the addition of Locke's solution, the active cilia could be observed for several hours at least. This was true throughout all phases of the cycle as well as during pregnancy. In the specimens from the uterus, however, cilia were never seen on the surface, but only in glands opening upon it, where the ciliated cells comprise perhaps one-fourth of all the epithelium. Significant variations in number and activity of the cilia were never observed.

In the sections of fixed material from the same uteri which were

---

*This and the following illustrations are taken from an article by G. W. Corner on "Cyclic Changes in the Ovaries and Uterus of the Sow, and Their Relation to the Mechanism of Implantation." (Carnegie Institute of Washington, Publ. No. 276.)

examined in the fresh condition, cilia were always found readily in the glands (Figure 2). In addition, the confusion of Beiling (1906), Stegu (1912) and others as to the irregular or frayed-out surfaces of many of the cells of the superficial epithelium, suggesting loss of cilia or even secretory activity, became more intelligible. The accompanying

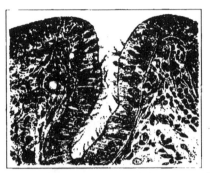

Fig. 2.—Neck of a uterine gland showing presence of cilia on the gland-cells and their absence from the surface cells, x300.

Figures (3, 4, and 5), taken from the paper of Corner (1921 a) demonstrate that during the phase of estrus (Figure 3) and the postestrus development of the uterine mucosa (Figure 4) the surface epithelial cells present smooth borders. During the stage of the 10th to the 15th

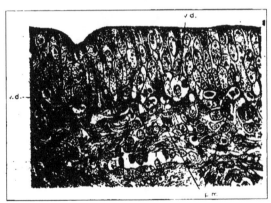

Fig. 3.—The uterine epithelium during estrus, x600.

day after ovulation, however, (at which time the embryos, if present, are becoming attached) the epithelial cells undergo a remarkable alteration of surface by the production of cytoplasmic processes, as illustrated (Figure 5). These processes occur, of course, on the same cells which a few days before have given appearances of a secretory function (Figure 4); they have nothing in common with ciliation, as evidenced above all by the absence of basal granules. We suppose that this surface roughening serves to facilitate attachment of the embryos. Similar processes can be observed in the living tissue in somewhat less detail; and they have also been clearly described in the human uterus and differentiated from the cilia by Geist (1913). There seems to be

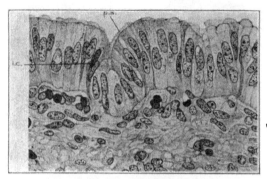

Fig. 4.—The uterine epithelium during the stage of 8 to 10 days after ovulation, x600.

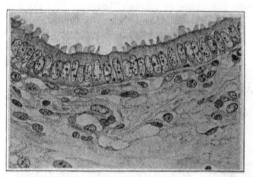

Fig. 5.—The uterine epithelium during the stage of 10 to 15 days after ovulation, x600.

no doubt that such appearances as these have helped to bring about the confusing disagreement as to the uterine cilia.

DISCUSSION

From the foregoing observations on the uterus of the pig it may be concluded that no cilia are present, at any period of the estrous cycle, on the cells of the surface epithelium. In the glands of the uterine mucosa, however, the cilia are always present and appear to be equally active and numerous at all periods of the cycle. Previous statements disagreeing with these conclusions are probably explainable, as we have seen, by the occurrence of histologic changes in the superficial epithelial cells, somewhat resembling ciliation.

In the uterus of the pig at least, the cilia thus seem less important for transport of the ova than has frequently been supposed in regard to many animals, as for instance in man where (as expressed by Grosser) "the chief driving power in the wandering of the ovum, in the uterus as well as in the tube, is the ciliary current." With regard to the uterus, we are led to the same viewpoint which Sobotta (1916) has taken as to the forces which carry the ova through the fallopian tube of the rodents.

The occurrence of cilia at all times throughout the cycle and not only during the few days in which ova are present, suggests that the ciliation of the uterus is adapted to other functions beside the transport of the ovum. In fact, as shown by the studies of Corner (1921 b) on internal migration of the ovum, when there is an excess number of unimplanted embryos in one cornu of the sow's uterus, some of the embryos usually pass into the opposite cornu, frequently traversing a considerable distance down one cornu and up the other before reaching the site of implantation. Thus, whatever be the direction of any currents produced by the uterine cilia, early embryos can certainly be transported against them. The presence of the cilia through all stages of the cycle hints at the possibility that among their functions is that of producing a current to carry away cellular debris or perhaps secretory products of the mucosa, or to guard against the upward passage of infectious microörganisms.

This evidence from the pig's uterus, therefore, indicates that it is at present unsafe to erect etiological hypotheses upon supposed cyclic alternations in number, activity or secretory state of the uterine ciliated epithelial cells, or even to regard them as of prime and sole importance for the transportation of ova into the uterine cavity.

SUMMARY

1. In the pig's uterus, cilia are not present on the surface epithelium at any stage of the estrous cycle; but in the uterine glands they are always present, without obvious fluctuation in number or activity.

2. There is no evidence for an alternation of ciliated and secretory (nonciliated) phases in individual cells of the uterine epithelium of the sow.

3. Upon the basis of this and other facts which have been cited it would seem that transportation of the ova and embryos is not necessarily the prime function of the uterine cilia.

4. It is suggested that various hypotheses explaining pathologic states of menstruation and of implantation by supposed variations of the uterine cilia are not sufficiently supported by complete knowledge of the cyclic changes of the uterine mucosa.

REFERENCES

Bayer, H.: 1906. Die Menstruation in ihrer Beziehung zur Conceptionsfähigkeit. Strassburg. Beiling, K.: 1906. Arch. f. mikr. Anatomie, lxvii, 573-637. Christ, F.: 1892. Das Verhalten der Uterusschleimhaut während Menstruation. Inaug. Diss. Giessen. Corner, G. W.: 1921, a. Publications of the Carnegie Institution of Washington, No. 276 (Contributions to Embryology, No. 64) pp. 117-146. Ibid.: 1921, b. Johns Hopkins Hosp. Bull., xxxii, 78-83. Ellenberger, W., and Gunther, G.: Grundriss der vergleichenden Histologie der Haussäugetiere, 1908. Geist, S. H.: 1913. Arch, f. mikr. Anatomie, lxxxi, 196-219. Grosser, O.: 1919. Arch. f. Gynäk., cx, 297-327. Hitschmann, F., and Adler, L.: 1908. Monatschr. f. Geburtsh. u. Gynäk., xxvii, 1-82. Hoehne, O.: 1908. Zentralbl. f. Gynäk., xxxii, 119-125. Ibid.: 1911. Zentralbl. f. Gynäk. xxxv, 340-343. Ibid.: 1917. Arch. f. Gynäk., cvii, 73-104. Jolly, R.: 1911. Arch. f. Gynäk., xciii, 69-86. Keller, K.: 1909. Anat. Hefte., xxxix, 309-391. Leydig, F.: 1852. Arch. f. Anat. u. Physiol., 375-378. Lott, G.: 1872. Zur Anatomie und Physiologie des Cervix Uteri. Erlangen. Mandl, L.: 1908. Ueber das Epithel im geschlechtsreifen Uterus. Zentralbl. f. Gynäk., xxxii, 425-429. Ibid.: 1911. Monatschr. f. Geburtsh. u. Gynäk., xxxiv, 150-159. Möricke, R.: 1882. Ztschr. f. Geburtsh. u. Gynäk., vii, 84-137. Morau, H.: 1892. Nouvelles Archives d'Obstetrique et de Gynec., 7, 422-427. Schaffer, J.: 1908. Monatschr. f. Geburtsh. u. Gynäk., xxviii, 526-542, 666-688. Schmaltz, E.: 1911. Die Struktur der Geschlechtsorgane des Haussäugetiere, Berlin. Sobotta, J.: 1916. Anat. Hefte., xliv, 361-444. Stegu, J.: 1912. Oesterreichische Wochenschr. f. Tierheilk., xxxvii, 399-400, 409-411, 419-421, 431-433, 442-443. Storch: 1892. Oesterr. Wchnschr. f. Tierh. (quoted by Mandl, 1911.) Wendeler, P.: 1895. Ztschr. f. Geburtsh. u. Gynäk., xxxii, 316-319.

THE RELATIONSHIP BETWEEN TOXEMIA OF PREGNANCY AND UTERINE SEPSIS FROM A STUDY OF 400 TOXEMIC CASES

By Foster S. Kellogg, M.D., Boston, Mass.

Assistant in Obstetrics, Harvard Medical School; Physician to Out Patients, Boston Lying-in Hospital

WHEN this paper was originally read before the Obstetrical Society of Boston, February 24, 1920, I prefaced it with certain observations regarding toxemia of pregnancy and uterine sepsis calculated to show my audience the temper in which I had approached the study of the subject. These observations were in effect that toxemia of pregnancy and uterine sepsis were the two most interesting and baffling problems in obstetrics today. I stated that we know little or nothing new about toxemia of pregnancy of clinical value; that we have run a circle for many years in its treatment, favoring methods of elimination; that in toxemia with convulsions we have no ground for a prognosis even; that in spite of the best of watching toxemia does occur; that in the majority of cases that die we do not know the exact cause of death. I recalled two cases recently observed, one a woman with eight or nine convulsions on whom I did a difficult vaginal cesarean section. She was in coma before and for some time after delivery, and made a good recovery. The other, the next day, was also in coma, having had one convulsion and a normal delivery, and died two hours after I had given a fair prognosis. I said that in no respect did these women differ so far as medical clinical observation went, yet one died and the other recovered. Even supposing at autopsy there was a difference, we cannot make our autopsy before the patient dies, and clinically we are at a loss for an intelligent prognosis.

I said that toxemia with convulsions occurs once in each seventy admissions at the Boston Lying-in Hospital, and that the mortality there for the last seven and one-half years was twenty-five per cent. I then read this quotation from a report of a physician in Texas who, after treating three cases of toxemia with chloroform and some alleged kidney stimulant, concludes that: "while toxemia may occur very rarely in cases who are having urine examinations, death never need occur if the case is properly treated," *vide supra*.

I then said that uterine sepsis was interesting also because we knew so little about it; especially that we knew nothing more of hospital sepsis in obstetrics, and its manner of spreading, than was known at the time of Holmes and Semmelweiss; in fact by many hospitals doing maternity work sepsis was held not to exist at all in modern times. I quoted from the report of another physician from Texas who reached the conclusion, after I know not how much experience, that uterine sepsis is always due to the operator or his assistants at the time of delivery, and that all uterine sepsis is therefore unnecessary. I said also that uterine sepsis is morbidly interesting to me because it had been the subject of so many fantastic lies in my experience. I then observed that whereas the matter of whether an individual physician called a given case, running a temperature a few days after childbirth, milk fever, or constipation, or blood poisoning, or uterine sepsis was a matter of individual conscience, and in a way, perhaps, salesmanship, and was for each man to justify for himself; but that, when we found a high percentage of temperatures running in a maternity hospital, or in the maternity part of a general hospital, we and the public then have the right to expect that this epidemic should be designated hospital sepsis. In the light of our present lack of knowledge regarding the spread of this, or often of the initial focus of infection, we have the right to expect that this or that given hospital shall shut its doors to further obstetrical patients until with lack of material, and cleanliness in all its forms, the epidemic shall have run its course. The reason is that it is safer, if less comfortable, to have a baby in the gutter than in an infected hospital.

I said further that I had seen in some detail five such epidemics of variable extent, in eight years, and in only one was the institution closed, and in that one alone were no lives lost. I said that the reason that this was not done in the others was either through ignorance on the part of lay boards of trustees or doctors (usually surgeons) in charge, or fear by them of admitting that hospital sepsis still existed in the community, or an unwillingness to accept financial loss due to closure. I said that the reason boards and doctors in charge were afraid to shut up was not only that "the public is not sufficiently educated in clean obstetrics," as is so often said and is true, but also that *the public is uneducated regarding uterine sepsis*. While much sepsis is due to dirty obstetrics, much also is due to other things. Evidence is accumulating all the time that autoinfection, especially in cases of difficult delivery, due to unavoidable causes, is a cause; for bacteriologic investigation has shown that the vagina in a certain percentage of pregnant women contains pathogenic organisms. Evidence also accumulates that a certain number of infections are respiratory in origin, or tonsillar; occasionally a uterine sepsis seems traceable to a tooth as much as some pyelitis cases. The accumulation of evidence regarding the mutability of strain of streptococci, etc., all tend to confirm the fact that a certain variable percentage of uterine sepsis is due to other causes than dirty obstetrics.

It is frequently said, and I think generally considered, that a patient with toxemia of pregnancy is more susceptible to infection than a patient normally pregnant. I have said, and heard other obstetricians say, that such and such a patient is septic because she was toxemic, meaning that the toxemia had reduced her resistance to infection so that she became septic when she otherwise would not have done so; or that she was not handling the sepsis well and was severely sick with it on account of her toxemia, when if she had not been toxic she would presumably have had only a mild sepsis. We mean that the toxemia is a large contributing factor in the sepsis.

Williams, *Obstetrics*, Second Edition, page 554, says: "In view of the marked liability of eclamptic women to infection, all operative measures must be conducted in the most rigidly aseptic manner, particular care being taken to avoid the contamination of the vagina and the hands of the operator by fecal material."

A further study of the text book literature in regard to this matter reveals that there is nothing on the subject in the *Year Books of Obstetrics* from 1916 to 1919; nothing in Reynolds and Newell's *Practical Obstetrics*, and nothing in *The Practice of Obstetrics* by Cragin. In the English Berkeley and Bonney, Second Edition, under "Sequelae of Eclampsis" is stated: "Patients who have had eclampsia are liable to the further complications of puerperal insanity, *puerperal fever* on account of operative manipulations, etc.," and later, speaking of operative evacuation of the uterus in eclampsia: "In our opinion the abdominal route is best as being quicker, easier, and more *aseptic*." (italics mine.)

De Lee, First Edition, 1913, page 355, after describing the series of convulsions of the typical eclamptic as accompanied or followed by fever, says: "A recrudescence of the fever usually means that sepsis is starting." On the other hand, "If the woman is going to die, the attacks usually increase in frequency and force; the temperature goes up to 103°, sometimes to 107°, or it sinks; the pulse increases, becoming weak and running." As a rule the case ends one way or another in three days. On page 361, "Infection is a common cause of death and eclamptics (he uses the term here for toxemics without as well as with convulsions if they have all the symptoms without the fits) show a decided susceptibility to it. Sepsis is common and usually runs a severe course since the liver and kidneys are already diseased." Speaking of abdominal cesarean section in eclampsia he says: "Sepsis is much more common." Again, "During the delivery of eclamptics extraordinary precautions against sepsis must be observed because they are particularly liable to infection, the liver and kidneys being thrown out of immunizing action. In spite of the most rigid precautions the author has seen fatal infection arise. One source of trouble is feces streaming from the anus, the result of the administration of cathartics and enemata before delivery. This danger is so great that the author withholds such practice until after the uterus is emptied. If the field of operation is constantly soiled by discharges from the rectum, the anus should be closed by a circular suture, *which is to be removed just before the child is delivered.*"

It will thus be seen that textbooks, where they have anything to say on the subject, back up our stated belief either directly or by implication, that toxemia of pregnancy is a contributing cause of puerperal sepsis.

My own experience has borne this out, both in my personal and consultation practice. More dissatisfied with this single feature of my work than any other, I chose two hundred consecutive cases of my own, in which the records were good, to see what the relationship was between toxemia of pregnancy and uterine sepsis.

Briefly analyzed the results were as follows: In 167 there was no sepsis and no toxemia except of a mild sort which readily yielded to medical treatment. There were present slight traces of albumin or elevated blood pressure which was either moderate in amount, or yielded quickly. There were fifteen cases of sepsis in nontoxic patients (it is to be remembered that these cases include consultation and delivery by other men as well as by myself). There were nine cases of toxemia unaccompanied by sepsis. There were nine cases of sepsis and toxemia. By percentage: 83.5 per cent were free from both sepsis and toxemia; 16.5 per cent were either toxic or showed sepsis; about 7 per cent showed sepsis unaccompanied by toxemia; and about 8 per cent were toxic, 50 per cent of which were septic. It will be seen by these figures that whereas the rate of sepsis in all cases not toxic was one in eleven, the rate of sepsis in toxic cases was one in two. Of the twenty-four septic cases, 38 per cent were toxic.

It would have been more desirable in this accumulation of data to have used only cases in my own practice where the percentage of normal sepsis would, of course, have been much lower than the cases of other men calling me in consultation, because I only saw from their practice cases which had gone wrong. This is somewhat balanced, however, by the fact that as a rule I saw the severe toxemias, at least, in the practice of the same men, and sufficient data was available only in this way. Having established the fact that the ratio of uterine sepsis in severe toxemias that I had seen was one in every two cases, as against one in every eleven cases that were not toxic, (irrespective of method of delivery) I determined to go through as many records of toxemias of pregnancy as possible, and by using a large control of nontoxemic records, establish the relative percentage of sepsis in toxemics and nontoxemics. Furthermore, I determined to attempt to settle finally whether toxemia of pregnancy does lower resistance to sepsis, and to what extent; and by comparison to demonstrate whether or not my results were worse than they should be. The purpose of a large series is to obtain both in the toxemic series and the nontoxemic control series, including enough cases delivered in the same manner so that we can throw out the method of delivery by checking one against the other, and have our comparison direct.

The series studied from the Lying-in Hospital records of 7,326 cases of admission are from April 20, 1912, to January 21, 1920—seven years and nine months. The reason for stopping abruptly at this time was that a severe epidemic of hospital sepsis ended on the earlier date, and it was felt that it was better to avoid these records in which there would be an undue amount of sepsis irrespective of toxemia.

During the period there were 7,326 admissions, which included 400 toxemias with or without convulsions; 103 with convulsions; 297 without convulsions. There was one toxemia with or without convulsions in each eighteen admissions, about 5 per cent. There was one toxemic with convulsions in every 71 admissions, or about 1.5 per cent. Toxemia without convulsions represents one case in every twenty-five hospital admissions, 4 per cent. Of the 103 with convulsions 27 died, a mortality of about 25 per cent. Of the 27 cases with convulsions that died, 23 cases died within thirty-six hours of entrance. Of these 23 cases, 20 died without further diagnosis than of "eclampsia." The other three complications were separated placenta, postpartum hemorrhage, antepartum pneumonia. Of the cases that died more than thirty-six hours after delivery, three in number, one died of terminal bronchopneumonia plus the toxemia, on the fifth day; and two of definite sepsis,—one a streptococcus septicemia, on the ninth day, and one a pulmonary embolism following uterine sepsis, on the fifteenth day. In the series of fatal toxemias with convulsions 9 per cent died of uterine sepsis; 83 per cent died of eclampsia without further diagnosis and within thirty-six hours of entrance. Of the series of 103 toxemias with convulsions, 27 died, reducing the number to 76, from which it is possible to study the question of sepsis. In one of these seventy-six the diagnosis is not certain and is therefore omitted.

The question of what constitutes sepsis is one capable of different interpretation, but for the purposes of this paper we have divided all cases in this respect into three groups: one called the Normal Temperature Group, in which the temperature never rose above 99° during the puerperium; two, the Group of Slight Elevation in which, though the temperature is elevated for one or more days, there is no evidence either in the lochia, the involution and feel of the uterus or lower quadrants, and no evidence on the discharge examination that uterine or pelvic infection is or has been present. In this group also, for the purposes of the paper, I include temperatures due to breasts, and one or two certain cases of gonorrheal salpingitis. In group three, cases in which there was definite evidence of uterine infection.

The result of study of these seventy-five cases of toxemia of pregnancy and convulsions which did not die showed that seventeen cases ran absolutely normal temperatures; thirty-nine cases showed slight elevation; nineteen cases were definitely septic. Roughly, 25 per cent were septic; 20 per cent ran normal temperatures throughout and 55 per cent showed slight elevation of temperature. If we include the cases that died, we find that in the whole series, 103 cases of toxemia with convulsions, something over 20 per cent, were definitely septic. If there is any error in these figures, it is on the side of conservatism, because, as my own records have shown, a certain number of cases running low degrees of temperature end with an enlarged tender tube which proves that they did have some degree of sepsis.

The series of 297 toxemias without convulsions, admitted to the hospital, is reduced in number by ten that were discharged against advice; seven that are thrown out by questionable diagnosis, usually the question of chronic nephritis, (all definite chronic kidney or cardiorenal cases were omitted in the beginning); and fifty-four that were discharged relieved before delivery. In addition to these, fifteen had no toxic symptoms at the time of delivery, but were delivered before leaving the hospital. *These figures show that of the toxemias without convulsions about 18 to 20 per cent improved enough under medical treatment to be discharged relieved, and about 25 per cent improved so that they were able to leave the hospital, or were symptom-free at the time of delivery.*

These figures reduce the series left for consideration regarding the question of sepsis and temperatures to 222. Of these 222, thirty were definitely septic, about 14 per cent. Fifty-three per cent showed slight elevation of temperature and 34 per cent showed normal temperature throughout.

Five cases died in the series of 222 toxemics without convulsions, giving a mortality of about 2.5 per cent. Only one of these five died of sepsis, a mortality from sepsis of less than 0.5 per cent in the series without convulsions, as opposed to a mortality of 9 per cent in the series with convulsions. The causes of death in this series, other than sepsis, were one necrosis of the liver, one bronchial pneumonia, one separated placenta, one ruptured uterus from delivery.

A study of 2200 unselected control cases taken from the records in sequence showed: normal temperature 44.5 per cent; slight elevation 53 per cent; septic 2.5 per cent. Table I shows the relative degree of sepsis in nontoxemics, in toxemics without convulsions, and in toxemics with convulsions, irrespective of method of delivery, as in Table I.

TABLE I

	NORMAL TEMP.	SLIGHTLY ELEVATED TEMP.	SEPSIS
Nontoxemics	45%	53%	2.5%
Toxemics Without Convulsions	34%	53%	14.0%
Toxemics With Convulsions	20%	55%	25.0%

It is interesting to note that the "Slightly Elevated Temperature" series is practically constant.

We now come to the more difficult task of checking up the above facts which are established *irrespective of method of delivery*, by studying the methods of delivery in each series in order to show the relative risk of sepsis in toxemics in delivery by the same method. I have divided methods of delivery into six headings as follows:

1. Normal delivery and low forceps after natural dilatation. 2. Bag dilatation in which the bag alone brings full dilatation, with any other form of delivery. 3. High forceps, breech extraction, and version after natural full dilatation. 4. Manual dilatation, with or without bag, followed by any method of extraction. 5. Vaginal cesarean. 6. Abdominal cesarean.

The numbers at the top of the accompanying tables indicate these different methods of delivery.

Table II demonstrates: (1) that in toxemics with and without convulsions normal deliveries and low forceps are about one-half as frequent as in all other cases; (2) that the Voorhees bag is used nine times as often in toxemics as in all other unselected cases; (3) that high forceps and version are twice as common in toxemics as in all other unselected cases; that some form of accouchement forcé is fifty times as common in toxemics as in other unselected cases; and that vaginal cesarean is used in toxemics very much oftener, while abdominal cesarean is slightly less frequent in toxemics than in all other

TABLE II
METHODS OF DELIVERY IN THE THREE SERIES

	1	2	3	4	5	6
Control Nontoxemics	86%	3%	4%	0.1%	0.1%	6%
Toxemias With Convulsions	40%	28%	7%	5.0%	5.0%	5%
Toxemias Without Convulsions	50%	20%	8%	5.0%	2.0%	3%
Toxemias With Convulsions That Died	40%	12%	0%	12.0%	8.0%	8%

unselected cases. It also demonstrates that when we are forced to accouchement forcé or abdominal cesarean, the mortality is higher than by other methods of operative delivery not *necessarily* from the form of delivery, but from the severity of the toxemia, since 46 per cent of the toxemias with convulsions that died were normal deliveries or low forceps.

It now becomes necessary to attempt some study of the rate of sepsis in these series according to *method* of delivery.

Table III shows in detail the amount of sepsis in the toxemics with *convulsions* that lived, according to method of delivery.

TABLE III

METHOD OF DELIVERY	1	2	3	4	5	6
Sepsis	7	3	0	5	2	1
Sl. El. Temp.	12	10	2	1	1	2
Normal Temp.	6	5	2	3	0	9
	25 cases	18 cases	4 cases	9 cases	3 cases	12 cases
Sepsis	38%	16%	0	55%	66%	25%

This table demonstrates that of the toxemics with convulsions that lived, 38 per cent of the normal deliveries and low forceps were septic; no cases in which the bag was used were septic; 55 per cent of some form of accouchement forcé were septic; 66 per cent of the vaginal cesareans and 25 per cent of the abdominal cesareans were septic. Of all sepsis in the series 38 per cent were normal deliveries; 27 per cent were some form of accouchement forcé; 11 per cent were vaginal cesareans; 5 per cent were abdominal cesareans.

Table IV shows in detail the percentage of sepsis in the toxemics without convulsions, and for comparison, the amount in cases with convulsions, according to method of delivery.

This demonstrates that sepsis is four times as common in normal deliveries and low forceps if the patient has had convulsions than if she has not: that allowing for the greater immediate mortality it is

TABLE IV

METHOD OF DELIVERY	1	2	3	4	5	6
Septic Without Convulsions	9%	21%	16%	9%	50%	35%
Comparison:—Cases With Convulsions allow 20 per cent Higher Mortality	38%	16%	0%	55%	66%	25%

still higher: that in any form of accouchement forcé it is very much higher in those who have had convulsions: that making this same allowance, it is higher in vaginal and abdominal cesarean sections and very high in these methods whether the patient has or has not had convulsions: that with other methods of delivery it is approximately the same.

Table V shows amount of sepsis in toxemics with and without convulsions according to method of delivery in detail showing number of cases:

TABLE V

METHOD OF DELIVERY	1	2	3	4	5	6
Sepsis	19	12	3	6	4	4
Sl. El. Temperature	12	31	12	12	3	6
Normal Temperature	59	24	7	5	0	1
No. of Cases	150	77	22	23	7	11
Per Cent of Sepsis	13%	16%	13%	20%	57%	36%

Table VI shows method of delivery in control series by per cent; rate of sepsis according to method of delivery in control, compared with rate of sepsis according to method of delivery in toxemics.

TABLE VI

	1	2	3	4	5	6
METHOD OF DELIVERY IN CONTROL SERIES	85%	3%	4%	.1%	.1%	7.5%
Rate of Sepsis Control	2.5%	4%	2%			13%
All Toxemics Rate of Sepsis	13.0%	16%	13%	26%	57%	36%
Toxemics With Convulsions allowing 20% higher mortality	38.0%	10%	0%	55%	66%	25%
Toxemics Without Convulsions	9.0%	21%	16%	9%	50%	35%

This table demonstrates that by similar methods of delivery, a toxemic with or without convulsions is five times as likely to be septic as a nontoxemic, unselected, if she has a normal delivery or low forceps; four times as likely if she has a bag delivery; six times as likely if she has a high forceps or version; very much more likely if she has an accouchement forcé or vaginal cesarean section; and about three times as likely if she has an abdominal cesarean.

Roughly all toxemics are *four* to *five* times as likely to become septic as nontoxemics, unselected, with similar methods of delivery.

Toxemics with convulsions that survive are *fifteen* times more likely to become septic with normal delivery or low forceps, than nontoxemics unselected. Toxemics without convulsions are three to four times as likely to go septic with normal delivery or low forceps as nontoxemics unselected.

It is of course as obvious to the writer as to the reader that these figures are not absolute, especially in the series with a few cases; but they are suggestive, particularly in the group of normal delivery and low forceps, the bag and the abdominal cesarean section series, which are not small.

The normal delivery, bag and abdominal cesarean section series are shown in Table VII repeated for simplicity.

TABLE VII

	NOR. DEL.	LOW FORCEPS	BAG		ABDOMINAL CESAREAN	
Control	2.5%	Sepsis	4%	Sepsis	13%	Sepsis
Toxemics With and Without Convulsions	13.0%	"	16%	"	36%	"
Toxemics With Convulsions	38.0%	"	16%	"	25%	"
Toxemics Without Convulsions	9.0%	"	21%	"	35%	"

SUMMARY

1. "Eclampsia" is not a "self-limited disease" except in the sense that "all things end in death" and so are self-limited. If 25 per cent of our eclamptics die, these usually coming to us moribund with the head on the perineum, the limit is somewhat too early for the patient's good. Whether treatment is active medical, or active surgical, or active both, it is always active and the term self-limited as applied to "eclampsia" should be dropped, for psychologically it leads to too much watchful waiting on the part of the general practitioner. Toxemic symptoms call for something to be done when discovered, be it medical or surgical. Some cases of everything get well if watched and let alone, but this should be forgotten in toxemia of pregnancy.

2. The mortality of toxemia with convulsions in hospital practice is 25 per cent; 90 per cent of these die within thirty-six hours of eclampsia,—whatever that is. It is, therefore, one of the most dangerous diseases from which people recover.

3. The mortality in hospital practice of toxemia without convulsions is 2.5 per cent which shows that best hospital care for these cases is none too good.

4. Uterine sepsis is responsible for 9 per cent of deaths of toxemias with convulsions that survive.

5. Uterine sepsis in toxemics without convulsions and in the nonseptic control show the same percentage mortality—0.5 per cent, but uterine sepsis is responsible for more deaths in toxemics than in nontoxemics because it is more frequent.

6. Two and five-tenths per cent of nontoxemics unselected become septic, 14.0 per cent of toxemics without convulsions become septic, 25.0 per cent of toxemics with convulsions become septic, *irrespective of method of delivery.*

7. Toxemics are about four times as likely to become septic *under similar methods of delivery* as nontoxemics, unselected. If they have convulsions, more; if without, slightly less. They are more likely to have difficult operative deliveries with a higher septic rate.

8. That these figures establish that toxemics are very prone to sepsis; that the quotation from De Lee regarding withholding salts until after delivery, or closing off the rectum if the patient has been under medical treatment and delivery is forced in the midst of it, is worthy of more attention than in general is given it.

9. That though we must be very cautious in applying these figures to methods of delivery, since sepsis is only one element in the situation, and the series of vaginal and abdominal cesareans studied here is very small, it speaks for normal labor or low forceps, and the Voorhees bag, and delivery from below after full dilatation, as against vaginal or abdominal cesarean. But certain cases are only deliverable by these methods. I, personally, believe at the present time that no toxemic with or without convulsions *making progress in dilatation,* either by her own pains, or with a Voorhees bag, should be operated to hasten the delivery, even in the presence of impending convulsions, or increasing symptoms, because of the increased danger of sepsis. I also personally believe now that a cutting operation, vaginal or abdominal cesarean, as the case may call for, should be done only in cases in which preliminary observations show an unwillingness of that cervix to dilate readily enough to take a large bag. With this exception, I think that bag induction—failing to start labor with catharsis—and allowing the patient if possible to deliver herself, or at least dilate herself fully and come to low forceps, is the choice of procedure in all toxemics with and without convulsions, controlling the convulsions as much as possible with morphia, and in selected cases in which repetition of convulsions is more to be feared than excessive hemorrhage afterwards, with blood letting. I do not believe that the amount of time saved by hurried, difficult operating through the undilated cervix is worth the risk of immediate shock and subsequent sepsis.

This conclusion should be qualified by stating emphatically that when an introduced bag fails to work, it should be removed and delivery completed in the most appropriate way, which may be either vaginal cesarean section, or completing dilatation manually.

10. We frequently hear that hospital figures do not apply in private practice; but in the relationship of toxemia to uterine sepsis, nothing in my own work or in what I know of the work of others leads me to believe that these hospital figures are worse than private and consultation figures. That they are worse than the careful specialist's own private work is not on account of any difference in the relationship of toxemia and uterine sepsis; but because he has learned the real danger of toxemia of pregnancy, and dallies not at all with these cases. It is this point of view which all practitioners of obstetrics should get, namely, that symptoms of toxemia of pregnancy call for quick action and good judgment.

19 BAY STATE ROAD.

LITHOPEDION FORMATION IN EXTRAUTERINE FETAL MASSES

BY RIGNEY D'AUNOY, M.D., AND E. L. KING, M.D., NEW ORLEANS, LA.

(From the Department of Pathology, Tulane University, New Orleans, La.)

IN EXTRAUTERINE gestation the greater number of embryos are destroyed during the first few weeks of growth. Mall[1] after an exhaustive study of extrauterine pregnancy, says that in tubal implantation most ova are destroyed by the hemorrhage superinduced for their own nourishment. He states that in some few cases the trophoblastic dam is sufficient to check this hemorrhage and that enough villi remain to nourish the ovum. If rupture of a gravid tube occurs on the free side, the embryo is thrown into the peritoneal cavity and its career usually terminated. If, on the other hand, the tube ruptures into the broad ligament, the outlook for continued embryonic life is good, as here considerable surface exists for implantation and resultant proper embryonic nourishment.

Mall's study showed that more tubes containing normal embryos rupture than do tubes containing pathologic ones. According to Schumann[2] 3.3 per cent of normal embryos implanted in tubes go on to full term, 10.5 per cent become pathologic and die, 2.2 per cent become monsters, the remainder undergoing absorption. Von Winckel[3] believes that one-half the fetuses in ectopic gestations are deformed. In eighty-seven collected cases, he found fifty-seven malformations, with twelve monsters. Cragin's[4] case of full term ectopic pregnancy, though mentally normal, showed some asymmetry of the head in addition to a congenital dislocation of the hip and an umbilical hernia. That such deformities are due to pressure has been suggested by Ballantyne.[5] Undoubtedly nutritional deficiencies induced by faulty placentation have considerable influence on such developmental abnormalities.

Many extrauterine fetuses go on to full development and by appropriate surgical interference can be removed. Schumann[2] mentions fifty such cases. When such interference is not carried out the fetus necessarily dies, and if the dead fetus is not then removed it must undergo one of several terminal changes. These changes are skeletonization, adipocere, suppuration and lithopedion formation.

Skeletonization occurs when disintegration and absorption of soft parts has taken place, with a result that only the bony parts remain to represent the fetal mass.

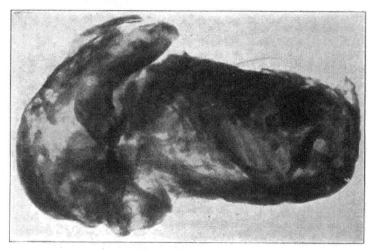

Fig. 1.—X-ray showing skeletal elements.

Adipocere consists in the apparent replacement of muscles and soft parts by a mass made up of a mixture of fatty acids, soaps and salts of palmitic and stearic acids. Such a product is resistant to putrefaction and will remain intact for many years.

The advent of suppuration naturally indicates the entrance of microorganisms. These, usually of the colon group, enter the sac wall by penetration from the intestines. From the sac wall the invading organisms spread to the fetus, setting up a low grade inflammation. As further changes, the fetal soft parts may undergo liquefaction necrosis; the bony parts may injure various internal organs and set up a peritonitis, or as is most usual a pelvic abscess may develop, with eventual discharge through vagina or rectum.

Lithopedion formation as the termination of a tubal or abdominal pregnancy takes place when the dead fetus is infiltrated with calcium salts, becoming as a result a more or less completely calcified and usually distorted mass. The first mention of this interesting termination of an extrauterine pregnancy occurs in Bauhin's[6] "Gynecorum." This is the classical lithopedion of Sens reported by Cordaeus in the sixteenth century. Since then Strauss[7] has collected 38 cases from

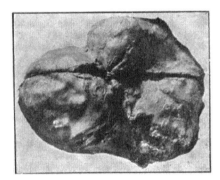

Fig. 2.—View of lithopedion as removed.

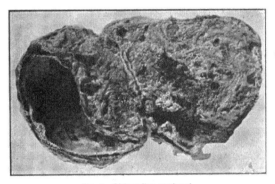

Fig. 3.—Lithopedion sectioned.

1880 to 1900. Bainbridge[8] added 36 cases to 1912. Our search of the literature from 1912 to date has resulted in the addition of 12 cases. These latter we desire to tabulate briefly.

Letoux[9] reported a calcified fetus removed by operation from a woman aged fifty-five. The patient had had two children before her ectopic pregnancy at twenty-one. She gave a history of typical signs of rupture at three months; growth continued and false labor occurred about the calculated date of delivery. The mass decreased, but did not disappear. The patient had two more normal pregnancies and labors. At operation, thirty-four years after rupture, the fetus was found to be calcified and the membranes were fibrocalcareous.

Smith[10] reported a specimen removed at autopsy from a woman aged eighty-eight years. The diagnosis was made before death by palpation through the thin abdominal wall. The right tube was embedded in the mass, which weighed 13½ ounces, and "was apparently of four or five months' development." Patient had passed through the menopause forty-three years previously, and the author thinks that the fetus had probably been retained for about sixty years.

Fox[11] exhibited before the Tennessee State Medical Association a specimen removed at operation eight years after a "missed labor". Patient was thirty-three years old and gave a history of pregnancy eight years previously, with amenorrhea for seven months, followed by labor pains which lasted "a number of hours, when they suddenly ceased without delivery." The mass was completely calcified, and was bound down by many adhesions. Patient recovered. No note as to other pregnancies.

Tilp[12] exhibited before the Alsatian Medical Society at Strassbourg, a lithopedion removed at autopsy from a woman fifty-six years old. It was embedded between coils of the small intestine, and was adherent to the omentum and to other organs. The mass was of a stony hardness, 25 cm. long, and the author thought that the fetus had developed to the fifth lunar month. From the history and the study of the specimen, he concluded that an ampullar pregnancy had ruptured, and that the fetus had been carried for at least twenty-one years.

Schweitzer[13] discussed in detail a specimen removed at autopsy from a woman sixty-eight years old. It measured 9x5x5.5 cm., and the fetal parts were clearly discernible. The author classed it as a lithokelyphos. Patient had had one normal pregnancy.

Von Campen[14] removed a lithopedion by laparotomy from a woman aged sixty-three, who had passed through the menopause at the regular time. From the history, the author concluded that her first (and only) pregnancy was ectopic, and had ruptured at four and one-half months.

Fraser[15] also removed a lithopedion by laparotomy, which had been carried for forty-two years. The patient had had three children prior to 1870. Early in that year she became pregnant, progressed apparently normally for six months, then fetal death occurred and a firm, hard mass persisted. The patient subsequently had four more children. The head, body, fetal parts, and placenta were easily distinguished when the specimen was removed and studied. Patient recovered.

Lamb[16] records a specimen in the Army Medical Museum at Washington, which was removed by Dr. J. B. Murfree. The patient had false labor pains at eight months in the first pregnancy. A tumor formed and persisted. She had five children and died at age of seventy-eight. The specimen was removed at autopsy, after being carried for fifty-four or fifty-five years.

Biener[17] described a specimen found at autopsy in a woman fifty-six years of age. It was connected only with the great omentum, and had apparently developed to the fifth month. Microscopically, bone, striped muscle fibers, and elastic fibers were found. Examination of the woman's genitalia showed that the fetus had been expelled from a ruptured ampullar pregnancy of the left tube. It had been carried about 20 years. The author classed it as a true lithopedion, after Küchenmeister.

McMurphy and Sellers[18] removed a lithopedion from a colored woman, age thirty-seven, with a clear history of a ruptured ectopic pregnancy seven years previously. One normal pregnancy nineteen years before operation. The right tube encircled the mass; the right ovary could not be found. The tumor was hard and bony throughout, measured 6½ x 3½ inches, and weighed three and one-half pounds. Fetal parts were easily made out. Recovery.

Luker[19] reports the removal of an extrauterine fetus covered by a bony shell, from a woman of thirty-three years. The patient had been married twelve years and had given birth to three stillborn fetuses. Three months after marrying she had suffered from a "complication of diseases." Luker believes this to have probably been the ectopic gestation from which the lithopedion resulted. The calcified fetus removed by laparotomy was 6 cm. long.

Kamoth[20] reported a calcified fetus removed by operation from a Hindu female aged thirty-five, which calcified mass had been carried for twelve years. False labor pains had supervened after ten months of amenorrhea, and the enlarged abdomen had decreased to the size of a seven months' pregnancy. The patient had had a child five years previously. The fetus was entirely calcified, was covered with a membrane (calcified also), was seven inches long, and weighed thirty-six ounces. The right tube was about 1 inch in diameter, was ruptured and was adherent to the side of the uterus. The author thinks the fetus had developed at least to the eighth month. Recovery.

Peterson[21] reported a case which, while not a lithopedion, showed a beginning calcareous change of interest. A full term ectopic gestation was carried eighteen years and was removed at operation. The fetus was skeletonized, but a portion of the cerebellum was calcified.

Schrenk[22] gives the occurrence of lithopedion in extrauterine pregnancy as eleven among 610 cases, or 1.8 per cent. Schauta[23] found nine among 626 cases or 1.5 per cent. Schumann[2] believes these figures to be too high. In his series of 207 cases there were no lithopedions. Futhermore he states that in a compiled series of 866 studied cases of extrauterine pregnancy from various sections of the country there were no lithopedions.

It thus appears that recognized or reported cases of lithopedions are uncommon, hence our excuse for reporting the present one.

CASE REPORT

Ellen F., colored, admitted 9-28-20 to Charity Hospital. Age ninety years. (This was age given by patient and family. She was apparently older in the opinion of the authors, and undoubtedly as old, this statement being made after subsequent correlation of various events concerning her early life.)

Chief complaint—dyspnea, "pain all over body." Family history—negative. Married; no children; no miscarriages; never pregnant. Past history—negative. Present illness—sudden onset, duration of five (5) weeks. Cannot eat, coughs a great deal. "Shortness of breath." Physical examination: (on admission) colored woman, well developed for age, poorly nourished. Heart—systolic blow best heart at apex. Marked arrhythmia with extrasystoles. Vessels—marked arteriosclerosis. Edema of both lungs with râles crepitant in character at base of both. Large mass felt on left side of abdomen, movable; connected with uterus and fixed in pelvis, probably a large fibroid. Sensitive, smooth, but present several nodules on surface, about 3-5 fingerbreaths above symphysis. (Says she has had this mass for last fifty years, and that it has given her no trouble.) Liver—slightly enlarged. Spleen—not palpable. Extremities—Edema with sensitiveness of long bones. Knee reflexes—diminished. Gyn. Exam.—Large mass lying posterior to uterus, and probably connected to it (leiomyoma). Temperature normal; pulse 84; respiration 24.

SUBSEQUENT COURSE

Patient became weaker day by day and was nourished very poorly. On 10-12-20 she died, fourteen days after entering ward, with diagnosis of senility, general arteriosclerosis, cardiac hypertrophy and dilatation, acute nephritis and uterine myoma.

Necroscopy was performed with anatomic diagnosis of: General arteriosclerosis. Cardiac hypertrophy and dilatation. Acute parenchymatous nephritis. Anasarca. Edema of lungs. Chronic passive congestion of liver. Chronic splenitis. Lithopedion formation.

The following salient features are quoted from the autopsy protocol.

"On opening the peritoneal cavity there appears an irregularly shaped nodular mass lying in the pelvis, principally to the left of the median line. This mass apparently is a fibroid uterus. Further examination reveals that it is thoroughly calcified, is anterior to the uterus and does not spring from this organ but is intimately attached to it and to the intestines by dense fibrous tags. The right tube and ovary are present, the ovary being small and sclerotic. Left tube and ovary cannot be definitely located, the latter being closely adherent to the posterior surface of the calcified mass. The external outline of this mass is somewhat suggestive of the position assumed by the fetus in utero. Upon removal and further study outline of lower fetal extremities can be determined with accuracy; the outlines of the nose, chin, and superciliary ridges are readily discernible. Section made by means of the saw through the long diameter of the mass reveals; *First* the calvarium, containing semigelatinous substance through which dense fibrous cord corresponding to the dural folds can be seen; *Second*, the upper extremities, which can be readily outlined; the humerus is present, the metatarsal bones evident. The musculature is represented by a soft brownish red material; *Third*, folds of the small intestine. *Fourth*, the bony parts of the lower extremities which can be outlined without difficulty. The mass measures 15x13x10.5 cm. and weighs eight hundred grams. Its calcified envelope varying in thickness from 8 mm. to 16 mm. shows extension of calcification into fetal parts at points corresponding to lungs and soft parts of lower extremities. It is impossible to trace the left tube farther than 1 cm. from its uterine attachment. There it becomes obliterated and evidently in some manner involved in the fibrous tags which cause adherence of intestines and calcified mass. From these findings it is assumed that an ampullar pregnancy of the left tube has ruptured, the calcified mass being a lithokelyphopedion according to Küchenmeister."

THEORIES OF LITHOPEDION FORMATION

Numerous theories have been advanced to account for the process by which extrauterine fetuses became calcified. Calcification occurs but rarely in normal tissue except as concerned in the formation of bone. As a general rule it can be stated that any portion of noninfected dead tissue which on account of its size or position cannot be absorbed will eventually undergo calcification. No matter where calcification is to occur the calcium salts must reach the site through the blood in which they are held in suspension by the proteins possibly in the form of a complex double salt-tribasic calcium carbon phosphate according to Barille. In tissues which will undergo calcification the circulation is very sluggish, plasma seeping through without any erythrocytes, thus preventing active exudative changes. In such areas deposition of calcium salts depends according to Wells[24] upon "one or more of the following conditions":

(1) "Increased alkalinity or decreased CO_2 in degenerating tissue

with resultant precipitation of inorganic salts in fluids seeping through.

(2) Utilization of protein of fluids by starved tissue with result that calcium cannot be held any longer in solution.

(3) Formation within degenerating areas of substance having affinity for calcium.

(4) Production of physical conditions favoring local absorption of salts, least soluble salts accumulating in excess.''

According to Lichtwitz,[25] changes in the proteins constitute the principal factor in the deposition of lime salts. These changes consist in colloidal precipitation in degenerating areas with a decrease in the amount of cystalloids which can be held in solution and a resulting precipitation of the least soluble salt (i.e.) calcium. That calcium binding substances are found in the degenerating areas is asserted by numerous investigators and given by them as the real factor influencing calcification.

Freund[26] endorses Kroemer's explanation, as to method of calcification of extrauterine fetal masses. According to them, the metamorphosis which primarily takes place in the fetus is induced by withdrawal of amniotic fluid and body juices. Adhesions between sac and fetus then take place with consequent fatty changes and calcium salt deposits at these sites. Küchenmeister,[27] though contributing little to the knowledge of the method of formation of these calcified products of conception, presents the most generally accepted classification: namely into lithokelyphos, lithopedion and lithokelyphopedion. His differentiation of these various types is as follows:

Lithokelyphos: Calcification of fetal membranes with fetal calcification only at points where adhesions between fetus and membranes have occurred during fetal life. Originates usually when fetus with its unruptured membranes is discharged into abdominal cavity.

Lithopedion: Originating by wrapping of membranes around fetus after the waters have escaped through a large tear. Calcification then begins in vernix caseosa, extending to membranes and finally to fetus.

Lithokelyphopedion: Found only in case of fetus adherent to membranes during fetal life.

Werk says that when decomposition of the products of pregnancy fails to occur, calcification supervenes as the final stage. Kieser[28] gives the most elaborate description of the calcification and as a result of his studies concludes that in lithopedion formation mummification of the fetus is the primary change with calcium deposition beginning in the maternal envelope and involving the fetus only secondarily. His explanation and further elaboration of Küchenmeister's classification is as follows:

Lithokelyphos: Fetus mummified; maternal envelope calcified and not adherent to fetus.

Lithokelyphopedion: Fetus adherent to envelope and involved in calcification process.

True Lithopedion: Fetus alone seat of calcification; deposition of lime salts being in vernix caseosa. Such masses invariably found free in abdominal cavity.

Kieser believes contrary to Küchenmeister that the type designated by this latter as lithokelyphopedion is the most common of all. As regards the course of the lime salts, Kieser holds that they are supplied from the maternal blood current, and that the deposition of calcium salts can occur only in areas readily within reach of maternal blood and tissue juices.

We desire to thank Dr. S. H. Nothacker and Mr. H. Buisson of the Department of Roentgenology for their kindness in preparing radiographs.

BIBLIOGRAPHY

(1) Carnegie Institute, Publication No. 221. (2) *Schumann*: Extra Uterine Pregnancy, 1921, D. Appleton & Co. (3) *Von Winckel*: *Handbuch der Geburtshülfe*, iii, Part I, Wiesbaden, 1904. (4) Am. Jour. Obst., 1900, xli, 740. (5) *Ballantyne, J. W.*: Manual of Antenatal Pathology and Hygiene, Edinburgh, 1904. (6) *Bauhin*: Gynaecorum sine de Mulierum Affectibus Commentarii, Basel, 1586. (7) Arch. f. Gynäk., 1903, lxviii, 3. (8) Am. Jour. Obst., 1912, lxv. (9) Gaz. Med. de Nantes, 1912, xxx, 1. (10) Jour. Am. Med. Assn., 1912, lviii, 1114. (11) Jour. Tenn. State Med. Assn., 1913, v, 351. (12) Deutsch. med. Wchnschr., 1913, p. 535. (13) *Schweitzer, Theodor*: Inaug. Dissertation. Berlin, 1912. (14) Nederl. Tijdschr. v. Geneesk., 1914, ii, 654. (15) Brit. Med. Jour., 1913, ii, 1624. (16) Washington Med. Ann., 1913, xii, 254. Brit. Med. Jour., 1914, i, 512. (Reported previously Transactions Tennessee State Medical Society, 1886, 88-85.) (17) Monatschr. f. Geburtsh. u. Gynäk., 1913, xxxviii, 428. (18) Southern Med. Jour., 1914, vii, 813. (19) Proc. Roy. Soc. Med., London, 1913, No. 14, vii, 253. (20) Indian Med. Gaz., Calcutta, lii, No. 8, p. 301. (21) Jour. Mich. State Med. Soc., 1917, xvi, 316. (22) *Schrenk*: Inaugural Dissertation 1893. (23) *Schauta*: Beiträge zur Casuistik, Prognose and Therapie der Extrauterin Gravidität, Prague, 1891. (24) *Wells*: Chemical Pathology, W. B. Saunders Co. (25) Deutsch. med. Wchnschr., 1910, xxxvi, 704. (26) Beitr. z Geburtsh. u. Gynäk., 1903, vii. (27) Arch. f. Gynäk., 1881, xvii, 153. (28) *Kieser*: Inaugural Dissertation, Stutgart, 1854, quoted from Bainbridge.

THE PREMATURE SEPARATION OF THE NORMALLY IMPLANTED PLACENTA

A. C. WILLIAMSON, M.A., M.D., PITTSBURGH, PA.

From the Department of Obstetrics, Western Pennsylvania Hospital Pittsburgh, Pennsylvania.

PREMATURE separation of the normally implanted placenta is a condition calling for the keenest judgment on the part of the attending obstetrician. Although it is true that in the majority of cases there is no need for interference because the degree of separation is so slight as to be followed by no serious effects, in a small group, however, the life of the patient may actually depend on accurate diagnosis and the procedure chosen to meet the situation. Each such event, therefore, must be considered as an entity and the treatment should wholly depend on the conditions to be met.

The cause of premature placental separation has not been definitely demonstrated but there seems to be a definite relationship between this condition and the toxemias of pregnancy. While there are unnumbered cases of toxemia of pregnancy in which there is no evidence of placental separation, it is rare to find a case of placental separation without toxemia.

It is rather commonly agreed that the condition is not an uncommon one, but the incidence varies markedly according to different observers. One clinic reports a frequency of one case in every one hundred and eighty-six deliveries while another clinic has reported only one case in every seven hundred and fifty-six deliveries. Doubtlessly, if obstetricians reported every case, in which, after an apparently normal delivery, they found evidence in the placenta of partial separation, the incidence would be much higher than is commonly believed. In a large proportion of these cases old retroplacental clots or blackened areas near the edge of the placenta indicate that some separation has taken place shortly before or during labor, although the portion detached may not have been of sufficient extent to threaten seriously either the life of the mother or child.

The placenta may separate at any time after its formation, with the curve of incidence rising sharply during the last six weeks of gestation. The accident is more common in multiparae than in primiparae and is apparently more prone to happen if successive pregnancies have been many and close together.

This article has been prompted by the observation of ten cases, three of which presented unusually extensive pathologic lesions. This is a small series of cases but it was felt desirable to place them on record, together with an analysis of the salient points in order that they may be developed farther or at least be given consideration in any more comprehensive study of this condition.

GENERAL CONSIDERATION OF ETIOLOGY

The causes suggested for accidental separation of the placenta are numerous but those given most consideration may be catalogued as follows: (1) a short cord; (2) a short and severe, or unduly prolonged labor; (3) direct or indirect trauma; (4) syphilis or any form of nephritis; (5) persistently high temperature from any cause; (6) certain toxemias of pregnancy.

Most writers are willing to concede that a short cord may be the cause of separation of the placenta in a few instances but it is generally believed that the importance of this factor has been greatly overrated. J. Whitridge Williams[1] refers to the fact that "in the classical specimen which is figured in the Atlas of Pinard and Varnier the accident was attributed to traction upon the placenta by a relatively short cord." It would seem, however, that if the short cord is to have much effect it must be at the expulsive stage because at that time only will traction be exerted, for at other times the uterus and fetus move synchronously together in the same common direction with each contraction. The possibility of separation occurring from this cause must, of course, be admitted but Essen-Moeller[2] found that traction on the cord will rupture it before it will loosen the placenta. It is probable that every obstetrician can remember one or more cases in which the cord was short enough to cause symptoms of fetal distress during labor as evidenced by the irregularity of the heart rate, although the traction on the cord failed to detach the placenta. It is apparent therefore that if the short cord plays a part in this condition it does it so rarely that for all practical purposes it may be disregarded as an etiologic factor.

In cases where the labor is of the fulminating type and the pains are severe, the fetal heart may noticeably increase in rate and cause some anxiety for the safety of the infant. On deliverance of the child the placenta may come away almost at once because it has been loosened with the first violent pains. Thus it is possible for it to have been separated, somewhat after the manner and mechanism of the Credè maneuver whereupon it would be promptly extruded. This may likewise occur after the administration of pituitary extract late in labor if, as so often happens, the contractions become severe or tetanic in character. Under such circumstances the baby is born with the placenta trailing along almost immediately behind. The infant is delivered in beginning asphyxia and the physician congratulates himself that he administered pituitary extract at the opportune moment, when as a matter of fact the infant's condition is due to partial separation of the placenta plus the shutting off of the blood supply caused by the severe contractions induced by the drug. Occasionally in unduly prolonged labors, the placenta will be found completely detached with no other cause to account for the condition but they may be with propriety excluded from those which are considered as definitely abnormal, rather than merely accidental.

A few cases may present all the signs of separated placenta who give a history of trauma. The story may be that they have been riding in a train or an automobile and thus jolted or shaken, or there has been direct trauma to the abdominal wall. It may be, as some of the older obstetricians think, that in these few cases chronic endometritis plays a part. Meyers, as quoted by Ahlsrom[8] believes that traumatism may initiate severe uterine contraction or even hemorrhage into the decidua thus causing placental separation. In many cases composing this relatively small group there is nothing else to account for the condition, so we are forced with such a history to accept this as a cause for placental separation although we do it with mental reservation.

In the outline of the causes given above, syphilis, nephritis, fever, and toxemias of pregnancy may be classified under the main heading "toxic type" of placental separation and as such will be discussed under the cases reported.

Considered from an etiologic standpoint, I believe there are only two types of placental separation, one of these may be called, for want of a better name, the traumatic type. In this group are included those cases which have a definite history of trauma, as well as those in which there is placental separation without demonstrable cause, as for example, the apparently healthy women who repeatedly abort. The other group, which is by far the larger and more important group is nearly always associated with toxemias and so may be termed the "toxic type."

It is immediately apparent that the general principles expounded and the theories advanced are not new, but such a strict limitation of the causes of placental separation is in marked contrast to the generally vague and indefinite ideas offered whenever the question arises in any given case as to why the accident occurred. I feel that sufficient evidence can be presented to indicate if not actually demonstrate, that practically such cases of separation are due either directly or indirectly to toxic processes. For example, the infarct is a result of an irritating process which finally blocks off a portion of the placenta and the sudden separation occurring in the severe toxemias is the same process from a standpoint of cause only carried out instantaneously. It is an accepted fact that fibrous tissue appears as a reaction to an irritative process and if a section be made through a placental infarct the vessels will be found to be quite completely surrounded by a thick coat of fibrous tissue while in some portions they are entirely thrombosed. It seems reasonable to assume that the reaction in the fulminating cases is the same, only carried out more swiftly.

J. Whitridge Williams[4] states that the primary cause of infarct formation in a great majority of cases is to be found in the primary endarteritis of the vessels of the chorionic villi, due to a coagulation necrosis of the portions of the villi just beneath the syncytium with the subsequent formation of canalized fibrin. As the process becomes more marked the syncytium likewise degenerates and is converted into canalized fibrin which is followed by the coagulation of the blood in the intervillous spaces. This results in the matting together by fibrin, of one larger or smaller groups of villi. Later the entire stroma of the villi degenerates so that eventually the infarct consists of a massive network of fibrin.

It will be commonly agreed that endarteritis is present in all cases and the arterial changes are identical with those observed in obliterating endarteritis in other parts of the body. Endarteritis pathologically is caused by some toxic agent, either mechanical or biochemical. In the case of the slow infarct the agent is working leisurely due to its low potency while in the termed fulminating type, a terrifically toxic agent is working almost explosively in the blood stream. It has been shown repeatedly that there is an easy transmission of blood soluble substances by virtue of the process of osmosis between mother and child, and if the toxic agent is a proteinogenous amin, transmission from the maternal to the fetal blood stream or vice versa, with its resulting destruction of end vessels, is definitely possible. Bigler[5] in commenting on the failure of the various tests of pregnancy remarks that it has been impossible to induce anaphylactic reactions in the maternal organism with serum from the fetus. He thinks that the pregnancy toxin is not a ferment but more of the nature of a proteinogenous amin. These amins he considers the product of an atypical proteolysis in the placenta itself. He feels that the problem of pregnancy toxicoses is to be sought for in chemistry rather than in immunology.

The query of course arises as to whether the endarteritic processes result from the inability of a defective kidney to eliminate ordinary waste products or whether the trouble is due to toxins eliminated by the fetus plus the defective excretory function. It cannot be insisted that it is purely a defective excretory function for in the fulminating cases there is no evidence of previous difficulty and after the acute illness is over no apparent permanent damage is left. The conclusions of Prutz as stated in Williams' Obstetrics[6] emphasize the point that we must not lay too much stress on the kidney as cause. He says "Notwithstanding the frequency of kidney lesions we are not justified even in the majority of cases in considering them as the anatomic substratum of eclampsia for in many cases they are too insignificant.'' Accordingly, it must remain a question as to whether they are not purely secondary in many cases. If we consider the slow infarct process as being of the same type as the rapid and fulminating, the question may also arise as to why separation occurs in one case when in another the placenta becomes so densely adherent as to be a part of the uterus itself. A section through the placenta and uterus will show how difficult it may be in these latter cases to distinguish the line of union between placenta and uterus. The most rational explanation of this is that, in cases of separation the infarct has been on the placental side and the hemorrhage has dissected its way between the uterus and placenta. In the type that has the firmer attachment the infarct has occurred on the uterine side and as a fibrous ball has sunk into the uterus, locking placenta to the uterine wall and making hemorrhage between the two as practically impossible.

GENERAL CONSIDERATION OF TREATMENT

The treatment of placental separation can be narrowed down to two, depending upon whether the patient is a primipara or a multipara and whether the hemorrhage be severe or moderate.

If the hemorrhage is not alarming, as is often the case, rest in bed with enough morphia for relaxation may be sufficient. If, on the other hand, the bleeding is at all severe whether appearing externally or not, it is at once necessary to empty the uterus speedily. Under such circumstances the baby need not be considered, for the majority of them are already dead and the mother's life is of prime importance. It goes without saying that accurate and early diagnosis is essential and seldom will earlier diagnosis fail to be made if the obstetrician is giving the patient proper prenatal care.

The method of delivery to be chosen is often influenced by the parity of the patient. If she is a multipara there is an opportunity afforded for somewhat more conservatism than if she were a primipara. It may be felt that in a given case, provided the patient is a multipara and in fairly good condition, that merely rupturing the membranes artificially will allow the uterus to contract sufficiently to control hemorrhage and at the same time hasten labor. This may also be an aid, if the labor is already progressing, but otherwise valuable time may be lost awaiting the outcome of such an uncertain procedure. The use of bags too may be slow and uncertain. Manual dilatation may be considered when the cervix is soft and lax, remembering always that manual dilatation usually means laceration and is therefore dangerous. The Rotunda method of vaginal packing has been well recommended but its benefit is questionable and at least in one case reported here valuable time was lost by the procedure. It goes without saying that the introduction of a gauze pack in the vagina for any time, means a definite increase in the chances of infection.

Kellogg of Boston states that cutting operations should be avoided whenever possible in toxemia, because there is a higher percentage of sepsis than in normal pregnancies, due probably to the lowered resistance to infections. There are times when section is the only safe and ideal method for emptying the uterus. In many primiparae, as well as some multiparae, the cervix is rigid and closed and there is no other method which permits rapid delivery. In cases where the infant is not over seven months and is not too large, where the cervix can be pulled down comfortably, vaginal section is the operation of choice. It should be done by skilled men in a hospital and when so carried out is ideal, for the patient may be delivered with little or no additional loss of blood. In other cases where the infant is too near term or too large to be delivered by vagina, abdominal cesarean is the operation of choice and in some cases the only choice because the uterus may be of the type which requires removal, a decision only that can be made when the abdomen is opened. Williams was the first to point out its advantages in his detailed reported results. They may be summarized by saying that abdominal cesarean affords a speedy and easy means of delivery and at the same time offers more information regarding local conditions than any other method of delivery. If the interstitial hemorrhage has damaged the uterine wall so extensively that the uterus cannot properly contract and thus stop the bleeding after the removal of the fetus, the exposure accomplished by section will immediately make this evident by both the appearance and action of the uterus. The organ will have a peculiar ligneous feeling, doughy in spots and will not contract well despite the use of pituitary extract or vigorous massage. Hysterectomy under these conditions is the only treatment and with the abdomen open the field is ready for such an emergency. The uterus can thus be removed immediately and the patient spared the risks of other slower methods of delivery termed "conservative" which really are not conservative but definitely dangerous. One case of this type is usually impressive enough to make the operator feel certain that abdominal section is the only way to handle such patients. There are of course a certain number of patients who do not survive the shock of section but it is usually because the diagnosis was made late and they would not have survived under any conditions. Supportive measures such as transfusion before operation are to be reserved as necessary, but here again the judgment of the operator must play the important rôle.

CASE REPORTS

CASE 1.—Mrs. K., multipara, thirty-six years old, in her third pregnancy, advanced to the latter part of the eighth month. She had reported every two weeks and nothing in the way of abnormality noted. At her last visit, two weeks before entering the hospital it was thought that there might be a twin pregnancy. Just before entrance she had gone to bed feeling quite well. About three o'clock in the morning she arose to urinate and after she had gotten back into bed noticed that she was bleeding. She bled moderately for two hours and then called a doctor. He was in doubt as to the accurate diagnosis but insisted that she enter the hospital. She hesitated for some time and during the delay the doctor noted that her uterus was becoming larger and more tender. The fetal heart had become irregular and had risen in rate from one hundred and thirty to one hundred and sixty. The patient's pulse had risen from sixty-four to ninety-six and she was complaining of pain in the left lower quadrant. She entered the hospital and a diagnosis of separated placenta was made. Since the cervix was soft, easily admitting two fingers, and easy to manipulate, it was decided to manually dilate and deliver. Two babies were born, one dead and one resuscitated with difficulty. During delivery a large amount of both clotted and fresh blood was evacuated. Since the uterus did not react promptly the hand was introduced into the uterine cavity and about half of the placenta was found to be free. When delivered half of the placenta was covered with old and new blood clot. The patient was discharged on the fifteenth day after an uneventful convalescence. Her blood pressure was 115/75 and there were no urinary findings to suggest a kidney lesion.

CASE 2.—Mrs. N., a primipara, twenty-seven years old, seven and a half months' pregnant. Her pregnancy had been uneventful and she was feeling well. She had travelled seven hundred miles by train and during the latter part of the journey had noted some vaginal bleeding. There had been no particular jarring or rough riding and she could assign no cause for the hemorrhage. On her entrance to the hospital she was in fairly good condition with a pulse of one hundred and twenty, respirations twenty, but she was pale and looked as though she had lost a good deal of blood. Her uterus was boggy and tender, well up under the costal margin while the fetus was palpated with difficulty and no fetal heart could be detected. There was a moderate amount of vaginal hemorrhage. Examination revealed full dilatation with the head lightly engaged. Internal podalic version was easily carried out and a large amount of fresh blood came away with the delivery of a dead baby. The placenta was completely detached but some membrane remained behind and as much as possible was removed manually. The uterus did not react well and pituitary extract and ergot were used intramuscularly. It still failed to react and after a hot douche was packed tightly. Because of her depletion she was given pectoral saline. She rallied well and her convalescence was uneventful. Forced feeding and iron given intramuscularly caused rapid improvement, so that she went home in fair condition although still somewhat anemic. She was seen four months later and was well although she had bled a little after leaving the hospital. Eighteen months later she was delivered of a full term child after an uneventful pregnancy and labor. During both these pregnancies she never showed any kidney disturbance and the urine was persistently negative.

CASE 3.—Mrs. T., primipara in the last month of her pregnancy. She had always been well and had no serious illness earlier in life. During her pregnancy she had been seen frequently by her physician and apparently was well.

For a week prior to entrance she had been troubled by swelling of the hands and feet together with some slight vaginal bleeding. During the thirty-six hours before entrance she had been having rather alarming vaginal bleeding with beginning tenderness in the lower abdomen. The baby had been noticeably more active for the last twenty-four hours but she had felt no movements for the last three hours. By the time she had arrived at the hospital the abdominal pain had become acute and almost unbearable. In addition she said that she had a headache which was driving her insane.

Examination showed a well developed woman with slight edema of the face, hands and feet. There was slight systolic murmur at the apex not transmitted. The pulse was ninety, the respirations twenty-two, and the blood pressure 130/82. The urine was loaded with albumin, and granular, blood, and occasional hyaline casts. The fundus of the uterus was just below the costal border and although tense and tender seemed to relax and soften at regular intervals. The fetal heart and position could not be made out. Vaginal examination showed three fingers' dilatation, a vertex presentation and a deal of clotted and fresh blood. A diagnosis of separated placenta was made and the membranes ruptured. Labor went on rapidly and the patient delivered herself of a dead fetus two hours later. The placenta was immediately expressed being free in the uterus. It was small and had numerous infarcts interspersed with normal placental tissue. There was abundant evidence of recent hemorrhage and no evidence of lues. Autopsy of the baby showed slight petechial hemorrhages over the lung coverings and subserous hemorrhages in the heart, brain, and kidney. The patient was given eliminative treatment with the usual diet for nephritics and she left the hospital two weeks later with a blood pressure of 112/72, a negative urine and nothing to indicate a kidney damage.

CASE 4.—Mrs. C., primipara, twenty-seven years old, in the eighth month of gestation, well until she began to bleed just prior to her entrance to the hospital. She had been properly cared for, having been seen by her physician every two weeks for general observation and for urinary analysis. Four weeks before this time her urine showed a slight trace of albumin and an occasional granular cast. She entered the hospital in active labor, the pains coming every five minutes. Her uterus was slightly tender and she complained that she was "sore," indicating the lower left quadrant. The uterus did not react particularly well between pains but the position was a left occiput anterior, the head well engaged, the fetal heart 136, strong and regular. There was nothing sufficiently abnormal to warrant active interference and she was allowed to go on under surveillance. Four hours later there was a sharp vaginal hemorrhage and her uterus became more tender while the fetal heart rose to 160, irregular. When the service was called in consultation no fetal heart could be made out and the uterus was tender and boggy. The cervix would barely admit one finger so the Rotunda method of packing vaginally was used and she was allowed to go on under careful watching. Three hours later she was delivered of a dead baby. The placenta was completely detached and a large amount of fresh and clotted blood followed delivery. The uterus reacted after pituitary extract and ergot was given intramuscularly but so slowly that uterine packing was deemed wise. During the first ten days of convalescence the uterus showed a tendency to relax and for that period fluid extract of ergot was given four times daily. The placenta showed two infarcts about nine centimeters in size together with numerous fresh and old clots. The patient was discharged apparently well on the eighteenth day still showing an occasional hyaline cast and a trace of albumin. Two months later the condition still persisted so it seems fair to assume that a permanent kidney damage resulted from this pregnancy.

CASE 5.—Mrs. G., multipara, thirty-eight years old, in the eighth month of her eighth pregnancy. Her pregnancies had been close together coming at intervals of approximately eleven months. She had not seen a physician during this pregnancy and had been doing her work and feeling well up to the present time. The baby had been active for the past month but during the last week she had felt no movement at all. She had been working hard and four hours previous to entrance to the hospital had felt a severe pain in her right side which was distressing enough to force her to bed and call a physician. The doctor made a diagnosis of separated placenta on his arrival and ordered her to enter the hospital at once. The delay ensuing was an hour and a half. Examination at the hospital revealed an unusually distended and tender abdomen. Neither position nor fetal heart could be made out. Her clothes were soaked with blood, her pulse was one hundred and thirty-six, her mucous membranes were pale and she was restless, perspiring and very thirsty. Vaginal examination revealed a completely dilated cervix with a head slightly engaged. Version was easily accomplished and a dead child delivered. A gush of blood came away at once and the placenta was born before the cord could be clamped. The placenta was small, and one-half of it infarcted while the other half was covered with fresh and old blood clot. Convalescence was uneventful, except that the patient passed small amounts of urine with a fixed gravity of 1.016. She insisted on her discharge the tenth day after delivery and at that time the urine still showed a slight trace of albumin with an occasional hyaline cast, while her blood pressure was 138/76. It would not be accurate to say that a kidney lesion existed, for the patient was never seen again and whether she would show symptoms of kidney degeneration for some time, two months for example, could not be stated.

CASE 6.—Mrs. M., multipara, forty-one years old, in her sixth pregnancy and due in two weeks. She said that she had always been well but admitted that her family physician had been taking care of her over a period of two years for kidney trouble. This pregnancy had apparently been normal until eight days before entrance when the baby had begun to be very active and she had developed severe frontal headache. Her doctor had seen her from time to time but had never examined her urine or taken a blood pressure. For the last four days her headaches had been more severe and the fetal movements had ceased. For the past two days coincident with the headaches had come "flashing lights." Her physician sent her to the hospital because he "could not hear the baby." On entrance careful questioning brought out the fact that for a week past her face, hands and feet had been edematous, and twelve hours prior to entrance she bled about a cupful of bright red blood, per vagina.

Examination showed a stout, well developed woman, markedly edematous. The fundus of the uterus was two fingers' breadth below the costal margin, the position was a left occiput anterior, no fetal heart could be detected. The blood pressure was 215/120 and the urine was practically solid with albumin, loaded with casts of all description. The eye grounds showed a few scattered hemorrhages with a slight blurring of both discs. A diagnosis of beginning separated placenta was made, and this together with the toxemia present made immediate induction of labor the logical procedure. A Voorhees bag was used and the cervix was so soft that it easily delivered in an hour, allowing a simple version to be carried out. The fetus was about eight months and macerated. The placenta was free except for a small porton and was quickly delivered. It was completely infarcted, except for a small portion about three centimeters square. After the usual eliminative treatment and bland diet for sixteen days the patient left the hospital with her eye symptoms well cleared up. Her urine still showed small amounts of albumin and an occasional hyaline cast. Her blood pressure was 150/80. Her phthalein function test was fifty-five per cent and her eyegrounds still showed the typical nephritic picture. In this case it was assumed that the patient had a previous kidney lesion.

CASE 7.—Mrs. C., multipara, thirty-eight years old, in her fifth pregnancy and at the beginning of the eighth month. She had always been well except that during the last two years she had been getting stout. Her previous pregnancies had been quite uneventful and this one had been normal up until her present difficulty. Her membranes ruptured and for this reason she called a physician. He made a vaginal examination, found her bleeding, decided that she had a placenta previa and recommended entrance to the hospital. Physical examination aside from the pregnancy was negative. Her uterus, however, was tender and tense in the upper right quadrant. Although she insisted that she was only seven and a half months' pregnant the uterus was well up under the costal margin. No fetal heart could be detected and abdominal palpation was unsatisfactory. Vaginal examination revealed a soft, easily dilated cervix, filled with blood clot, this probably accounting for the diagnosis of previa. A diagnosis of separated placenta was made and because two fingers could easily pass through the soft, easily dilatable, cervix, it was decided to dilate slowly and deliver, The thick abdomen made external manipulation difficult. In bringing down a foot the right side of the cervix was torn deeply into the vault. A dead baby of seven and a half months was delivered and the placenta was found completely detached. A large amount of both fresh and old blood clot was expressed and the uterus was packed for safety's sake. The patient was put back to bed in good condition and her pulse promptly dropped from one hundred and thirty to eighty-four. Her blood pressure was 118/75. A red count showed 2,860,000 erythrocytes with a hemoglobin (Sahli) of 55 per cent. For the first seven days she had an elevation of temperature to 101° but finally recovered and was discharged in good condition on the eighteenth day. The results of her cervical repair were satisfactory. At discharge the urine showed a very slight trace of albumin with a few scattered hyaline casts and her blood pressure was 142/78. It was assumed in this case that a previous kidney lesion existed.

CASE 8.—Mrs. S., a primipara, twenty-one years old. She had been carefully followed throughout her pregnancy and had reported every two weeks for observation and urinalysis. She was last seen ten days previous and at that time the urine was negative and the blood pressure 114/76. She was feeling well, had no complaints and the baby was active, this being the last month of her gestation. On the morning she entered the hospital she had arisen at the usual hour and was preparing breakfast when suddenly she had an uncommonly sharp pain in the abdomen. The pain continued to grow worse and she was forced to go to bed. Shortly after retiring she noticed a slight amount of vaginal bleeding. Two hours later she began to feel faint and realized that her abdomen was becoming larger and more tender. Examination showed a well developed woman, distinctly pale, holding her abdomen and complaining of constant and violent pain. Her blood pressure was 98/76, pulse 140, and respirations 28. The uterus was well up to the costal margin and quite tender and tense. No fetal heart heard. The diagnosis of separated placenta was apparent from the history and the findings, and the condition of the patient plus the fact that she was a primipara made abdominal cesarean the operation of choice.

When the uterus was opened the baby literally floated out with a gush of blood and the placenta was completely detached. Grossly it showed no marked changes. There were a few hemorrhagic changes in the uterus, especially in the anterior wall, but it reacted so readily that hysterectomy was not considered. The patient had an uneventful convalescence except that for the first five days she showed a slight degree of jaundice and some tenderness over the hepatic region. Her urine at entrance contained a large trace of albumin with various casts but two weeks later it was completely cleared up and when examined two months after delivery was still negative. It is fair to assume that this patient did not sustain any permanent kidney damage.

CASE 9.—Mrs. B., multipara, thirty-six years old, in her sixth pregnancy, at the beginning of the eighth month. Her past history was uneventful, the first four pregnancies terminating normally, and the fifth resulting in a miscarriage at the tenth week. She said that she had never seen a doctor until the present trouble. At the beginning of this pregnancy she was bothered with severe nausea and vomiting but it cleared up at the third month. She had been troubled with headaches and constipation at frequent intervals. Four days before arrival at the hospital she had a violent attack of vomiting with severe headache and her hands, face and feet began to swell. For the last thirty-six hours she had been bleeding from the vagina. Fetal movements had been quite violent twenty-four hours before entrance but she had noticed none for the last twelve hours. She said that her abdomen had grown distinctly larger and for the last three hours she had been feeling faint. A diagnosis of separated placenta was made on the history and findings but operative procedure was postponed because of the rather precarious state of the patient. She was put on toxemia treatment, her stomach washed out, the colon irrigated, and glucose given by mouth and proctoclysis. This was done because of the marked trace of albumin in her urine, despite the fact that her blood pressure was only 112/78. Twelve hours after entrance she was decidedly a better operative risk. Her abdomen had increased in size meanwhile and was more tender. The uterus had the peculiar ligneous feeling spoken of by Williams, and as a result the abdominal route was chosen for delivery so that hysterectomy could be carried out in case the uterus failed to react. Classical cesarean was done and the uterus was found filled with blood. The placenta was completely detached and a dead fetus, approximately eight months' gestation, was delivered. The uterus was plum colored, felt like a wet sack and would not react even when pituitary extract was injected directly into the uterine wall. The operator felt that he was dealing with the typical hemorrhagic uterus and immediately decided upon hysterectomy. For eight hours following the operation the patient was in precarious condition and finally transfusion was resorted to as a means of combating shock and loss of blood. She rallied well, became mildly septic, but finally was discharged six weeks after entrance. When she left the hospital there was no evidence of kidney lesion and she seemed well in every way, despite the ordeal she had been through.

Sections through the uterus showed hemorrhages widely scattered in the musculature, more marked anteriorly than posteriorly. Some of the hemorrhages were massive enough to separate the muscle and produce clots. There was a marked edema of all tissue and in some places an extensive infiltration of leucocytes suggested an infection or injury by a toxic agent with beginning repair.

CASE 10.—Mrs. O., primipara, twenty-six years old, considered herself between six and seven months' pregnant. She said that she had never had any serious illness, nor had she been troubled with either throat or dental infections. From the beginning of her pregnancy up until five weeks before entrance to the hospital she had been well except for occasional nausea and vomiting. Then she noticed that her hands, face and feet were swelling. Two days before coming to the hospital she began to develop severe frontal headache with flashing lights before her eyes. She was markedly edematous and although she said that she only weighed one hundred and sixty pounds, the edema made her appear to weigh much more. She was complaining bitterly of flashing lights before her eyes and frontal headaches. There was a faint systolic murmur over the apex of the heart, not transmitted. The fundus of the uterus was just above the umbilicus and the position an L.O.A. with the fetal heart 144. Vaginal examination revealed a soft, easily dilated cervix, admitting one finger. The blood pressure was 178/110 and the urine loaded with albumin and all manner of casts. Immediate delivery was considered, but because of religious prejudices and the fact that she was a primipara it was compromised and she was allowed to go on for twenty-four hours under careful observation. Meanwhile she was given copious colonic irrigations of sodium bicarbonate solution, her stomach washed out, an ounce of magnesium sulphate given every four hours, morphia grain ¼, and seventy-five grammes of glucose in three hundred cubic centimeters of normal saline was given intravenously, allowing thirty minutes for it to run in, while in addition two ounces of ten per cent glucose was given every two hours by mouth and all other food stopped. When seen the next day, eighteen hours after entrance, she said that she was much better and she looked and seemed better. Her bowels were moving freely, the headaches gone, and the eye disturbances had practically disappeared. Her blood pressure remained at the entrance figure and her urine was unchanged. She was so decidedly better that it seemed to be fair to wait a little longer because she was anxious for a living baby. She was given a second dose of glucose and at this time 150 c.c. of blood was withdrawn, the blood clotting so rapidly that no more could be withdrawn. The glucose solution had hardly been started when it was noticed that the patient was cyanotic. An hour and a half later she had a chill which lasted for twelve minutes and her temperature promptly rose to 103°. She quieted down after a little time and the symptoms were attributed to glucose. Not long afterward she complained of epigastric pain. When seen she was propped up in bed, grunting with each breath and attempting to belch gas. She remarked that she had had similar attacks before and had always been relieved by vomiting. No definite tenderness could be made out and after washing out her stomach and giving a quarter of a grain of morphia she seemed relieved and quickly fell asleep. She slept throughout the night and the next morning at eight o'clock, fifty hours after entrance, the interne was called by a nurse who said that the patient had a temperature of 95° and looked bad. Fifteen minutes later the patient was in severe shock. Her pulse was 136, of poor quality and easily obliterated. Her blood pressure was 130/70 and for the first time there was a little external bleeding. The abdomen was tense and tender, the uterus well above the umbilicus and much larger than at entrance. The diagnosis of separated placenta was at once made and a hurried delivery attempted. The patient died before the anesthetic was started. The fetus was delivered dead and the placenta was found completely separated but showed no gross infarcts or changes. When the abdomen was opened a moderate amount of bloody fluid was free in the peritoneal cavity. The uterus was soft, pulpy and plum colored with many small hemorrhagic areas throughout. In addition the kidneys, adrenals and small intestine showed widely scattered petechial hemorrhages. The liver itself was riddled and there was scarcely any normal tissue left. The end vessels with their endothelial linings were destroyed and it seemed as though some substance had suddenly ruined the vessel walls and allowed the hemorrhage to go through them. Autopsy of the baby presented a similar picture in brain, kidney, spleen, adrenal, lung and intestine.

ANALYSIS OF CASES

The cases as presented group themselves rather strikingly into two main classes. Cases one and two fall into the first or "traumatic group" and cases three to ten comprise the second or "toxic group." This latter group may be subdivided according to the rapidity of the process. In cases three to seven inclusive, the toxic action was gradual but nevertheless increased in speed and steadily, while in cases eight to ten inclusive the process was rapid enough to be termed fulminating.

In case one it is difficult to find a cause for the accident unless it be that the twin pregnancy caused an overdistention of the uterus and so brought about the separation. In the second case, no demonstrable cause can be assigned unless the trauma of the train journey can in some way account for it. It may be as Morse[7] suggests that here there was torsion enough of the uterus, due to its mobility, to cause a venous interference, with stasis, back pressure, hemorrhage and the consequent loosening of the placenta. The argument that there is definite obstruction in cases where by multiparity, for example, undue mobility of the uterus, together with torsion, might account for the few otherwise apparently inexplicable cases of separation. It certainly does not apply, however, to those cases where hemorrhages are found not only throughout the uterus, but also throughout the liver, adrenal, kidney, brain, spleen and intestine.

In cases three to seven inclusive, a definite kidney lesion apparently has some relationship to the condition. All these cases excepting number three, show a definite and permanent kidney damage which was not an acute affair. It preceded rather than followed the placental infarction. The placentas of all showed infarcts ranging in size from a half inch up to what was practically an involvement of the entire placenta. The portions of the placenta not infarcted showed a definite increase of fibrous tissue suggesting an irritative endarteritis which would in time involve the whole placenta.

If it is acceptable that nephritis may be secondary to the irritative effects of toxins, this same type of process may be thought of as taking place slowly in the infarction of the placenta or very swiftly in cases of abrupt placental separation. A slight irritation and then the plugging of the delicate end vessels is begun. Thrombosis very speedily follows by reason perhaps of the enclosure of fetal cells or the reparative formation of connective tissue. It is possible that in the cases reported by Morse[8] in which there was an increase in connective tissue that this was merely an attempt at a reparative process following the toxic irritation.

In patients where the so-called placental apoplexy has taken place there may be a combination of hemolysis throughout the blood vessels due to toxins together with the bursting of the end vessels from a sudden rise in blood pressure. With the evidence thus far collected the most rational explanation which can be offered for the simultaneous hemorrhages in the uterus, brain, liver, spleen, kidney, adrenal, intestine and other organs, is that there is a sudden accumulation in the blood stream of violent toxins which directly injure the delicate endvessels of the structure affected, so that this, with a change in the viscosity and coagulability of the blood which they likewise produce, may bring about the mechanical and biochemical conditions necessary to permit these widely scattered hemorrhages. The organs affected are those in which the terminal vessels consist of practically nothing but endothelial vessels with a slight amount of connective tissue. Furthermore these local hemorrhages are not peculiar to the condition with which the paper is particularly concerned, but resemble strikingly the petechial hemorrhages produced by the violent septicemias and the lesions produced by the venom of rattlesnakes or cobras. It is fairly well known that the venom of the snakes mentioned speedily destroys the cells of the liver, spleen and kidney, acting especially upon the endothelial cells lining the vessels. It has the property of digesting coagulated blood, destroying the coats of vessels, penetrating muscle and raising blood pressure. Neurotoxin is one of the chief components of the poison and raises the blood pressure probably because of its irritative effect upon the nerve centers in this way being again comparable to the action of the toxins of the disturbances in pregnancies. In the last three cases something of this sort apparently happened.

It is of interest in this connection to note that Prusak-Tuna[9] have shown recently that the blood of pregnant women suffering from nephritic conditions will hydrolyze normal placenta and liver to a striking degree, kidney and adrenals to a lesser degree.

SUMMARY

1. The premature separation of normally implanted placenta is more frequent than is commonly believed.

2. Complete separation of the placenta is a grave condition calling for both skill and good judgment on the part of the attending obstetrician.

3. Etiologically classified, there seem to be two main groups of cases, (a) a small indefinite group which for the want of a better name may be called the "traumatic group"; (b) the "toxic group" so named because the patients usually show varying degrees of toxemia,

which is so considerable that it could not be merely termed mild but may always be spoken of as moderate or severe.

4. Mild toxemias may act slowly and be responsible for the partially separated placentae or even those which separate almost entirely with all the warning that is given by days of moderate bleeding and other symptoms. These placentae show more or less infarction which apparently seems to be the result of attempted connective tissue repair of the end vessels after the irritative toxic effects.

5. The causes of abruptio placentae or placental apoplexy show the same process raised to the nth degree. The process is fulminating because the toxin is rapidly formed and poisonous. Its action may be compared to that of snake venoms or the toxins of violent septicemias. There is apparently a corrosive action on the endothelial blood vessels, the coagulability of the blood is disturbed and hemorrhages are still further favored by the sudden rise of blood pressure. Hemorrhages occur not only in the uterus but also in all other organs containing vessels of the endothelial type.

6. The treatment is expectant if the disturbance is only moderate, whereas the patient should be delivered promptly if the condition is at all serious. A method of delivery should be chosen which seems to offer the patient the greatest security, cesarean section usually being given the preference in fulminating cases where one suspects an unresponsive uterus because it not only gives a speedy method of delivery but because it gives more information regarding the prospects of the patient and permits hysterectomy if necessary.

(Since the preparation of this paper we have seen seven more cases all of which fall under the toxic group, three of which were fulminating in character and the four of the slow infarcting type. The histories in each case together with the findings add additional weight to the view presented in this paper.)

I wish to express my thanks to Dr. Franklin S. Newell, of Boston, for the privilege of reporting two cases seen by me during a service at the Boston Lying-In Hospital.

REFERENCES

(1) Surg., Gynec., Obst., xxi, 541. (2) Surg. Abst., xviii, 61. (3) Surg. Abst., xxix, 208. (4) Johns Hopkins Hospital Reports, ix, 455. (5) Schweiz. Med. Wchnschr., October, 1920, 1, No. 43, 968. (6) *Williams:* Obstetrics, Chapters on Toxemia and Eclampsia (7) Surg. Gyn. Obst., xxvi, 133. (8) Surg. Gyn. Obst., xxvi, 133. (9) Surg. Abst., xix, 279.

805 HIGHLAND BUILDING.

GYNECOLOGIC OPERATIONS UNDER LOCAL ANESTHESIA*

By Robert Emmett Farr, M.D., F.A.C.S., Minneapolis, Minn.

THE sensory nerve supply of the pelvis is fairly accessible. The sacral plexus and the pelvic plexus of the autonomic system furnishes with sensory nerves the organs with which we have to deal. The blocking of these nerves, therefore, allows the performance of operations upon the whole of the vaginal mucous membrane and the labia, but not upon the clitoris, without blocking the nerve supply from above. All except these nerves may be reached by an infiltration block, or by the induction of caudal anesthesia. The uterus and adnexa receive additional sensory innervation from the pelvic splanchnic nerves of the autonomic system.

The interception of the sensory nerve supply to the pelvic organs is simple and comparatively certain in all cases in which adequate exposure of these structures can be obtained. The securing of this exposure anticipates complete abolition of the reflexes of the abdominal wall with resulting negative intraabdominal pressure and the use of gravity to carry the intestines away from the field. In order to successfully block the sensory nerve supply of the pelvic organs after the abdomen has been opened it is obviously necessary to visualize the points at which the blocking is to take place. There are a number of conditions which interfere, in varying degrees, with this visualization. The presence of uterine myomata, or other tumors with abbreviated pedicles may interfere because it is impossible to move them out of the field without causing the patient pain. Acute or subacute inflammatory processes may render peritoneal surfaces so sensitive that a negative intraabdominal pressure cannot be obtained, and the field be obscured by the presence of coils of intestine. Gaseous distension is a common cause of embarrassment, and in some cases even the most perfect blocking of the abdominal wall will not prevent an involuntary expulsive effort on the part of the patient, giving a condition which will be best met by the use of mixed anesthesia.

We have, as a rule, used direct infiltration in anesthetizing the abdominal wall. With the pneumatic injector anesthesia may be established in from two to three minutes, and with almost no margin of error. The solution is, by the infiltration method, brought directly into contact with the ultimate arborizations of the sensory nerves, where it is most efficient, and the edematization of the tissues interferes neither with the performance of the operation nor with healing. Sen-

---

*Read at the Thirty-Fourth Annual Meeting of the American Association of Obstetricians, Gynecologists, and Abdominal Surgeons, St. Louis, Mo., September 20-22, 1921.

sitive cases should have the abdominal wall lifted by means of towel clips in order to avoid pressure upon the viscera while making the incision. While entering the abdomen, muscle spasm should be watched for, as an evidence of incomplete anesthesia, rather than complaint of the patient. Complete abolition of the reflexes should be aimed at, and, as stated, perfect anesthesia will usually show a pelvis free of small intestines when the abdomen is opened. As an additional aid we have made use of pneumoperitoneum, the gas being introduced just before opening the abdomen, and we believe that this will prove to be an aid in emptying the pelvis. In case of marked ptosis, or bony deformity, we have not hesitated to turn the pelvic intestines out upon a rubber towel during the performance of the operation. If this is carefully done, avoiding tension upon the mesentery, and extremes of temperature, it is not a painful procedure. Provision should be made for placing the patient in extreme Trendelenburg, and for tilting the table laterally, without causing the patient discomfort. Provided a preliminary caudal has been made one may not find it necessary to reinforce the anesthesia after opening the abdomen. Where transsacral anesthesia has been employed reinforcement is not necessary. Reinforcement, when necessary, may be made by the use of an anterior splanchnic at the pelvic brim, or by an infiltration block along the lines which the nerves are known to follow, and depending somewhat upon the operative procedure which is to be carried out.

In simple operations, such as suspension, blocking of the round ligaments will suffice. This should be done as follows: Vertical retraction of the abdominal wall exposes the round ligament near its distal end, where it may be steadied while the point of a long needle is inserted into it. In some instances the ligament may be best approached by passing the needle through the abdominal wall. In any case it is to be thoroughly edematized. The same procedure is then carried out on the other side, with the operator making the retraction and the assistant the infiltration. Work upon the ovaries requires an infiltration of the ovarian pedicle. Complicated tubal disease, in many instances, requires transsacral or splanchnic anesthesia, but, with a perfect exposure, sharp dissection and the avoidance of traction it is surprising how much may be done with direct infiltration only. Abdominal hysterectomy may be done under sacral, transsacral, or direct infiltration. The uterine cervix should be surrounded by a subperitoneal infiltration, and the fluid should be used liberally between the cervix and the bladder, and the cervix and the rectum. This has the effect of separating the cervix from these hollow viscera, and simplifies the dissection.

As stated above, the main obstacle to success is inadequate exposure from any cause. Incomplete anesthesia of the abdominal wall, too vigorous retraction with rigid instruments, marked ptosis, gaseous distension, hypersensitiveness of the intraperitoneal viscera due to acute or chronic inflammatory processes, the presence of large tumors with short pedicles, or even a full bladder may make the completion of the operation under local anesthesia impracticable.

Ovarian cysts of any size may be evacuated by suction, and we have for a number of years operated upon all of our cases under local anesthesia. Dermoids, intraligamentous cysts and subperitoneal fibroids may be handled by the same technic, provided the tumor can be grasped and sharp dissection made. Adhesions, contrary to the general belief, have only occasionally been the cause of failure. Perfect exposure, vertical retraction, and sharp dissection along the white line shows a marked contrast to the orthodox method of introducing the gloved hand and breaking up these bands by the use of the tactile sense alone.

The presence of abscesses and infective processes, while increasing the difficulty of using local anesthesia, serve well to illustrate the advantages of the method, providing operations can be performed under its use. Perfect repose of the viscera, the "silent abdomen," so-called, and the absence of engorgement, is in marked contrast to the condition which is apt to occur when general anesthesia is employed. This quiescence of the viscera not only permits of a more refined technic, but is an important factor in preventing the spread of infection. The rapid excursion of the viscera when a patient is under general anesthesia, the trauma produced by gauze packs, the distortion and displacement of the viscera which must take place during the recovery from general anesthesia, and the retching and vomiting incident thereto, must, in a certain percentage of cases at least, increase the possibilities of disseminating infection with its immediate and remote sequelae, and must, to a certain extent, upset the order in which the viscera were arranged before the abdomen was closed.

Pelvic abscesses which demand vaginal drainage do not lend themselves well to the use of local anesthesia. Many of these patients are in an extremely nervous and septic condition, and unless heavy preliminary hypodermic medication is employed, suffer more or less psychic shock. This is one of the conditions in which psychic incompatibility may be sufficiently marked to contraindicate the use of local anesthesia. Technically, the method also has objections. Nothing less than a transsacral will insure sufficiently complete anesthesia to allow one to drain multiple collections of pus in the pelvis by bluntly rupturing the abscess walls, which is necessary in a certain percentage of cases.

Practically all other gynecological operations which may be performed through the vaginal route are possible under the use of local anesthesia. The peritoneum may be anesthetized by an infiltration block of the pudic nerves. The uterus may be completely anesthetized, allowing the performance of operations upon the cervix, and endometrium, after an infiltration block of the uterine ligaments through the vaginal vault. The anterior vaginal wall is best anesthetized by a circumferential infiltration. The same is true of the labia and clitoris. Vaginal hysterectomy and interposition operations, as well as vaginal hysteropexy, require sacral, transsacral, or an infiltration block of the peritoneum, and the broad and round ligaments. If only direct infiltration is used it is necessary to eliminate traction as far as possible, and to infiltrate the round ligaments high up as soon as their exposure has been accomplished.

One of the most common causes of complaint in sensitive individuals is due to stretching of the vagina with retractors. It is, in most cases, well to anesthetize the introitus before introducing the retractors, thus insuring more easy dilation of the vaginal canal, and eliminating discomfort from this cause.

We have in many instances, performed vaginal operations upon unmarried women, and occasionally upon young girls, under local anesthesia. Perfect anesthetization of the vaginal canal is especially important, even though only an intrauterine operation is to be performed. The relaxation, resulting from perfect local anesthesia, as evidenced by the easy dilatation of the vaginal canal, is most surprising, and permits one to perform operations upon these classes of cases with much less difficulty than might be anticipated.

The great advantage of the use of local anesthesia is manifest when both vaginal and abdominal operations are required in the same individual. In these cases the patient is inhaling no anesthetic during the period that must elapse between the operations, and before the abdomen is opened, anesthetization of the internal genital organs may be fairly well established from below. Cesarean section under local anesthesia is a comparatively simple procedure, and in a certain percentage of these cases, it is desirable to avoid the use of general anesthesia.

Large or firmly fixed tumors, malignant disease, or marked immobility of the pelvic organs from any cause, are the most difficult conditions with which we meet. Transsacral anesthesia will effectually prepare a patient for any of these operations, so that a reinforcement of the anesthesia will be found unnecessary. However, the technic necessary for the induction of transsacral anesthesia is complicated, it is difficult to acquire and difficult to execute. Patients who are very large or very fat place an additional handicap upon the method, as, in these cases the pelvis is usually deep, and the fat not only increases the distance of the organs from the surface, but, by its presence, is apt to obscure the view which is so essential when working under local anesthesia. It has been our plan to open the abdomen under local anesthesia, and where complicated pathology is anticipated, to precede this by the induction of sacral anesthesia. The operation is carried as far as practicable, and is completed, when possible, under local anesthesia. Should conditions that in any manner interfere with the carrying out of the procedure in a satisfactory manner present themselves, mixed anesthesia is employed. The rapid, smooth and peaceful manner in which these patients respond to light inhalations of gas or ether, when one's limit has been reached is in such marked contrast to the manner in which people usually submit to inhalation anesthesia, that one might almost feel like using local anesthesia as a preliminary to general anesthesia, in order to facilitate the induction of the latter. This method is so practicable, and its practice enlarges, with such rapidity, the scope of local anesthesia for the individual who employs it, that I feel no hesitation in recommending it. While the merits of mixed anesthesia, as recommended by Crile, are not to be doubted, its superiority over efficient local anesthesia alone is yet to be proved. Whether psychic trauma will be sufficiently reduced as patients develop the faith which will result from the performance of painless operations under local anesthesia, so that surgeons will consider it less of a menace than the inhalation of gas or ether, the future must decide. Surgical results are dependent upon many factors besides those relating to anesthesia alone, and excellent judgment and a highly refined surgical technic must be considered in tabulating results. At any rate, even admitting that mixed anesthesia is the method of choice at present, it must depend largely for its efficiency upon the completeness with which the local anesthesia is employed. Poor local anesthesia demands a greater amount of general anesthesia, and vice versa, and there would seem to be no question but that the method recommended above will much more effectively develop good local anesthesia than would be the case if consciousness is eliminated before local anesthesia is begun. Anoci association may be most effectively employed by the surgeon who has learned to do painless operations under local anesthesia before attempting it.

The use of local anesthesia in the tissues, even in cases in which complete anesthesia cannot be established, so greatly reduces the amount of general anesthesia and mixed anesthesia, as used by Crile and others and furnishes such excellent results, that it would seem desirable to begin at least a certain percentage of gynecologic operations under local anesthesia, or to use local anesthesia combined with a reduced amount of gas or ether, rather than depend entirely upon inhalation anesthesia as a routine procedure. Beginning operations under local anesthesia, and adding inhalation anesthesia as soon as one's limit is reached in any particular procedure will be found to be the means of developing the technical ability of the operator, and general anesthesia will be found necessary less and less often. On the other hand, should the patient be anesthetized with gas or ether before the local anesthetic is injected the opposite tendency is more likely perhaps to be noted, and one's ability to develop a local anesthesia technic is apt to be somewhat retarded.

In conclusion, I would state that the most ideal condition which has presented itself to us for the performance of surgical operations has been brought about by the preliminary use of morphine, combined with magnesium sulphate, and the establishment of perfect local anesthesia. By this means psychic incompatibility is practically eliminated, although in a large percentage of cases the psychic element has seemed to us to be of minor importance. Mixed anesthesia has many points of advantage. My feeling is that local anesthesia alone, or combined with gas, or with the judicial use of morphine and magnesium sulphate, offers special advantages over other forms of anesthesia now in use.

2435 BRYANT AVENUE SOUTH   (*For discussion, see p.* 431.)

URETERAL OBSTRUCTION*

THE FAILURE TO RECOGNIZE URETERAL OBSTRUCTION A FREQUENT CAUSE OF UNNECESSARY OPERATIONS

BY K. I. SANES, M.D., F.A.C.S., PITTSBURGH, PA.

BEFORE taking up the subject of the paper let me describe briefly the anatomy of the ureter and the etiological factors of ureteral obstruction.

The ureter is an extraperitoneal organ. Its walls are thin and collapsed when empty; but, under pressure, are capable of great dilatation. It is loosely connected with the underlying structures, especially, in its abdominal portion. At the brim of the pelvis the ureter lies directly on bone, while above and below the brim it is in contact with soft structures. It has three constricted areas. The first and most constricted one is at about the ureteropelvic juncture, accentuated by the renal fascia passing over it; the second, the least constricted area, is at the pelvic brim, and the third at the ureterovesical juncture. The nerve supply of the ureter is derived from the renal, mesenteric, spermatic and hypogastric plexuses, which supply the intestinal and the greater part of the genitourinary tracts.

---

*Read at the Thirty-Fourth Annual Meeting of the American Association of Obstetricians, Gynecologists, and Abdominal Surgeons, St. Louis, Mo., September 20-22, 1921.

In its course from the pelvis to the bladder the ureter lies in close contact with organs which not uncommonly are the seat of operable pathology. At its beginning the right ureter is covered by the third portion of the duodenum. The abdominal portions of ureters are situated immediately to the inner side of the colon. At the pelvic brim, on the right, the ureter lies just to the inner side of the base of the appendix, and, not infrequently, is crossed by it; on the left, the ureter is crossed by the first portion of the rectum. The pelvic portion of the ureter in the female, lies posteriorly to the ovary and, on its way to the bladder, passes through the base of the broad ligament to the side and front of the cervix and vagina; in the male, it is crossed by the vas deferens and enters the bladder immediately in front of the seminal vesicle.

ETIOLOGIC FACTORS OF OBSTRUCTION AND THEIR RESULTING PATHOLOGIC CHANGES

Not uncommonly obstructed areas are found along the course of the ureter. They are of different types, and are caused by various etiologic factors. The causes may be extraureteral, including constricting bands, cicatrices, and sclerosed cellular tissue, which may either result from operative procedures or follow such inflammatory processes as tubo-ovarian, appendiceal, parametritic, colonic (diverticulitis), etc. Here belong also uterine, broad ligament and ovarian tumors, pregnant uteri, scoliosis, anomalous blood vessels, etc. Obstructing causes may be intraureteral. Such are the impacted calculi, blood clots, and pus plugs, congenital stenosis, strictures from ureteral ulceration, etc. An obstruction may also be the result of such irregularities in the course of the ureter as kinks, angulations, and high insertion into the pelvis.

These various etiologic factors give rise to many pathologic changes in the urinary tract. In a general way, we may say that a normal ureter, obstructed by any of the causes mentioned, becomes dilated above the site of constriction, the degree of dilatation depending upon the length of time and the extent of the obstruction. If the obstruction is bad and lasting, the dilated ureter may become elongated and kinked, the kidney may become hydronephrotic, and, if infection supervenes, there may develop a pyoureterosis and pyonephrosis.

If an obstruction takes place in an inflamed ureter, the character and extent of its pathologic changes will depend greatly on the origin, nature and severity of the preceding inflammation, i.e., whether the inflammation was ascending or descending; extra or intraureteral; tubercular or nontubercular; acute or chronic; ulcerative or nonulcerative. In any case, however, in the inflamed obstructed ureter the destructive changes are much greater and pyoureteronephrosis more common than in the obstructed ureters without a preceding inflammation.

We see from the above that the ureter lies in close proximity to organs which are frequently the seat of surgical lesions, and that the etiologic factors of ureteral obstruction and the pathologic changes they induce are various and complicated. Before we discuss the causative influence of these facts on our frequent failure to recognize and properly treat ureteral obstruction, I will cite three cases that came under my observation recently.

CASES OF URETERAL OBSTRUCTION MISDIAGNOSED AND UNNECESSARILY OPERATED UPON

CASE 1.—Miss B., age twenty-one, Western Pennsylvania Hospital, No. 1729. History, upon admission Aug. 10, 1920, as follows: For the last five years the patient has been subject to attacks of pain in the right lumbar region, radiating to the front of the abdomen and bladder. No urinary disturbances accompanied the attacks. For these complaints an appendectomy was performed three and one-half years ago. As the attacks recurred, she was operated upon eight months later, the stump of the appendix was removed and an operation for a Lane's kink was done. No relief followed the second operation, and a year later the patient was subjected to a third operation; this time for obstructing adhesions. As this also failed to give relief, a fourth operation for adhesions was performed a year ago. The data obtained from the history suggested an investigation of the urinary tract. Repeated explorations of the right ureter showed an obstruction four cm. above the right ureteral meatus, which was finally passed. The urine obtained from the right kidney showed a few leucocytes; otherwise it was normal. A pyeloureterogram was taken, which demonstrated a dilatation of the ureter above the site of obstruction. A diagnosis of stricture of the ureter was made.

CASE 2.—Mrs. B., age 25, Western Pennsylvania Hospital. No. 4694. She was admitted to the hospital Dec. 4, 1919, with the following history. For nine years she has been suffering from a constant dull pain in the right lumbar region, with frequent acute exacerbations requiring morphine. The pains when severe, radiated to the right iliac fossa and down the thigh. She had frequency, nocturia, and, at times, hematuria. For this, six years ago, an appendectomy and a right salpingooophorectomy were performed. No improvement followed. An x-ray examination three years ago showed a right-sided renal shadow, and an operation for nephrolithiasis was undertaken. No stone, however, was found, but a renal cyst was incised. Her condition remained unchanged except for the added chills and fever. Upon admission the urine showed pus; but the cystoscope revealed no pathology in the bladder. Repeated catheterization of the right ureter demonstrated an obstruction about 10 cm. above the ureteral ostium, which was finally passed. The specimen of urine obtained from the ureter was loaded with pus. A ureteropyelogram showed a dilated, kinked ureter with a large renal pelvis and obliterated major and minor calices. A diagnosis of a right ureteral kink with a pyonephrosis was made.

CASE 3.—Mrs. S., age 28, Western Pennsylvania Hospital, No. 7603. After the delivery of her first child, six years ago, patient developed a backache, worse on the right side. During her next pregnancy, four years later, the backache somewhat improved, but after the delivery the symptoms became worse than ever. As the complaint was attributed to a lacerated perineum and cervix, a perineorrhaphy and trachelorrhaphy were performed two and one-half years ago. The pain, however, grew gradually worse. Six months later, in addition to the backache, she developed a pain in the left groin which annoyed her so much that she consented to a second operation. The uterus was fixed and the appendix was removed. No relief followed; in fact, her symptoms became worse. Chills and fever began to accompany the attacks of right lumbar pain.

She was admitted to the hospital May 1, 1917. Her urine was found to contain many red and white blood cells. Upon catheterization of her right ureter, its upper third was found blocked. Repeated attempts to pass the obstruction failed. A specimen of urine from the right kidney showed pus. An x-ray plate of the right urinary tract demonstrated a stone at the tip of the catheter and a ureteropyelogram showed the ureter dilated below the obstruction. No opaque fluid was found above the stone. A right ureteronephrectomy, May 28, 1917, confirmed the diagnosis of an obstructing ureteral calculus with pyonephrosis.

CAUSES OF DIAGNOSTIC ERRORS IN URETERAL OBSTRUCTION

The anatomic relations of the ureter and the complicated pathology of the obstructed ureter, described above, explain, to a great extent, our frequent failures to recognize and interpret disturbances of ureteral origin. Not infrequently symptoms, that are due exclusively to lesions in the ureter, are ascribed to that of the adjoining organs; and, when pathology in the ureter and its adjacent organs coexists, the symptoms resulting from such combined pathology are attributed entirely to the neighboring organs, and the ureter is ignored in the diagnostic consideration. Sometimes, even after the surgical removal of adjacent organs, the ureteral disturbances that persist after the operation are attributed to postoperative adhesions for which surgical procedures are recommended and carried out.

Of all the abdominal organs, the appendix, in our observation, is most commonly involved in such diagnostic errors. As we mentioned above, the ureter, at its second constricted area, is situated immediately to the inner side of the appendix, and, in some cases is crossed by it. One can easily see how, for instance, an acute right-sided ureteral pain from an impaction of a calculus in this constricted area may be interpreted as an appendiceal pain; how a ureteral inflammation, resulting from extention of an appendiceal inflammatory process, may be overlooked, and how the symptoms of ureteritis or ureteral strictures secondary to an appendectomy may be ascribed to postoperative abdominal adhesions.

The pelvic organs in the female are next in frequency involved in such diagnostic errors. The intimate relation of the ureter to the pelvic organs and the not uncommon exacerbation of ureteral disturbances during menstrual periods lead us, when not sufficiently on guard, to interpret ureteral obstructive symptoms as those produced by the pelvic organs, to ignore them when they are secondary to pelvic pathology, and to ascribe them in postoperative cases to pelvic adhesions. For similar reasons disturbances caused by ureteral obstruction are incorrectly attributed to pathology of the rectum, colon, ileum, seminal vesicles, etc.

INDICATIONS FOR INVESTIGATION OF THE URINARY TRACT IN CAREFULLY TAKEN HISTORIES

Cases of ureteral obstruction always give in their clinical histories, if carefully taken, data indicating pathology in the urinary tract. With the great varieties of location, etiological factors, structure, and complications of ureteral obstruction, one cannot expect to obtain symptoms sufficiently characteristic, as to make a definite diagnosis; but a good history almost always gives data that suggest the investigation of the urinary tract, which usually lead to such diagnosis. These data include:

1. Continuous ache or pain localized at some definite part of the urinary tract, the order of frequency of such locations being the kidney, bladder, and ureter.

2. Intermittent attacks of severe pain in lumbar or ureteral region with radiations, usually, downward toward the bladder and thigh, and, occasionally, upward toward the kidney, such attacks being frequently accompanied by gastric disturbances, chills and fever.

3. Urinary disturbances such as frequency, dysuria, and urgency (amounting at times to incontinence), which may be continuous or occur only during the intermittent acute attacks, the most common of these disturbances being frequency of urination.

With such a history a urinalysis (in females, of a catheterized specimen) should be made; but while the presence of pus or blood in the urine, especially if it is known to be intermittent, is of unquestionable diagnostic value, negative findings can by no means exclude ureteral pathology.

If the data obtained so far suggest an investigation of the urinary tract, a physical examination of the kidney and ureter should be made first. By first percussion over the lumbar region and by bimanual pressure over the lumbar and hypochondriac regions we look for renal tenderness. At the ureteropelvic junction and at the brim of the pelvis by pressure and palpation, we try to make out the tender, dilated ureter if such be present. By vaginal we can examine the lower third of the ureter. This last examination is of particular importance, for by it the terminal three inches of a pathological ureter can be felt as a cord-like, tender tube along the anterior and lateral fornices of the vagina as it runs backward, upward, and outward to the pelvic wall. As a part of the physical investigation an examination of the pelvic organs and the appendix should be made on account of their anatomic relationship to the ureter and the influence of their pathology on ureteral obstruction.

METHODS OF INVESTIGATION OF URETERAL OBSTRUCTION AND THEIR RELATIVE IMPORTANCE

The patient is cystoscoped and a careful inspection of the ureteral orifices is made. We may find the cause of the obstruction right at the ureteral meatus, may see a stone presenting at the orifice, or an edematous and inflamed meatus, suggestive of a calculus, immediately above it. We may notice a stenosed, prolapsed, dilated, or ulcerated ostium; we may find the meatus obstructed by a papillomatous growth or, in bad cystocele cases, by extensive folds of the mucous membrane.

After careful cystoscopic inspection of the orifice, an opaque graduated catheter is introduced as far as possible into the suspected ureter, preceded, if required, by ureteral meatotomy for stenosis. A specimen of the kidney urine is then obtained for culture, chemical and microscopic analysis, and, if tuberculosis is suspected, guinea pig inoculation.

Whether the catheter is passed up into the kidney or, on repeated attempts, is stopped at a definite point below it, the question of absence or presence of obstruction is not definitely settled. Such obstructing factors as calculi, angulations, or constrictions from external pressure, may be present; and yet the catheter may pass up into the kidney. Even bad cicatricial strictures resulting from ulcerations may, at periods of greater patency, permit the passage of a catheter. On the other hand, in the absence of obstruction in the ureter, the catheter may be prevented from going up into the kidney if caught in a small diverticulum, valve, or in the wall of a somewhat dilated and freely movable ureter. In certain conditions, however, the catheter does give us very suggestive information. A "hang" during the withdrawal of a catheter speaks in favor of a stricture; a rapid collection through the catheter, with the aid of a syringe, of more than 15-20 c.c. of urine, suggests a hydro- or pyonephrosis; and the finding of scratch marks on a waxed tipped catheter used for ureteral examination diagnoses a calculus. If an x-ray picture is taken with the catheter in position, the catheter shadow may also demonstrate the location and size of the stone.

The most valuable aid, however, in the diagnosis of ureteral obstruction is given by ureteropyelograms. The opaque fluid injected into the ureter and renal pelvis gives us x-ray shadows which, if properly interpreted, supply us with valuable information that cannot be obtained by any other means. It shows such cases of ureteral obstruction as kinks, strictures, etc.; it demonstrates constrictions resulting from extraureteral pathology; it discovers such diagnostically difficult conditions as obstruction by an anomalous renal vessel; it distinguishes the simple inflammatory stricture from tubercular and both from noninflammatory obstruction; it proves definitely the presence of the obstruction by demonstrating the dilatation of the ureter and pelvis above it; it gives quite a definite idea about the extent of pathologic changes, and, not infrequently, about the prognosis and treatment of ureteral obstruction. True, ureteropyelography entails some technical difficulties and, if not carefully done, is liable to cause pain and injury to the patient; but this applies just as well to many other diagnostic and therapeutic procedures. In our judgment a great deal of these difficulties may be avoided if we use smaller catheters, inject smaller quantities of opaque fluid, and drain away the fluid through the catheter after taking the ureteropyelograms. This has been our experience in several thousand pyelograms.

I have called attention in this paper to the frequent failures to diagnose ureteral obstruction, gave as reasons for them the anatomic relationships of the ureter and the great variety of obstructive factors; I brought out the point that good histories and careful physical examinations could be relied upon to give us the indications for investigation of the urinary tract; and, finally, discussed the diagnostic value of cystoscopy, ureteral catheterization, and ureteropyelograms in the cases of ureteral obstruction.

If the studies suggested above were conducted in doubtful urological cases, many a patient could have been saved the trouble of unnecessary treatment or operative procedures, and could have their pathologic lesion corrected before it became irreparable. The unfortunate results of the neglect of such investigations are seen in almost every clinic. Attention of the profession, especially the surgical, should be called to it. True, such investigations require a great deal of effort. It demands a carefully taken history, a complete urinalysis, an examination of the abdominal and pelvic organs, a cystoscopic examination, a catheterization of one or both kidneys, an x-ray study of the urinary tract; and, not infrequently, of such abdominal organs as gall bladder, colon, stomach and duodenum. Such a study is time consuming, expensive, and requires a close cooperation of well organized cystoscopic, pathological and roentgenologic departments. All this is true, but let us not use such arguments against diagnostic methods of procedure that are intended to save many lives and much unnecessary suffering.

519 JENKINS BUILDING. (*For discussion, see* p. 432.)

THE INDICATIONS FOR AND THE DANGERS IN THE USE OF SPINAL ANESTHESIA IN OBSTETRICS, GYNECOLOGY AND ABDOMINAL SURGERY*

By R. R. Huggins, M.D., F.A.C.S., Pittsburgh, Pa.

TWENTY-TWO years ago Bier, of Kiel, developed the technic of spinal anesthesia and demonstrated its value as an aid in surgical procedures upon the lower extremities. It was at once popularized by Tuffier who extended its application to operations upon the pelvic and abdominal organs. During this time it has been used with various degrees of satisfaction by surgeons all over the world. Some are enthusiastic about it, others denounce it in no uncertain terms. A study of the literature shows that the indications and contraindications are not clearly understood. Even those who are most enthusiastic have not made clear exactly why it is to be preferred to other methods of anesthesia under certain circumstances; nor has an earnest effort been made to educate the profession as to its advantages or dangers. That its use has slowly grown more popular and that those who have taken the trouble to develop a reliable technic and who have a healthy respect for its dangers still continue to use it, would suggest that it has earned a permanent place among anesthesia procedures.

When a new therapeutic or a new surgical procedure is discovered we are very prone to expect the unusual and sometimes the impossible. For this reason they are used as a last resort after all other means have been employed with failure or given without knowledge either of their true indication or physiologic action. If one attempts the use of spinal anesthesia only when some other anesthetic is contraindicated, unless he has had a good experience with it, he may be greatly disappointed and the experiment may be accompanied by disastrous results. We believe that no anesthetic has yet been discovered that is free from mortality either immediate or remote. A certain number of deaths occur suddenly on the table from all forms of inhalation anesthesia, whether it be ether or nitrous oxide. The percentage of deaths depends upon the skill of both the anesthetist and the operator. That there is a mortality and morbidity with which all forms of inhalation anesthesia have much to do, which occurs after the patient leaves the operating room is equally true. There is an interval here that still needs much study and careful observation in order to deter-

---

*Read at the Thirty-fourth Annual Meeting of the American Association of Obstetricians, Gynecologists, and Abdominal Surgeons, St. Louis, Mo., September 20-22, 1921.

mine how the credit must be shared between the shock and exhaustion incident to the anesthetic and that due to the surgical procedure minus the event of anesthesia, in patients who die from so-called exhaustion and shock within two or three days after an operation. Here lies one of the main points in the indication for spinal anesthesia in selected cases, and in a comparison of the dangers of its use this must not be overlooked. That death does not occur for forty-eight hours after operation in no way absolves a certain responsibility for any form of inhalation anesthesia.

The stimulating action of ether in the first half hour of anesthesia is readily observed in the flushed face, the rapid respirations, the increased pulse rate and the hot, moist skin. In patients who take the anesthetic badly, there is in addition, the suffused cyanotic skin of the face, the engorged veins, the stiff muscles and the forced respirations due to increased mucus, laryngeal spasm or obstruction as a result of falling back of the tongue, so that ether anesthesia produces a condition of activation and stimulation at first, which is followed later by the exhaustion which is certain to follow long continued overactivity. The later stages of prolonged anesthesia are characterized by lowered temperature, absence of the flushed skin of the early stages, skin drenched with perspiration, respirations that are shallow, and evidence of exhaustion. Many patients are not sufficiently supplied with a reserve force of energy to withstand an hour or two of such activation without exhaustion. Add to these effects of the anesthetic *per se*, the increased trauma on the part of the surgeon in overcoming the tense abdominal muscles, the tendency of the patient's respiratory movements to extrude the intestines through the incision, the increased amount of hemorrhage as a result of the stimulation, the overventilation of the lungs due to rapid breathing, the loss of fluid from sweating and postoperative vomiting, and we have the elements that contribute to shock. It is readily apparent that the increased heart action incident to the stimulation and rapid breathing during the stage of excitement leads to cardiac exhaustion and in a patient with a weak cardiac muscle the result is the same as it would be under forced exercise.

In spinal anesthesia, the blood pressure falls, the respirations become slow, the pulse rate is reduced, the heart is working slowly as a result of the lowered blood pressure against less peripheral resistance and the skin remains dry and warm. In no possible way could the heart be given a better rest for a certain definite period. If the patient has been properly prepared by the previous administration of scopolamine and morphine, she comes to the operating room indifferent and oblivious to her surroundings. There is no psychic trauma and consequently no expenditure of nervous energy. A patient with the combined "Daemmerschlaf" and spinal anesthesia presents the appearance of one in hypnotic sleep, so that after an operation of one and one-half hours with all bodily activities subnormal and all traumatic impulses blocked, the patient has expended less energy than under normal conditions. In addition, there is perfect relaxation of the abdominal muscles and the contracted intestines lie quietly in the abdominal cavity. As a result of the low blood pressure, bleeding and troublesome oozing is much less. The conservation of energy that may be applied and which is often needed in the stress of postoperative recovery, the good condition of the patients after extensive severe operations, the lessened postoperative shock and discomfort with rapid recovery of strength, are all factors that lead to enthusiasm in the interested observer. It is by such a method that shock is reduced to the minimum and in our experience it has not only resulted in a lower mortality in certain cases, but it has led to a more rapid recovery with lower morbidity.

With the above important facts in evidence, certain groups of cases are at once suggested where spinal anesthesia is especially indicated. They include severe pelvic infections with dense adhesions, where the removal of the diseased structures is accompanied by profuse bleeding and an unusual degree of shock, and in fibroid tumors where the heart and entire musculature is weakened as a result of toxemia and hemorrhage. A similar condition is found in chronic gall bladder infections. In such patients there is usually a weakened heart muscle and often the general condition is much below par as a result of the infection and associated toxemia. In obesity accompanied by fatty degeneration of the heart muscle and where operation is often followed by pneumonia; in the early stages of an acute spreading peritonitis before the patient becomes saturated with the toxins of infection; the mortality of such a series of cases is still sufficiently high in every clinic to cause concern, and it is here that we have derived the greatest benefit from spinal anesthesia. That we have been able to operate safely many cases which die under the use of ether, leads to our enthusiasm and earnest effort to bring out if possible the advantages and dangers of this method, and lend what aid we can in placing it upon a safe and sound basis. It is in the above class of patients, the majority of whom are young or in middle life that should be operated without mortality. The heart muscle temporarily weakened from infection will entirely recover its normal if the cause is removed. It is definitely indicated in pulmonary tuberculosis and asthma.

It is dangerous where there are permanent changes in the arterial system which interfere with the normal elasticity of the vessels. It has been repeatedly stated that it is contraindicated after the age of sixty-five. It is dangerous here because of the drop in blood pressure in arteries which do not have the power to adapt themselves to the changed condition on account of their inelasticity. It is not a matter of age. This may happen in one much younger if there is marked disturbance of the arterial tone, and on the other hand it can be given to a person much over sixty-five if the walls of the arteries are healthy. For this reason we avoid its use in patients with a high blood pressure, and where there are signs of the above mentioned arterial changes. For this same reason we avoid its use in patients who have an extremely low blood pressure. A blood pressure of eighty-five or ninety usually indicates a low vital resistance and it may be uncertain how much fall in blood pressure the patient may safely withstand. We must constantly bear in mind that surgery is contraindicated in some patients on account of the low vital resistance and that no form of anesthesia can be given without risk. We believe that a careful study of the arterial system together with a knowledge of the vital resistance is an important element in the successful use of spinal anesthesia because it is here the danger lies rather than in a sudden effect upon the respiratory center. With our present method, there seems little danger from this standpoint. We have avoided its use in patients desperately sick such as in general peritonitis and those in severe shock. The experience of those who used it during the late war would indicate that results were better in a comparative way than in other forms of anesthesia. Patients who are psychopathic or extremely nervous should not be given spinal anesthesia. Where there is a history of chronic headache its use is contraindicated for the reason that the patient may get the idea that this symptom has been aggravated. In syphilis especially when it in any way involves the nervous system spinal anesthesia should not be used because all symptoms which follow the operation are usually attributed to the operation and no doubt, in cases where paralysis of various forms have been reported following this method of anesthesia, careful study would have revealed syphilis as a cause instead of the anesthetic. We have made every effort to prevent accidents because we believe no unnecessary prejudice should be established against a method of such great value if given properly and with due regard for its dangers.

Spinal anesthesia is not free from danger, neither is any other anesthetic, even the simplest if not given with intelligence. It requires the greatest care always with attention to detail which includes careful study of the patient before its administration and constant attention by some one who is trained to observe the patient throughout the period of anesthesia. Unless, one is willing to subscribe to all these details, after having acquired a working knowledge of the method he should never be responsible for its administration. We have used it with the above principles in mind over a period of years. We believe that it is a special method which will eventually become part of our armamentarium and will be used under special indications. It is folly to use it generally or to expect it to succeed when there are certain definite contraindications to its use or as a last resort. Surely we have reached the place where it is well known that we have no anesthetic which can be applied indiscriminately and that will meet all requirements. Many charts might be exhibited showing the marked difference in the reaction of the pulse and temperature following this method as compared with inhalation anesthesia. This would consume time and fill valuable space and after all would in no way convince any one who may be skeptical. This is all strikingly demonstrated at the bedside. In our last 1000 major gynecological operations exclusive of five deaths of peritonitis which were caused by imperfect sterilization, in one instance contaminated water, in another improperly prepared gloves, our mortality has been seven-tenths of one per cent. This included many bad risks, some of whom could not possibly have been operated safely by any other method. We are pleased with the result and feel that our mortality has been distinctly lowered.

We have had two fatalities in a series of 1500 cases. The first occurred in a case of eclampsia in a primipara with contracted pelvis where cesarean section was necessary. The patient had several convulsions before the operation and was seized with a convulsion almost immediately after the anesthetic was introduced. Death occurred suddenly from cessation of respiration in spite of all efforts of resuscitation. While the condition of the patient was not good and there may be a possibility that she died from the convulsion, I have no doubt that the death was due to the sudden change in the spinal fluid which carried the anesthetic immediately up the canal to the medulla. Little is known about the spinal fluid at best, but that it is greatly disturbed in the paroxysm of a severe eclamptic convulsion is undoubtedly true. I would say that spinal anesthesia is definitely contraindicated in the presence of any form of convulsions. The second case was a patient who had been ill for ten weeks with a severe puerperal infection, where operation was undertaken as a last resort and where one would be almost certain of death with any method of procedure. She had a blood pressure of only 80 before blood transfusion which brought it up to 90. It may be recorded as a foolhardy attempt at the impossible. It was interesting from the standpoint of emphasizing the danger where there is low vital resistance with extremely low blood pressure. Before giving the anesthetic, we had placed a cannula in the vein and had given a solution of adrenalin almost immediately. As soon as anesthesia came on, the blood pressure fell and continued to fall without any response to all stimulation. It was a striking example of death from fall in blood pressure in a patient who had no reserve force in the vessel walls upon which to draw in such an emergency.

These deaths in no way change our views about spinal anesthesia. It should never have been given to either of these patients. We learn from mistakes and they should be recorded. It is the only way progress may be attained, but these deaths should not be charged against the method without reference to the condition of the patient at the time of operation. We are entirely satisfied that we have been able to operate upon patients successfully where it would have been impossible under any other form of known anesthesia today, and that our mortality has been materially lowered in the class of cases above mentioned among the indications for its use. We are so thoroughly convinced of this fact that we desire to throw every safeguard about it and offer our experience in such a way that those who may be interested may approach it in a sane manner and without prejudice.

We have always used novocaine because it is the least toxic of all effective local anesthetics. We give 2 c.c. of an 8 to 10 per cent solution in water which has been trebly distilled. To this is added 4 minims of absolute alcohol. The solution is made fresh and boiled just before its introduction. All instruments used are also boiled in distilled water so that all danger of chemical irritation is avoided. We believe it is of the greatest importance to be sure about the technic and all details in order to avoid the danger of infection. If this practice is carefully followed, headaches will seldom occur. This is a sequel often mentioned and given as a criticism of the method. Wherever headaches have occurred, it has been due to some error in technic. At one time a number of headaches in a series of cases caused us to make a thorough examination which revealed the fact that we were using distilled water which was contaminated with some inorganic matter from a defective still. Since that time, we have used a small glass still and this water is always freshly distilled just before use. Some dissolve the novocaine in the spinal fluid. We have hesitated on account of the danger of infection from imperfectly sterilized novocaine. No other untoward symptoms such as local paralysis have been observed. We aim in every way to avoid psychic shock and all mental excitement or disturbance by careful preparation of the patient for anesthesia. Two hours before operation, a hypodermic of scopolamine gr. $\frac{1}{200}$ and morphia gr. $\frac{1}{8}$ is given. Thirty minutes before the scheduled time a second hypodermic of morphia gr. $\frac{1}{8}$ is administered. The patient is then brought to the operating room in a comfortable sleepy condition which renders even the most nervous individual free from fear and excitement. Ears are plugged with cotton and the eyes blind-folded and all unnecessary talk and noise forbidden in the operating room. With the additional fall in blood pressure, the patient often goes to sleep and does not regain interest in her surroundings until the operation is ended. All "grandstand" performance such as allowing patients to witness the proceedings, reading, smoking, etc., are not allowed. Before they are sent back to the ward another hypodermic of morphia is given to control the pain, the onset of which is somewhat sudden and may be severe after the effect of the anesthetic passes away. We never place our patients in the Trendelenburg position because we believe it increases the danger. We do not as yet know exactly what may happen in the spinal fluid under all circumstances and I have seen trouble in the hands of other men which I thought was caused by the extreme Trendelenburg position.

CONCLUSIONS

Increased experience leads us to the same conclusions stated in a paper before this Society five years ago. The freedom from nausea, abdominal distention, postoperative weakness and other disturbances so common with other forms of anesthesia recommend it as an improved method for cases when given under proper supervision and with full knowledge of its danger. We believe this method to be worthy of careful consideration on the part of every progressive surgeon who is willing to spend the time and care which are necessary in order to achieve success. Spinal anesthesia is the best anesthetic known today for certain operations in the lower abdomen. It should be given only after careful study of the patient. If it is not properly employed by one possessing sufficient skill, it may have a large mortality. There is no form of anesthesia which is altogether free from danger either immediate or remote. There are well defined contraindications to the use of all anesthetics in certain instances, and the operator must exercise considerable judgment as to which anesthetic should be employed in a given case.

1018 WESTINGHOUSE BUILDING. (*For discussion, see* p. 433.)

OXYGEN IN THE PERITONEAL CAVITY, WITH REPORT OF CASES*

By William Seaman Bainbridge, M.D., New York, N. Y.

IF IT seems necessary to offer an explanation of a paper on the intraabdominal use of oxygen, at this time, may I say that my attention was recently redirected to the subject by a number of physicians who spoke of this method of using the gas as new in surgery. Besides a reawakened interest in the subject, because of the clearer concept resulting from the use of oxygen in war surgery, there is an added interest in the comparatively new use of oxygen in connection with radiography.

Doctors Stewart and Stein, in a recent number of the *Journal of Roentgenology*, describe the methods and results of introducing oxygen in the abdominal cavity ''to make visible a number of organs, tumors and abdominal areas which heretofore have been more or less inaccessible to the Roentgen ray examination. The liver, spleen, and region of the gall bladder, pyloric end of the stomach, the wall of the stomach and large intestine with gas contents and the bladder filled with urine can all be distinctly outlined by gas inflation.'' The authors state ''that the oxygen method is not a competitor of the opaque meal method, as the latter concerns the hollow organs, while oxygen inflation of the peritoneal cavity shows the solid structures but, in conjunction, the two methods are ideal and, when the oxygen method has been perfected to a greater degree, the gas inflation for an obscure condition may save many patients exploratory laparotomies.''

During the years 1908, 1909, and 1913, I published three articles on the intraabdominal use of oxygen. The first paper was written with the purpose of stimulating interest in the subject, reviewing the literature, reporting illustrative cases and mapping out fields for further investigation. In this paper were reported experiments made upon animals with the purpose of discovering the beneficial effects, as well as the possible dangers, of the introduction of oxygen in the abdominal cavity. The tests were conducted to determine the absorbability of oxygen when injected into the abdominal cavity; the effect upon blood pressure, pulse, respiration, degree of anesthesia and the time of recovery after the anesthetic was discontinued; to determine the danger point of intraabdominal pressure, as expressed by a fall in blood

---

*Read at the Thirty-fourth Annual Meeting of the American Association of Obstetricians, Gynecologists, and Abdominal Surgeons, St. Louis, Mo., September 20-22, 1921.
Reported in part in the New York State Journal of Medicine, June, 1908, Ann. Surg., March, 1909, and Am. Jour. Surg., October, 1913.

pressure, respiratory difficulty and cardiac failure and the effect of oxygen upon the formation of adhesions. Although I reported many of these experiments upon animals in my earlier paper, a brief résumé of the purpose and results of the experiments, in which I was assisted by Dr. Harold D. Meeker and Dr. James T. Gwathmey, may prove of interest at this time.

In the experiments to determine the absorbability of oxygen, when injected into the abdomen of a cat, the following technic was employed: a cat was anesthetized, the abdomen shaved, and a small incision made down to the peritoneum. A small trocar was introduced through this tissue at a sharp angle, while the peritoneum was lifted away from the intestines. The trocar was secured by a purse string suture of silk. The arrangement of the apparatus made it possible to determine the amount, the temperature and pressure of the oxygen used. The gas was introduced at a temperature of 38° C. A number of animals were distended with 200 c.c. of oxygen at 60 mm. water pressure, others with 300 c.c. at 100 mm. pressure and still others with 400 c.c. at 200 mm. pressure. After withdrawal of the trocar and closure of the wound, the cat was partly immersed in a jar of water to determine possible leakage. The animals were observed at frequent intervals and apparent reduction in the size of the abdomen noted. When the abdominal girth approximated the normal, the cat was again anesthetized, the abdomen punctured under water, and any gas bubbles expressed were collected and measured. Summary: the oxygen was completely absorbed in all cases left undisturbed thirty-six hours. In six of the cases no trace of the gas could be found after twenty-four hours, and in two none after eighteen hours. The increased intraabdominal pressure had but little influence in hastening the process of absorption.

In the second series of experiments the effect of the intraabdominal introduction of oxygen was noted upon the following: (1) blood pressure, (2) pulse, (3) respiration, (4) degree of anesthesia, (5) time of recovery after the anesthetic was discontinued.

A cat was anesthetized, a carotid artery exposed, and connected in the usual manner with a mercurial manometer and kymograph. The oxygen was introduced into the abdomen in the manner described above. The following observations were made: (1) a slight increase in pulse rate. This was probably due to a certain amount of oxygen reaching the heart and stimulating the process which causes contraction of the heart muscle. (2) A slight increase in respiration, probably due to a stimulation of the respiratory center, dependent upon an increased production of carbon dioxid. (3) A slight rise in blood pressure, which returned to normal in two or three minutes. The rise was due to pressure on the splanchnic vessels, thus assisting the venous flow to the right heart, and obstructing the arterial flow. The return to normal was probably due to a compensatory dilatation of other vessels and to diminished diaphragmatic excursions which would cause a lessened amount of blood to flow from right to left heart through less distended lung tissue. (4) In all cases the immediate effect upon the degree of anesthesia was marked, the animal showing a tendency to come out from under the anesthetic almost immediately. In cases where the anesthesia was profound, reflexes quickly became active. (5) Animals into which oxygen had been introduced were able to stand in two to ten minutes after discontinuance of the anesthetic.

In the third series of experiments a number of cats were distended with air, the same technic, quantity and pressure of gas being used as in the oxygen experiments, the object being to effect a comparison with the second series of experiments with regard to the points in question. The effect on the pulse and respiratory rate was less marked, the blood pressure showed essentially the same result as in the second series. The influence of the introduction of air upon the degree of anesthesia was practically nil. The time of recovery from the anesthetic after it was discontinued was from fifteen to twenty-five minutes.

In the fourth series of experiments a number of animals were distended with oxygen under high pressure in order to determine the danger point of intraabdominal pressure, as manifested by a full blood pressure, respiratory embarrassment and cardiac failure. The gas was introduced in the same manner as in the previous experiments, but the pressure measured by a mercurial manometer. The pressure was raised to the equivalent of 1,500 to 1,800 mm. of water, and in all cases the abdomen was exceedingly tense, so that it was scarcely possible to make any indentation with the finger tip. It was observed that the blood pressure rose steadily until the intraabdominal pressure reached a point varying between 1,500 and 1,800 mm. of water, when it suddenly dropped. The heart action became more rapid and less regular and respiratory embarrassment primarily, and cardiac failure, secondly, caused death in a short time. Autopsy revealed no microscopic damage to the viscera. The effect on the animal of the high intraabdominal pressure demonstrated that the danger from the mechanical pressure of the gas may be practically disregarded. There was but slight rise in blood pressure, and no marked respiratory or cardiac disturbance until the pressure became extreme, i.e., reached a degree far in excess of that to which any human abdomen would likely be subjected either by accident or intention. In any case the respiratory embarrassment would give warning of the approach of a danger point.

In the fifth series of experiments the object was to determine the effect of the intraabdominal introduction of oxygen upon the formation of adhesions. Abdominal section was performed in a number of cats. In some the parietal and visceral peritoneum was scarified, the abdomen moderately distended with 200 to 300 c.c. of oxygen, according to the size of the animal, and the wound closed. In others the same operative procedure was performed but no oxygen introduced into the abdomen. In still other animals, in order to make the approximation of the scarified surfaces a certainty, a portion of small intestine three inches long was anchored to the transverse colon by two silk sutures. The approximated surfaces between the sutures were generously scarified, the abdominal cavity distended with oxygen, and the wound closed. This procedure was repeated on other animals and the wound closed without the introduction of oxygen. The animals used in this series were left for two and four days respectively. The contrast observed on autopsy between the cats in which oxygen had been used and those in which no gas had been injected was striking. Of the six treated with oxygen, two had a few cobweb adhesions close to the anchoring sutures, one had a few fine adhesions between approximated intestines; all other cases were free from adhesions of any sort. In every instance, however, where oxygen was not employed, abundant adhesions were found, both intervisceral and parieto-visceral. The difference between the adhesions found on the animals autopsied on the second and those autopsied on the fourth day was one of density rather than number.

The deductions would seem to be: (1) that the oxygen mechanically held the scarified surfaces apart until new cells were formed; (2) that the oxygen increased the activity of the individual cells, thus hastening a new growth of epithelium to replace the destroyed peritoneal cells, the denuded areas being thus covered over; (3) that the increased peristalsis caused by the oxygen was unfavorable to the production of adhesions.

In addition to the observations already recorded, a striking change in the color of the blood was noticed upon the introduction of oxygen into the abdominal cavity of cats intentionally put into a state of partial asphyxia. The dark blood quickly changed to scarlet. It was also observed that intestinal peristalsis was increased by the atmosphere of oxygen. In no case was there microscopic evidence that oxygen was an irritant to the peritoneum or any of the abdominal viscera.

From the above experiments one may deduct the following: (1) Oxygen is completely absorbed in the abdominal cavity. (2) It is a slight respiratory stimulant. (3) It is a slight cardiac stimulant. (4) It has but little effect upon blood pressure when the pressure of the gas is moderate. (5) It tends to bring an animal quickly from deep anesthesia. (6) It hastens the recovery of an animal after discontinuance of the anesthesia. (7) A pressure of more than 1,500 mm. of water may cause collapse. (8) Oxygen tends to prevent the formation of adhesions. (9) It quickly changes a dark blood to scarlet in cases of anoxemia. (10) It stimulates the intestinal peristalsis. (11) It is not an irritant to the peritoneum or the abdominal viscera.

After many months of experimentation upon animals, I introduced oxygen into the peritoneal cavity, following laparotomies on patients. So far as I was able to learn at the time of publishing my earlier papers on oxygen, the gas had not been introduced and allowed to remain *in situ* until absorbed, previous to my own experiments in this line, though Thiriar and others had employed the gas in a continuous stream for flushing out the abdominal cavity after laparotomies and after evacuations of ascitic fluid in tuberculous peritonitis.

In more than two hundred and fifty laparotomies, I have used oxygen in the peritoneal cavity with uniformly favorable results. The method has been to balloon the abdomen with pure gas (94.3-97 per cent oxygen) at a temperature of from 90-100 degrees F., close the wound and allow the tissues to absorb the oxygen. In conditions of abdominal distention with ascitic fluid, in certain forms of tuberculous peritonitis, and in some cases where large tumors were removed, the gas was introduced to the point of distention caused by the fluid or tumor.

The following cases are reported to illustrate the action of oxygen in the abdominal cavity.

1. C. V., age thirty-nine, married. This patient consulted me January 12, 1904. She was anemic, had intestinal indigestion, prolapsed and cystic ovaries and chronic appendicitis. May 20, 1904, the right ovary, tube and appendix were removed. Many tuberculous nodules were found, especially on the broad ligament and left ovary. Immediately following the abdominal introduction of oxygen, the blood became of brighter color, and the pulse and respiration distinctly improved. The oxygen was absorbed in thirty-six hours. The pathological report was: "Follicular ovarian cyst; acute miliary tuberculosis of the peritoneum covering the ovary and appendix." September, 1921, the patient was reported well and strong and with no evidence of tuberculosis.

2. B. L., age thirty, single. Admitted to the hospital suffering from diffuse tuberculous peritonitis, cystic ovaries and chronic appendicitis. Operation was performed April 20, 1906, and included curettage, removal of the appendix, right ovary and portions of the left ovary. There was considerable cyanosis present, which disappeared upon the introduction of oxygen into the peritoneal cavity. The pulse immediately became stronger, respiration deeper and the patient's condition greatly improved. In forty-eight hours there was no evidence of the presence of the oxygen. The intraabdominal administration of the gas unquestionably had a distinct tonic effect in this case. A letter from the patient, June, 1921, states that there has been no return of the tuberculous condition.

3. J. H., age twelve, male. This patient was operated on April 8, 1919. The boy was greatly emaciated. Marked tuberculous peritonitis and considerable fluid were found in the abdominal cavity. The small intestines were matted together with adhesions and were separated with great difficulty. When the adhesions were freed, the intestine for more than four feet was denuded of all peritoneum—leaving a raw, bleeding surface. The appendix was removed and the abdomen dis-

tended with oxygen and closed. September 12, 1921 the mother of the boy reports that the lad weighs 140 pounds, gain of thirty-five pounds, and is absolutely well.

4. W. E., age sixty-eight, female. I was called in consultation, April 14, 1908, for patient suffering with abdominal carcinosis and kinking of the intestine, with obstruction. The case was so extreme that operative procedure was warrantable only upon the ground of attempting to control the vomiting which was persistent and almost fecal in character. A large amount of fluid was removed from the abdomen and an attempt made to straighten the kinked gut. The patient was practically pulseless. The intraabdominal administration of oxygen was followed by prompt improvement in pulse, respiration and general condition. The patient rallied from shock, vomiting ceased, and she did as well as could be expected as long as the oxygen remained in the abdomen, but when the gas was all absorbed, she succumbed from asthenia four days after the operation. In this case the supporting effect of the oxygen was remarkable.

5. M. B., age twenty-nine, single. Patient was operated on November 6, 1908, for fibroid tumors of the uterus, cystic ovaries, chronic appendix and tuberculous peritonitis. Following this operation, warm oxygen was introduced into the abdomen, and the wound closed. A second operation was performed July 18, 1912, for intestinal stasis. The small intestine, for about two feet from the junction with the large, was kinked at an acute angle, and fastened against the abdominal wall. After eliminating the kinks and suturing the intestine, a careful search was made for evidence of tuberculosis, of which not the slightest trace was found, not even the retroperitoneal glands being enlarged. The large intestine showed no ulceration, proving that the patient had been completely cured of the intestinal tuberculosis.

6. M. O., age fifty-three, married. At operation, November 18, 1908, this patient's right ovary was found to be the seat of a very large cyst which had become adherent to the stomach and other viscera in the upper abdomen. There were multiple uterine fibromata. Panhysterectomy was performed, only the tip of the cervix being left. The entire mass weighed sixty-one (61) pounds. Several pints of ascitic fluid were evacuated from the peritoneal cavity. Shock was very great. Oxygen was introduced until the abdomen was ballooned to very nearly its size previous to operation. The patient's condition immediately improved. During the entire time the oxygen remained in the abdomen, between thirteen and fourteen days, the face was somewhat flushed, the lips more than ordinarily moist and red. There was no nausea, no vomiting, and no paralysis of the intestine in spite of the previous intraabdominal pressure. The patient's recovery was uneventful and in 1920 she was alive and well.

In surgical shock, blood transfusion, intravenous injection of gum arabic, oxygen inhalation and oxygen per enema are methods now in use. Air is occasionally employed to secure intraabdominal pressure but the pulse and respiration do not react as quickly under air as under pure oxygen. Saline solution introduced into the abdomen and hypodermoclysis are both stimulants for respiration. However, the saline solution is very quickly absorbed and is but a temporary stimulant, often followed by a greater fall in blood pressure.

In the World War the subject of shock was very much to the fore and various theories as to its primary cause were advanced. Crile's deduction is that of adrenal and nerve exhaustion. Cannon's explanation—an accumulation and stagnation of blood in the capillaries, so that the blood is removed from currency—and Bayliss' theory of lack of adequate blood supply at the vital organs and nerve centers, are factors, doubtless, in the causation of surgical shock.

In the last analysis, however, shock probably is a multiplex condition and, among other causes, it seems evident that it may be produced by an engorgement of the blood vessels, especially in the abdomen, either from the removal of a large tumor or the withdrawal of a considerable amount of fluid. Years ago, surgeons realized the importance of supporting the organs of the abdomen, the vessels, etc., after operations for abdominal tumors. McBurney, following severe laparotomies, strapped the abdomens of his patients with bath towels to keep, as he said, the blood from centering in this region. Of course, we know now that, for obvious reasons, this procedure did not accomplish the desired result but the idea had a very important and far-reaching inference.

The introduction of oxygen in the peritoneal cavity, after the removal of a large abdominal tumor or a considerable amount of fluid, permits the abdominal viscera to resume their normal positions gradually. Without this oxygen pressure, or its equivalent, collapse of the organs usually follows the removal of the mass. The walls of the vessels are accustomed to the intraabdominal pressure and, when the support is removed, the walls become flabby and give way quickly. Any method which produces postoperative intraabdominal pressure lessens the engorgement, prevents dilation and a resulting tendency to paralysis of the vessels of the splanchnic viscera. Therefore, it would seem evident that when oxygen is introduced into the peritoneal cavity after operation, it is an agent of distinct value in *prevention* of shock or in the *treatment* of shock when such a condition exists.

Clinically, oxygen has been utilized in innumerable ways. As early as 1799 Beddoes employed oxygen for the cure of ulcers of a "mauvaise" nature. In 1861 Mauiere and Gimbernat used injections of sterilized air in the treatment of hydrocele, and Marcane and Demarquay, in 1865, announced the cure by oxygen injection of a case of senile gangrene. Other authors cite the local use of the gas in furuncles, renal fistulas and psoas abscesses.

In an earlier paper, June, 1909, I reported cases of tuberculous ulceration of the intestine, tuberculous peritonitis and other infective processes cured by oxygen injection.

In cirrhosis of the liver, with ascites, where frequent withdrawal of the fluid was necessary, I found that the intraabdominal introduction of oxygen often increased the length of the intervals between the necessary tappings. The patient himself frequently mentioned the tonic effect of the oxygen. In flabby abdomens, where extensive operative manipulation had taken place, or where there had been great abdominal pressure from a large tumor or considerable fluid, the introduction of the oxygen, with the mechanical supporting effect of the gas, seemed to act as a distinct factor in the prevention of ileus.

The beneficial influence of oxygen inhalation upon the digestive system is fully recognized and its bactericidal and antiseptic properties are conceded. However, from the results already secured, it is evident that there are still unrecognized therapeutic uses for the gas and a large field for further intensive research where the clinical and surgical possibilities of oxygen are to be considered.

34 GRAMERCY PARK.   (*For discussion, see* p. 434.)

RHYTHMIC ELECTRIC WAVES IN GYNECOLOGY*

By G. Betton Massey, M.D., Philadelphia, Pa.

ONE of the recent advances in the use of electricity in gynecology is the development of apparatus for the rhythmic stimulation of muscular tissue, both smooth and striated, and of the neurons supplying such tissues. By the action of these machines the current used is turned on by the mechanism smoothly and painlessly to the strength desired to produce a single muscle and nerve response, and is then turned off with equal smoothness and painlessness, followed by a period sufficiently long for repose before the next wave is turned on. By the older method this alternate contraction and repose was difficult to produce by hand, and the continuous excitation of an unvaried current was rather fatiguing than helpful to muscular tissues, though still useful in action on nerves.

The waves produced by the modern apparatus may be called rhythmic if the frequency of the waves is made to correspond, or approach near to, the normal rate of contraction of the neuromuscular parts stimulated, or are not so frequent as to interfere with the normal tonal impulses. For instance: it is probable that the semivoluntary muscle bundles of the pelvis would be quickly fatigued if compelled during a prolonged treatment to contract much oftener than about 25 times per minute, while contractions at a rate from 10 to 25 per minute do not seem to fatigue the patient, are not unpleasant, and are a valuable remedy in relaxed conditions.

Confining myself to this one subject in the broad field of electricity in gynecology, I shall discuss in this brief paper the two kinds of rhythmic waves of electric power available in this work, and indicate the differing action they exert on the semivoluntary muscles of the pelvis; on uterine tissue; and on the muscular coats of the intestines. It should be understood that these waves are all of low frequency cur-

*Read before the New York Electrotherapeutic Society, November 2, 1921.

rents, and are in no way similar to high frequency currents, and that the indications for their use are the strengthening by exercise of atrophied, torn or relaxed muscular tissue, both striated and unstriated.

The action and value of diathermy and nonrhythmic currents in gynecology is quite another and a most important subject, and is best considered separately.

There are but two rhythmic waves now available in pelvic applications: the slow galvanic sinusoidal wave and the slowly-surging alternating current wave.

The galvanic sinusoidal wave is, as seen in Fig. 1, a direct or galvanic current, or what might be called a continuous stream of elec-

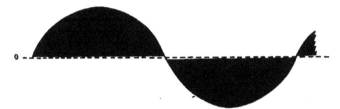

Fig. 1.—16 watt galvanic sinusoidal waves.

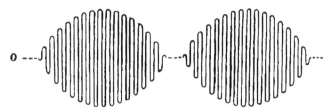

Fig. 2.—3 watt alternating current surges.

trons, that is smoothly turned on and increased by the machine as it passes through the patient to the strength selected, at which point it recedes to zero at the same rate of time and smoothness, the direction of the current being then mechanically reversed and the procedure repeated with changing polarity in each wave as long as desired.

The surging alternating current wave, (Fig. 2), is created by the surging by the machine of a current that is already alternating from 4000 to 7000 times per minute. To get the slow wave effect essential to rhythmic contractions it is mechanically surged into a rhythmic wave, which may be as slow, or even slower, than that produced by the galvanic apparatus.

Granting that we may obtain waves of the same periodicity suitable to our work from both of these machines, the question arises in what way do they differ as articles of the materia medica in their gynecologic applications.

The answer is: that their chief clinical difference lies in the *duration* of the individual stimuli in the two waves. Take waves, for instance, of 30 per minute. The apex of such a wave or surge would last about a second. In the galvanic wave each wave constitutes an individual stimulus, lasting the full second.

In the alternating current surge this apex of the surge (a second in duration) contains about a thousand or more distinct stimulations, and, more important still, each stimulus exceedingly brief in its own duration, something like the one-fourhundredth of a second. To lengthen the surge would not increase the duration of any one of these brief stimuli.

Now physiologists have long since shown us most positively that the brevity of an induction impulse or wave fits it only for stimulation of normal neurons and normal striated muscular fibers, and that a much longer stimulus is required for degenerated voluntary muscles and normal involuntary muscles.

The therapeutic indications are, therefore, that in the stimulation of organs containing unstriated muscle fibers the galvanic wave is more effective in both health and disease. In organs made up of striated muscle, on the other hand, the alternating current wave is just as effective as the galvanic wave in the absence of true degeneration of the muscle. Whether pelvic muscles torn at childbirth present this degeneration depends on whether their motor neurons were also injured during parturition, causing Wallerian degeneration and the Reaction of Degeneration, in which case the galvanic wave will be most effective.

But I should not fail to mention that an important advantage of the galvanic reversal waves over the alternating current waves in weak muscles, with or without reaction of degeneration, is the fact that galvanic waves following each other in alternate reversed directions not only give sluggish muscles a long enough time to contract and relax fully, but time for each polarity to impress itself on the muscle or neuron so fully that the next polarity impressed in the same spot is doubled in efficiency by the release of stored energy—stored in the muscle by chemical change exactly as happens in a storage cell, and that the release of this stored energy occurs with the next wave, being in the same direction. This the physiologists have verified in most laborious experiments, calling it electrotonus, accompanied by explanations so far fetched and mentally confusing that all practical clinicians have tried to forget the whole subject. But the facts of the accentuation of response after reversal of a galvanic current have been fully verified, and only needed modern electrical conceptions to interpret them.

There are certain practical disadvantages attending the use of the machines producing galvanic waves. They are less perfect in construction and more likely to give shocks by poorly acting moving parts. A motor generator is required to produce the galvanic current for their operation when the street supply is alternating. A slight electrolytic effect is produced on nickel plated vaginal or uterine electrodes but no lasting electrolysis or irritation of the tissues, and an indifferent pad with a better contact than generally used is to be advised when large currents are to be used with comfort to the patient.

The slight corrosion of the internal electrode is best met by the use of a copper ball or short cylinder (one by two inches, with an eight inch insulated stem) for the vagina that is kept amalgamated with quicksilver, and appropriate sized intrauterine copper sounds also amalgamated with quicksilver, the mercury surface readily absorbing any irritants temporarily formed during the waves and before the next wave has neutralized it. Kaolin pads form the best dispersing electrodes.

The alternating current wave generators are more fool proof, and may be turned over to an intelligent office nurse after the first treatment to a given patient. This wave is more soothing to the patient's nervous system, and seems to be fully effective in restoring tone to the voluntary muscles.

A few words should be said of the uterine muscle specifically in relation to these two waves. According to Morgan (Electrophysiology, New York, 1868, p. 701), T. Korner discovered through experiments on animals that the uterine muscle contracted most energetically when waves of the direct current were used. As to the proper periodicity of such stimulated contractions, it is possible that tonal impulses occur in the unimpregnated uterus at the same rate as the "pains" of childbirth.

Concerning the intestinal muscle, all physiologists agree that these muscles contract more energetically under galvanic waves than under the briefer induction waves. If this be true when the metal electrodes are applied directly to the muscular layers of the intestine how much more must it be true of currents through the abdominal wall. Yet, on the other hand, I am sure that the large wattage of the Morse type of alternating wave generator does increase peristaltic action, the only possible explanation being the very great wattage of the waves of this generator as compared with the old faradic currents, this great wattage overcoming the effect of the slight duration of the inductions of which the waves are composed. At any rate, many patients have quickened bowel movements after strong Morse surges, applied by large pads to the back and abdomen, those with thin abdominal walls being compelled at times to go to stool shortly after the application. This is true of these patients with both forms of rhythmic waves. How much is due in either case to the powerful contractions of the abdominal walls inducing peristalsis and how much to direct action on the intestinal muscles remains to be determined.

It is evident that we have in rhythmic waves of wattages of about 12 to 16 watts galvanic and 2 to 3 watts alternating current, a means of restoring function of the pelvic muscles after perineal tears, either with or without operative repair, if the applications are persistently given for weeks or a month or so.

In all degrees of uterine prolapse rhythmic currents are useful and at times curative, reposition preceding each application. Either wave may be employed.

In subinvolution of the uterus the galvanic wave is indicated. In both prolapse and subinvolution the vaginal electrode may be used instead of an intrauterine electrode, a distinct advantage when it is recalled that these applications must be made daily or tri-weekly for a considerable period. The dispersing pad is on the abdomen. Unlike intrauterine applications, the vaginoabdominal applications give some sense of relief at once, without the temporary discomfort attending intrauterine interference.

An hypertrophied cervix, on the other hand, needs intrauterine rhythmic applications at intervals of one week, preferably powerful galvanic waves, interspersed with more frequent vaginoabdominal applications of the Morse waves. The quick relief from discomfort and early shrinkage of the elongated cervix is most marked under these applications, and it has been my experience that greater after-comfort is experienced by patients so treated than by those in whose cases the cervix has been amputated.

Probably the most frequent indication for the vaginoabdominal application of either form of rhythmic wave is the neuromuscular impotence of multiparae who have relaxed pelvic muscles from several slight muscle tears, too slight and too multiple for effective joining of the torn ends; or who have general muscular weakness without tears. Here the effect of routine applications on the power and completeness of the contraction of all the muscles of the pelvis, at the slow rate of 10 to 25 waves per minute, can be readily judged by the grasping effect on the vaginal instrument, and the progressive increase in muscle power during the weeks or months of treatment.

In conclusion I wish to repeat that this paper is confined to the consideration of the rhythmic wave of electric power as a neuromuscular stimulant and tonic in gynecology, and does not cover the extensive surgical and medical fields of nonrhythmic currents.

1823 WALLACE STREET.

Society Transactions

AMERICAN ASSOCIATION OF OBSTETRICIANS, GYNECOLOGISTS, AND ABDOMINAL SURGEONS. THIRTY-FOURTH ANNUAL MEETING HELD AT ST. LOUIS, MO., SEPTEMBER 20, 21, AND 22, 1921

(*Continued from the March issue.*)

Dr. JAMES E. SADLIER, of Poughkeepsie, N. Y., read a paper entitled **A Study of the Cases of Carcinoma Mammae Operated upon by Myself and the End Results Obtained.**

This paper appears in full in the current volume of the official transactions, Vol. xxxiv, 1921.

Dr. ROBERT E. FARR, Minneapolis, Minn., read a paper entitled **Gynecological Operations Under Local Anesthesia.** (For original article see page 400.)

DISCUSSION

DR. GEORGE GELLHORN, ST. LOUIS, MISSOURI.—I am filled with admiration of the ingenuity which led to the perfection of all these methods. To my mind the development of local or any anesthesia that is apt to restrict inhalation anesthesia is a great step forward in the safety and success of our operations. I have learned a great deal this morning and shall begin to emulate, as far as possible, the work of Dr. Farr. I have been using local anesthesia in the work upon the cervix and have found it very simple. I have, however, been unsuccessful in working upon the perineum and would ask Dr. Farr to touch upon this in his closing remarks. I have tried to block the perineal nerve where it curves around the spina ischii, but my efforts have thus far been unsuccessful.

I am particularly impressed with the procedures that take the comfort of the patients into consideration, such as their being lifted about.

DR. A. J. RONGY, NEW YORK CITY, N. Y.—There is no question but that Dr. Farr has worked out local anesthesia very beautifully, but I believe the operator is not quite free to discuss the advantages and disadvantages of the operation when the patient is fully conscious, and that robs it of its usefulness in teaching when the patient is in the operating room. I have had some experience with sacral anesthesia in varous operations and, it seems to me, that some trophic disturbance takes place and the wound union is not so good as it might be. In one case a rectovaginal fistula developed. I would like to know what Dr. Farr's results are. Is his percentage of primary unions as good under local as under general anesthesia?

DR. WILLIAM SEAMAN BAINBRIDGE, NEW YORK CITY.—Referring to Dr. Rongy's remarks, it has been my custom to do practically all goiter work under local anesthesia. I have been unable to detect any difference in healing when the patient is given local anesthesia or placed under a general anesthetic, neither have I found local anesthesia of any great disadvantage in teaching. A preliminary dose of morphine usually dulls the general sensibilities sufficiently. A touch of psychic anesthesia is of value, tell the patient that what she is doing is of great service to humanity; tell her a little of what is going to happen, and I think you will find that she will respond by helping the operator.

Regarding the addition of magnesium sulphate, I can only speak from experience with a few cases, but it seems that Gwathmey has added something to anesthesia —prolonging the effect and lessening certain disagreeable results.

DR. FARR, (closing).—With regard to the perineum, I would say that we use caudal anesthesia or an infiltration block. By going well out to the side there is nothing that can be injured, and by keeping the needle point on the move one may put in an ounce or two of the solution. In this way the nerve supply is sure to be reached.

My experience agrees with that of Doctor Bainbridge. This can be made an absolutely painless operation. Infiltration can be done in two minutes and it is so simple that I have for many years used only local anesthesia in these cases.

Charity cases are not good subjects for the use of local anesthesia, unless one has a reputation with this class of people for doing painless operations. I tried to develop my technic for local anesthesia upon this class of cases at the time I was teaching in the University of Minnesota. In 1914 I resigned so as to devote myself entirely to my private practice, for I found that I could get along so much better in the work when operating upon patients with whom I was acquainted.

We never talk to our patients before operation, if we can avoid it. If the patient brings up the subject, I ask her whether she is not willing to leave the details to me, and, as a rule, patients will say ''Go ahead, and use your own judgment.''

We have done approximately seventy-five abdominal hysterectomies, 25 per cent of which included the removal of the cervix. We have also done twelve or fifteen vaginal hysterectomies. We, therefore, believe that with a little experience men should do at least the simple things under local anesthesia, on account of its safety and other advantages.

We have had no difficulty with healing of wounds.

DR. WILLIAM EDGAR DARNALL, of Atlantic City, N. J., read a paper entitled **Suppurating Uterine Myomata**.

This paper appears in full in the current volume of the official transactions, Vol. xxxiv, *1921.*

DR. K. I. SANES, of Pittsburgh, Pa., read a paper entitled **Ureteral Obstruction**. (For original article see page 405.)

DISCUSSION

DR. JOHN O. POLAK, BROOKLYN, NEW YORK.—The paper of Dr. Sanes brings out something of considerable interest to the gynecologist. All of us who are operating in teaching hospitals find great numbers of these surgical derelicts who have been operated two, three, or four times for appendicitis, adhesions and the like; and we have learned that the department of gynecology must include a department of urology in order to make the diagnosis in these pelvic cases, for the reason that most of the cases give a history of starting during pregnancy or after labor. All of us know that there is considerable trauma during labor and that parametritis is much more frequent than any one supposes unless one is making examinations in a postpartum clinic. When one opens the abdomen and finds the pelvic veins obstructed and the ovaries adherent in every case where a parametritis has been present, one can see how this same scar tissue can constrict a ureter and produce sufficient stasis in the ureter to cause intermittent hydroureter. A great many of these cases, as the doctor said, have these strictures. They are more frequent than stones and cause intermittent hydroureter and hydronephrosis.

DR. E. GUSTAV ZINKE, CINCINNATI, OHIO.—How do you differentiate between a shadow that represents a stone and a shadow that is created by some other body not in the ureter, perhaps beneath it, above it or to one side of it?

DR. SANES, (closing).—Dr. Polak's remarks are correct. We have frequently found these patients giving a history of preceding pelvic inflammation. An inflammation of the pelvic organs may, by extension, affect the periureteral and ureteral tissues, causing constriction and ureteritis. Dr. Zinke's question I think is answered in the paper. One of the slides showed a shadow of a calcareous substance outside the ureter, demonstrating the x-ray catheter. If we find a shadow outside of the ureter we know that it is not caused by a stone. We do not diagnose a stone unless it is in the ureter, in immediate contact with the ureteral x-ray catheter.

DR. R. R. HUGGINS, of Pittsburgh, Pa., read a paper entitled **The Indications for and the Dangers in the Use of Spinal Anesthesia in Obstetrics, Gynecology and Abdominal Surgery.** (For original article see page 412.)

DISCUSSION

DR. GEORGE GELLHORN, ST. LOUIS, MISSOURI.—I want to endorse what Dr. Huggins has said. I believe firmly, as he does, that spinal anesthesia forms one of the most valuable aids to our operative procedures. Have you noticed how inconsistent we are? We preach to the profession and laity about the right of the patient to be considered individually and claim that every case should be treated on its merits, and then we calmly go ahead and carry out our routine. Thus, there are operators who operate on all kinds of patients under ether. They would not change from that habit for anything in the world. Conversely, there are others who do everything under the sun under spinal anesthesia. I am at this point at variance with a well-known surgeon in the east, who advises spinal anesthesia for everything. He does curettages, hysterectomies, and hemorrhoidectomies under spinal anesthesia. That looks to me like training a big cannon on humming birds. Spinal anesthesia must be reserved for major operations. I have used spinal anesthesia for more than eleven years on something like 600 cases, and would not give it up. The absolute contraindications are hypotension and kyphoscoliosis or other deformities. There are also relative contraindications, such as a neuropathic disposition, a tendency to headaches, and skin eruptions at the site of injection. I cannot, however, agree with Dr. Huggins as to hypertension being a contraindication. On the contrary, I feel that such cases are eminently well suited for spinal anesthesia. Ether would be most dangerous, whereas in spinal anesthesia, the blood pressure will be reduced immediately. To prevent too rapid a fall of the blood pressure, adrenalin may be injected when the drop becomes manifest.

I regret the fact that our professional anesthetists, as a rule, limit themselves to one or two methods of inhalation narcosis. In order to be true specialists, they should be experts in *every* kind of anesthesia or analgesia used in surgery.

DR. WILLIAM SEAMAN BAINBRIDGE, NEW YORK CITY.—Some years ago, when spinal analgesia was first brought before the profession, I put it to a thorough test, having special opportunity to do so at the New York City Children's Hospital and Schools at Randall's Island and at some other institutions. I employed it in 1600 cases of all kinds under varying conditions, using the method for operations below the clavicle. Many of the patients were poorly developed, undernourished children, and some were cases in which one would hesitate to use any form of anesthesia. The ages ranged from three months up to seventy-five years. The three months old child had a congenital cardiac disorder and a hypostatic pneumonia; it recovered perfectly except for the heart condition, which still remains. An interesting fact of the case is that during the entire operation the child nursed from a bottle.

I believe spinal analgesia has a place in surgery but is not without its dangers and should be very carefully employed.

DR. HUGGINS, (closing).—There have been two methods of preparing the solution, the heavier and the lighter. When alcohol is used it makes the solution lighter than the spinal fluid and we then elevate the head of the bed, thus allowing the fluid to drift toward the base of the column rather than toward the medulla. We have felt that this is more effective, that alcohol slowly introduced gives us a better anesthesia.

One thing in regard to high blood pressure, as brought out by Dr. Gellhorn. I am thoroughly convinced that is where we get into trouble sometimes. A man will give one or two or three hundred spinal anesthesias and then a patient will die suddenly and they will throw the method up. That is what happened in the genitourinary clinics down at Baltimore, they would not give it because some old men died. In such cases the patients should not have been given spinal anesthesia for they had inelastic arteries and they do not withstand the change.

We must be careful about that one thing, and if we are careful about the fundamental principles I think we will keep out of trouble.

DR. JOHN W. KEEFE, of Providence, R. I., read a paper entitled **A Plea for Routine Examination upon the Operating Table as a Preliminary to Abdominal Operations.**

This paper appears in full in the current volume of the official transactions, Vol. xxxiv, 1921.

DR. WILLIAM S. BAINBRIDGE, of New York, N. Y., read a paper entitled **Oxygen in the Peritoneal Cavity with Report of Cases.** (For original article see page 424.)

DISCUSSION

DR. A. J. RONGY, NEW YORK CITY.—My experience with the introduction of oxygen into the peritoneal cavity is practically limited to a study of the patency of the fallopian tubes. When Dr. Bainbridge began the study of oxygen he had no way of measuring accurately the quantity he had introduced into the abdominal cavity. Now we have instruments by which we can accurately measure the quantity used. Not a great deal of oxygen need be introduced into the abdominal cavity to cause pain. A column of oxygen forms between the liver and the diaphragm as soon as the patient assumes an erect position which causes painful pressure on the diaphragm. One of my patients went into syncope on the table. It is safer to use carbon dioxide on account of its rapid absorption. It takes twenty-four to forty-eight hours for oxygen to be absorbed and during that time the patients have a great deal of pain in the abdomen and also in the right shoulder. They feel as they usually express it, that "they are almost paralyzed on the right side."

DR. STEPHEN E. TRACY, PHILADELPHIA, PENN.—I would like to know whether Dr. Bainbridge obtains better results with the use of oxygen in his cases of tuberculosis of the peritoneum than he did in cases not treated with oxygen. My experience has been that if the source of infection is removed and the abdomen closed the results are good. We have used oxygen in the treatment of tuberculous sinuses, and it seemed that they healed in a much shorter time than those treated by other methods.

DR. H. J. SCHERCK, ST. LOUIS, MISSOURI.—I wish to say a few words on the question of pneumoperitoneum, not so much from a therapeutic as a diagnostic standpoint. I would like to say that the technic worked out by me and my associates has served to make the diagnosis between intraabdominal and extraperitoneal tumors perfectly clear without exception. The method is very simple. A large block of wood is placed under the thorax and underneath the pelvis, allowing the abdominal contents to sag, and after this the abdomen is distended, using air. Oxygen is introduced under pressure from the tanks and we produce our own pressure. If a tumor is situated retroperitoneally the clear prevertebral space can be seen impinged upon by the tumor mass, and you can make a diagnosis at once between the intraabdominal and retroperitoneal growths.

I have not observed in our series a single alarming symptom. I have noticed the pain in the shoulder referred to by the last speaker. We did have a certain amount of emphysema following but since we have adopted a little apparatus designed by Dr. Sante placing between the tube and the needle, a manometer from an ordinary blood pressure apparatus, we can determine whether the needle is in the abdominal cavity or in the gut or tissue. If pressure is registered we know we are up against an obstruction.

There was another experiment of particular interest to me and that was some other work that we have been doing in reference to fluoroscopy in conjunction with the pneumoperitoneum and the injection of the ureters and pelvis of the kidney. We have introduced 15 to 25 per cent bromide of soda when the pneumoperitoneum was made. We get a much better view in that way than without the distention of the abdomen. I think we were the first to suggest this. If the air in the abdomen is in the way it is easy to remove it before the patient is put back to bed by leaving the needle in and simply pressing it out.

We had a type of case not mentioned by the essayist, an intraabdominal hemorrhage due to traumatism. In this case we were unable to tell whether or not there was a rupture of the gut. So we took a picture to determine whether there was a rupture, believing that there would be enough gas admitted into the abdomen from the bowel to show whether the gut had been ruptured. In this case there was enough gas to determine this point. In the next case we found no pneumoperitoneum and upon laparotomy found a rupture of the kidney and then after operating on the case we distended the abdomen with air in order to sustain intraabdominal pressure. As soon as the intraabdominal pressure is reduced, the hemorrhage will start again in many of these cases.

DR. BAINBRIDGE, (closing).—Dr. Rongy has had experience with the adulteration of oxygen. I, too, have spent much time in testing the quality of oxygen on the market. We must be just as careful in regard to the purity of the oxygen we use as we are with digitalis, atropin, or any other drug.

I have not had the experience mentioned by Dr. Rongy in regard to syncope and invalidism. In my reports on this subject, the first one published in 1908, you will find that very few patients have any annoying effects whatever from this procedure. One woman I tapped 134 times and usually introduced oxygen into the peritoneal cavity, at her request. After a few hours she was always able to return to her work as Probation Officer in a suburb of New York. I have had scores of cases markedly benefited through this means. I believe we have here a therapeutic agent in selected cases.

Dr. Tracy has spoken of tuberculous peritonitis; I think oxygen is just another element of help. We have all seen these cases get well with only a laparotomy.

The point about hemorrhage is a very good one, and you will find that in my paper published in 1908 I speak of the prevention of secondary hemorrhage by the pressure of the volume of gas.

THE NEW YORK OBSTETRICAL SOCIETY. MEETING OF DECEMBER 13, 1921

THE PRESIDENT, DR. RALPH H. POMEROY, IN THE CHAIR

DR. RALPH WALDO read a paper on **Abdominal Drainage.**

Dr. Waldo referred to the wide differences of opinion still existing in the minds of experienced abdominal surgeons regarding this procedure, although if a thorough appreciation existed of a limitation of abdominal drainage, such differences in opinion would be less. He stated that except for the relief of ascites, either of local or general origin, there is no such thing as general abdominal drainage.

Drainage does not take the place of surgery, but on the other hand, if properly employed, assists very materially in the cure of many serious abdominal diseases. It will not remove a pus tube, a gangrenous appendix, or gall bladder. In a very limited number of cases where the offending organ has been practically removed by an abscess, it may be good surgery to only drain the abscess, especially if the patient's general condition is bad.

In all of these cases it is regional and not general abdominal drainage that is employed.

Dr. Waldo advised drainage where there is a markedly infected area or where there have been extensive adhesions from which there is more or less oozing of blood and from which there is likely to be an exudation of serum for several days. In the last instance quite a large amount of blood and serum is apt to accumulate, which would act as a culture medium for the few infecting germs that are sure to be present and which under ordinary circumstances would be taken care of by the peritoneum. This infected blood and serum is sure to result in general infection that may cause the patient's life. A properly applied drain will prevent this by not allowing a culture medium to collect. The drain in this class of cases is called upon to do two things. The first and possibly the most important is to hold the abdominal contents (intestine, omentum, and mesentery) as much as possible away from the infected area. The second is drainage. A drain does not directly cure sepsis; but on the other hand in properly selected cases, it prevents the addition of septic poison to a patient who is usually more or less infected.

During Dr. Waldo's early work in abdominal surgery, glass tubes, rubber drainage tubes with lateral perforations and then strips of gauze, usually iodoform were used. It soon became apparent that these methods drained only a very small area and that very imperfectly. Many times, when tubes were used, intestinal fistulae resulted.

About twenty years ago, he had many cases of severe pelvic infection to treat, and also quite a number of adherent tumors to remove by abdominal section. In a limited number of cases, there was much bleeding and packing with iodoform gauze as recommended by *Mikulicz* was used. In some of these cases there had been severe infection with the presence of more or less infected pus. In other cases there was no infection.

To the surprise of all who observed these cases, the infected patients did as well as the noninfected cases. With a prejudice against placing iodoform gauze in contact with the peritoneum, the large piece of gauze in the Mikulicz abdominal tamponade was replaced by plain sterile gauze. Strips of iodoform gauze are still used as a middle packing. No silk thread is attached to the middle of the large piece of gauze as advocated by Mikulicz. The drain is at least one to one and a half inches in diameter where it passes through the abdominal wall and great care is taken to see that it is not constricted at that point. On the fourth or fifth day after the operation, the interior packing of iodoform gauze is gently loosened and usually partially removed. Each day thereafter, a little more is taken until at the end of the week after the operation, it is all removed. In two or three days after, the remaining large piece of gauze is easily removed and as this frequently leaves a fair sized opening, a strip of gauze, or piece of rubber tissue is introduced and changed daily for a few days until the opening is entirely closed, which is usually two or three weeks after the operation.

Where the drain is left in as long as here recommended, there is never any protrusion of intestine or omentum, and hernia in the abdominal wound very rarely follows. Three months after the operation, from the appearance of the wound, it is very difficult to detect that the abdomen has been drained. This method keeps the abdominal contents away from the infected region and also prevents the accumulation of blood and serum. It drains the infected region. It is not a drain to the general abdominal cavity. A strip of gauze, small cigarette drain or tube, either glass or rubber, does not drain the general abdominal cavity, nor does it effectively drain a region. A tube is liable to injure the neighboring structures.

DISCUSSION

DR. HOWARD C. TAYLOR.—An experience of the past I value very highly is that in connection with abdominal drainage and I think it is an experience that those of us who have been practicing surgery for many years have had, which the younger men can never have. My first training in surgery was at Roosevelt Hospital and practically no abdominal work was done without some drainage. Even a simple appendectomy would be drained down to the stump. The result was a large number of sinuses because of the packing and drainage employed. After training on the surgical service I went over to the gynecological service of Dr. Tuttle, and it was strange that conditions could be so different in two services in the same institution. The plan of Dr. Tuttle at that time was this: if we had a double pyosalpinx or anything where there was need of drainage, a glass tube put down to the bottom of the wound, that was cleaned out until the discharge lessened. Then two or three silkworm gut sutures which were left in place were tied and the abdominal wall was closed entirely though a certain amount of fluid was left in the peritoneal cavity. Those cases did perfectly well. In other words, the method pursued by Dr. Tuttle was a very marked advance over the constant packing and drainage as practiced by Dr. McBurney. It seems to me that what Dr. Waldo has said is true in regard to the question of the necessity of drainage. We cannot drain the peritoneal cavity, you simply drain the condition that is left at the end of the operation, and not the condition that was there at the beginning. If there is any infected tissue left, it must be drained and taken care of; otherwise a general peritonitis will result. If everything is left clean, drainage is not necessary. I very rarely drain through the abdominal wall, because it is much better to drain through the vagina.

DR. WILLIAM E. STUDDIFORD.—I have gone through about the same experience as Dr. Taylor on the subject of drainage. One important fact that we have learned is when to operate. Formerly we invaded the "acute" abdomen and operated on a good many cases that might have recovered or had partial resolution and less severe operation if they had been let alone. Studies of infected tubes show that, in the majority of cases, they are sterile, even in the presence of large collections of pus, and the majority of such cases are to be drained through the vagina.

The cases in which I use drainage, but more as a safety valve, rather than for the principle of drainage itself, are the cases in which there have been a great many adhesions, in which there is a good deal of oozing into the culdesac from the peritoneal surfaces. I think in that particular type of case a puncture of the posterior vaginal wall and a packing with a cigarette drain, or even iodoform gauze into the culdesac at least, gives an outlet to the accumulation which may be present and very rarely does any harm.

I can recall only one case in the past two years in which I used abdominal drainage, in which there was an adherent tube and ovary between the bladder and the peritoneum of the anterior abdominal wall. When I completed the operation there was a raw bleeding surface between the bladder and the anterior wall, and instead of the old fashioned drainage gauze, I simply introduced a little rubber tissue drain through the lower angle of the wound going to the bleeding surface, which was left in for about forty-eight hours and then withdrawn.

Dr. Waldo's description of the Mikulicz pouch reminded me of my first experience with it, when I was a house surgeon at Bellevue Hospital. Dr. Lusk, who was the attending surgeon, had been abroad that previous summer, and came back, having seen Mikulicz use his pouch. It was packed into the culdesac and a long strip of iodoform gauze was packed through the middle of it. I remember in those days we used silk ligatures in the broad ligament and rather heavy silk at that. We got the gauze out of the pouch and then came the day to remove the outside pack, which Dr. Lusk did himself. With the pack in the case to which I am referring came both the ligatures from the ovarian arteries, then a stream of blood shot up, and the woman immediately went into collapse. Dr. Lusk immediately repacked the wound. The woman got well, but she was not so fortunate as Dr. Waldo's case, because she developed a large ventral hernia. I have always been skeptical about the Mikulicz pouch ever since that experience.

DR. RALPH WALDO (closing).—I fully approve of that telltale drain about which Dr. Taylor and Dr. Studdiford have spoken.

I don't want to create the impression in anybody's mind that I drain very frequently. I formerly used to drain quite frequently. I don't drain now unless there is a good reason for it.

Another thing about the acute cases: I was criticized quite severely a few years ago because I would not operate on acute infections of the pelvis, tubes and ovaries. At the present time there is no abdominal surgeon who would operate on acute cases.

Dr. Frederick C. Holden read a paper entitled: **Are the Operations for Absence of the Vagina Justifiable?**

The question of operation for the construction of an artificial vagina has been brought rather forcibly to my mind on several occasions during the past few years. At an autopsy held recently at the City Mortuary the specimen shown was removed. It illustrates, perhaps, the most frequently used operation, the so-called Baldwin operation, or ileac substitution. This subject was operated upon in a small New York hospital and I submit the following quotation from the autopsy report of Dr. Charles Norris, to whom I am indebted for the privilege of presenting it.

"Small intestines: Mucous membrane normal with the exception of a few reddish areas in lower part of ileum. A loop of ileum is adherent to the vagina and when separated there is found an opening about ½ inch in diameter. Part of the mesentery has been removed at operation, in which place there are sutures. There is a lateral anastomosis of the ileum near the cecum, sutures being present, the communication being free, the lumen being somewhat narrow. There is an opening connecting the pelvic cavity with the vulva. Bladder is normal, there being infiltration with blood in front of it. There is an ovary on each side about normal in size, and internal to it on either side connecting with the broad ligament, there is solid tissue somewhat elongated, about 1 inch in length by ⅝ to ½ inch in width and thickness, which on section is firm. Microscopic section of this tissue shows it to be typical uterine structure."

To my mind an operation is not justifiable if it carries too great a mortality rate, and it must substitute a reasonable degree of improvement in the anatomical and physiological state. There are, at present, three types of operations used for the formation of an artificial vagina. First and most commonly the substitution of a section of the ileum, the Baldwin operation; secondly the substitution of a portion of the rectum, Schubert's operation; and lastly a plastic procedure using the skin of the vulva and thighs as devised by Graves. With Schubert's and Graves' procedures I have had no experience and from collected reports they are apparently little used.

By personal communication with our confreres in this city, I have noted seven cases operated within the past few years with a mortality of three. I have, however, communicated with Baldwin and he reports fifteen cases with a mortality of one. From personal observation and communication I have arrived at the following conclusions:

1. The Baldwin or any other type of operation for construction of an artificial vagina is not justifiable in an unmarried woman who desires the operation that she may marry. The prime object of marriage is to beget children, and this type of woman surely can never conceive; her married life is bound to be unhappy and marriage upon her part should be discouraged and the operation not performed.

2. The Baldwin operation is justifiable in a woman already married, who finding the consummation of her marriage is impossible desires relief through operation and who thoroughly understands the mortality risks and the fact that the relief obtained is often decidedly unsatisfactory.

3. It is my opinion that the plastic operation of Graves and the rectal substitution of Schubert are very seldom justified, for they substitute at best a de-

cidedly unsatisfactory vagina, although undoubtedly they carry a much lower mortality rate.

DISCUSSION

DR. HIRAM N. VINEBERG.—I have done the Baldwin operation once with only partial success so far as the vagina was concerned. The patient made a very good recovery from the operation but the result was such that I did not consider it a very successful vagina, although it served the purpose fairly well. She was a married woman and desired to have some relief for otherwise she was going to be divorced. For the first few months it seemed to be fairly satisfactory, then I lost track of her. There is, however, in the absence of the vagina one condition which must be considered, namely, the absence of the lower third of the vagina. In those cases there is usually a rudimentary uterus and there is a vagina higher up. Those cases are very successfully operated upon; in fact, I have had occasion to do several myself. One dissects between the bladder and the rectum from below as far as possible and then does a laparotomy, pushes down the bladder away from the rudimentary uterus, finds the upper part of the vagina and introduces an instrument through the upper vaginal pouch until it reaches the space created by the dissection from below. A strip of gauze is left in the opening in the vaginal pouch and serves as a guide to connect the vaginal pouch with the skin outside. In one case that I did this operation, it was very successful. In this case there was only a small nodule the size of an almond representing the uterus. There is apparently no vagina present, but if you examine these cases *per rectum* you will find there is a small uterus and usually this upper part of the vagina is developed sufficiently to be brought down to the external skin and sutured to it, forming a very satisfactory and permanent vaginal canal.

DR. GEORGE G. WARD, JR.—I recall a case similar to those under discussion, one in which there was a rudimentary vagina present, but it was so small that its calibre was about that of a lead pencil. I operated on this patient in the Woman's Hospital. She had been previously operated on by an incision with an attempt at suturing the reverse way, without any satisfaction. I was able to get a flap from the labia minora, leaving it attached, and turned it in, thereby increasing the calibre of the vagina. The result was perfectly satisfactory, so I was informed by the patient.

I agree with the conclusions that Dr. Holden has drawn. In these cases of total absence of the vagina I doubt very much if any of them are really satisfactory and there is no question about the very grave risk that these cases must undergo.

DR. GORDON GIBSON.—I can add one Baldwin case to the record. This girl had been in several hospitals in Brooklyn and finally came into the Long Island College Hospital. She was most unhappy and wanted an operation done. She had the risk explained to her, knew what the proposition was and really demanded operation. The findings were surprisingly like those of Dr. Holden's specimen in that there was no vagina, rudimentary uterus and no fusion of the ducts.

The operation is not difficult at all, but the margin of error is tremendous. In the first place, you must get that part of the ileum so well mobilized that there is no tension on the mesentery; second, you must get the right length so that none of it hangs in the abdominal cavity after you get through.

This case which we did lived fourteen days. There was no reaction so far as the abdomen was concerned, but she had a terrific vaginal discharge. She died on the fourteenth day of sepsis. In the last few days we dilated up this artificial tract and evacuated the pus which had collected in a little loop of ileum which was left at the top of the sinus. I would very much question the advisability of this operation and think I can subscribe to Dr. Holden's remarks that an operation of this kind is unjustifiable.

DR. J. RIDDLE GOFFE.—I had a case a number of years ago like that which Dr. Ward referred to in which the vagina had the caliber of a lead pencil. The clitoris was about 2½ inches long. This pseudohermaphrodite was in love with a man and wanted to get married, and came to me to have that organ removed and to be put in condition to be married. I studied the case for some time and finally decided that I could make an incision along the side of the vagina on either side and through the vagina until it would reach the proper capacity, and then make an incision along the dorsal side of the clitoris, or the penis, and then on the ventral side. After doing this I dissected off two flaps laterally and removed the clitoris and then carried these two flaps into the vagina in order to fill up the spaces on either side. The flaps adhered and when I discharged the patient she had a vagina of perfect functional capacity. I understood that she was married about six weeks afterwards and I learned that everything was satisfactory.

DR. FRANK R. OASTLER.—I can add one more case to the record. She was operated on in Vienna. An external flap operation had been performed. The result was functionally good, except that the pubic hair had continued to grow in the vagina to such an extent that the new vagina was always partially blocked, so that the ultimate result of the operation was not very good. I am in accord with Dr. Holden's statement that this operation should not be done unless under extreme circumstances.

DR. FRANKLIN A. DORMAN.—I recollect a case at the Post-Graduate Hospital, a young Italian woman, of the thin, poorly-nourished type, who was very unhappy because her husband had told her that if he was not able to have intercourse with her he would leave her.

On examination of this woman no sign of a vagina was found although she seemed to be a normal female. I decided to try to make a vagina for her. We succeeded in getting an opening between the rectum and bladder and did the flap operation. The patient left the hospital after a reasonable time with a fairly adequate vagina, but it looked as though it was not going to stay. There her history ended until a year or two later, when she came back to the clinic with a friend. She looked well, happy and contented.

NEW YORK ACADEMY OF MEDICINE. SECTION ON OBSTETRICS AND GYNECOLOGY. STATED MEETING, HELD NOVEMBER 22, 1921

DR. HAROLD BAILEY IN THE CHAIR

DR. MILTON A. SHLENKER reported a case of **Hydatidiform Mole.**

Although this condition is supposed to occur only once in every 2400 cases, I have had occasion to present two other specimens before this Section within the year. I am presenting this case because of its typical symptomatology and the great difficulty we experienced in coming to a conclusion.

The patient, R. L., thirty-five years of age, an Austrian, came under observation on July 18, 1921. Her father died of carcinoma of the stomach at the age of forty-five years. She had been married fourteen years, had had four children and no miscarriages. Her husband is well. Her first menses occurred at the age of fourteen years, were of the 8-day type, usually every thirty days. The last menstrual period was April 2, 1921. Appetite poor, and she is habitually constipated. She has had stomach trouble for the past ten years, and states that the doctor told her she had gallstone attacks. Her weight was 134 pounds which is ten pounds lighter than a year ago. She presented no bladder symptoms and denied history of venereal disease. She stated that about June 1, she began to bleed and at the same time suffered with cramps in the lower abdomen, and passed large clots. During the latter part of June she contined to pass clots but did not experience any cramps or abdominal pain. She was admitted to the Gouverneur Hospital on July 18, looking critically ill. Her teeth were poorly kept and many were missing. Her tonsils were enlarged and cryptic. The heart sounds were regular and of good quality, with a faint systolic murmur at the base, and a thrill in the precordial region. The fundus of the uterus was four inches above the symphysis. The abdominal wall was relaxed. There was no tenderness or tumor. Vaginal examination revealed a lacerated perineum, rectocele and cystocele, and bilateral laceration of the cervix. The uterus corresponded to a three months' pregnancy and was in the normal position. Palpation of the adnexa showed a small round hard mass the size of hickory nut on the left side, which was very tender on palpation.

On July 21, the patient complained of an abscessed tooth which was removed. On the following day she seemed much better. The bleeding had stopped. The uterus was still enlarged and the cervix firmly closed. The diagnosis was threatened abortion. The patient insisted in leaving the hospital against advice. On August 29, she was readmitted. She stated that after her return home she began to bleed and to pass clots more or less continuously, but she did not experience any pain whatsoever. About three weeks before she noticed that she began to sweat, and complained of backache, headache, and difficult vision. She stated that she passed dark colored urine freely. Had a bad taste in the mouth. She had not yet felt life. Examination showed the abdomen enlarged and prominent, with edema of the lower abdominal wall. The uterus was large, globular, and extended a little above the umbilicus. No fetal heart was heard, nor was ballottement present. There was also marked edema of the vulva and lower extremities. The blood pressure was 178/90. The specific gravity of the urine was 1034; albumin 4-plus, and many leucocytes and granular casts and red blood cells were present. The temperature was normal. On September 2 interruption of pregnancy was decided upon for a supposed toxemia. The cervix, which admitted one finger, was packed with iodoform gauze. Three days later the patient was bleeding profusely and was removed to the operating room and the cervix dilated. Grapelike bodies could be felt, but no evidences of a fetus. With the use of a sponge forceps large quantities of this material were removed from the uterus. The uterine cavity was thoroughly evacuated. The patient began to bleed profusely and caffeine and camphor in oil were given plus a hypodermoclysis of normal saline solution. After complete evacuation of the uterus it contracted down to about one-fourth its previous size.

The pathologic report stated that fragments of cyst wall and chorionic villi were found. The diagnosis was hydatidiform mole. The patient made an uneventful recovery, and was discharged September 18, apparently well.

On October 25 this patient was admitted to the surgical division of the hospital with a history of bleeding more or less at times since she left the hospital in September; the bleeding was of negligible quantity. On the morning of her admission she had bled profusely and complained of pains in her back and both sides of the lower abdomen. Her temperature was normal, pulse 62.

On October 26th she was operated on by Dr. Ladin and a large amount of tissue resembling placenta was removed. There was no evidence of products of conception. A laparotomy was performed and both ovaries found to be cystic, the right being the size of an orange, while the left was much smaller. A bilateral salpingooophorectomy was performed.

The pathologist reports that the scrapings were simply hypertrophied endometrium and that the ovaries had undergone a simple cystic degeneration.

DR. SHLENKER also reported the **Death of a Fetus in Twin Pregnancy Due to Twists in the Cord.**

Death as a result of this condition is supposed to occur within a few days prior to the delivery of the child. In our case the patient complained of excessive fetal movements about two weeks before her delivery, but had scarcely felt any life whatsoever after this period. The dead fetus was a male and decidedly more robust than the female child which was delivered alive and in good condition. The first child to be delivered was the dead male. The membranes were ruptured artificially, and much meconium was discharged with the amniotic fluid. On delivery the fetus did not breath, nor was there any beating of the heart, and all efforts to establish respirations were without avail. The second child was delivered by a breech extraction and without difficulty.

The specimen shows a single placenta with two cords, each coming from the opposite sides. Each child was contained in separate amniotic sac. The dead child was attached to the large half, which in the fresh state was pale in color and tough to the feel, and there was more or less of a demarcation line from the other half of the placenta which was apparently normal in consistency and otherwise.

DISCUSSION

DR. H. C. WILLIAMSON.—The toxic symptoms in the case of hydatidiform mole interested me. The patient had a low blood pressure and the urine showed albumin and casts, a kidney toxemia which was cured when the hydatid mole was removed. This I believe is an evidence that toxemia of pregnancy is due to syncytiotoxins.

DR. WILLIAM P. HEALY.—The case of hydatid mole has several very interesting features about it. Dr. Shlenker in his remarks drew attention to the unusual experience of having had three of these cases within a year, the specimens of which he has presented here. That indicates that he is more or less on the alert in regard to the diagnosis of cases of this kind, and in this instance the symptoms were not sufficiently definite to enable him to make the diagnosis. In other words, the symptoms were those of impending abortion. There was only one possibility of avoiding error and that might have justified his making the diagnosis of hydatidiform mole when the patient first came under observation, that was he mentioned that the fundus was four inches above the symphysis pubis. That would indicate a uterus somewhat larger than it ought to be at that period. However when the woman came under observation later, after she had been home for a time, it was evident that she had a very large uterus, larger than it should be and there were no fetal heart sounds. With these symptoms and the history of bleeding the diagnosis became an easier matter. Dr. Shlenker then removed the hydatid mole and cleansed out the uterus being careful not to use a sharp instrument. The patient then passed out of observation in absolutely good condition, the toxemia having subsided. The question that comes up is whether when she was first seen she had the hydatid mole or whether the hydatid mole developed in an incomplete abortion. I do not see how we can answer that question, but we do know that a careful examination of the secundines microscopically has shown a very high percentage of hydatid degeneration. It is more than possible that the patient may have incompletely aborted and later developed the hydatid mole.

DR. BAILEY.—Perhaps some of you may remember that Dr. Vineberg reported before the New York Obstetrical Society a case of hydatid mole in which after leaving the hospital the patient had frank hemorrhage. She was brought back and the uterus was removed without further examination, and that uterus proved to have a chorioepithelioma in the fundus. The case brought up some discussion as to the advisability of going ahead and removing the uterus with only a history of bleeding following the removal of a hydatid mole. You may recall that some 13 per cent of women having hydatid moles die in the first place, and 15 per cent of the remainder develop chorioepithelioma. For this reason it is questionable whether the treatment should not be removal of the uterus. I have always done what Dr. Shlenker did, that is, dilate the cervix and attempt with the finger and sponge forceps to remove the hydatid mole. This woman should have had at the second operation a laparotomy and removal of the uterus. There were bilateral cysts of the ovaries which were simple cysts, but nevertheless it would have been better for the woman to have had the uterus removed for it is probable that a chorioepithelioma is growing there. Dilatation of the cervix and removal of the mole by sponge forceps is the usual, but cannot be considered as satisfactory, treatment for this condition.

DR. BAILEY.—It is exceedingly remarkable that the child in the case of cord dystocia should have grown to full size and did not die until a short time before birth.

DR. SHLENKER.—The fetus was slightly macerated. From the history of the case it would seem that the fetus had been dead for two weeks. It is still remarkable that the child should have grown all through the fetal period and obtained sufficient nourishment from that twisted cord.

Replying to Dr. Healy's inquiry as to the period of gestation when this mole occurred, this could have, in a degree, been determined by a microscopic examination. We know that after the third month of gestation, the layers of Langhans and the syncitium become fused into a single layer.

Answering Dr. Bailey as to the removal of the uterus for a hydatidiform mole, I would consider a panhysterectomy for this condition a rather radical procedure. It is our plan to carefully evacuate the uterine cavity, and thereafter keep the patient under careful observation for quite a long period. Had this patient been returned to our service, I would have, under the existing condition, performed a panhysterectomy, especially since this patient had bilateral ovarian cysts. We know that lutein cysts are now an etiologic consideration in chorioepithelioma. The pathologist reported these tumors of the ovaries as simple cysts.

I was deeply interested in this case of twisted cord with death of the fetus because of its extreme rarity. I have been unable to find any great number of similar cases reported. I noted where one case was reported in which there were 348 twists in the cord. This fetus while in fair state of preservation showed some evidences of postmortem changes.

Department of Reviews and Abstracts

CONDUCTED BY HUGO EHRENFEST, M.D., ASSOCIATE EDITOR

Collective Review

FEAR OF THE FETUS: AN ANCIENT CAUSE FOR THE CESAREAN SECTION

BY ALFRED ELA, BOSTON, MASS.

"THE fear of the spirits of the dead appears to have been one of the most powerful factors, perhaps, indeed, the most powerful of all, in shaping the course of religious * * * development from the lowest to the highest; and for that reason it is not specially characteristic of any form of society."[1, 2] Linked with this was the jealousy toward living mankind felt even by the Olympian gods[3] which they manifested by causing premature deaths.[4] This too was felt by demigods, the belief in whose jealousy, the world over, gave rise to hero-cults, that is, "appeasement of souls cut off by misadventure in their prime and believed to be envious of their survivors."[5] Similar were the cults of martyrs[6] and of criminals;[7] and the like belief may have caused the "murder-stones" and cairns of loose rocks where some one had died by violence.[8] Most envious of all, however, were the spirits of fetuses who, not having had any fair chance for life on earth, were naturally resentful toward those enjoying better fortune, manifested especially by inflicting disease upon some relative, "because, not having lived long enough on earth to form attachments to their living relations, they were less likely to show mercy."[9] Far away from modern New Zealand[10] is ancient Egypt's gilded mummy which Pierre Loti graphically describes thus: "On a table in the middle of one of the rooms, a thing to make you shudder gleams in a glass box, a fragile thing that failed of life some two thousand years ago. It is the mummy of a human embryo, and some one, to appease the malice of the born-dead thing, had covered its face with a coating of gold—for, according to the belief of the Egyptians, these little abortions became the evil genii of their families if proper honor was not paid to them. At the

---

[1] The Golden Bough (J. G. Frazer) ed. 3, viii, 36-37; ibid., ix, 93, 98.
[2] Dread of evil spirits is generally gone from modern culture, see Proceedings of Charaka Club, 1916, iv, 5; why, a problem for psychologists, (E. C. Parsons), Psychoanalytic Review, 1916, iii, 291.
[3] (J. A. Scott) Classical Journal, 1914-15, x, 271-272; ibid., 1918, xiii, 372.
[4] (T. Reinach) note in Revue Critique, March 18, 1916, p. 192.
[5] Folk-Lore, 1917, xxviii, 279-294, at 285-286.
[6] Compare Tertullian's Invidia of the Martyrs, Expositor, July, 1919, at 33, end.
[7] Cult of Executed Criminals at Palermo (E. S. Hartland) Folk-Lore, 1910, xxi, 167-179, at 178.
[8] Passim in Notes and Queries (London), e.g., 12 Series, v, 188. And so generally, Golden Bough, ix, 21; Popular Religion and Folk-Lore of India, (W. Crooke, 1896 ed.) i, 235.
[9] Maori Religion and Mythology (E. Shortland), 31, 107-108. Compare, as to spirits of own family, Golden Bough, vi, 188.
[10] (E. Tregear) Journal of the Polynesian Society, 1917, xxvi, 87-88.

end of its negligible body, the gilded head with its great fetus eyes, is unforgettable for its suffering ugliness, for its frustrated and ferocious expression."[11] The same fear, which Loti sets out, doubtless caused the preservation of a prehistoric (probably paleolithic) fetus in a Syrian grotto.[12]

The Maori's (New Zealand) belief in the malignant evil spirit of the dead fetus may arise from the latter having had no soul and so being especially liable to carry off souls of survivors;[13] the disastrous consequences of its death while in this soulless condition were avoided in Old Calabar, by giving abortives as tests, early in the pregnancy.[14] "Saxon Leechdoms"[15] also gave directions for removing a dead fetus; but removing a living fetus, for uses in magic, seems still to be frequent in India.[16] That the fetus has a will of its own was believed in France not long ago[17] and forms the basis of obstetrical practice in China,[18] and in sundry places where (it is thought) the time of delivery is at the option of the fetus and where it must be starved, or frightened, out.[19] The Maori belief that the parent of such an ill-shaped creature (as a fetus) is a shark or lizard,[20] appears in more extended form among some of our own countrymen, their belief having been written upon by a Massachusetts lady.[21] A similar fear of the fetus is extant in Europe today; for instance in Maestricht where one of "the names to fearen babes withal"[22] is that of "Gerritje ongeboren" (little Girard who has not been born);[23] so in the Shetlands, from a parallel cause, work is suspended on St. Thomas' Day, December 21;[24] it of course not being now understood there of whom Thomas was a twin,[25] and that one of twins, as also a prematurely-born fetus, in various parts of the world should be exposed for destruction, while special purification is required by the mother.[26] That she (after miscarriage or delivery of a stillborn child) is dangerous in high degree, many primitive peoples believe; if she conceals it,[27] disaster is brought to her family or to the whole tribe,[28] doubtless because the fetus-demon can then not be duly exorcised. The methods of preventing such "revenants" cover too much ground for discussion here, except in the cases of *fetus in utero*; viz.,

---

[11]Egypt (La Mort de Philae) (by Pierre Loti, translated . . . . W. P. Baines) at 49; in the original, 54-55.
[12]L'Anthropologie, 1900, xi, 781, quoting Lyon Médical, (no date).
[13]See Golden Bough, viii. 97 and 102; ix, 261-262. Compare (s. v. Abortions) Semitic Magic (R. C. Thompson, 1908) 20, 21, 23; and Tales * * * Eskimo. (Rink, 1875) xlv, 439f, cited in Encyclopaedia of Religion and Ethics (ed. Hastings, et al., 1914) vi, at 55, end.
[14]Labor among Primitive Peoples (G. J. Engelmann, 3d. ed.) 2.
[15]Leechdoms, Wortcunning and Starcraft of Early England (ed. O. Cockayne) i, 27, 39, 362-363.
[16]Omens and Superstitions of Southern India (E. Thurston) 224-229.
[17]Labor among Primitive Peoples (G. J. Engelmann) 7.
[18]Ibid., 6-7 (as translated and ed. by Rodet) 335-359.
[19]Ibid., 6, 20, end.
[20]Maori Religion and Mythology (E. Shortland) 18.
[21]Hawaiian Shark Aumakua (M. A. Beckwith) American Anthropologist, 1917, xix, 505-517.
[22]Names Terrible to Children, a long but incomplete series, in (London) Notes and Queries, at and prior to, 11 Series, ii, 133.
[23]Revue des Traditions Populaires, 1917, xxxii, 223.
[24]See Folk-Lore, 1917, xxviii, at 304.
[25]That is, Jesus; see Boanerges (J. R. Harris) 245-246, *et passim*; but the intended elaboration thereon in India, was interrupted indefinitely in consequence of the learned author's being submarined twice.
[26]Golden Bough, iii, 286, and 286-7, note⁶.
[27]"If the woman should conceal from the other people that she has had a premature birth . . . the standard of conduct is shifted from a natural to a supernatural basis; . . . the will of God tends to supercede the wishes, real or imaginary, of purely natural beings." Golden Bough, iii, 213-214.
For confession is like a spiritual purge, ibid., 214-219.
[28]Ibid., iii, 140; 152-155, 211.

"Among the Kei Islanders, if a woman dies in child-bed, they kill the unborn babe, to prevent the woman becoming a *Pontianak*, in which case she would haunt her husband and emasculate him."[29] Far nearer to us, in every way, is "The universal belief of Galician Jews that no dead pregnant woman should be buried with child within. That would mean a great danger to the town in which it happened. So when such a case occurs, all means are taken to abstract the child from the body of its mother."[30] This cause-and-effect I felt sure about but never expected to find it thus exemplified; it seems to bring into today's life the reason for that operation among the ancient Hebrews[31,32] which has long stood unexplained in the history of the cesarean section. This history has been written in a skeptical spirit, possibly as a consequence of the heavy percentage of cesarean mortality, almost into our time. In view of the numerous representations in the arts[33,34] and of incidental notices,[35] it seems probable that the Greeks and Romans were more successful in performing the cesarean section than were our ancestors; this is the more likely because of the surprising finds of such operations in Africa.[36,37] That the child was extracted from the dead mother on magical grounds was doubtless the reason for the Roman *Lex Regia* which comes to us from very early times.[38] This law puzzled a famous surgeon-theologian-inquisitor of the Church in explaining in his *Sacra Embryologia*[39] how the practice as to baptism, as set out in the *Rituale Romanum*,[40] coincided in effect with that coming "*ab antiquis Romanis, quamquam Idololatris et nihil de Baptismate cogitantibus.*" This can properly be explained by remembering that ancient Rome was a regular fossil-bed of primitive beliefs and practices;[41] so (the Romans of all epochs being singularly conservative) it would be strange indeed if so important a practice should not have survived. Only a small shift in view was needed and this in line with other analogues to "Sin-eating" as noted by Frazer: "The original intention of such practices was perhaps not so much to take away the sins of the deceased as to rid the survivors of the pollution of death."[42]

All necessary was to fix the time for the soul's entering the fetus (say at forty or eighty days of pregnancy),[43] and to direct attention

[29] Mystic Rose . . . . (A. E. Crawley), 73.
[30] Translation of (S. Rubin) Der Urquell, 1897, n.f. i, 270.
[31] "Nothing more or less than the classical Cesarean section:" Embryology and Obstetrics in ancient Hebrew Literature (D. I. Macht) Johns Hopkins Hospital Bulletin, 1911, xxii, 143-146 at 145.
[32] But see more extended discussion in Biblisch-talmudische Medizin (J. Preuss, 1911) at 490-498, 698-700.
[33] L'operation césarienne dans l'art, Chronique Médicale, 1910, xvii, 1785; (and 1908, xv, at 149-150).
[34] Der Kaiserschnitt nach den ältesten Überlieferungen unter Zugrundelegung von 18 Geburtsdarstellungen, (F. Weindler) Janus, 1915, xx, 1-40.
[35] E. G., Across a Gap of 2,000 Years (A. Ela) Jour. Am. Veterinary Med. Assn., 1916, n. s. i, 650.
[36] Notes on Labor in Central Africa (R. W. Felkin) Edinburgh Med. Jour., 1883-4, xxix, 922-930, at 928-929, and plates.
[37] L'âme d'un peuple africain, les bambara (Joseph Henry) 225, (non vidi); Mit Emin Pascha ins Herz von Afrika. (F. Stuhlmann, 1894) 82, 184, 391, 625, 674, 724.
[38] Numa Pompilius; "Negat lex regia mulierem, quae praegnans mortua sit, humari, antequam partus ei excidatur: qui contra fecerit, spem animantis cum gravida peremisse videtur." Digesta, i, xi, t. 8 (ed. T. Mommsen, 1902, i, 158).
[39] Theologie und Geburtshilfe nach F. E. Cangiamila's Sacra Embryologia (editio Latina, MDCCLXIV) mit aktuellen Bemerkungen (L. Knapp, 1908).
[40] Ibid., at 72: "Si mater praegnans fuerit, foetus quam primum caute extrahatur, ac si vivus fuerit, baptizetur."
[41] See Golden Bough, ix, 234; and Religious Life of Ancient Rome (J. B. Carter) 5.
[42] Golden Bough, ix, 46, footnote[2] end.
[43] Archiv für Kriminal-Anthropologie und Kriminalistik, 1914, lx, 330; this question has a very great literature (J. Preuss in Biblisch-talmudische Medizin at 450); discussion, with some new light thereon, is postponed.

toward saving this immortal soul rather than toward what injury it might do the survivors. This gave rise to the new[44] theory of the rights of the unborn child as a separate creature,[45] which were discussed in connection with abortion, cesarean section and, later, in "the great debate as to intrauterine baptism."[46] The doctors of the Sorbonne finally decided that such baptism even by midwives is valid,[47] and special apparatus to administer such was made and can be seen depicted.[48,49] As the Church is opposed to craniotomy[50] and other killing of the unborn,[51] so (for the purpose of the child's baptism) it enjoined performance of the cesarean section if the mother be dead; this command was enforced on the physician, by the Civil Arm, under penalties even reaching death. Whether it is his duty to operate on the living mother (who has had the sacraments) with or without her consent, is still a matter of controversy.[52]

45 BROMFIELD STREET.

[44]Infant-baptism was not usual among the early Christians (M. Höfler in Archiv für Religionswissenschaft, 1909, xii, at 353, end), before the fifth century (Evolution of Infant Baptism, Tymms, 1912, non vidi), after the Roman influence had loomed larger in comparison with the Jewish and Greek.
[45]See Encyclopaedia of Religion and Ethics, vi, 56; Medical Record, Jan. 8, 1919, 108, end; Alienist and Neurologist, 1911, xxxii, 262-273.
[46]Die Medizin in der klassischen Malerei (E. Holländer), 240, end.
[47]L'Art d'Accoucher (J. Astruc, 1785) 336-341; 327-335.
Fuller details in Histoire des Accouchements chez tous les peuples (G-J-A. Witkowski, 1887 ed.) 141-144.
[48]Ibid.: Appendice: L'Arsenal Obstétrical, 47-48; text, 145-146.
[49]An instrument for the baptism of children before birth (H. M. B. Moens) Med. Rev. of Rev., Oct., 1919, xxv, 622-624, seems to be the result of a ghastly hoax gulped by a traveler blinded by religious prejudice; see L'Arsenal Obstétrical, 29-35, devices depicted under heading: Accouchement prématuré artificiel et avortement provoqué. Investigation is under way, at the place of the alleged occurrence, to ascertain whether his error was the result of such a hoax, of his misunderstanding explanations in a tongue unfamiliar to him, or of what.
[50]Ecclesiastical Review, 1895, xiii, 128; see its index as to all the points herein touched, as also Das Kind (Ploss-Renz), and Das Weib (Ploss-Bartels) passim.
[51]Ethics of Medical Homicide and Mutilation (A. O'Malley), passim; this book, published under archepiscopal sanction after this article was typed, agrees with many details herein.
[52]See, as to this whole part of the subject, these good items: Histoire des Accouchements ... (Witkowski) 147-148; Address on the administration of baptism, delivered before the Guild of Sts. Luke, Cosmas and Damian. . . . (A. J. Schulte, 1915); Med. and Surg. 1917, i, at 143-144; Discussion on legal aspects of postmortem Cesarean section (C-W. Whiteside) Am. Jour. Obst., 1916, lxxiii, 1051-1058, 1126-1127; Postmortem Cesarean Section (O. G. Pfaff), ibid., 1916, lxxiv, 967-970, 970-972; Same in Tr. Am. Assn. Obst. and Gynec., 1916, xxix, 42-45, 45-47; (G. Linzenmeier) in Med. Klin., 1920, xvi, 439-442.
The diminishing chances of the child's survival and its lessened legal rights (and especially such of the widower), if extraction be delayed till death of the mother, are questions, interesting indeed, but not germane.

Selected Abstracts

General Problems of Obstetrics

Herbert R. Spencer: William Harvey, Obstetric Physician and Gynecologist. British Medical Journal, 1921, No. 3173, p. 621.

The author gives a brief sketch of William Harvey and some of his work. He also considers the contribution of 16th century Paduan teachers of obstetrics and gynecology, discussing the status of obstetrical work in the 16th and 17th centuries. The paper contains interesting pictures of the frontispiece of Harvey's "De Generatione Animalium"; the facade of the university building at Padua; the title page of Mercurio's "La Comare", and the illustration of a Cæsarean Section from the same work. There is also a print of the Canterbury portrait of William Harvey. Quotations are given from the Medical Observations of Harvey which deserve careful consideration at the present time. Following some remarks on the management of ordinary labor in which he advocates patience and gentleness in imitation of Nature, which "is a perfect operatrix" Harvey says, "if you carefully ponder Nature's works, you shall find none of them made in vain, but all directed to some end and some good".—F. L. ADAIR.

Keukenschriever and Doorenbos: Parturition in Javanese Women. General Tijdschrift voor Nederlandsch Indie, Abstr. Nederlandsch Tijdschrift voor Geneeskunde, 1922, i, 403.

It is always of interest to compare labor in women who have been under the influence of civilization for only a short time with the same process in European women. It is for this reason that the above authors made careful notes of 1,000 native women delivered in a hospital in Java.

In the series there were three deaths, two from eclampsia and one from malaria. In only four cases were forceps applied. The number of stillborn children amounted to 3.73%. Twins occurred once in every 180 cases. In only two out of 400 patients in whom the urine was examined were traces of albumin found. Placenta previa occurred only three times and in these, delivery was spontaneous after rupturing the membranes. In 16% of the patients the temperature rose above 38°C. due to malaria or infections, none of which were serious. Pyelonephritis and phlebitis were not encountered. Since all syphilitic patients are registered in the islands, syphilitic mothers are treated early, therefore there were no syphilitic children.

The average weight of the infants was 2,797 gm. as against 3,500 in European children. The authors found that the infants' weight was greater in those cases where the women spent some time in the hospital previous to delivery.

The internal pelvic measurements corresponded closely to those of European women, while the external measurements were less, owing to the finer bone structure of the Javanese.—R. E. WOBUS.

Salesby: The Antenatal Factors of Life and Death—Genetic, Toxigenetic, Gestational and Obstetrical. New York Med. Journal, 1921, cxiv, 413.

The author subjects to a critical review the theory of a certain school of eugenists, who maintain that infant mortality is an illustration of natural selection, that it weeds out the unfit and that to attempt to correct it, is to arrive at racial degeneracy. A study of the causes of death among infants reveals the fact that the solitary instance in which true heredity may be considered a factor—in which death is due to the intrinsic transmission of something in the germ-cells—is hemophilia. The disease, aside from being so rare that it is of no statistical importance, runs contrary to the principle of natural selection, since the female who transmits the disease does not die, but survives to transmit it to her own sons. While true heredity then is negligible in infant mortality and the natural selection theory is baseless, there are a number of antenatal factors of the greatest importance. These include the racial poisons, alcohol and syphilis. Upon the protection of youth and adolescence from these, and upon perfect nutrition and the complete and continuous protection of the expectant mother from intoxication and infection must depend our efforts to save the baby and improve the race.—MARGARET SCHULZE.

Ley: Difficulties Encountered in Pregnancy, Labor and Lactation in Working Class Mothers and Those of the Educated Classes. New York Medical Journal, 1921, cxiv, 412.

The author finds that the minor discomforts of pregnancy are noted far less by the educated classes; probably largely because they observe more carefully the rules of hygiene. They also approach labor and endure its earlier stages with more equanimity, but later demand an anesthetic. The lower classes usually approach labor with fear and do not realize the possibility of relief. Minor difficulties in labor are more common among the upper classes, while major difficulties are extremely rare, since pelvic deformity is almost unknown among the upper classes. Inability to nurse the child due to an insufficient supply of milk is far more common among the upper classes although the mother may desire to nurse it.—MARGARET SCHULZE.

Taylor: Prenatal and Obstetric Care. Pennsylvania Medical Journal, 1921, xxv, 39.

The author presents a considerable group of well selected statistics to show the fallacy of considering pregnancy a harmless physiological process. That the majority of deaths incident to childbirth are preventable by proper prenatal and obstetric care has been proved. The routine employed in the prenatal clinic of the Altoona Hospital is given in detail. The physician gives each prospective mother a booklet containing the information about her care that should come from him instead of the babbling neighbors.—H. W. SHUTT.

Cumpston: The Effect of Legislature Control on the Incidence of Antenatal Syphilis. Medical Journal of Australia, 1921, ii, 133.

Only through a study of accurate statistical data can the effects of legislation for the control of venereal diseases be determined. Reliable statistics are available only so far as antenatal infection is concerned. Two tables are presented showing the mortality figures for a period of ten years, during which the statutes have been in operation. The tables deal with the mortality in the first month and in the first three months respectively.

Scrutiny of these tables demonstrates that no State shows any improvement throughout the period. This would seem to show that either the mortality at the ages under discussion is not the result of venereal infection or the measures now in operation against venereal diseases are not favorably affecting mortality from congenital venereal infections. To better this situation the author suggests the following administrative measures: (1) Routine examination of the wife (or husband) and children of the syphilitic; (2) Routine examination of every pregnant woman (which involves compulsory notification of pregnancy) and a proper origination to insure antenatal examination; and (3) The provision of facilities, at strategic points, for effective prophylaxis for immediate application after exposure to infection.—NORMAN F. MILLER.

Couvelaire: A Dispensary for Syphilis as Part of a Maternity Service. Gynécologie et Obstétrique, 1921, iv, 9.

The necessity of some provision for the proper care of syphilitics seemed evident to Couvelaire when he found that in the Maternité Baudeloque lues seemed evidently responsible for at least one half of the fetal deaths after the sixth month of pregnancy, and for about 20 per cent of the deaths of feeble infants within the first ten days of life. He created a special dispensary under the joint supervision of a syphilographer and an obstetrician who in 1920 cared for 700 syphilitic mothers and 125 babies. The efforts of the dispensary to a large extent are also educational, and most tactfully contact is established with the rest of the family of every syphilitic baby met in the service—R. T. LAVAKE.

Sequiera: The Dangers and Treatment of Antenatal Syphilitic Environment. New York Medical Journal, 1921, cxiv, 415.

Syphilis is a most important factor in the production of premature births, still births and infant mortality. The statistics of Williams, of the Royal Commission on Venereal Diseases of England, of Watson at Glasgow and of Epstein at Prague all emphasize this point. Yet the treatment of the mother by salvarsan and its allies while the fetus is still in utero is remarkably efficient. Statistics vary from 90% to 100% of healthy babies born to treated syphilitic mothers. It is, therefore, most important to impress upon the public that no person who has contracted syphilis, should marry while likely to infect the other partner. Energetic treatment of the syphilitic pregnant woman must begin at once, no matter what the stage of the pregnancy. If a child is brought to a clinic suffering from congenital syphilis, the parents should be seen and, if necessary, treated, and if possible, all the other children should also be examined. In this way, we may hope for the gradual disappearance of a grave menace to life and health.—MARGARET SCHULZE.

Bell, W. Blair: Some Common, but often Unrecognized, Obstetrical Difficulties. British Medical Journal, 1921, No. 3171, 545.

The author calls attention to occipito-posterior positions and emphasizes the possibility of their manual correction. He discusses postmaturity and advises the induction of labor when it is definitely evident that 40 weeks have elapsed. For this purpose he advises intramuscular injection of infundibulin, night and morning, for three days. If this is unsuccessful he uses uterine bougies. The milder grades of pelvic deformities are the ones most frequently overlooked, nonrachitic, flat, generally flat and funnel pelves. He mentions the possibility of diagnosing atonicity of the uterus before labor by failure to react to manipulation during the latter weeks of pregnancy; also by a systolic blood pressure of 110 mm. or less in the latter weeks of pregnancy. This may be overcome and primary uterine inertia avoided by the administration of calcium. He advises a preparation containing pure lactic acid (200 grains), precipitated calcium carbonate (75 grains), and chloroform water (8 ounces). Two ounces of this should be given every night. In addition infundibulin (0.5 c.cm.) may be injected every night and morning for a couple of weeks.—F. L. ADAIR.

Arnold: A Brief Review of Recent Obstetrical Progress. New York Medical Journal, 1921, cxiv, 405.

The science of obstetrics, and perhaps the practical part as done in the better class of institutions throughout the country, shows very decided gains in the last twenty-five years. Yet the great proportion of practical obstetrics is not done in suitably equipped institutions and the mortality and morbidity rates the country over have shown practically no improvement during this period. Statistics for the country at large show that among women of child bearing age, childbirth is second only to tuberculosis as the cause of the greatest number of deaths, that one woman of every 140 who become pregnant dies as a direct result of pregnancy or labor and that one child of every twenty-five dies during the process of birth or as a direct result of that process. The great need is for the application of our knowledge in the domain of practical obstetrics.

Eclampsia may be largely prevented by careful prenatal care. Fetal mortality and maternal morbidity may be greatly reduced by careful diagnosis of the exact relationship in presentation, position and size of the child and the birth canal and by the systematic use of the labor stethoscope. In the treatment of asphyxiated babies, vigorous and violent methods of resuscitation have been replaced by the aspirator, which is all that is needed except in asphyxia pallida. The routine use of pituitrin in the third stage of labor is helpful as blood saving procedure.

Morphine and scopolamine lessen the severity and usually the length of the first stage of labor. The second stage is then terminated artificially under anesthesia, either by the Potter version or a prophylactic forceps operation. A wide episiotomy is done to save the pelvic floor, and is later accurately repaired. This method of delivery conserves the mother's strength. It shortens convalescence, saves the pelvic floor and avoids the dangers of prolonged compression to the baby's brain.—MARGARET SCHULZE.

McKeown: Present Day Obstetrics. Journal of the Kansas Medical Society, 1921, xxi, 320.

The writer advocates advice to mothers; aseptic surgical technic; proper diagnosis; great care of the newborn and special care in all pathological cases, and also discusses episiotomy, version, and cesarean section.—W. K. FOSTER.

Rucker and Haskell: The Dangers of Pituitary Extract: Some Clinical and Experimental Observations. Journal American Medical Association, 1921, lxxvi, 1390.

Supplementing the observations of other obstetricians, Rucker and Haskell find that the use of pituitary extract is responsible for occasional uterine rupture, and definitely increases the frequency of perineal lacerations even in cases where its use is indicated. In the child, asphyxiation and intracranial hemorrhage are more frequent. In experimental animals and, at times, in human beings, the drug causes tetany of the uterus.

In view of the definite danger of even "safe" doses, they feel its use should be discouraged.—R. E. WOBUS.

Schmitt: The Conduct of Labor in Contracted Pelves. Zeitschrift für Geburtshilfe und Gynäkologie, 1921, lxxxiii, 366.

The author considers the conduct of labor in the 538 cases of contracted pelves observed in the second 10,000 deliveries in the Würzburg clinic from 1907 to 1919. Direct measurements by Bylicki's method were employed. Since this is no longer applicable following engagement of the head, many cases of spontaneous labor with mild degrees of pelvic contraction necessarily are omitted from these statistics. This explains the rather low percentage of spontaneous deliveries, 215 or 54.9 per cent of 392 cases of head presentation with a fetal mortality of 4 or 1.02 per cent. Two mothers died, following spontaneous delivery from causes which could not be related to the pelvic contraction.

Breech presentations were encountered in 19 cases or 3.6 per cent of the total number. Three children, or 15.7 per cent of this series died but there was no maternal mortality. Transverse presentations were found in 98 cases or 18.8 per cent of the total number. Three were in primiparae, the rest in multiparae. Sixteen children died or 16.3 per cent. One mother died of dysentery three weeks after labor.

One hundred seventy-seven cases, or 45.1 per cent, were delivered by operation. Version and extraction was employed 28 times, or in 7.1 per cent of cases. Twelve children died, or 47.1 per cent. High forceps were used 24 times with a fetal mortality of 20.8 per cent. The maternal mortality in both these series was 0. Premature labor was induced 63 times. Thirteen children died, 11 were stillborn, the other 2 died within 2 weeks. One mother died 3 weeks postpartum, the case of dysentery mentioned under transverse presentation. Perforation was employed 32 times; twice on the living child, 22 times on the advancing, 10 times on the after-coming head. Two mothers died, both cases of uterine rupture which had occurred before entry; 92 cesarean sections were performed; 32 of those were repeated cesareans; 23 were performed after rupture of the membranes, in 15 cases shortly after, in the rest from 24 hours to 8 days after rupture of membranes. Two cases were Porro operations which survived, of the others, clean cases were operated by the transperitoneal cervical section, infected or suspicious cases by the extraperitoneal section. There were 2 deaths or 2.17 per cent. There were no complications in any of the other cases, not even a wound infection. All the children were born alive, but 3 died in the first few days, or 3.3 per cent.

Bone-splitting operations were employed in only 4 cases, of which all the children and all the mothers lived, but one mother had a thrombosis and a fistula leading to bone, with a very protracted convalescence.

Prolapsed cord occurred in 28, or 7.27 per cent, of the cephalic presentations as opposed to the general incidence of 1.08 per cent in the total of 10,000 cases. 57.1 per cent of these children died.

The total maternal mortality was 7, or 1.33 per cent, the corrected maternal mortality 3, or 0.57 per cent, of whom one woman died of sepsis after a normal labor and 2 died of sepsis after cesarean section. The total fetal mortality was 10.2 per cent at birth, 11.21 per cent including the cases which died in the first few days after labor.—MARGARET SCHULZE.

Browne: Stillbirth: Its Causes, Pathology and Prevention. British Medical Journal, 1921, No. 3161, p. 140.

The article is based on a study of 200 consecutive cases of stillbirth (120) and neonatal death (80). There were 19 craniotomies, 3 on the aftercoming head. Of the stillbirths 49 or 40 per cent were attributed to antepartum asphyxia. Also in 15 of the craniotomy cases death was probably due to asphyxia. The corrected figures would be 64 cases or 53 per cent. The contributory causes of death were placenta previa, accidental hemorrhage, and eclampsia. The chief causes of intrapartum asphyxia were disproportion between the head and the pelvis, primiparity, prolapsed cord and difficulty with the after-coming head. Of the 38 cases of intrapartum asphyxia 11 were breech presentations. Postmortem findings are described in detail. Cerebral hemorrhage was present in 29.5 per cent. Of these 20 were breech and 39 were vertex cases. In the cases of hemorrhage tearing of the tentorium cerebelli was present in 37 per cent, 63 per cent of these were breech cases. There were 22 cases with intraventricular hemorrhage. Of all the cases with tears of the dural septa 60 per cent were unassociated with cerebral hemorrhage. There were 35 cases of syphilis including 14 macerated fetuses. Pneumonia during the first week accounted for 26 per cent of the neonatal deaths. The author describes the pneumonia as acute hemorrhagic pneumonia of infants. He found 18 cases of suprarenal hemorrhage. Out of 200 babies 95 were born prematurely. The causes for it in order of frequency were: syphilis 28; multiple pregnancy 16; induction of labor 12; eclampsia 11; placenta previa 8. Of the premature infants 56 died in the neonatal period. Causes were: cerebral hemorrhage in 22 cases; syphilis in 12; syphilis with pneumonia in 6. The author attributes 3 deaths to twilight sleep. There were also other miscellaneous causes. The author emphasizes the necessity for expert supervision during pregnancy. Only 3 per cent of the 200 cases had received adequate antenatal care. He advocates either voluntary or compulsory notification of pregnancy.—F. L. ADAIR.

Polak: The Defects in Our Obstetric Teaching. Journal American Medical Association, 1921, lxxvi, 1809.

While the mortality from practically all diseases has been reduced, Polak finds that the statistics not only do not show a decrease but a very definite increase in the mortality from childbirth in the U. S. from 1902 to 1919. There have been approximately three times as many deaths from sepsis, four times as many from eclampsia, and twice as many from other obstetrical causes as seventeen years ago. This, he thinks, is due to the relatively poor training of the medical student in the practice of obstetrics. He feels there should be more uniformity in the teaching of the fundamentals of obstetrics and that greater emphasis should be laid upon the responsibility of the obstetrician for the lives of both mother and child.—R. E. WOBUS.

Bourne: The Causation and Prevention of Puerperal Sepsis. The Clinical Journal, (London) 1921, 1, 456.

Despite the apparent advance of sepsis in obstetrics the proportion of deaths from septicemia was exactly the same in 1917 as in 1857. Two factors enter into the production of puerperal fever, (1) the implantation of microbes directly on the placental site; (2) the diminished resistance of the patient against their growth and spread. Sporadic cases of sepsis occur even when all precautions have been used, and when no examinations have been made. Out of 43 cases with a severe, purulent vaginal discharge prenatally, 15 cases had a febrile puerperium, 2 cases being serious. This would lead to the conclusion, that in about a third of the cases with a preexisting infection of the cervix as evidenced by the vaginal discharge, the organisms may ascend into the uterus and cause puerperal fever. Of the last 15 cases of septicemia, at the Queen Charlotte Hospital, London, 8 cases had severe postpartum hemorrhages and in 6 cases the placenta had been removed manually. This means that two of the most favorable conditions for leading to sepsis were present, namely, lowered resistance from hemorrhage and the possibility of direct transference to the placental site of organisms by the hand of the operator. Of 154 cases of manual removal of the placenta 54, or 35%, developed some form of uterine sepsis. The prevention of puerperal sepsis consists in the adequate preparation of the patient and operator, a prenatal attempt to clear up any vaginal discharge, care against postpartum hemorrhage, judgment in manually removing the placenta, and the immediate suturing of perineal wounds.
—A. C. WILLIAMSON.

Bell, W. Blair: The Prevention and Treatment of Puerperal Infections. British Medical Journal, May 14, 1921, i, 693.

According to the Registrar-General's statistics the mortality from puerperal infection now is greater than for any previous year for fourteen years. The author thinks the cause of this is due partly to unnecessary interference. He deplores the too frequent use of forceps. Natural defences against infection are: (1) The general condition of the patient, (2) the normal acid secretion of the vagina, (3) the so-called physiologic leucocytosis occurring toward the end of pregnancy. The points of entry of infection are the placental site and any laceration of the tissues. The promotion of healing by first intention of all lacerations, especially of the perineum, should be secured by appropriate suturing.

His general conclusions are as follows: (1) Puerperal infection must be recognized as largely an avoidable disease. (2) The remedy is in the better application of principles of asepsis and antisepsis. (3) Rectal examination should be substituted for vaginal examination of parturient women in so far as is possible. (4) All lacerations of the perineum should be carefully sutured. (5) Care should be taken in maintaining the natural defences of the patient. In regard to the treatment of puerperal infection the author advocates (1) the early removal of large pieces of placenta with antiseptic irrigation of the uterus; (2) autogenous vaccines and polyvalent serums for general infection; (3) major operations such as ligation of veins in puerperal thrombo-phlebitis. He also suggests (1) the investigation of general and local defences of infection; (2) more appropriate institutional care of the cases of puerperal infection in special wards; (3) the supply of sterile obstetrical outfits for the poor; (4) better organization for the handling of obstetrical cases.—F. L. ADAIR.

Schmitt: The Prevention of Puerperal Fever. Zeitschrift für Geburtshilfe und Gynäkologie, 1921, lxxxiii, 335.

The author gives the morbidity statistics for the second 10,000 labors in the Würzburg clinic, from 1907 to 1919 The list includes 4492 primiparae and 5508 multiparae. Of these cases 17.08 per cent required operative intervention of some type or showed severe obstetrical complications.

The total morbidity was 8.8 per cent, including all cases in which the axillary temperature touched or exceeded 38° C. The "puerperal morbidity" was 3.49 per cent and included all cases in which the fever could not definitely be ascribed to some extragenital cause. The author does not regard bacteriological examination of the lochia as of value in determining which cases of fever are due to puerperal infection, since it is impossible to determine which organisms are pathogenic and which are saprophytic.

Severe disturbances, including cases in which the fever reached or exceeded 39° C., are recorded in .71 per cent, and of these, 15 or .15 per cent died. Only 5 of the labors of these 15 cases were conducted entirely in the clinic, and in 2 of the 5 cases, postmortem examination indicated that the sepsis was of tonsillar rather than puerperal origin. Of the 3 cases in which a fatal infection was acquired in the clinic, one followed a manual removal of the placenta and two a normal labor.

Cases in this clinic are conducted with repeated vaginal examinations by physicians, students, and midwife students, with a careful aseptic technic, though in most cases without gloves; and the author believes the results justify a continuation of the procedure rather than an adoption of routine rectal examinations. Routine preliminary vaginal disinfection is also employed, since it is impossible to determine whether or not the vaginal organisms present are pathogenic. The author does not state what germicidal agent is employed. In a short space of time from October 1, 1909 to April 1, 1911, in which this preliminary vaginal douching was omitted, two cases of fatal sepsis following normal spontaneous labor occurred, and although these were presumably of tonsillar origin, it was deemed wise to return to the old routine.—MARGARET SCHULZE.

Pagge: Circumcision. The Clinical Journal, (London) 1921, 1, 593.

The routine circumcision of every male child is condemned. An occasional death from sepsis or hemorrhage cannot be prevented. The writer feels that insufficient evidence has been presented to prove that circumcision prevents enuresis, hernia, convulsions or any of the other numerous ills attributed to the foreskin. He has never seen any figures to shows that there is less venereal infection or masturbation among the circumcised than the uncircumcised. The foreskin does not naturally retract from the glans until at the time of puberty, and merely because it will not retract before that time, due to adhesions, is no reason for removing it. If the prepuce is redundant so that there is definite uncleanliness; if there is a phimosis or definite interference with urination, circumcision is justifiable and should be done as carefully as any other surgical operation.—A. C. WILLIAMSON.

Book Reviews

Diagnostische und therapeutische Irrtümer und deren Verhütung in der Frauenheilkunde.—Herausgegeben von Professor Dr. J. Schwalbe, im Verlage von Georg Thieme, Leipzig.

This new publication, appearing in the form of small monographs, is based on the truism that a great deal of our most valuable knowledge and experience we acquire through proper appreciation of our mistakes. A group of prominent German gynecologists have expressed their willingness to discuss selected obstetrical and gynecological topics from this novel point of view. They set forth the most common errors in diagnosis and therapy and suggest the means of preventing such mistakes. So far five of these monographs have appeared: Common Errors in the Management of Labor, by Professor Fehling; Diagnostic Mistakes and Their Prevention in the Management of the Puerperium, by Professor Zangemeister; Diseases of Vulva, Vagina, Bladder, Ureters and Urethra. Gonorrhea, Syphilis and Tuberculosis of the Female Genitalia, by Professor Henkel; Diseases of the Uterus, by Professor Reifferscheid; and Diseases of Ovaries, Tubes, Ligaments, Cellular Tissue and Peritoneum, by Professor von Jaschke.

There is no attempt made in these essays to cover the entire subject in a systematic manner as is done in every standard textbook. They rather supply a large amount of valuable information customarily omitted from the textbook.—H. E.

Les Hémorrhagies Méningées Sous-Dure-Mériennes Traumatiques du Nouveau-Né.—By Pierre Lantuéjoul, Interne des Hôpitaux. Paris, Amédée Legrand, Editeur, 1921.

In this monograph of more than 160 pages the author discusses very thoroughly the problem of intracranial birth hemorrhages of the newborn infant. His conclusions are based on 35 observations of injuries of this sort and a careful study of the entire literature on the subject.

Heart Disease and Pregnancy.—By Sir James Mackenzie, M.D., F.R.C.P., Hon. Consulting Physician to his Majesty the King in Scotland; Director of the Institute for Clinical Research, St. Andrews; Consulting Physician to the Victoria Hospital, Burnley, and the London Hospital, London, Henry Frowde and Hodder & Stoughton. 1921.

It will suffice to call the attention of obstetricians to the fact that this lucid exposition of the inter-relation between heart diseases and pregnancy has appeared in form of a monograph. Readers of our Journal have been offered an exhaustive review of this important contribution by Mackenzie in December, 1921, ii, 659.

The American Journal of Obstetrics and Gynecology

Original Communications

DIFFUSE ADENOMYOMA OF THE UTERUS: CONDITIONS INFLUENCING ITS DEVELOPMENT*

BY OTTO H. SCHWARZ, M.D., AND F. POWELL MCNALLEY, M.D.,
ST. LOUIS, MO.

From the Department of Obstetrics, Washington University School of Medicine.

ADENOMYOMA forms one of the most interesting chapters in gynecologic pathology. Its distribution and classification, both uterine and extrauterine, have recently received much attention. Of all types of adenomyoma there is none so common as diffuse adenomyoma of the uterus, and the frequency of the lesion can only be realized by those who study uteri from a microscopic standpoint. When one examines a stained section of uterine wall in which there are present numerous penetrating islands of uterine mucosa several questions immediately present themselves. Several of these are most important. First: What is the origin of the glands? Secondly: What is responsible for their presence in this abnormal situation? Thirdly: What is the nature of the diffuse thickening of the uterine wall and what are its chief characteristics? Fourthly: Is it a tumor, or how should it be classified?

The question as regards the classification of the lesion, particularly whether it deserves the name of tumor or whether it should be considered as a type of hyperplasia has received considerable attention. As a result of various views, apparently the same lesion has been assigned several different terms. Frankl, in 1914, points out that adenomyoma is frequently confused with so-called adenometritis,

---

*Read at a meeting of the New York Obstetrical Society, January 10, 1922.

NOTE: The Editor accepts no responsibility for the views and statements of authors as published in their "Original Communications."

adenomyositis, adenomyometritis and adenoma diffusum. He suggests that the term adenomyoma should be reserved for those lesions which are definitely circumscribed and contain glands; adenometritis for those conditions in which the diffuse thickening with its contained glands is associated with inflammation, which Robert Meyer feels is the basis of explanation for most cases. Frankl states that he has seen cases in which there was absolutely not the slightest evidence of inflammation and suggests the term adenomyosis for such cases.

Strong, of New York, in a recent paper, discusses the same question and points out similarly the shortcomings of the term adenomyoma, and although the title of his paper is adenomyometritis, not adenomyoma, he does not suggest adenomyometritis for general application. Strong also refers to irregular penetrations of the uterine glands of the basalis into the myometrium. He tells us that these are quite common and are most important because they have a distinct bearing on the causation of so-called adenomyoma. These penetrations according to this author, are present to a greater or lesser degree in all uteri, and are extensive in proportion to the amount of inflammation, hyperplastic, or sometimes atrophic change that is present in the endometrium or the myometrium. It has been our experience also, that the endometrium has a very definite tendency to penetrate the myometrium in a large percentage of cases. This is strikingly brought out in the routine microscopic study of uteri removed at operation. Our experience has been that this occurs to a more marked degree in uteri of women that have borne children. Just how extensive this penetration should be, as to whether it should be disregarded or the lesion classified as a so-called adenomyoma is difficult to say. Perhaps an additional factor to consider would be the reaction of the myometrium in the vicinity of this penetrating tissue, in other words, the degree of the myometrial hyperplasia.

It is not our purpose in this paper to review the various theories as regards the origin of the glands in adenomyoma. First, because Lockyer has done this so ably in his recent monograph, and secondly, because we are not dealing with adenomyoma as a whole, but have confined our study only to the diffuse type of the uterine wall.

Although earlier there was a good deal of discussion as regards the origin of the glands in diffuse adenomyoma of the uterus, at the present time the mucosal origin which was first suggested by Cullen and definitely proved by him, is generally accepted. Frankl, in 1914, states other sources of origin for this type of lesion need scarcely be considered. Lockyer in his recent comprehensive review of adenomyoma, discusses at great length the etiologic theories which have been suggested and emphasizes particularly Cullen's mucosal theory. Of particular interest in this connection is the abstract which he gives of

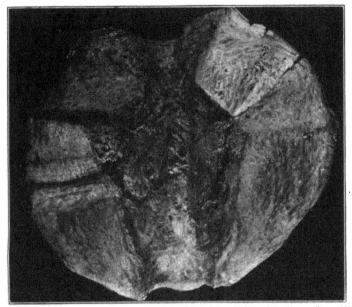

Fig. 1.—Diffuse adenomyoma associated with hyperplasia of the endometrium. Case 1299. Nulliparous uterus, supravaginal portion. Marked diffuse thickening of uterine wall—numerous dilated glands present in uterine wall in upper right portion. Only slight penetration in lower half. Marked hyperplasia of the endometrium.

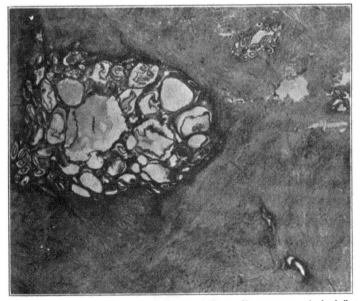

Fig. 2.—Section taken from upper right portion of Fig. 1. Shows numerous glands similar to glands in hyperplasia of the endometrium, which was very striking in this case.

Robert Meyer's latest views regarding the causation of uterine adenomyoma. Meyer tells us that the mucous membrane sends hyperplastic and hypertrophic glands into the uterine muscularis. While the surface layers as a rule are not hyperplastic, and frequently even atrophic, according to Meyer these bits of invading mucosa follow the muscular interstices and the lymph vessels, but do not penetrate the lymph spaces. The invasion, he states, is postfetal, and is a disease of the adult uterus. In this connection Meyer studied one hundred uteri from fetuses, newborn, and girls up to fourteen years of age, and stated that the mucosal projections are seldom seen, and when they do occur it is only singly. We, personally, have examined a great number of similar uteri but have never been impressed with any definite tendency of the endometrium to penetrate the myometrium in such cases. It is quite characteristic of the endometrium of the fetal uterus of about thirty-six weeks' gestation to show only a few layers of cells lining the cavity, from which are differentiated the endometrium, both stroma and uterine glands. There is usually at this time of development no evidence of gland formation. Meyer feels that the invasion of the mucosa is favored by the absence of a true submucosa in the uterine wall and suggests that as a result, mechanical lesions such as might occur after therapeutic means, gestation and inflammation, the intrafascicular connective tissue is incapable of resisting the entrance of the mucosal element.

Cullen, in his elaborate monograph of 1908 on uterine adenomyoma, discusses the question of the causation of diffuse adenomyoma in one short paragraph. He mentions that probably pregnancy with its incident extensive stretching of the uterus might leave crevices in the uterine wall into which the mucosa could later flow. He states, however, that fifteen out of forty-nine patients were never pregnant, and with pregnancy as a possible factor, other causes must be considered for the appearance of the lesion in the nulliparous uteri. Cullen remarks that a number of cases gave a decided impression that the diffuse myomatous growth was the primary factor. He refers to this as a myomatous tendency by the almost constant presence of discrete myomatous nodules in these cases. He emphasizes the fact that the only pathological change in some cases lies in the extension of the normal glands into crevices throughout the diffuse myomatous growth.

Novak, in a recent paper, mentions the fact that hyperplasia of the endometrium is frequently associated with myoma of the uterus, but even more frequently with adenomyoma. Novak's statements made in a discussion of Dr. Cullen's latest paper on the distribution of adenomyoma are of considerable interest in connection with conditions influencing the occurrence of adenomyoma. Novak has been struck with the relationship which appears to exist between adenomyoma of the

SCHWARZ AND MCNALLEY: DIFFUSE ADENOMYOMA   461

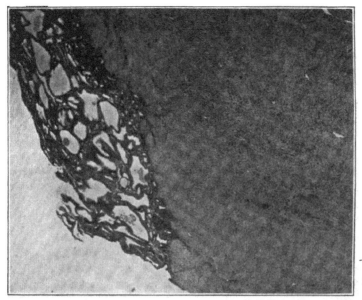

Fig. 3.—Section taken from lower left portion of Fig. 1. Marked hyperplasia of endometrium, shows only a slight tendency to invade. Hypertrophy of myometrium.

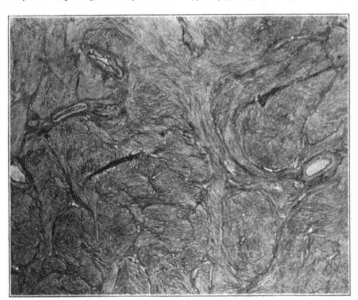

Fig. 4.—Myometrium, higher power; same area of myometrium from which Fig. 3 was taken; orcein-Van Gieson stain. Shows nulliparous distribution of elastic tissue. The internal elastic membrane of the arteries stands out well in this picture. The connective and muscle tissues show prominently. The connective tissue is the fine darker tissue between the lighter muscle bundles.

uterus and the condition known as hyperplasia of the endometrium. He points out that hyperplasia of the endometrium was first accurately described by Cullen in 1900. In many cases of adenomyoma of the uterus, according to Novak, the mucous membranes, both of the surface and deep down in the muscular tissue, show the characteristic pattern of hyperplasia. He mentions that both these conditions are characterized clinically by extensive menstruation, and the apparent connection between the two conditions suggests various interesting possibilities. Hyperplasia of the endometrium, as the term indicates,

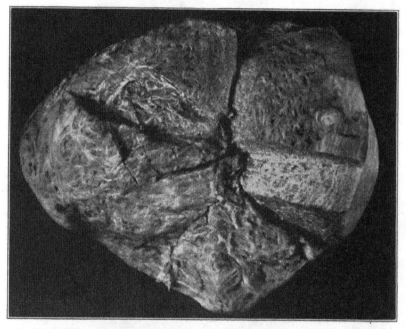

Fig. 5.—Diffuse adenomyoma associated with hyperplasia of the endometrium. Case 1323—similar to Case 1299 except for one full term pregnancy. No evidence of subinvolution. Marked hyperplasia of the endometrium. Marked diffuse thickening of the uterine wall throughout. Lowest portion of the uterus to right—fundus to left.

is characterized by a genuine increase in epithelial and stromal elements of the endometrium, while adenomyoma, in a broad sense is a hyperplasia of the muscular element. Novak feels that both may be produced by the same underlying cause. He calls our attention to the fact that in recent German literature the inflammatory theory of origin is by far the most popular. This is particularly emphasized as regards the causes of adenomyoma of the recto-vaginal septum. He closed by stating that he merely mentioned these facts in order to lure

Dr. Cullen into a discussion of the cause of these interesting lesions. In closing Dr. Cullen merely stated that the cause of adenomyoma is unknown and that there is no evidence that it is due to inflammation as has been suggested by numerous observers.

We feel rather strongly, that on account of the fact that there has been considerable confusion as regards our knowledge of pathological lesions of the uterine wall, that conditions, if any, favoring the development of diffuse adenomyoma would likewise be more or less confused. In our opinion, however, the recent work of Shaw has definitely cleared up certain types of lesions of the uterine wall. Shaw discusses

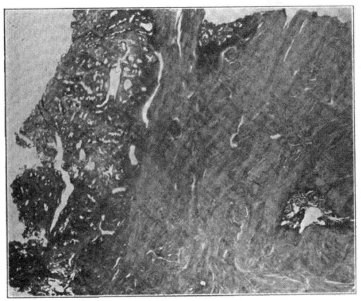

Fig. 6.—Case 1323—low power; showing hyperplastic endometrium and penetration of glands. Structure of myometrium similar to Case 1299, except separation of muscle bundles are more prominent and myometrium coarser looking in the gross.

three lesions, namely, chronic subinvolution, chronic metritis and hypertrophy. Briefly, chronic subinvolution consists of subinvolution of the circulatory system characterized by a diffusion of dead elastic tissue around the walls of the arteries. This material in addition contains unabsorbable portions of the old vessels, a smaller and newer vessel having developed within the old lumen. The veins, particularly the larger ones in the middle third, show a marked increase in this diffused elastic tissue, which has a tendency also to be present between the muscle bundles directly adjacent the veins. Reduplications of the internal elastic membrane in the larger arteries are also a striking

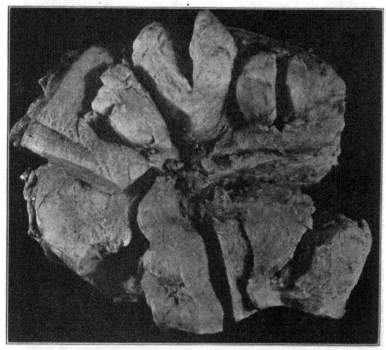

Fig. 7.—Case 1790. Diffuse adenomyoma associated with myomata. Nulliparous uterus. Note the diffuse thickening in the extreme upper portion of the picture.

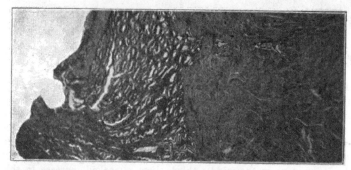

Fig. 8.—Case 1790. Section from area of diffuse thickening in upper portion of Fig. 7. Includes endometrium, which shows definite hyperplasia, and myometrium with several invading glands. Note the definite separation of the muscle bundles.

feature. In the outer third of the uterus between the muscle bundles there is present also a definite increase of this black stained tissue, which, in some instances, is quite excessive. More or less edema is also constantly present. Chronic metritis is a lesion which results from previous active inflammatory process within the uterine wall, and is characterized by a definite increase in connective tissue and small round cell infiltration in the myometrium. If this lesion is present of itself the uteri in most instances are not particularly enlarged and the walls are usually quite firm and cut with considerable resistance. Hypertrophy of the uterine wall is characterized by an increased thickness due to both hypertrophy and hyperplasia of the muscle cells and connective tissue of the uterine wall. This condition is in the nature of a work hypertrophy and, perhaps, is somewhat analogous with hypertrophy of the myocardium under certain conditions. Hypertrophy is chiefly associated with hyperplasia of the endometrium, myomata and also forms a part of the lesion of adenomyoma even to a more marked degree.

Three years ago one of us confirmed the work of Shaw, except that we felt that there was more overlapping of these conditions than his descriptions lead one to believe. Shaw, in a personal communication, referred to this article not as a criticism of his work, but stated that there was very little difference between this work and his, and suggested that it was due rather to the difference of conditions under which the articles were written than to any real difference of view. At the time Shaw wrote his article he used one heading, namely, chronic metritis, and placed the three above mentioned lesions under this one title. He mentioned the fact that the rigid classification which he adopted was due to the fact that he had to emphasize these very distinct types, but realized that there was frequently distinct overlapping. In our opinion Shaw clears up a rather confused subject which should result in the abolishing of a large list of terms referable to lesions of the myometrium.

We know that myomata and hyperplasia of the endometrium frequently accompany diffuse adenomyoma. We felt that a study of a series of cases in which particular attention would be paid to the presence of the conditions described by Shaw, in addition to the presence of myomata and hyperplasia, might lead us closer to an explanation of why the mucous membrane of the uterus penetrates the uterine wall in the lesion of so-called adenomyoma. We, of course, consider that the mucosal origin of the glands in this type of case is proved. This has been shown by serial section, and has been particularly emphasized by Dr. Cullen. Further, because in the early lesions it is very easy to see the connection with the mucosa in almost any single section. We have recently modeled the penetrating islands of mucosa in order to

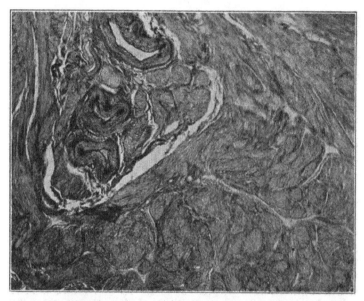

Fig. 9.—Case 1790. Myometrium (orcein-Van Gieson stain) higher power; shows a loose structure, muscle and connective tissue both prominent; nulliparous distribution of elastic tissue. The internal elastic membrane of the arteries stands out clearly; no other elastic tissue evident in the picture.

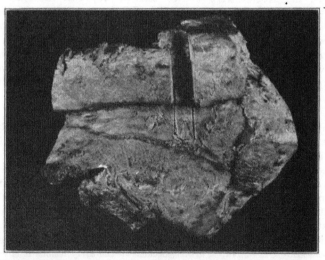

Fig. 10.—Diffuse adenomyoma of the uterus associated with chronic subinvolution. Case 480. Supravaginal uterus—wall 22 mm., thick, endometrium 1 mm. Diffuse thickening not prominent. Penetration of glands over 1 cm., in myometrium in places.

definitely show the relation to one another and also to the endometrium. Mr. Wm. D. Dieckmann prepared this model in the Obstetrical Laboratory. The model shows very clearly the tendency of the mucosa to invade the myometrium; it also shows how the islands communicate with one another. A large portion of the model, however, could be connected to the endometrium only by a very small strand of mucosa, and we have refrained from publishing this work hoping to use a case which shows the connecting links to a more marked degree.

The fact that we rather frequently made a diagnosis of early adenomyoma of the uterus in routine work caused us to become particularly interested in these early cases. We were also particularly interested in the circumstances under which these lesions started, and in the chief characteristics of the myometrium in these cases.

This paper includes the study of forty-nine uteri in which the lesion of adenomyoma exists, apparently, of itself, or coincident with other lesions. The material for this study was chiefly obtained from the Barnes Hospital. However, we are indebted to H. S. Crossen, Lee Dorsett and George Ives for a considerable number of cases. These were divided into two groups. The first group were those cases in which a definite diagnosis of adenomyoma could be made, the lesion, however, still comparatively early. The second group were those cases in which the lesion was well advanced. In the first group there were twenty-three cases and in the second group there were twenty-six cases. These cases were carefully described in the gross, and celloidin sections were studied, stained with hematoxylin and eosin and also with orcein and Van Gieson's stain. The clinical histories were available in all but four of these cases. Careful attention was paid to the presence of hyperplasia of the endometrium, chronic subinvolution, chronic metritis, hypertrophy and myomata.

The hyperplastic myometrium which is present more or less marked in most cases of adenomyoma attracted our attention first. We shall briefly mention some of the impressions that this study made. In the first place the tissue involved has more the characteristics of hyperplasia than of new growth. These lesions of themselves do not reach the limitless growth that the ordinary discrete myomata do. If they reach any considerable size it is due to a dilatation of the contained glands rather than the result of any enormous hypertrophy of the uterine wall. The hypertrophy of the wall is due both to hypertrophy and hyperplasia of the connective tissue and muscle tissue of the uterine wall. This in the gross appears very much coarser than the normal, and in the gross the individual muscle bundles appear much larger. The amount of connective tissue varies. In almost all cases it is definitely increased. This is most striking, perhaps, in the cases in which intramural myomata are associated with the lesion.

This is prominent in both parous and nulliparous uteri. It is also quite marked in cases which are accompanied by hyperplasia of the endometrium. With this condition the connective tissue content of the wall seems to be more prominent in cases in which the patient had

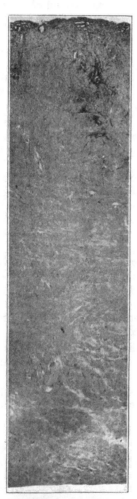

Fig. 11.—Case 480. Entire wall—low power—Hematoxylin-eosin stain. Shows an atrophic endometrium with glands penetrating one-third of the distance to the serosa.

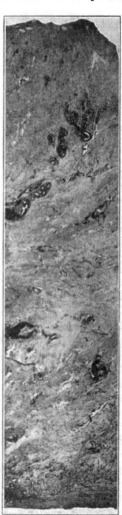

Fig. 12.—Case 480. Same field as Fig. 11. Orcein-Van Gieson stain. Marked evidence of subinvolution throughout wall, collars of diffused elastic tissue about arteries of inner third, marked amount of diffused elastic tissue between muscle bundles of outer third.

had no children, or, perhaps only one. The same fact may be noted in ordinary hypertrophy of the uterine wall in the absence of adenomyoma. The connective tissue increase is less conspicuous in cases which have had numerous pregnancies and where the invasion of the glands is not particularly marked. In such cases also the entire thickness of the uterine wall may not be markedly increased. It is also quite clear that the increase in connective tissue is in no way referable to the inflammatory process such as we see in chronic metritis because we see no accompanying round cell infiltration in this hyperplastic tissue. We do not recall a clear cut case of chronic metritis which

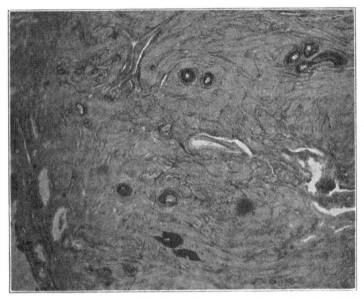

Fig. 13.—Same as Fig. 12. High power. Extreme upper left portion. Shows black collars about numerous arteries; also prominence of connective tissue associated with hypertrophy of the wall.

did not show some definite round cell infiltration in the myometrium.

The individual cells of both muscle and connective tissue are usually somewhat enlarged but are in no way suggestive of being atypical or tumor cells. We have never observed any evidences of degeneration in this tissue. This is in striking contrast to ordinary discrete myomata. This increased connective tissue relation is present in the early lesions and the point which differentiates this tissue from that of early myomata which are noted for their lack of connective tissue in early stages of their development. We have had the opportunity recently to observe the uterus of a nineteen-year-old girl which was riddled with countless small myomata, from microscopic size to as large as 5 mm., none larger. The absence of fibrous tissue in the smaller tumors was quite striking. Comparing these young tumors with the myometrial hyperplasia of ordinary adenomyoma suggests very strongly that their origin has nothing particularly in common and suggests an origin outside of the muscle or connective tissue of the uterine wall. This strongly suggests the origin from blood vessels, as some writers point out. Our case also points strongly to this source. Dorsett and one of us will report this case in detail at a later date.

In short the condition of the myometrium is a definite hyperplasia of all its constituents quite similar to the lesion of ordinary hypertrophy of the uterine wall. This hyperplasia may be present primarily as a result of the presence of discrete myomata, or due to an accompanying hyperplasia of the endometrium; it may be considered a work hypertrophy. In other instances the glands may invade the myometrium primarily and the hyperplasia result from the presence of the glands, and may be considered an expression on the part of the uterine wall to rid itself of the invading tissue. This involves particularly cases in which subinvolution is the only accompanying lesion.

In classifying the forty-nine cases which were selected in this study, seven groups were arranged. They consisted of groups in which chronic subinvolution, hyperplasia of the endometrium and myomata existed alone; the remaining four groups representing various combinations of these lesions. In the group where subinvolution was present alone there were placed twelve cases. The striking feature of the chronic subinvoluted uterus was very marked in all of these cases with one exception in which it was quite definite. Chronic subinvolution occurred in combination with hyperplasia of the endometrium in eleven cases; in five instances chronic subinvolution and myomata were present and in six instances there was a combination of chronic subinvolution, myomata and hyperplasia. There were four cases in which hyperplasia occurred alone—in each of these instances the hyperplasia was very striking. Two of these cases were classified as early adenomyoma (one perhaps questionable) and the other two were very well advanced cases. Hyperplasia occurred in connection with myomata in five instances—in four of these cases it was quite striking and very definite in the fifth. Myomata occurred alone in six cases. The cases of the last group as a whole were uteri which were studded with numerous small myomata, many nodules being between ½ and 3 cm. in diameter, just the type of uterus in which the accompanying hyperplasia of the myometrium is most strikingly seen. In thirty-four instances subinvolution was present of itself or with these various combinations. Hyperplasia was present of itself or in combination with other lesions in twenty-six cases. Myomata were present of

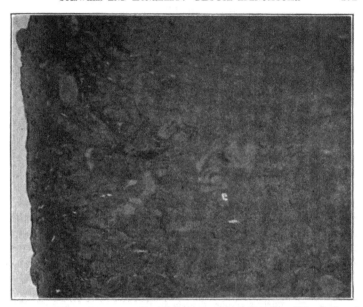

Fig. 14.—Diffuse adenomyoma with marked chronic subinvolution. Case 1984. Section of inner third of uterus—low power—hematoxylin-eosin stain. Endometrium atrophic. Note the marked irregularity of the endometrium with very marked penetration of strands of mucosa in numerous places; also the numerous blood vessels with thickening walls.

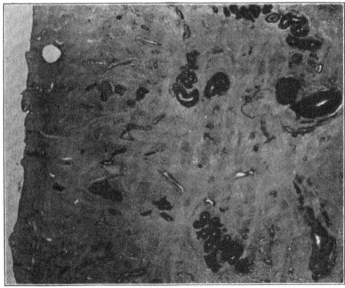

Fig. 15.—Same as Fig. 14. Orcein-Van Gieson stain. Almost every artery in the field shows the characteristic black collar of chronic subinvolution. No hypertrophy of myometrium.

themselves or in combination with other lesions in twenty-one instances. In every one of the forty-nine cases it was possible to place the case under one of these headings. It is readily seen that subinvolution and hyperplasia are by far the most frequent accompanying lesions in this series, subinvolution alone and in combination with hyperplasia occurring in twenty-three cases, and in forty-three cases either one or the other of these lesions existed. In six cases myomata alone were present and in five out of these six cases the patient had borne children. There was not sufficient evidence microscopically of chronic subinvolution but enough to stamp them as parous uteri.

Clinical histories were obtainable in all but four cases; in two or three others it was incomplete. We were particularly interested in the frequency of menorrhagia. In these forty-nine cases there was a definite history of menorrhagia in thirty-one instances. In the chronic subinvolution cases alone out of the twelve cases there were eleven with complete histories, of which six gave a history of menorrhagia. In the cases where subinvolution and hyperplasia existed, histories were obtainable in eight out of eleven cases; in six cases there was a definite history of menorrhagia, in one case the information was doubtful and in another it was negative. In the case of doubtful history the hyperplasia was fairly striking, whereas in the case which was negative there was only a moderate hyperplasia. In five cases of subinvolution and myomata the history was complete in four, of which two were positive for menorrhagia and two were negative. In the cases where all three lesions occurred there were four positive histories and two negative histories as regards increased menstrual flow. In one of these cases the lesion was quite moderate and in the other it was not particularly striking. In the cases of hyperplasia alone there was marked menorrhagia in all four, two of these being nulliparous women, one uniparous and the fourth having had two full term children. In the five cases in which hyperplasia and myomata were present together the history was complete in four cases and showed menorrhagia in all four instances. Where myomata occurred alone four out of six cases had menorrhagia and two gave negative histories.

This résumé as regards the frequency of hemorrhage associated with cases of adenomyoma seems to us to show that those cases which are combined with hyperplasia of the endometrium are most apt to show a definite history of menorrhagia. This is so in our series of which there were twenty-six cases, in all but three instances. In two of these instances the lesion was not particularly striking and in the third instance in which it was fairly striking there was some doubt about the history. It also shows that the cases associated with subinvolution alone or in combination with myomata may quite frequently not be associated with menorrhagia. Two cases with myomata alone showed no increased bleeding.

So we feel we can say that adenomyoma of the uterus may or may not be accompanied by profuse menstruation. The largest percentage of adenomyoma which consistently gave a history of menorrhagia are found to be accompanied by hyperplasia of the endometrium. We feel that this series shows very strikingly that adenomyoma is very clearly accompanied by other uterine lesions. We thought, however, that a series of forty-nine cases, a few of which were quite early, could not be considered too seriously. We, therefore, thought it a good plan to go over the cases of diffuse adenomyoma of the uterus in Cullen's monograph and see how many could be placed more or less definitely according to the accompanying lesions. This, of course, was difficult because one could not study cases of subinvolution with a special stain. However by placing all cases which showed no other lesion and had a definite history of having had full term children under the heading of subinvolution fairly accurate conclusions could be drawn.

In going over the cases in Cullen's text book, there were forty-seven cases of diffuse adenomyoma, which we reviewed. The placing of these cases in definite groups as in the series just described is obviously difficult and perhaps in a few instances inaccurate, but we felt, perhaps, some comparison and some conclusions could be drawn. There were four cases which were not classified according to this scheme:—Three of these gave no history, and the fourth will be considered by itself. The remaining forty-three cases were placed as follows: Subinvolution alone, five; subinvolution and hyperplasia of the endometrium, four; subinvolution with myomata, five; subinvolution with both myomata and hyperplasia, four; hyperplasia alone, four; hyperplasia and myomata, ten; myomata, eleven. These groups showed that hyperplasia of the endometrium occurred eighteen times of itself or in combination; myomata occurred in all combinations thirty times. The inferential diagnosis of subinvolution in all combinations was made in eighteen cases. This series showed a definite increased incidence of myomata, while the frequency of hyperplasia was slightly less striking and the subinvolution incidence was also less. In these forty-seven cases there were a greater number of nulliparous women. In the hyperplasia cases only one out of the four had no children; in two cases there was no available data. In the hyperplasia-myomata cases there was a definite history of no pregnancies in seven cases, while in the cases of myomata alone two had had children, one case none, and in the remaining cases the clinical data was incomplete.

It was quite evident that menorrhagia was present to a more marked degree than in our series. It occurred in thirty-one instances in Cullen's cases. It was negative for menorrhagia in eight instances and in the remaining cases no history was obtainable. In the cases of hyperplasia alone it occurred in fifteen instances, one case negative and two gave no histories. In the six subinvolution cases alone, all showed increased bleeding; and in the myomata alone, six out of eleven were positive, three negative and two gave no information. There was a striking difference as regards the frequency of nulliparous women in the series. Nine cases with no pregnancies and ten cases where this information was not obtained—only six cases in our series were nulliparous. We might add that the age incidence of our series compares very favorably with Cullen's series—our youngest patient was nineteen, as was his. He states disease is most prevalent between thirty and sixty years; chiefly near or just past forty is the most frequent time our series shows.

Cullen's case 5768, is quite remarkable. In this case the patient was single and was thirty-eight years of age. The menses at fifteen were regular, profuse and accompanied by clots. She has had a severe dysmenorrhea as long as she can remember, this being more pronounced during the first three days. The uterus amputated at the cervix measures 8 x 9 x 8 cm.; the endometrium is of normal thickness and seems unaltered; the increase in thickness of the uterine wall is due entirely to the diffusely thickened myometrium. No discrete nodules were present. The invasion of mucosa in this case was very marked and was literally falling in the uterine wall through clefts in the myometrium.

This case suggests, first, that myometrial hyperplasia might have occurred before the invasion of the glands. Then the question comes up: what was the cause of the hyperplasia? It seems to us that it is reasonable to assume from the fact of the history of profuse bleeding with this case, that it represents a case of hyperplasia of the endometrium in a young girl which caused this myometrial hyperplasia to develop as a work hypertrophy, the hyperplasia of the endometrium subsequently disappearing. On the other hand, long continued dysmenorrhea may be explained in this case, on mechanical grounds, or to an increased density of the compact portion of the endometrium. In either case there would result a definite increased effort on the part of the uterine wall, which in turn would result in a work hypertrophy.

SUMMARY

Our study of forty-nine cases of diffuse adenomyoma of the uterus brings out a few rather definite points. In the first place it shows that diffuse adenomyoma of the uterus in almost every instance is present coincidently with one or more other lesions. That these lesions are fundamental in influencing the development of this condition is quite apparent. It is rather difficult to say which one of these exerts a greater influence. It is quite evident that it rarely, if ever, occurs in a normal wall.

The lesion is explained chiefly on mechanical grounds. A parous uterus, or more particularly a uterus which shows the lesion of chronic subinvolution, favors the invasion of the mucosal elements. This invasion immediately causes a reaction on the part of the myometrium due perhaps, either to local irritation or an attempt on the part of the myometrium to withstand this invasion; in some cases this results in a marked hypertrophy of the wall and in other instances this hypertrophy is not particularly striking in this selected group. The explanation that this lesion does not occur in the subinvoluted uterus may rest in the fact that in these cases of subinvolution the endometrium is frequently atrophic and does not have the same tendency to penetrate that a more active endometrium might exercise. The mechanism in cases of hyperplasia alone is explained on an entirely different basis. In this instance the hyperplasia of the endometrium is the primary lesion; subsequently, as a result of the persistent hyperplasia of the endometrium, a work hypertrophy results in the uterine wall which gives it its coarse structure and allows the mucosal elements to penetrate between the widened interstices. In cases of myomata alone the thickened uterine wall exists before the invasion of glands and results from work hypertrophy in an attempt on the part of the uterine wall to rid itself of discrete nodules. That there may be an occasional case in which the explanation of the hypertrophy must be sought elsewhere is shown by the case in Cullen's series, and perhaps our explanation for these may prove satisfactory. As a whole, however, diffuse adenomyoma of the uterus occurs in almost every instance as a result of the presence of some pathological lesion of the uterine wall favoring its development.

That inflammation in the uterine cases is a definite factor in the production of the lesion as in the cases of tubal adenomyoma cannot be substantiated. Cullen has repeatedly remarked the same. In our series it was so inconspicuous that the number of cases was not even tabulated.

CLINICAL CASE HISTORIES

LABORATORY NO. 480.—*Typical case of subinvolution associated with diffuse adenomyoma.* No other lesion in uterine wall. Endometrium 1 mm. thick.

Patient forty-seven years of age, has had eight children, the last two years ago. Since her last pregnancy a partial prolapse of the uterus developed, with more or less constant pelvic discomfort and a marked increase in the menstrual flow. She menstruated every two weeks for the past two years, the flow lasting three to four days at a time. Vaginal hysterectomy was performed.

The uterus was considerably enlarged and measured 12x6x5 cm. There was no evidence of pelvic inflammation. The uterine wall at its thickest portion measured

21 mm.; the endometrium 1 mm., and was normal. There was no general increase in connective tissue but its presence was quite striking in the inner third. Blood vessels of the inner third show in most instances a very marked collection of diffuse elastic tissue around the outer portion of the new vessel wall. The vessels of the middle third, particularly the veins, show an immense amount of this diffuse elastic tissue. The elastic tissue between the muscle bundles and the outer third was also markedly swollen.

This case was reported previously as a typical case of chronic subinvolution which, to be sure, it is. The adenomyoma was discovered subsequently in studying further sections.

CASE NO. 1299.—*Diffuse adenomyoma of the uterus associated with marked hyperplasia of the endometrium in a nulliparous woman.*

Patient was thirty-four years of age. Menses had been three to four days in duration and appeared every 28 days up to about three years ago. Since then the flow has been increased, of long duration, frequently lasting two weeks. The last period has been three weeks in duration and there is still some flow on admission.

Supravaginal uterus is globular in shape and measures 10x10x8 cm. Uterine wall measures 4½ cm. in thickness in the left upper portion. The endometrium in the upper cavity has a shaggy, stringy appearance and is from 1 to 1½ cm. in thickness all over; the tissue hangs in shreds from a base and there are blood clots hanging to the shreds. Microscopically there are numerous glands present in the thickened uterine wall surrounded by a definitely hyperplastic myometrium. Section from the right uterine wall shows a very definite hyperplasia of the endometrium, with only a very slight tendency to invade.

CASE NO. 1323.—*Diffuse adenomyoma associated with a marked hyperplasia of the endometrium in a parous uterus which shows not the slightest evidence of subinvolution.* Specimen presented by Lee Dorsett.

Patient a married woman 48 years of age. One child seventeen years ago. Menses began at twelve and were profuse until twenty, normal to thirty, profuse after thirty, with flooding spells for the last five years. Specimen consists of a symmetrical uterus diffusely thickened throughout, removed by supravaginal amputation. The uterus measures 12x12x10 cm. The uterine wall measures 4.5 cm., in thickness and has a very coarse appearance. No discrete nodules present. Microscopic section shows a very marked hyperplasia of the endometrium, endometrium being 7 mm., thick. The muscle wall is 40 mm. thick. Glands are embedded in the myometrium 1.5 cm., from the base of the endometrium.

CASE NO. 1790.—*A nulliparous uterus with numerous small myomata, hyperplasia of the endometrium, diffuse thickening of the uterine wall and an early adenomyoma.*

Outside case, no history available but patient is single. The uterine wall is studded with numerous interstitial nodules, the largest 5 cm. in diameter. The uterine wall itself, outside these nodules, is very coarse and much thickened. The endometrium is thrown into numerous folds and is greatly thickened. Microscopically the endometrium shows definite hyperplasia and definitely invades the myometrium for a distance of 7 mm. Muscle bundles show a very definite tendency to separate.

CASE NO. 1984.—*An early penetration of the endometrium in the wall of a markedly subinvoluted uterus*

The patient forty-four years and has had twelve pregnancies, the last, a full term, three months before admission.

Specimen consists of a large subserous tumor 21x7x8 cm., attached by a small pedicle to the posterior wall, and a supravaginal uterus measuring 7x6x4 cm., which was entirely distinct from the myomatous mass. The uterine wall measures 18 mm. in thickness; the endometrium is thin but smooth. Microscopically the endometrium shows a very definite tendency to invade the myometrium and by special staining shows very marked evidence of subinvolution throughout the wall.

REFERENCES

Frankl, O.: Liepman's Handbuch, ii, p. 40. *Strong, L. W.:* AM. JOUR. OBST. AND GYNEC., *June,* 1921. *Lockyer:* Fibroid and Allied Tumors, London, 1918, MacMillan Co., p. 287. *Cullen:* Adenomyoma of the Uterus, Philadelphia, 1918, W. B. Saunders Co. *Novak, E.:* Jour. Am. Med. Assn., July 31, 1920. *Cullen, T. S.:* Bull. Johns Hopkins Hosp., 1920, xxxi, p. 246. *Novak, E.:* Bull. Johns Hopkins Hosp., 1920, xxxi, p. 248. *Shaw, F.:* Eden & Lockyer, System of Gynecology, London, 1917, MacMillan Co., ii, 117. *Schwarz, Otto H.:* Am. Jour. Obst., January, 1919.

40 N. NEWSTEAD STREET.   (*For discussion, see p. 537.*)

NEOPLASIA OF THE KIDNEY[*]

WITH REPORTS OF FIVE PRIMARY CASES: 1. PAPILLARY EPITHELIOMA, 2. HYPERNEPHROMA, 3. MALIGNANT TERATOMA, 4. SQUAMOUS CELLED CARCINOMA, 5. LYMPHOBLASTOMA.

BY JAMES E. DAVIS, A.M., M.D., DETROIT, MICH.

THERE is no part of the body where developmental complexes are better illustrated than in the urogenital system and the nephridial division is more intricate than the genital. Felix[1] says the kidneys do not have a gradual but rather a saltatory development (the word "saltatory" is derived from the Latin "saltator," a leaper or dancer). Others have used the term "nephridial successions" or "dynasties" in referring to this interesting phase in renal development. It is noteworthy that this rapidly moving divisional change has to fit into a definite period of one entire development and as a part of this accomplishment there occurs not only the formation, but also the disappearance of the entire pronephros and the greater part of the mesonephros. The period of development for the excretory system in most vertebrates reckoning from its formation until its completion, occupies an interval, says Felix,[2] that is long in comparison with that shown by other organs. The pronephros begins to appear in embryos of 1-7 mm., when there are but 9 to 10 primitive segments. All its tubules have developed and the primary excretory duct is nearly complete in 2.5 mm. embryos. At 4.25 mm. the duct has reached the cloaca and fused with it, establishing the outlet for the celom.

This first kidney is both[3] vestigial and rudimentary for it is a disappearing structure, but it is also an appearing imperfect organ. While it is true the pronephros functionates in amphioxus and certain lamphreys, it must be regarded as a very limited excretory organ in an imperfect representation of its species.

It is important for the purposes of this contribution to refer at this time to the relation obtaining between the vestigial-rudimentary kidney and its primary or primitive cell units since the pathology may be postulated or the histogenesis determined for neoplasia from just such premises as may here be laid down.

The considerations are of the facts involved in (1) rapid growth, (2) rapid degeneration, (3) growth and degeneration in the same organ at the same time, with constant conformity to a general body growth impulse, (4) cell and organic immaturity held in abeyance to

---
[*]Read at the Thirty-fourth Annual Meeting of the American Association of Obstetricians, Gynecologists, and Abdominal Surgeons, St. Louis, Mo., September 20-22, 1921.

larger growth impulse, (5) a three phase evolution from dissimilar component units. The import of the foregoing is made clear by the briefest review of the morphological development of the first of the two primary kidneys. A description of one adequately answers for both primary organs and also covers the essentials of each in the formation of the metanephros.

In the general course of normal development the blastoderm produces its layered divisions of ectoderm, mesoderm and entoderm providing differentiation, proceeds in the orderly way. From the mesoderm of the intermediate cell mass is derived the nephrotome. But in some animals a differentiation of the germ cells occurs before the blastoderm is formed.[4]

From the nephrotomes seven pairs of rudimentary pronephric tubules are formed as dorsal sprouts. These grow dorsally, also laterally, bending so as to unite and form a long collecting duct from the seventh to the fourteenth segments. The first tubules in the seventh segment degenerate before those of the fourteenth have developed.

The free end of the collecting duct extends in a caudad direction beneath the ectoderm and lateral to the nephrogenic cord until it reaches and perforates the lateral wall of the cloaca.

The higher number of nephridial structures occur only in the amniotes. All three are closely related in development and structure whether they are parts of an original continuous organ[5] (holonephros) extended the length of the body cavity and which has broken into separate parts or are they three separate organs or, are they not strictly homologous but superimposed structures has not yet been decided.

The plan of repeating one part after another (metamerism) is said to have its origin in the mesothelial structures and has been secondarily impressed on other systems. The mesothelial walls dispose their parts in three zones of each coelom—the muscle plate zone (epimere), the lower or lateral-plate zone (hypomere), and between the foregoing plates a middle plate zone (mesomere). All three plates form in the trunk. Constriction or segmentation forms the series of hollow cubes (myotomes) each with a part of the coelom (the myocele) within.

The myotome grows between the ectoderm and the somatic wall of the hypomere. Each myotome has a somatic and a splanchnic wall. From the latter or splanchnic wall there is derived the musculature (from the upper part) and the skeletal tissue (ventral part).

The mesomeral (middle plate) part is largely concerned in the formation of the excretory (nephridial) system and it has both excretory portions and the skeletogenous parts (these are called nephrotomes and sclerotomes, the nephrotome cavities being the nephrocoeles).

The foregoing brief discussion may set forth with some degree of clearness the more important essentials to be considered in relating the vagaries of kidney neoplasia with the histogenetic conditions of its development. The latter has yet many unknown problems for elucidation and this is equally true concerning the neoplastic changes developed in the kidney.

The benign tumors of the kidney are usually small, unimportant, and rare, but neoplastic growths constitute approximately 2 per cent of all malignancies. The difficulties connected with their diagnosis, removal, size and vascularity are well understood. The gross appearance in neoplastic tumors of the kidney is fairly characteristic. In the majority of specimens the tissue consistency is soft, resembling degenerating brain structures. Areas of hemorrhage are very constant and blood cysts may occur.

The tumors vary in size according to their age, but ordinarily when discovered they are large and occupy almost the entire kidney area. Some portion of the kidney outline is usually recognizable. Examination of a cross section will frequently show the kidney tissue compressed between the new growth and the capsule. This is most commonly observed in papillary and sarcomatous growths. It is also seen with the very rapidly growing tumors.

Five reports of primary kidney tumors illustrating striking contrasts in histopathologic changes are herewith presented in detail.

CASE 1.—*Papillary Epithelioma.* This type of tumor in the kidney is rare. Knack[6] reported one case in 1918 of a man of seventy-three years of age in whom the growth was found at autopsy and had developed from the ureter. He discussed the scarcity of such cases and found but nine reported in the German literature up to that time.

Hirsch[7] reported one case of papillary carcinoma of the kidney with metastasis in the brain which was found at autopsy in a patient 58½ years of age. The tumor was soft, cellular and with scant stroma. There was a radial arrangement of the cells about thin-walled blood vessels. Capillaries were clearly defined, forming rosette-like structures in the villi. Numerous necrotic and hemorrhagic areas were found. Hirsh quotes Wohl as having collected 12 cases of this type and Kretschner and Moody 11 cases.

McCown[8] reported one case of papillomatous epithelioma of the kidney pelvis, and stated he was able to find but 10 cases in American literature and 38 cases from foreign sources, making 48 in all. Kelly, Babcock, Watson and Cunningham, Lower, Hyman and Beer, Burford, Parmeter, Mayo and Judd are listed as reporters in American literature.

Braasch[9] has reported that 5 cases were seen in the Mayo Clinic up to Oct. 30, 1920.

Patient, a married woman; aged fifty-one years; mother of five children, who had no history of abortions or miscarriages. *Chief complaints*, frequent urination, pain in the left hypogastric region, and bloody urine. *Present illness* began 7 months ago. A painful area together with a mass the size of a hen's egg developed in the posterior portion of the left side. This apparently did not increase in size. A backache with some burning sensation occurred when urinating. At times blood clots passed in the urine. The patient believed she had passed bloody urine for five years. Nocturia and albuminuria were absent. *Clinical data:* Operation was done in October, 1920, by Dr. C. T. Root seven months after the tumor mass was recognized by the patient. Aug. 28, 1921, Dr. Root reported the patient able to do her own housework and that she was without pain or distress and had gained 25 pounds in weight.

Gross description of the tumor mass: The specimen exhibited an irregular form of a kidney with a partly obliterated marginal line in the pelvic portion. Projecting from the slight concavity of the kidney margin there was seen the pelvic portion and its ureter. This resembled the formation usually seen in hydronephrosis,

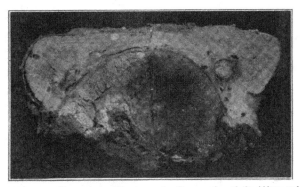

Fig. 1.—Malignant papilloma of the kidney, case 1. Cross section of the kidney and tumor mass made 3/4" from the pelvis.

the ureter being dilated to a diameter of 2 cm. This dilation of the pelvis and uppermost part of the ureter was caused by the new growth. The poles of the kidney were quite definitely outlined and projected independently of the tumor mass for a distance of 3 cm.

The new growth had enlarged ventrally and laterally. Complete encapsulation was evident. The surface was roughly nodulated. This was caused in part by the projecting poles of the kidney and in part by irregular bulging incident to the enclosed new growth and hemorrhagic changes, for on cross section just beneath the capsule there were seen areas of hemorrhage and areas of vigorous new growth, causing definite thinning out of the capsule.

On section ventrally from pole to pole at a distance of 1 cm. from the midpoint of the pelvic margin of the kidney, the capsule of the new growth was found at the center on the medial side to be 1 cm. and in the poles 3-4 cm. thick. (Fig. 1.)

The margin of the new growth was sharply defined but in the upper pole there was a separate papillary projection at a distance of 5 mm. external to the margin of the tumor. This occupied the position of an obliterated calyx. Multiple vertical

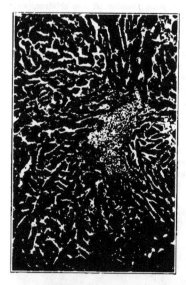

Fig. 2.—(Case 1.) Low magnification showing the papillomatous structure and arboreal arrangement. X-110. Note the areas of hemorrhage and degeneration.

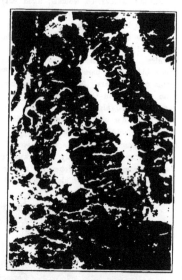

Fig. 3.—(Case 1.) High magnification showing the papillomatous projections. Note the marked anaplasia of epithelial cells irregularly arranged on papillary forms.

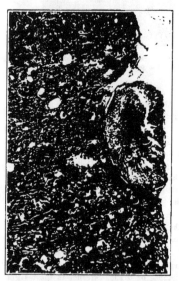

Fig. 4.—Adrenal rest tissue in the kidney capsule from a patient age 69 years.

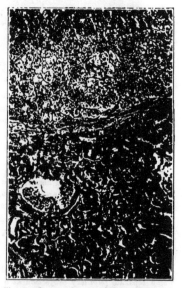

Fig. 5.—Contrast between kidney cortex and adrenal rest tissue. Magnification X-430.

sectioning revealed a varying thickness of capsule down to 1 mm. upon the lateral surface.

The central portion throughout exhibited numerous recent and old hemorrhages. A tracery of fine light-colored seams could be followed throughout the growth. The older portions of the growth were centripetal and the new portions centrifugal.

The entire new growth portion was of light color except where changed by hemorrhage and necrosis. When torn apart the surfaces presented a minute polypoarboreal appearance. The fatty capsule was thick and its fat lobules firm and resistant.

Histopathology: The sections taken from parts of the kidney not involved in the new growth change showed compacted tissue with consequently deformed tubular and glomerular units. The poles of the kidney which had the greatest depth of uninvolved structure showed dilated tubules suggesting hydronephros and mild hydropic cellular change. An extensive, fairly well focalized lymphocytic cell infiltration was observed in the pelvic and corticular kidney tissues. Many scarred glomeruli, some interstitial connective tissue increase and considerable pressure atrophy was present. (Figs. 1-5.)

The new growth tissue was predominantly cellular with a delicate stromal supporting structure giving a papillary plical or arboreal assembling. The widest and most distinctive portions of these stromal supports were outgrowths from the epithelial layer of cells in the kidney pelvis. At the interpapillary positions on the epithelial border there were many intact cells. Each papillary form had multiple laterally projecting irregularly shaped arboreal forms of different lengths, which were richly fruited with epithelial cells, not very remotely differentiated from the same type of cells upon the normal epithelial surface of the pelvis.

The growth of the papillary forms was quite uniformly outward in a fungus-like form from pelvis to the outer convexity of the cortex. A marked compactness of the structure was observed in the entire upper portion of the growth. The epithelial cells in the upper portions had not the same systematic positional arrangement observed in the pelvis and there was marked disassociation of their nuclei. Anaplastic changes were not marked.

The capillaries of the tumor were clearly defined at different places and endothelial cells were frequently observed widely detached from vascular structures. The growth was not markedly vascular. There were numerous areas of moderate hemorrhage and some small places of necrosis. Localized areas of small round cell infiltration were frequently observed within the tumor mass.

Diagnosis: Papillary epithelioma of the kidney. A primary growth from the epithelium of the pelvis.

CASE 2.—*Hypernephroma with Metastasis to the Liver, Lung and Spleen.* This type of neoplasm is by far the most frequent of kidney tumors. A clear distinction should be made whether the tumor originated in adrenal or kidney structure. If from the kidney, sex changes never arise. This has been clearly pointed out by Glynn[10] and emphasized by Bowlby and Andrews.[11]

These tumors are of a sulphur yellow color and remarkably soft in consistency. They can become very large and sometimes are sharply outlined or they may be diffused through the renal substance and by rapid growth attain a malignant character. Their cells are large, many-sided and richly filled with fat.[12]

Patient, Mrs. J. S., aged fifty-six, mother of nine children, seven of whom were living and well. Last illness was indefinite in relation to kidney tumor. Ill health began about one year before her death, being initiated with a severe cold which was followed by a bronchial infection and gastrointestinal disturbances, constipation and loss of weight. General weakness was her constant complaint. *Clinical data:* A palpable tumor 4 by 4 inches in size was observed in the right upper abdominal quadrant. The liver was enlarged and hard, but was movable. The hemoglobin was 65 per cent. Slight hyperexia prevailed and there was cachexia. There were no kidney symptoms discovered and there was no record of blood in the urine. Death occurred 13 months after the onset of her ill health. Gross examination of tissues at autopsy included kidneys, liver, lung, spleen and detached tumor mass. The right kidney was 12 cm. in length, 7 cm. in width and 3½ cm. in thickness. The left kidney was 19 cm. long, 12 cm. broad and 7½ cm. thick. Its cortex varied

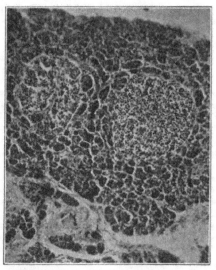

Fig. 6.—Hypernephroma, case 2. Section of pancreas adherent to the tumor mass; note the hypertrophy of the islet structures and areas of fibrosis showing proliferation of islet tissue.

in thickness from 2 mm. to 10 mm. In the area of the lower pole there was approximately 5 cm. of kidney structure with well-defined hypertrophic pyramids. A sharp line of demarcation separated this part from a new growth mass of a soft, yellowish, fatty character in which were band formations. In places necrotic, cystic and hemorrhagic changes were observed. The right kidney was hypertrophic. The liver tissue was hard and contracted excepting an area of new growth change comparable to the mass in the kidney. In the lung and splenic tissues localized changes were observed.

Microscopic examination: A partially encapsuled new growth structure of epithelial character was found with large, irregular, usually polyhedral, light-staining cells attached loosely to a delicate endothelial and connective tissue stroma suggesting the architecture of the adrenal, zona fascicularis. The cell nuclei were usually single, but often multiple. When single their position was usually at or near the center of the cell and when multiple they were eccentrically placed. The nucleoli were prominent and the nuclear substance was granulated and stained deeply with hematoxylin. A marked prevalence of cell vacuolization was observed, especially in the older portions of the growth, leaving almost a naked capillary framework. In many places old and recent hemorrhages were observed. Tubule forms were not observed in the new-formed tissue. In one section a part of the pancreas was attached to well-preserved actively growing tumor tissue. The pancreatic islet tissue was actively proliferating and its connective tissue was increased. The sections from the liver, lung and spleen showed metastasis of tumor tissue identical with that of the kidney. (Figs. 6-8.)

Diagnosis: Hypernephroma of the left kidney with metastasis to the liver, lung and spleen.

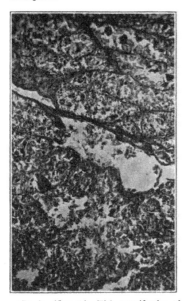 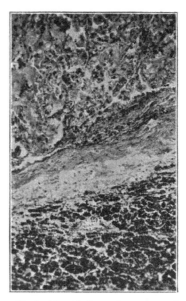

Fig. 7.—(Case 2.) High magnification of new growth tissue. X-430. Note the connective tissue reticulum giving an areolar arrangement of the new growth cells. The vacuolation of the anaplastic cells is best seen in the upper part of the field.

Fig. 8.—(Case 2.) Contrasting pancreas and contiguous hypernephroma structure. Note the anaplasia of new growth cells with giant cell formation to the left.

CASE 3.—*Malignant teratoma.* The derivation of this type of tumor is difficult to trace because of differentiation and developmental unknowns. It is most satisfactory to recall that myotome may give striped muscle fibers, scleratome may yield cartilage, mesenchyme may produce connective tissue including smooth muscle and possibly vessels and the intermediate cell mass the glandular or epithelial formations. It is also to be considered that the intermediary cell mass middleplate in the myotome and in the mesenchyme may yield mixed tumors.[13] Junkel[14] says these cells of undifferentiated tissue have failed to take part in the ulterior cellular differentiation and for some unknown reason begin to grow and differentiate themselves in the grown-up organism. It is useless to attempt a summary of the literature of this type of tumors, there being but few cases reported in detail and all differ in interpretation of essentials.

Patient, Miss E. G., aged sixty years. *History:* About six months before her demise there was general malaise, loss of weight and appetite. Three months later occasional pain of a dull, aching character was felt in the left lower quadrant and back. This gradually increased in frequency and severity until it was almost unbearable. A mass just above the iliac crest appeared with the onset of pain and increased to a large tumor which was palpable over the entire side. Palpation or pressure over the area was painful. Micturition was frequent and painful.

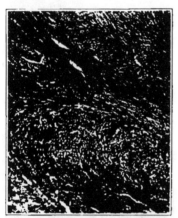 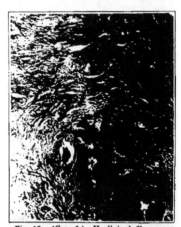

Fig. 9.—Malignant teratoma of the kidney, case 3. Connective tissue portion of the tumor. Low magnification X-110. Note the fascicles and interlacing fibers of connective tissue and muscle cells, the marked cellularity of tne structure, and the vascular spaces.

Fig. 10.—(Case 3.) Hyalinized fibrous portion of the tumor. Low magnification X-110. Note the vascular spaces, the dense acellular type of architecture, and the deposits of calcium salts in the lower right corner.

Clinical data: Repeated urinalyses were negative. Kidney efficiency tests were negative until later when the output from the left was 12 per cent in 15 minutes. Catheterization and roentgenogram showed the left ureter displaced medially and the presence of an irregular homogenous mass. The total white cell count was 17650 and the polymorphonuclear cells were 80 per cent. Operation by Dr. Ray Andries revealed a retroperitoneal tumor mass involving the lower pole of the left kidney and extending medially across the spinal column to the right side and adhering to the surrounding tissues. The postoperative shock was severe. Death occurred 27 days following her operation. Autopsy was not obtained.

Gross description: The specimen was an irregular hunter's horn shaped mass of tissue with a well-defined upper pole, preserving a fairly normal kidney outline. The dimensions of the mass were 15 cm. long by 9 cm. wide across the lower pole, and 6 cm. thick. A portion of the mass at the lower pole, including the capsule was torn away. When vertically sectioned the tumor mass was shown to be 8 x 8 x 6 cm. in size. A well-defined encapsulation was seen along part of the upper surface. The substance of the new growth mass was partially soft, and light-colored, the structure was partially fibrous and cartilaginous in character. Evident extension through the capsule had occurred at the lower pole and outer lower convexity.

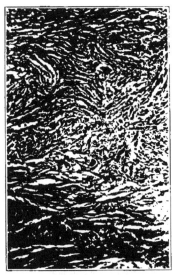

Fig. 11.—(Case 3.) Fibrous tissue portion of the new growth. Low magnification X-110. Note the irregular diffuse arrangement of new growth tumor cells and the atrophy and anaplasia of cells.

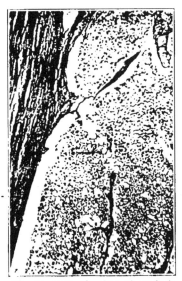

Fig. 12.—(Case 3.) Area of anaplastic epithelial new growth cells. Low magnification X-110. Note the solid mass of large epithelial cells showing abundant cytoplasm and round or oval nuclei.

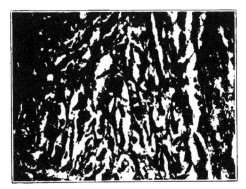

Fig. 13.—(Case 3.) Fibrous portion of the tumor. Note the hyalinized tissue in the upper part of the field, the thin-walled blood spaces at the line of demarcation, and the anaplasia of new growth connective tissue cells.

At the upper border of the tumor mass what appeared as capsule was identified as distended displaced pelvic wall. The ureter was not seen.

Microscopical examination: The kidney tissue not involved by the new growth exhibited early albuminous degenerative changes with irregular tubular dilatation and some blood casts, also slight local interstitial tissue increase, a few scarred glomeruli and small round cell infiltration, particularly in the pelvic tissues. In sections from the hilum of the kidney there was a partially walled-off tumor mass which in places flattened out the calyces and compressed the contiguous kidney structure. The structural units of connective tissue, muscle and epithelium were clearly definable. In parts where fibrosis, hyalinization and calcification were prominent, cartilage was in question. There were places where atypical tubules were recognized. In the more acellular tissues very prominent lacunar spacings were found. The parts of the tumor constructed from connective tissue and muscle elements had a prominent fasciculated and interlacing architecture. The cells in the connective tissue structure were distinctly more anaplastic than in either the muscle or epithelial tissues, but the two later types were better differentiated. The connective tissue cell nuclei were very irregular in size and shape and many were multinucleated. The muscle cells were fairly uniform. The epithelial areas of the tumor had rather small and almost uniform sized cells, many of which were vacuolated. The stroma was very scanty and vascularity was not marked. A fatty degeneration was observed in certain areas. (Figs. 9-13.)

Diagnosis: Malignant teratoma of the left kidney.

CASE 4.—*Squamous and spheroidal celled carcinoma of the kidney.* Primary carcinoma is rare in the kidney. Ewing[15] speaks of these tumors as remarkable and of large size and of their relation to leukoplakia and calculi. Bowlbey and Andrews[16] mention carcinoma of the kidney, though rarer than sarcoma, as not uncommon in adults and that it may originate in the pelvis and be of the squamous type. More frequently it originates in the cortex and is spheroidal or columnar-celled.

Patient, Mrs. M. LaT., aged sixty-two, mother of 3 children. *Last Illness:* Duration approximately 4 months. The onset of symptoms was characterized by aching in the left hip and, when severe, radiation down the leg. In 6 months there was a loss of 35 pounds in weight, but no urinary disturbances occurred.

Clinical data: A large, hard nodular mass was palpable in the left lumbar region. The urine examination was negative and the blood picture indicated a moderate secondary anemia. At operation the left kidney was removed by Dr. Geo. E. Potter. It was found to be 8 inches long, 4 inches wide and 5 inches thick and showed that extensive degenerative changes had occurred throughout the entire organ. The patient died in 23 days after her operation.

Gross examination: The specimen was not intact and fragmentation of the tumor in its pelvic portion was evident. The thickness of encapsulation by the compressed displaced renal tissue varied from 2 cm. to 2 mm. The tumor areas were of whitish color and of fairly firm consistency and occurred as multiple areas when viewed from the cut flat surfaces. Extensive involvement was evident and the pelvis showed the older growth of tissue.

Microscopic Pathology: In sections from the pelvis of the kidney the new growth tissue was composed of compact squamous and spheroidal, closely arranged cells with but little or no intercellular substance. The formation was an irregular stratified layer replacing the pelvic epithelium while the tissue from the cortex exhibited marked compactness of structure with a rich deposition of intercellular substance. The blood vessels of this part were few in number and small, but in the pelvis they were numerous, thin-walled and dilated. There was no positive alveolar arrangement of new growth structure, but infiltration of tumor cells in columns replaced the renal structure. In the greater part of the entire new growth coalescing of the cell groups prevailed and the involvement extended quite generally to all parts of the kidney. The tumor cells showed a most pronounced anaplasia and unusual cell division changes. The cell nuclei were exceedingly irregular in shape and number. Epithelial pearl formation was not prominent. The kidney structure was rapidly and diffusely undergoing tumor cell metaplasia. In the pelvis and medulla chronic infection and hemorrhage were marked. In the cortex compression changes were prominent and many scarred glomeruli were found, but no evidence of calculi was observed. (Figs. 14 and 15.)

Diagnosis: Rapidly growing squamous and spheroidal celled carcinoma, originating in the kidney pelvis.

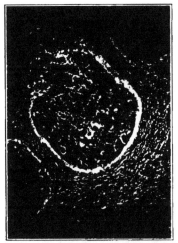 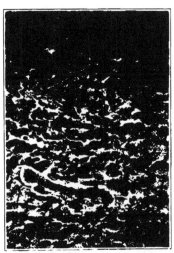

Fig. 14.—Primary carcinoma of the kidney, case 4. Low magnification of kidney tissue showing the invading epithelial new growth. (X-110.) Note the few isolated kidney tubules in the lower right corner and the solid masses of flat new growth epithelial cells.

Fig. 15.—(Case 4.) High magnification of new growth cells. X-430. Note the marked anaplasia of cells.

CASE 5.—*Lymphoblastoma.* The literature upon this type of kidney tumor illustrates an unsettled classification and careless nomenclature. (Longhuame.[17]) The occurrence of this type of tumor in children under 5 years is relatively frequent. Its size is sometimes very large, reaching ½ the weight of the child. In renal tumors of infancy the round and spindle cells are nearly always found.

Patient, Philip S., aged seven months. The tumor was unnoticed until a few days before death. During the last five days the abdomen had become greatly distended and the patient appeared exsanguinated. A tumor mass extending from the costal margin to the lower border of the pelvis and three finger-breadths to the left of the median line was easily recognized.

Clinical data: Abdominal exploration was done by Dr. Jas. A. MacMillan, but removal of the tumor was deemed impossible. Severe hemorrhage followed the removal of some tissue from the tumor mass. Death occurred a few hours later.

Autopsy Examination: Revealed a tumor mass filling the entire right half of the abdomen, extending from the dome of the diaphragm to the inner aspect of the ileum and extending transversely 6 cm. to the left of the umbilicus. The ascending colon crossed the tumor mass obliquely, ascending from the right outer margin

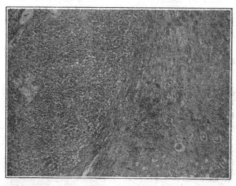

Fig. 16.—(Case 5.) Malignant embryomata of the kidney from a child 7 months old. Low magnification showing the line of demarcation between new growth and kidney tissue. (X-110.) Note the pressure changes in the kidney tissue in the upper part of the field.

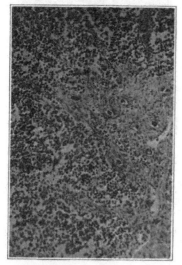 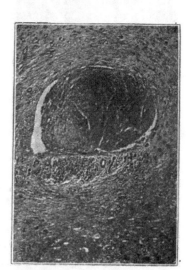

Fig. 17.—(Case 5.) Section of new growth tissue with kidney tubules at the right. Low magnification X-170. Note the marked pressure atrophy of the kidney tubular structure, the irregular line of demarcation between kidney and new growth.

Fig. 18.—(Case 5.) Section of kidney showing thrombosis of a blood vessel. Low magnification X-110. Note the focal aggregations of tumor cells below the blood vessel.

of the lower pole across the mass to the median line, carrying the hepatic flexure toward the median line. The capsular surface of the tumor was thickened, distended and nodulated. The ureter was free and the adrenal was uninvolved. Two

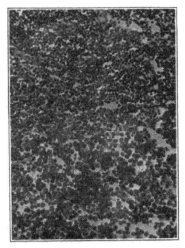

Fig. 19.—(Case 5.) New growth metastasis in a contiguous lymph node X-430. Note the marked anaplasia of cells. The larger cells in the lower half of the field are the anaplastic cells.

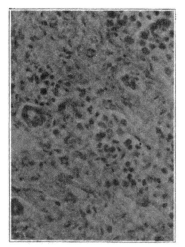

Fig. 20.—(Case 5.) Line of demarcation between kidney tissue and the new growth cells on the right. X-430. Note the degenerative changes in the kidney tubules, the interstitial tissue increase, and the extension growth of anaplastic cells in the center and right portion of the field.

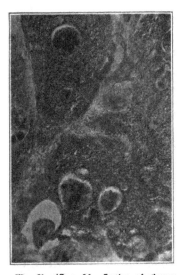

Fig. 21.—(Case 5.) Section of thymus gland showing premature ageing. Note the hypertrophic Hassel's corpuscles and fibrous tissue increase in the septae.

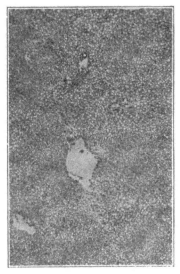

Fig. 22.—(Case 5.) Section of liver showing marked fatty degeneration.

lymph glands were involved, but with this exception the new growth appeared entirely intrarenal.

The tumor mass was firm and appeared indistinctly lobulated. Considerable hemorrhage had occurred within and without the tumor. The left kidney showed slight hypertrophy and moderate cloudy swelling. The liver was very pale and yellow, suggesting hemorrhage and fatty degeneration. The right adrenal was firmer and somewhat smaller than normal.

Histopathology: The sections from the ovary, thymus, thyroid and adrenal tissues showed advanced ageing of these structures. The liver was uniformly undergoing fatty degeneration. The tissue of both kidneys was markedly advanced in development. The characteristic narrow cortex crowded with small glomeruli was changed to correspond with a development of eight or ten years. The renal interstitial tissue was irregularly increased.

The new growth was extensively infiltrated through the greater part of the right kidney by cells indefinitely comparable to lymph cells, but the majority of the tumor cells were, however, more than double their size as shown in the photomicrograph of the invaded lymph gland. A considerable number of these cells were morphologically like very young connective tissue forms. All of the neoplastic cells were hyperchromatic and anaplastic. A fine stroma of capillaries prevailed in all parts of the new growth. Cell division forms were numerous and giant cells were seen. Multiple hemorrhage occurred throughout the mass and many thin-walled dilated vessels were evident. (Figs. 16-22).

Diagnosis: Lymphoblastoma of marked malignancy in the right kidney and mesenteric lymph gland metastasis.

SUMMARY

1. The developmental history of the renal tissues is yet incomplete and at many points theoretical. 2. The histogenesis for tumor tissue of the kidney is intricately involved by existing obscurities in both ontogenetic and phylogenetic development. 3. The frequency of renal neoplasia occurrence is again emphasized as selective of young and old age periods of life. 4. The diagnostic symptomatology is frequently exceedingly indefinite. 5. Clinical and pathological investigation of renal tumors should be carefully made and reported in the literature. 6. The five cases are here reported as primary renal tumors. All have been carefully studied to exclude metastatic origin.

BIBLIOGRAPHY

(1) *Felix, W.:* Keible and Mall, Embryology, p. 753. (2) Ibid., p. 753. (3) *Ryder, J. A.:* Proc. U. S. Nat. Mus., 1886, p. 80. (4) *Schafer, E. A.:* Text Book of Microscopic Anatomy, p. 4. (5) *Kingsley, J. S.:* Comparative Anatomy of Vertebrates, ed. 2, p. 337. (6) *Knack:* Deutsch. med. Wchnschr., 1918, xliv, 982. (7) *Hirsch, E. T.:* Arch. Int. Med., xxi, 231. (8) *McCown, P. E.:* Jour. Am. Med. Assn., Oct. 30, 1920, lxxv, 1191. (9) *Braasch:* Ibid. (10) *Glynn, E. E.:* Quart. Jour. Med., Jan., 1912, v. (11) *Bowlby and Andrews:* Surgical Pathology, ed. 7, p. 419. (12) *Thierry:* Aus der Privatklinik von Hofrat Krecke in München, May 27, 1921, p. 638. (13) *Buerger and Lautman:* Am. Jour. Surg., 1914, xxviii, 453. (14) *Junkel:* Arch. f. klin. Chir., 1914, ciii, 940. (15) *Ewing:* Neoplastic Diseases, 1919, p. 743. (16) *Bowlby and Andrews:* Surgical Pathology, ed. 7, p. 421. (17) *Longhuame, F. McG.:* Brit. Jour. Surg., 1914, ii, p. 77-91.

111 JOSEPHINE AVENUE. (*For discussion, see p. 501.*)

TRANSPERITONEAL NEPHROPEXY*

By Thomas B. Noble, M.D., Indianapolis, Ind.

THE normal position and relationship of the abdominal viscera depend, primarily, upon the integrity of the abdominal wall. Of secondary importance is to be considered their ligamentous attachments and their variations in specific gravity. All the abdominal viscera float more or less freely within a cavity having a fixed and rigid back and base, with a highly elastic cap, sides, and front.

Through their ligamentous attachments must, naturally, come their blood and nerve supply. The solid viscera are rather firmly attached by short supports in fixed localities, while the hollow viscera with much longer supports have a more indefinite topography or position. It is obvious then that anything which tends to disturb the normal position of any one of the abdominal organs will have a distorting influence on all the others. And as a physical proposition those organs of shortest attachments will be, naturally, the first to have nerve irritation and to present symptoms. It is a logical sequence then that, among the first viscera to cry out against the disturbing features of visceroptosis, is the kidney. The right one is most frequently involved. This occurs more often in women than in men. Men rarely have it.

We have in common use the terms, movable or palpable; motile or hypermotile; floating or wandering kidneys; all of which refer to the degree of motility but bear no relationship to symptoms. They serve their purpose in nomenclature, but aid us little in practical therapeutics.

Subjective symptoms are not in accord with the degree of mobility or displacement. Some cases of slight distortion have many symptoms while others of great displacement have none. There is nothing pathognomonic of this condition. Objective signs may be confused with pathologic processes of the gall bladder, stomach, duodenum, colon—including the appendix and teratomata. While subjective symptoms may be associated with most everything. All sorts of secretory, sensory and motor disturbances of the gastrointestinal tract, disturbances of circulation and urinary output, pelvic symptoms, headache, vertigo, general exhaustion with dragging pains in the loins are a few of the many symptoms associated with this disease. And while they may be properly associated with this disease, many of them may be just as properly associated with other pathologic conditions in and near to this region.

---

*Read at the Thirty-fourth Annual Meeting of the American Association of Obstetricians, Gynecologists, and Abdominal Surgeons, St. Louis, Mo., September 20-22, 1921.

No operative treatment, therefore, should be undertaken without a most careful and painstaking investigation, and should be made with an incision which gives the widest field for observation and pathologic differentiation. Such an incision is logically in front and not in the back. As a result of unsatisfactory experiences with the lumbar incision I abandoned it fifteen years ago, and during these years have confined myself wholly to a method which may be described as follows:

Open the abdomen by an incision a fingerbreadth below the costal border, extending from the median line to near the tip of last rib. Elevate the liver and gall bladder by means of a broad retractor in the hands of the first assistant, while the second assistant with a gauze pad introduced into the abdomen holds downward and inward the hepatic flexor of the colon. Proper traction by the two assistants makes taut the peritoneal reflection lying in front of the kidney and brings it well into view. The peritoneum overlying the kidney is now incised for the distance of about four inches. Through this incision the hand is introduced around the fatty capsule and after free dissection, the kidney and its capsule are lifted outside of the abdominal wound. Looking into the bed from which it has been removed, there will be seen some loose areolar tissue lying upon the reflection of the diaphragm, the transverse fascia and the quadratus lumborum muscle. With a pledget of gauze in the jaws of forceps, this should be wiped well away from these structures, so that the fascia is perfectly clean. If this be carefully done no hemorrhage or oozing will occur and the pocket which the kidney is to occupy will be dry.

Turning now to the kidney itself which lies outside of the abdominal wound, the fatty capsule is completely removed from its posterior aspect, exposing the fibrous capsule underneath. Hemorrhage may occur from a few small vessels which should be carefully ligated.

Next, incise the fibrous capsule from the upper to the lower pole carrying the incision close to the hilum. Separate now, the fibrous capsule from the kidney substance, denuding the entire posterior aspect of the kidney of its fibrous capsule so making a fibrous flap everywhere free except at its base, where it still remains attached to the major curvature or convex surface of the kidney. Care should be exercised in removing the fibrous capsule lest wounding of the kidney substance and troublesome oozing occur.

A suture of No. 2 chromic catgut 20 inches in length is now carried through the upper end of the flap of fibrous capsule which still remains outside of the abdomen and is next caught in the fascia transversalis or quadratus lumborum high up in the bed from which the kidney has been removed.

A second suture of the same character is likewise introduced through the lower end of the fibrous capsule and carried down and made to catch up a second portion of the fascia or the quadratus muscle in the lower aspect of the cavity. A third suture is again introduced through the same structures but midway between the two former sutures. Clamps are attached to either end of these sutures as they are introduced.

The kidney is now restored to its normal position by being dropped back into the abdomen through the incision in the posterior peritoneal reflection. Clamps are removed from the ends of the sutures and they are securely tied. Thus the kidney is suspended with its denuded posterior aspect lying against the quadratus lumborum muscle to which it has been attached by three sutures through a flap of its fibrous capsule. Under the eye of the operator it has been restored to its normal position with no distortion of its blood and nerve supply and with a free ureteral drainage.

A running suture of plain catgut next closes the wound in the peritoneum overlying the kidney. The edges of this wound should be turned in so as to prevent the formation of adhesions. The abdominal wound may be closed in the usual manner.

I have been fixing the kidney by this method for fifteen years. I have had no case return to me with failure. In two cases infection necessitated drainage for a time. Two cases were relieved who had been operated by the lumbar route with low fixation and increase of symptoms.

I feel warranted in recommending this operation: 1. Because it establishes regional and general abdominal diagnosis. 2. Because through its primary incision much other work can be done on other abdominal viscera, if necessary. 3. Because it permits the operator to place the kidney where it belongs. 4. Because the lapse of time since its inauguration has been sufficient to prove its value.

1008 HUME-MANSUR BUILDING. *(For discussion see p. 531.)*

TRANSUTERINE INSUFFLATION, A DIAGNOSTIC AID IN STERILITY*

By A. J. Rongy, M.D., F.A.C.S., and S. S. Rosenfeld, M.D.,
New York, N. Y.

IN a previous paper, I stated that the subject of sterility was not only important from a medical standpoint but also from a social aspect. I am now more than ever convinced that early environment and mode of living, especially in metropolitan districts, must be taken into consideration in our study of the subject. Our social structure, in recent years, has undergone great changes. It is a question whether the so-called "Woman Equality Movement," now permeating the entire civilized world and, of necessity, bringing the adolescent girl into various industrial fields, is not having its deleterious effects; so that a great many girls, who are of an inferior constitutionality, do not develop properly; with the result that the entire cycle connected with menstruation and ovulation is, to a great extent, interfered with.

Every gynecologist who has been in active practice for a score or more years knows that, primary as well as secondary, sterility is constantly on the increase; and that, in the majority of instances, he is unable to relieve or cure the condition. The two years preceding August 1, 1921, I saw in my office 403 patients who consulted me because of their sterility. The male aspect was in every instance investigated either by us or through other laboratories, and I was pleased to find that sterility due to the husband is on the decrease. I believe that the educational campaigns, conducted by the medical profession and various Public Health Agencies, are now just beginning to bear fruit. The average intelligent young man has been, practically, frightened into the practice of continence before marriage and the result is that gonorrhea and all its complications are on the decrease. In previous years, in fully 25 per cent of cases of sterility, the cause could be ascribed to the male; now it is not more than 10 per cent.

In this paper I shall not attempt to discuss the general subject of sterility, or even make a complete study of the material at hand. I shall confine my remarks only to one phase of it and that is fallopian tube patency. And here I wish to state that the present practice followed by the profession at large, and also by some specialists in ascribing stenosis of the cervical os as a cause of sterility, is entirely fallacious in fully 95 per cent of cases and I am certain that not only do operations on the cervix fail to cure the patient, but, in a number

---
*Read at the Thirty-fourth Annual Meeting of the American Association of Obstetricians, Gynecologists, and Abdominal Surgeons, St. Louis, Mo., September 20-22, 1921.

of instances, cause mild and insidious infections which finally involve the tubes and the patients become permanently sterile. Dilatation and curettage as practiced by the general practitioner; the stem pessary and cutting operations on the cervix, as practiced by the specialist, have cured very few patients. That this contention is true is proved by the fact that over 300 of my patients had cervical operations ranging in number from one to six. One of these patients had her cervix dilated four times by general practitioners, once a stem pessary operation by a specialist; not having been cured by these five operations she again consulted a gynecologist. He performed a Dudley operation on the cervix and she is still sterile. I have always held that, if a woman has a cervical canal sufficiently large to discharge the menstrual blood, the canal is roomy enough for a spermatozoon to pass through. In all but two cases I succeeded in introducing a fairly large cannula into the lumen of the uterus without any discomfort to the patient, proving that cervical stenosis is, usually, a myth and practically does not exist.

I believe that the time is ripe for the teachers in our medical colleges to point out to the future members of the profession the erroneous conception heretofore held regarding the mechanical aspect of sterility and, in that way only will be eliminated useless and obsolete operations which in a great many instances are a cause for permanent sterility. I maintain that in the few instances, where pregnancy followed such procedures, these patients would, eventually, have become pregnant even if they were not operated upon. Operations on the cervical canal without definite knowledge as to the condition of the fallopian tubes are obviously incomplete procedures. Heretofore we had no means by which we could definitely establish the patency of the tubes. All of us have realized that in a great number of patients the involvement was so slight, that no matter how skillful and astute the examiner was, that very often he was unable to detect these pathologic changes, and yet they were sufficient to cause complete closure or obstruction in the tubes.

The recent work of Stein and Stewart in this country, reawakening interest in peritoneal gas inflation, followed by Roentgen examination, has evidently stimulated Rubin of New York to adopt this procedure in order to study the patency of the fallopian tubes. To Rubin must be given the credit of really adding a new diagnostic point which is definite and certain if properly carried out and which is of great aid in our study of sterility. We feel that at present the treatment of sterility is incomplete unless the patient is examined for patency of the tubes. Unfortunately, however, there are a great number of cases whose fallopian tubes are patent and, notwithstanding treatment, remain sterile. These cases must be grouped under the heading of sterility of constitutional origin which may be temporary or permanent in nature. The menstrual history of the patient must be thoroughly studied as to time of onset, frequency, duration, and quantity of blood lost with each menstrual period. This, with the findings elicited by vaginal examination, will often help to decide whether the sterility is of a permanent or temporary nature.

In recent years to the glands of internal secretion have been ascribed marvelous curative properties in the treatment of sterility and menstrual disorders. The literature abounds with enthusiastic reports of the successful treatment of sterility by various combinations of glandular extracts. In my series of cases, the majority of patients have, from time to time, been treated by some of our most enthusiastic advocates of glandular therapy but still remained sterile. I have also attempted to treat these patients along the same lines and, with but few exceptions, the results were not good. Endocrinological treatment has its place in some of the milder menstrual disorders, but it certainly fails to cure the more severe types of menstrual disorders and is of little avail in the treatment of sterility. I make this statement advisedly; for the 403 women who have consulted me regarding their sterility have, from time to time, consulted many other gynecologists, some of whom practically limited their entire conception of human derangement to some endocrinologic disturbance and who have fed them on various combinations of gland extracts and still the women remained sterile. It seems to me that sterility is not caused by ovarian, thyroid or pituitary disturbance, but by that something which causes that disturbance in these various glands. In other words, glandular disturbance is a terminal condition and is only secondary in nature to some processes in the human economy which alter the normal physiologic functions of these glands. And, it seems to me, that the mysteries associated with functional disturbances will only be solved by a thorough understanding of the biochemical processes of the body.

In December, 1920, after familiarizing myself with the work of Rubin as reported by him and, also, after a personal visit to his clinic by Dr. S. S. Rosenfeld in order to study the technic of this procedure in detail, I instituted this method of examination at the Lebanon Hospital. The patients were carefully selected and were thoroughly examined clinically before they were subjected to this examination. During the past ten months we made one hundred examinations.

TECHNIC

The examination must be carried out under the most rigid aseptic precautions. The patient's clothing is removed and she is dressed in an operating gown. She is placed in the lithotomy position. The vagina and cervix are carefully cleansed and the latter is grasped, preferably, by a sponge holder. The cannulae employed are of the Keyes-Ultzman type with a perforation at the tip and several along the sides. The caliber of the cannula used will depend on the size of the cervical canal. The introduction of the cannula will often be facilitated by first determining the direction of the uterine canal with a sound. The apparatus consists of a glass blown cylinder enclosing a glass siphonometer. This and its attachments can be obtained from Machlett of New York. Before introducing the cannula into the uterus I make sure that there is no obstruction in the cannula itself. This is usually determined by immersing the cannula in a sterile solution and watching for the gas to bubble through. The cannula is then introduced into the uterine cavity and the gas turned on slowly so that it takes about 15 seconds for the column of mercury to rise from zero to 100 mms. The amount of gas consumed is determined by the reading of the siphonometer which is incorporated in the apparatus. Each "bubble" approximately represents 37 c.c. of gas. Regurgitation of the gas through the cervix is prevented by the use of a rubber urethral tip, which is fitted over the cannula and snugly inserted into the lumen of the external os. The rise of the mercury in the manometer is carefully watched. In this series, the average rise in the "patent" cases was 118 and in the "closed" cases the average rise was 176. If oxygen is used not more than 300 c.c. should be introduced since oxygen is slowly absorbed and, therefore, is likely to produce pressure symptoms in the right upper quadrant of the abdomen causing pain in the right shoulder. When carbon dioxide is used a greater quantity can be introduced because of the rapidity with which it is absorbed. The patient is then fluoroscoped in the erect posture in order to see whether gas is present in the abdominal cavity. Usually the gas is seen in the right upper quadrant under the diaphragm separating it from the liver. A smaller quantity is also visible in the left subphrenic space. With increased experience one is usually able to foretell by the manometer reading, studying the rise and fall of the mercury column, whether the tubes are patent or not. However, in order to establish a positive diagnosis the fluoroscope must be employed. I have had several instances where the mercury rose to comparatively low levels, nevertheless, the fluoroscope failed to reveal the presence of any gas and vice versa, I have had cases where the mercury rose to over 200 mm. with very little fall and yet the fluoroscope showed the presence of gas. I do not allow the pressure to rise above 220 mm. of mercury; however, on two occasions the mercury rose to 250 and 260, respectively, without any complications. In patients in whom the tubes are closed the gas will usually escape through the cervix as soon as overdistention of the uterine cavity has taken place. In doubtful and negative cases, it seems to me, that it would be a good rule to have the patients re-examined a second and even a third time in order to definitely establish the diagnosis. Two of my patients, in whom the first examination proved negative, were found to have air in the abdominal cavity on the second examination. I believe that it is possible for the gas to either dislodge or pass by the mucogelatinous substances which very often partly clog the tubes, and at times, it will even overcome a kinking of them. This may be the reason why in many of the patients the mercury column rises very high before the initial fall takes place. In my series of cases 58, or 58 per cent, were positive, i.e., air present in the abdominal cavity; 42 cases, or 42 per cent, were negative, i.e., no air present in the abdominal cavity.

CONTRAINDICATIONS

This method of examination must not be used in the presence of acute infections of the vagina or pelvic organs. The danger of spreading infection under such conditions is obvious. It also must not be used in the presence of chronic infections if the patient complains of pain. In these cases it is best to defer examination until the pain has subsided, indicating that any irritation about the pelvis has disappeared. It should not be performed at the time when the menstrual period is about to appear. Patients who have heart disease, especially when myocardial changes are suspected, should not be subjected to this examination because the pressure of the gas by raising the diaphragm may seriously embarrass the heart action.

In this series the only complications we had were: (1) a severe syncope in a patient who was quite obese. Apparently, as soon as the gas lifted the diaphragm, the heart action was interfered with. The patient became cyanosed and the pulse barely perceptible. However, she rapidly rallied and I was able to continue with the fluoroscopic examination; (2) the same, to a lesser degree, happened to another patient; (3) in one case, previously operated upon for acute appendicitis and later for intestinal obstruction, and who had adhesions in the left pelvic region. In this patient I evidently caused sufficient irritation by our manipulations so that the patient developed an acute inflammatory condition in the left fornix which lasted about two weeks and subsided under palliative treatment. Ordinarily patients will complain of pain in the right side of the abdomen and right shoulder which lasts anywhere from twelve to forty-eight hours when oxygen is used; but this pain can be minimized by the use of carbon dioxide.

A close study of this procedure convinces me that this method of examination should be utilized in every case in which the cause of sterility is of doubtful origin. It is important that the patency of the tubes should be established before any form of treatment is undertaken. It is especially useful in patients who have had a unilateral infection of the fallopian tube or in patients who have had one tube removed. Heretofore we had no means by which we could ascertain the patency of the other tube except by abdominal operation. Our conclusions in such cases were that the other tube was also involved, but the involvement was not sufficiently great so that it could be detected by the examining finger and, therefore, many of these patients were advised to undergo a plastic operation on the tube in order to cure sterility. Patients who are suffering from fibroid tumors of the uterus, and who are sterile, should be examined in order to ascertain whether the continuity of the genital tract is not interrupted and if, on examination, we find the tubes occluded, there should be no hesitancy on the part of the surgeon to advise removal of the tumor, for pregnancy in such patients is almost impossible. It is a very useful procedure in patients who have had myomectomies performed. It will disclose whether the continuity of the genital canal has not been disturbed. This was very well illustrated in one of my cases: Mrs. A. G., twenty-eight years, married $2\frac{1}{2}$ years, never pregnant, was one year ago operated upon by a well-known surgeon for multiple fibroids. She made an uneventful recovery and on vaginal examination the uterus and adnexa were apparently normal. She menstruated regularly and clinically there was no reason for her sterility. However, in attempting to "insufflate" this patient, we found complete obstruction to the passage of gas.

Patients who have had plastic operations on the tubes for the cure of sterility should be examined in order to determine whether the tubes remained patent. This procedure will, eventually, help us to make a proper evaluation of all plastic operations on the fallopian tubes for the cure of sterility; because it will make it possible to definitely tell in what percentage of patients we succeeded in overcoming the obstruction in the tubes. Until now plastic operations on the tubes for the cure of sterility resulted unfavorably in my hands as far as the correction of the obstruction was concerned. That this is so, I became more convinced since examining a number of patients who were operated upon by us as well as by others and when I tried to "insufflate" these patients I found their tubes closed.

The therapeutic value of this method of examination must, for the present, be left in abeyance. However, three of my patients became pregnant after they were insufflated. One is now in the seventh month of her pregnancy, the other in the fifth month and the third is pregnant six weeks. It is possible that the entrance of gas into the tubes under pressure will expel mucus plugs from them and also straighten out kinking which might have taken place along their course.

In conclusion I wish to state that this procedure has been used in a sufficiently large number of cases by three or more investigators to warrant its universal adoption as a routine method in the diagnosis of and treatment of sterility. I hesitated to institute this examination fearing that untoward complications might take place and in that way, not only endanger the lives of my patients, but also expose myself to legal complications. In my hands this procedure has been found to be safe and I utilize it in every patient in whom I think it is indicated.

345 WEST EIGHTY-EIGHTH STREET.   (For discussion see p. 554.)

END RESULTS IN OBSTETRICS*

By C. J. ANDREWS, M.D., F.A.C.S., NORFOLK, VIRGINIA

THAT the end results from obstetric practice are not all that could be desired, is a generally accepted fact among all who have investigated this subject.

According to the records of the provisional birth registration area of the United States, one mother dies for each 154 babies born. The United States is the fourteenth in mortality statistics for puerperal sepsis, only two, Switzerland and Spain, showing higher rates per hundred thousand. Sweden is best, with one maternal death to 430 labors. Seventeen thousand eight hundred is the estimate of maternal deaths in the United States in 1919. This is probably somewhat too high, but the fact remains that the number is very large. While these figures seem large for the maternal deaths, the infant mortality is much larger. As to the morbidity figures following labor, we have little accurate information. Brothers found stillbirths in New York City in as high as 8 per cent of all labors. Various European clinics show 4 to 7 per cent. Williams' figures show 705 fetal deaths in 10,000 labors, 283 probably due to labor. These are classified as follows: dystocia, 124; placenta praevia, 22; ablatio placenta, 13; toxemia, 46; prematurity, 6; unknown, 74.

The following statistics for Norfolk for 1920 have been furnished me by Dr. P. S. Schenck, Director of Public Welfare: Labors, 3,104; white 2,013, colored 1,091, stillbirths 337, white 164 and colored 173. These figures show that including colored, the percentage here is about 10 per cent stillbirths. It is my belief that this is also somewhat large because of the fact that many premature cases are included in this according to the regulations in this State. Nineteen mothers died—8 white and 11 colored. These are classified as follows: accidents of pregnancy 4, 1 white and 3 colored; puerperal hemorrhage 4, 2 white and 2 colored; sepsis 5, 2 white and 3 colored; eclampsia 5, 3 white and 2 colored; ill defined 1.

---

*Read before the Seaboard Medical Society, Norfolk, Virginia, December 7, 1921.

This shows that in Norfolk one woman dies for each 163 labors. It is further interesting to note that 108 babies die under one month, 57 white and 51 colored, and 251 die under one year. Holmes, in a paper read before the American Gynecological Society at its last meeting, made the statement that the death rate for women in hospitals is as great today as it was one century ago, this he attempts to prove by statistics. He also quotes the vital statistics of Newark to show that it is safer to be delivered by a midwife than by a doctor in a hospital. He concludes that this state of affairs is due to too frequent use of modern obstetric operations, such as induction of labor, forceps, cesarean sections, versions, etc. Holmes recognizes the wonderful diminution in mortality rates for infants and women in private practice.

This suggested to me that some light might be thrown on the subject by a study of our records in private practice, and if found to be better than those in other work, to consider the essential differences which cause the improvement. I decided to go a step further and consider the records of the discharge examination in order that we might also consider the end results as to morbidity. For the purposes of this comparison, I have selected 150 private case records. These are not selected in any sense other than the requirement that they must have been seen more or less regularly during pregnancy. In this series no mothers died. There was no stillbirth. One baby died of cerebral hemorrhage six hours after delivery. It was rather surprising to me to find that twenty of these cases showed a retroverted uterus. Three were known to be old cases, probably others were. Two were cured by simple replacement. Sixteen were corrected by the hard rubber pessary. Two were not relieved, one an old case with adhesions. Ten cases had toxemia to a degree which was regarded as threatened eclampsia. No case developed eclampsia. In eleven cases the perineum was relaxed, nine of these were in multipara and were old lacerations. One cervical polyp was found. Eight needed treatment for laceration or erosion of the cervix. Two were potential prolapse cases.

This report is not made for the purpose of proving superiority for any method of treatment. The methods used, in a large measure, were such as are generally accepted as conservative and safe. Almost every method of delivery was used. One case only had a cesarean section and this for central placenta previa and toxemia. There were no high forceps operations and only one at the superior strait. Low forceps were used in a considerable number of the primipara. Practically all were delivered under anesthesia. Induction of labor by bags was done on four cases. In a number of others, labor was induced by the castor oil and quinine method either for toxemia or a disposition to go over time. The number of cases is very small, but no doubt furnishes a fairly accurate cross section of this work. The results are practically the same as those of many others who are giving thought to this matter. I have not included in this report clinic cases, or those not having been seen before admission. It is this class which furnishes the high mortality rate. All cases of eclampsia which I have seen have been in this class. Certainly so far as our present knowledge is concerned, we cannot hope by adopting any method of treatment now available to make a very great change in the mortality rate in eclampsia. We cannot make very much change in the death rate in cases of placenta previa, which have been admitted after having been exsanguinated and possibly infected. We cannot show the best record in cases of contracted pelvis when they have been long in labor and also probably infected. It seems unnecessary for our present purposes to consider our records of these emergency cases. We will admit that they are unsatisfactory and probably as bad as any under similar conditions. Our own mortality statistics suggest this. Certainly our records in private work show a very striking contrast with the mortality statistics of the country in general.

Now, let us see what the essential differences in the management of these two classes of cases are. It is my belief that there is no essential difference other than prenatal care and a nearer approach to aseptic technic in delivery. In the private cases we have practically no deaths from eclampsia or sepsis, and rarely a fatal hemorrhage. It is these conditions which roll up such large death rates. In my own series ten cases were certainly potential eclamptics. They were treated by methods well known to all and none developed eclampsia. If we have any number of cases of eclampsia, we can expect a fairly definite mortality. So I conclude that our only method of diminishing this item, is to prevent the eclampsia, which certainly seems to be quite possible in practically all cases. Nearly all of my cases were delivered in hospitals. It seems an error to charge to our hospitals bad results in cases which have already been infected or allowed to become eclamptics before admission.

I do not believe we can charge the present high mortality rate to any particular operation or choice of methods of delivery, for reasons which I have already pointed out. As to placenta previa, certainly the greater number of these patients give warning before the fatal hemorrhage.

If we admit that the above is true, we cannot hope to greatly improve our mortality statistics in obstetrics until we have given the advantage of suitable prenatal care to all pregnant women and the same degree of aseptic technic during delivery, which is now generally practiced in general surgery. As to the midwife, it seems unnecessary to consider her results. The midwife should have no mortality, as the case gets into the hands of a doctor as soon as trouble comes.

Apparently in the past, very little attention has been paid to discharge examinations after labor. The comparatively large number of retroverted uteri in this series is not pleasing to me. Knee-chest and face positions have been used as routine to prevent this. I am aware that many symptoms have been attributed to the retroverted uterus which were really caused by something else. Apparently some regard the retroverted uterus as deserving little consideration. Probably no one will argue that a woman is better for having it. It is generally admitted that some pathology is due to it. Personally I believe that it is well worth our effort to see that obstetric cases are not finally discharged until the uterus is in position, if this can be done by simple office treatment.

For replacing the uterus, I use a method which was suggested by J. C. Hirst. The double tenaculum is first placed on the anterior lip of the cervix and the fundus released by gentle traction. The tenaculum is then held by an assistant, while the fundus is lifted and held forward by two fingers in the vagina. The assistant now shoves the cervix downward and backward, and thereby assists the other hand on the abdomen in catching the fundus and bringing it forward. This little maneuver makes it unnecessary to use the knee-chest posture and is much more effectual and satisfactory. After the uterus is replaced, it is in some cases let alone, in others the Smith or other hard rubber pessary is used.

In the event that this should fail to relieve the retroversion, we can advise the patient of the condition in order that she may return later for further treatment, if symptoms should arise.

Our attention has often been called to the train of symptoms following chronic irritation and infection of the cervix. Evidence seems to show that it has much to do with the development of cancer. We know that the cancer of the cervix is nearly always a disease of the parous woman. Is it not possible that one of our most effectual weapons against cancer may be the early treatment of these conditions of the cervix, which are found at the time of the discharge labor examination? It seems probable that at least one case in twelve needs some treatment of the cervix after labor. The condition of the uterine supports which is found after labor, together with the condition of the perineum, is information which will be of great advantage in the subsequent management of the patient. It seems unlikely that many old cases of prolapsus uteri, cystocele and rectocele will be found if the patient is acquainted with conditions following her labor which will probably give this result in later life.

REFERENCES

Williams, J. W.: Jour. Am. Med. Assn., 1915, lxiv, 95. *Bacon, C. S.:* Jour. Am. Med. Assn., 1915, lxiv, 2048. *Kosmak, G. W.:* Med. Rec., 1918, xciii, 417. *Levy, J.:* Am. Jour. Obst., 1918, lxxvii, 41. *Miller, C. S.:* Am. Jour. Obst., 1917, lxxvi, 615-622. *Thomas, L. W.:* Month. Bull. Dept. Health, N. Y., 1918, viii, 205. *Wing, L. A.:* Am. Jour. Obst., 1917, lxxv, 471-479. *Dublin, L. T.:* Am. Jour. Obst., 1918, lxxviii, 20-37. *Meigs, Grace L.:* Bull. Children's Bureau, Washington, 1917, Govt. Print. Off. Editorial, The Mortality from Childhood, Am. Jour. Obst., 1917, lxxvi, 1016. *Baughman:* Virginia Med. Month., 1920-21, xlvii, 495. *Browne, F. J.:* Internat. Clin., 1920, 30 s. ii, 280. *Harrar, J. A.:* Am. Jour. Obst., 1918, lxxvii, 41. *Davis, C. H.:* Surg., Gynec. & Obst., 1920, xxx, 288.

512 TAYLOR BUILDING.

THE INDICATIONS FOR THE MANAGEMENT OF THE CORD STUMP AFFORDED BY STUDY OF THE PHYSIOLOGY OF THE NAVEL IN THE NEWBORN

By PRENTISS WILLSON, M.D., WASHINGTON, D. C.

THE human infant shares with the young of all the other mammalia the necessity of avoiding certain dangers inherent in the severance of its vascular connections with the placenta, the separation of the remnant of the umbilical cord, and the healing of the wound left at the navel. In the present paper it is proposed to consider only the normal navel and cord, and to disregard the developmental defects of this region, such as Meckel's diverticulum, patent urachus, umbilical hernia, amnion navel, etc., all of which may threaten the child's life. Normally, then, the dangers to which the infant is subjected from the nature of the processes going on at its navel are hemorrhage and infection. For the prevention of each of these Nature has provided a physiologic mechanism, which, I believe, it may be profitable to examine before considering the ideal technic to be made use of by the obstetrician in his management of the umbilicus.

In all animals the separation of the cord from the afterbirth involves the tearing through of the umbilical vessels and opens up a channel for possible bleeding, venous, arterial, or both. Since, with the possible exception of some of the domestic animals, the bleeding vessels are not tied, except in the case of the human infant, it is obvious that the natural provisions for hemostasis here have stood the test of time as to their efficiency. In the case of lower animals, however, it must be pointed out that the means by which the severance of the cord is effected tend to favor hemostasis by occlusion of the vessels. In many species the cord is bitten through by the mother, in others, the dropping of the fetus from the mother's body results in its being torn through at a varying distance from the navel, or the mother or young animal, in struggling to get up from the recumbent position, produces the same result. In either event, instead of a clean-cut incision of the umbilical vessels with a sharp instrument, we have vessels which are crushed or torn through, and well-known surgical principles teach that hemorrhage under such circumstances is reduced to a minimum.

It would be interesting to know to what extent the wellnigh universal practice of tying the cord of the human baby had its origin in necessity for controlling hemorrhage from vessels severed by the unphysiologic use of a sharp instrument. It intrigues the fancy to imagine some primitive, prehistoric, Neanderthal midwife resorting to a ligature of deer skin to control a hemorrhage produced by her use of the razorlike edge of a flint skinning knife to which she had been prompted by the urge of a vaguely felt esthetic repugnance to more primitive, if better tried, methods. In any event, ligation is at present the accepted procedure in both the civilized and the savage. Engelmann, however, in his interesting work, "Labor among Primitive People," does state that among a few savage tribes the mother still severs the cord with her own teeth.

That these many centuries of cord ligation have not served to rob the baby of its ability to secure itself from death from hemorrhage are shown by the many instances in which precipitate labor with rupture of the cord has failed to produce it. Harrar has reported 3 cases in which the cord was torn through from 6 to 10 inches from the body, without hemorrhage, and 1 case in which the mother cut the cord, without ligature, in which the baby died from hemorrhage. I recall a case in my own practice where a woman was delivered precipitately as she was preparing to go to the hospital. The baby fell to the floor as the mother was walking across the room. When seen an hour later the cord was found torn through about eight inches from the naval. The baby was uninjured by its fall, and there had been no bleeding. Several of my friends have reported similar incidents to me. In another case in which the cord had been clamped some distance from the body, pending the transfer of the baby and mother to the hospital, I cut the cord off flush with the navel, without preliminary crushing, about four hours after birth. There was no bleeding. A sterile dressing was applied and the result left nothing to be desired. Negative evidence to the same effect is afforded by a study of the literature. The volume of the second series of the Index Catalogue of the Surgeon General's Library, containing the references to umbilical hemorrhage, covers the years 1893 to 1914 and gives 39 references to the subject. Study of all these articles discloses only one in which cases of primary hemorrhage from the umbilical vessels are reported. This is the Paris Thesis of Leriget, 1908, entitled, "Study of Umbilical Hemorrhages of Mechanico-Physiological Causation." This author reports 20 cases, 11 fatal, which he considers as properly classified under this title. He concludes that hemorrhages of this type are rare, and that they are due to absence of ligation or more frequently to improper ligation. The clinical data necessary to form an adequate conclusion as to the true character of the bleeding are, in the majority of the cases, entirely lacking. I am of the opinion that most of them are simply unusually early cases of secondary hemorrhage.

What, then is the physiologic mechanism for the control of umbilical hemorrhage which is shared by the human infant and the lower forms? The factors concerned in the usual biochemical phenomena of blood clotting are of course operating here and need receive no further consideration. The mechanical factors involved, however, differ for the arteries and the vein and merit separate consideration.

According to Cullen, the large development of the longitudinal muscular fibers of the arterial wall is the main mechanical factor in controlling arterial bleeding. Under the influence, presumably, of thermic and mechanical irritation following the birth, the contraction of these fibers causes a retraction of the vessels and a thickening of their walls which serve to occlude their lumina. The perfection of this physiologic ligation is shown, according to Demelin, by the fact that these arteries will, after birth, remain impermeable under pressures up to 120 to 160 mm. Hg. whereas the normal systolic pressure in the newborn is only 60 to 65 mm. Hg. If, therefore, the texture of the umbilical arteries is normal, they will have a retractile and contractile power sufficient to resist the most vigorous cardiac impulses.

In the case of the umbilical vein no such anatomic arrangement is present, and hemostasis is secured through the action on the circulation of the newly established function of respiration. Under the influence of vigorous and normal breathing, the aspirating power of the thorax is entirely sufficient to drain the umbilical vein into the internal viscera and maintain it in an empty and collapsed condition, most favorable for the initiation of the thrombotic and organizing processes which render it rapidly impervious.

Having escaped the danger of hemorrhage, the second hazard to be passed by the newborn is that of umbilical infection. The local conditions would seem to be most favorable for its occurrence. The gangrenous remnant of the cord, moist and kept warm by the adjacent living tissues, and containing freshly thrombosed vessels in direct communication through the navel with other recent thrombi would seem to fulfil all the requirements for bacterial invasion. Yet umbilical infection, at least in serious form, is a comparatively rare condition. And if we are too prone to attribute this fact to our modern aseptic technic, we should bear in mind that the young animal, born under conditions which are the very antithesis of sepsis, escapes infection in the vast majority of cases. This is not invariably true.

Necrobacillosis of the navel and joint ill are two conditions affecting domestic animals in the first few days of life. Both, however, usually occur epidemically, the former having caused the death of 1500 lambs out of 5200 born on one ranch in one season. Here again we see an analogy to human conditions, for the literature shows that umbilical infection is very prone to occur epidemically in maternity hospitals. What, then, is the secret of the comparative immunity to infection possessed by the young animal, despite the local conditions at the navel which apparently favor it? Of course the usual mechanisms for the control of bacterial invasion are operative here and need no further elucidation in this connection. To my mind the local factor mainly responsible for control of infection is one which, under normal conditions, rapidly turns the apparently favorable local situation into a very unfavorable one, namely rapid dehydration of the cord. If the navel of the newborn kitten, puppy, or lamb be examined in the first few days of life, the remnant of the cord will be found to merit the term navel-string applied to it in popular parlance, for it is represented by a withered, absolutely dry and almost brittle string-like body, usually of considerable length in comparison to the size of the animal. Technically the cord is undergoing a process of dry gangrene, and because of its almost complete dehydration is a practically impossible medium for bacterial development.

Let us now examine the usual method of dealing with the cord and navel in the light of the physiologic processes detailed above. This method may be fairly summarized as follows: When pulsation has ceased, or become much weakened, the cord is ligated from 2 to 5 cm. from the navel and severed with scissors distal to the ligature. It is usually then treated with some antiseptic, frequently iodine, and securely wrapped in sterile gauze, frequently a roller bandage being applied, and this dressing is tied in place and left to drop off with the cord. This technic I believe to be open to the following criticisms: An unnecessary amount of dead tissue is left, probably about 2 gms. There is no drainage provided, except back into the body of the infant, for the ligature effectually seals the distal, cut end. This lack of drainage, together with the thick dressing, inhibits evaporation and by preventing the physiologic process of rapid dehydration tends to convert what should be a process of dry gangrene into one of moist gangrene, thus favoring rather than inhibiting infection, and undoubtedly delaying the occurrence of separation. Such conditions can only increase the incidence of infection and, therefore of secondary hemorrhage. In this connection it may be pertinently asked whether the delayed separation of the cord interferes with the contraction of the umbilical ring sufficiently to be a factor in the production of the frequently observed umbilical hernias of young infants. Naturally the argument immediately suggests itself that the accepted method of procedure gives satisfactory results all over the world. To this it may be replied that we are dealing with the condition which of all others most frequently receives surgical care, and that, while the physiologic mechanisms involved may ordinarily overcome a handicap imposed upon them by an error in our art, if they fail to do so in only 0.1 per cent of the cases, the resulting variation in the mortality rate would not be readily detected and yet would cause the unnecessary annual loss of 2500 babies in the United States alone.

The literature on the ligation and care of the umbilical cord is voluminous; that in opposition to the accepted methods is the reverse. A. F. A. King had privately printed in 1867, "An Essay on the Ligation and Management of the Umbilical Cord at Child Birth," in which he advocated leaving the cord unligated in order to promote free drainage, prompt desiccation, and rapid separation. Dickinson has advocated the immediate complete amputation of the cord stump and the closure of the wound with a suture ligature. Flagg, Buckmaster, and Ballantyne have suggested similar procedures. Operations of this character will undoubtedly yield satisfactory results in competent hands. It would seem, however, that they substitute for physiologic processes which can be so handled as to render them perfectly safe, a surgical procedure capable of doing damage in the hands of the unskilled or careless. The article of Rendleman and Taussig bears on this point. These investigators compared the results in two series of 225 cases each, using the Dickinson technic in one and the ordinary ligation technic in the other. They noted a temperature of 100 or over in the first ten days in 37.7 per cent of the operated cases, as against 22.7 per cent in the ligated cases. The initial weight loss was also greater in the operated series, although compensated by a more rapid gain after the fifth day. These phenomena were attributed to the greater shock and infection of the operated cases at first, followed by quicker healing and less drain on the infant's vitality from prolonged attachment of the cord. Cook advocates tying the cord as close to the skin margin as possible in order to secure free drainage. With this technic he reports separation of the cord on the third day in 70 out of 75 cases. There was fever in 20 per cent of 50 cases in which the cord was ligated 2 cm. from the skin margin, as against fever in 3 per cent of the 75 cases treated according to his own technic.

For the past few years I have been employing a technic in the management of the cord stump and navel which appeals to me as being based on sound physiologic principles and has afforded me uniformly satisfactory results. It is in no sense original, as my attention was first called to it by the statement of a nurse that it was being successfully employed at a Philadelphia maternity. It is carried out as follows: When the respiratory function has been normally established, and pulsation in the cord has ceased or become limited to the fetal end, traction is made on the cord perpendicularly to the body surface, in order to draw the skin-cuff out to its full extent, and, after painting with 50 per cent tincture of iodine, a clamp is placed immediately adjacent to the skin margin and locked in place. Care is exercised to avoid catching the skin edge in the bite of the forceps. The cord is then cut through as close to the distal side of the forceps as possible and a few turns of a sterile gauze bandage are thrown around the clamp and stump in the ordinary figure of eight applications. After having been left in place for one hour the clamp is gently and carefully removed by the nurse. At this time the cord stump is represented by a narrow zone of congested cord tissue about $\frac{1}{8}$ inch in thickness, surmounted by a transversely compressed translucent zone, of paper thickness, the width of the jaws of the clamp. The stump is again touched with 50 per cent tincture of iodine and covered with a dressing of sterile gauze, held in place by a binder. Unless soiled this is not disturbed until the fourth or fifth day. The baby is not tubbed. Twenty-four hours after birth inspection of the navel discloses the remnant of the cord as a small, dry scab in the bottom of the depression. In the great majority of the cases this scab has separated and comes away when the dressing is changed on the fourth or fifth day. I have now employed this technic in over 300 cases without any mortality or morbidity referable to the cord stump or navel.

The first question to be asked, of course, will be as to the efficiency of the hemostasis, both primary and secondary. This has been entirely satisfactory. In most cases there is a small amount of oozing from the cord stump, sufficient to make a small blood stain on the gauze dressing. This has been alarming to nurses and internes occasionally and has been controlled by reclamping or compression with a gauze sponge. Personally I doubt if further interference was necessary except in one case. In this case there was quite decided and persistent venous hemorrhage after the removal of the clamp, which was easily controlled, however, by reclamping. This was a baby delivered spontaneously after a long, tedious, R.O.P. labor, with the cord tightly drawn twice around the neck. There was marked cyanosis, which persisted for several days, respiration was established with difficulty, and there were protrusion of the tongue and nystagmus, pointing to cerebral irritation. The baby, however, made a perfect recovery. This type of case, I now believe should have the cord ligated as close to the navel as possible, as the uncertainty of the aspiring action of the thorax predisposes to venous hemorrhage. (The suggestion of King, that in these cases of cyanosis the cord be cut and allowed to bleed, in order to relieve the embarrassed right side of the heart, would seem to be worthy of trial and investigation.) There was no case of secondary hemorrhage. In one case a small granuloma of the umbilicus had to be removed when the baby was five weeks old. In only one case was treatment for a dilated umbilical ring necessary.

This method of treating the cord stump seems to me to possess the following advantages: (1) The technic is simple and readily employed by anyone. (2) The cord is practically entirely removed, leaving a minimum of devitalized tissue to drain toxins into the infant's circulation. (3) Drainage from the minute amount of cord tissue remaining is facilitated. (4) Rapid dehydration is assured, thus preventing infection and insuring early separation. (5) In normal infants efficient hemostasis is secured by means which are entirely physiologic. In "blue babies" ligature close to the umbilicus is probably indicated. (6) The aftercare of babies thus treated is greatly facilitated.

In looking over the literature I find that Liebman, Hirsch, and Stoll in their "Inaugural Dissertations" have published statistics of a practically identical technic employed at Freiburg. This is described by Stoll as follows: "The cord is cut between two Kocher clamps, and the child rubbed with sterile oil. The cord is then clamped with a third clamp immediately at the umbilicus. This clamp is allowed to remain for ten minutes and is then removed and the paper-thick stump dressed with sterile gauze. The child is not bathed." In 3060 cases in which this technic was employed there was no mortality or morbidity attributable to the navel; bleeding in only 0.16 per cent; and the cord stump had separated by the seventh day in 73.72 per cent. In 264 cases treated by the old ligation method there was a morbidity from the navel of 0.87 per cent; a mortality of 0.87 per cent; no bleeding; and the cord stump had separated by the seventh day in only 51.72 per cent.

REFERENCES

Ballantyne, J. W.: Brit. Med. Jour., 1909, i, 944-946. *Cook, C. P.*: Jour. Am. Med. Assn., 1908, li, 917. *Cullen, T. S.*: The Umbilicus and Its Diseases. W. B. Saunders Co., 1916. *Demelin*: Rev. Obst. Internat. de Toulouse, 1897, iii, 261-264; 265-272. *Dickinson, R. L.*: Am. Jour. Obst., 1899, xl, 14. Ibid., Tr. Am. Gyn. Soc., 1916, xli, 713-717. *Flagg, E. B.*: New York Med. Jour., 1901, lxxiii, 1086. *Harrar, J. A.*: Bull. of the Lying-In Hosp. of the City of New York, 1907, iv, 48-53. *Hirsch, C.*: Über die Behandlung des Nabelschnurrestes. Inaug. Diss., Freiburg i. Br., 1911. *King, A. F. A.*: An Essay on the Ligation and Management of the Umbilical Cord at Childbirth. Washington, D. C., 1867, 37 pp. *Leriget, A.*: Etude sur les Hemorrhagies Umbilicales de Causes Mecano-Physiologiques. Thèse de Paris, 1908. *Liebman, D.*: Neuere Methoden in der Behandlung des Nabelschnurrestes. Inaug. Diss., Freiburg i. Br., 1910. *Rendleman, G., and Taussig, F. J.*: Jour. Am. Med. Assn., 1917, lxix, 1963-1966. *Stoll, A.*: Neuere Methoden in der Behandlung des Nabelschnurrestes. Inaug. Diss., Freiburg i. Br., 1913.

STONELEIGH COURT.

USE OF LUTEIN SOLUTION HYPODERMICALLY FOR THE CONTROL OF NAUSEA AND VOMITING OF PREGNANCY*

BY TITIAN COFFEY, M.D., F.A.C.S., LOS ANGELES, CAL.

FOLLOWING the suggestions of Hirst, in September, 1919, I began the use of hypodermic injections of Hynson and Westcott's J.C., solution of corpus luteum. To date sixty-two selected cases have been treated by this method. The total number of injections given in the sixty-two cases was four hundred and ten, making a general average of about six and a half injections per patient. The least number of injections received was one and the highest number given to a single patient was twenty-five. The following little table shows how they averaged:

cases	each	cases	each	cases	each
2	1	4	6	3	12
4	2	4	7	1	16
2	3	4	8	1	17
6	4	3	9	1	21
21	5	2	10	1	25
		1	11		

It will be noted that the greatest number of patients received five, the highest number of injections was twenty-five.

Fifty-five cases of the series improved more or less rapidly after beginning the injections, giving a total of 88.6 per cent improved, about the same average as Hirst reports. Six of the series aborted; one from overexertion four weeks after all gastric symptoms had ceased and injections stopped; one from a rough auto ride; two therapeutically, the first on account of active tuberculosis with hemorrhage and the other on account of uncontrollable vomiting. The fifth brought the abortion about herself, and I retired from the case, and the sixth aborted following an injection. The last is the only one in which I thought there might be a connection between the injection and the miscarriage and I will speak of it again with the case reports. In only one case was failure absolute, the one of uncontrollable vomiting mentioned above and to which reference will be called later.

The technic is to prepare the site of injection, using the deltoid preferably, with green soap followed by alcohol with enough friction to create redness of the skin. The solution is injected deeply into the muscle and the patient, if ambulatory, is instructed to return home and keep quiet for the following twenty-four hours; also if there be

*Read before the Santa Barbara County Medical Association, March 28, 1921.

any soreness at the site of injection to apply a compress of equal parts of alcohol and water.

If the discomfort is severe, patient losing all meals and nausea constant, the injections are given daily but usually they are given every other day, using the deltoids alternately. If the injection is given subcutaneously the reaction is quite severe but if given deeply in the muscle the discomfort is trifling. Occasionally a patient complains of dizziness after the injection and some state the following twenty-four hours their nausea is increased but by the second morning they are "feeling fine."

It is interesting to note the rapid clearing up of the distress and the return of appetite, usually after the second injection. Many patients state they feel much less languid and much more vigorous after the injections. So far I have seen no case of anaphylaxis or any alarming symptoms following the treatment.

As a summary of the results obtained it may be of interest to review briefly in outline some of the more interesting cases.

CASE 1.—Para i, age twenty-nine, about six weeks' pregnant, constipation and nausea severe, with considerable vomiting. Received eight injections in all and did not improve materially until after the sixth. This case delivered later by cesarean section, on account of generally contracted pelvis and nonengagement of head after labor began. Baby had spina bifida involving the last two dorsal and all the lumbar vertebrae and died three weeks later with a well developed hydrocephalus.

CASES 2 AND 3 received nine and eight injections respectively, and steadily improved.

CASE 4.—Para ii, age twenty-eight, one previous accidental abortion between the fourth and sixth week. Seen in consultation at the sixth week of pregnancy, nausea and vomiting severe for past two weeks. Patient given daily injections of 1 c.c. lutein and began to improve after the third injection, but it was only after the tenth that she was in condition to take solid food and the vomiting entirely ceased. She received twelve injections in all and left the hospital on October 9 in a very satisfactory condition. Three weeks later on October 31 she aborted spontaneously after having done some heavy housework. I could see no connection between the use of the lutein and the abortion.

CASE 9.—Para i, age twenty-one, received twelve injections. She was vomiting all her meals at first but slowly improved after the first injection.

CASE 11.—Para ii, age twenty-one, had four injections, headache followed first injection and after this was given one-half c.c. instead of the full ampule for the following three injections. Rapid improvement.

CASE 12.—Para ii, age twenty-three, had four injections and rapidly improved but it was necessary to do a therapeutic curettage at the end of the third month on account of active tuberculosis with hemorrhage.

CASE 19.—Para iv, age twenty-eight. This case is of interest because during three previous pregnancies it had been necessary to put her in the hospital from the sixth to the twelfth week on account of hyperemesis. Her case three times previously had been of extreme severity necessitating rectal feeding and large doses of bromides. At her third pregnancy she aborted spontaneously at the eighth week undoubtedly on account of her extreme toxemia. At the fourth pregnancy she reported when six weeks advanced, with beginning severe nausea and vomiting. This patient received six injections at three day intervals with improvement after the first and passed through the next few weeks with no distress at all. She was the most brilliant and satisfactory case of the series.

CASE 23.—Para ii, age twenty-six. Was vomiting all meals when she came under observation; six weeks advanced but immediately began to improve after the first injection. She received seven injections in all.

CASE 33.—Para ii, age thirty-one, had had stormy pregnancy two and one-half years previously in Arizona. Labor was induced at the end of the eighth month on account of albuminuria, severe vomiting and preeclamptic symptoms. Baby weighed five and one-half pounds. She reported to me when about two months pregnant and was suffering with persistent nausea and vomiting. Her improvement, though gradual, was not so satisfactory as I had anticipated. She received sixteen injections in all from May 18th to June 12th and she got through the summer fairly well, but in November, vomiting returned accompanied by pain. A diagnosis of duodenal ulcer was made and confirmed. Her condition became so grave on account of persistent bloody vomitus that preparations were made for termination of the pregnancy but fortunately the night preceding the expected operation she went into labor spontaneously, five weeks before her date of confinement and was delivered of a six pound baby. From then on her improvement was steady and satisfactory.

CASE 34.—Para iii, age thirty-one, received ten injections and was improved but miscarried spontaneously following a rough automobile ride. Six months later she was operated upon for a large ovarian cyst which may also have been a factor in her abortion.

CASE 36.—Para ii, age thirty-five. This is the one case of my series in which the injections though helpful at first were a complete failure. This woman received the highest number of injections, twenty-five in all with no improvement. I had seen the patient two years previously in consultation. She was then about three months pregnant and was in desperate straits, suffering with a severe hyperemesis, accompanied by profound acidosis. Her stomach had rejected everything for days. She was greatly emaciated, very weak, had rapid pulse, and subnormal temperature. I advised an immediate emptying of the uterus which was done, and the following day and in fact for the next week the patient was in great danger. She then slowly improved and finally made a complete recovery. In the second pregnancy nausea and vomiting began about the sixth week. It was not severe and at first she seemed to be improved by injections of lutein. There was a psychic element in this case that had to be taken into consideration. Her first experience had left a bad mental impression, also she had recently received a severe shock caused by the sudden death of a member of the family. At first her condition improved after receiving the injections and she was able to hold and assimilate food fairly satisfactorily. Suddenly one morning the nausea and vomiting returned, the urine became loaded with acetone and diacetic acid, albumin and casts appeared and the patient began vomiting blood. Her condition became so alarming within the next forty-eight hours it was necessary to terminate the pregnancy immediately. Severe hemorrhage accompanied the operation and the succeeding twenty-four hours her condition was bad, but she eventually made a slow recovery.

CASES 37 TO 53 inclusive, improved under treatment.

CASE 54.—Para i, age twenty-one. This patient when three months' pregnant came under my care. One hour following her second injection she began to flow and three days later aborted spontaneously. It is a question as to how much the injection had to do with the abortion. Patient after leaving office walked a considerable distance to visit a friend and while there was taken with uterine cramps. Sedatives were given without avail. I have been inclined to believe overstimulation of the uterus from the injection, together with fatigue following the long walk, was responsible for this abortion.

CASES 55 TO 62 inclusive improved steadily, without comment.

CONCLUSIONS

1. My experience with dry extracts of corpus luteum and placentæ tissues by mouth have been unsatisfactory. These substances are probably changed during the process of digestion and do not attain the goal desired.

2. In hypodermic medication with lutein for the relief of the nausea and vomiting of pregnancy, I believe we have a remedy that will prove of great benefit in a large number of cases. Those not actually cured are at least considerably benefited and the distress is held under control.

3. Satisfactory results are obtained in a majority of cases.

4. The earlier the injections are begun the more gratifying the results.

5. The drug is apparently harmless, easily administered and leaves no unpleasant after effects.

6. There seems to be no increased tendency to abortion if the patient remains quiet following the injections.

REFERENCES

De Lee, Joseph B.: Principles and Practices of Obstetrics, Third Edition. *Hirst, J. C.*: Jour. Am. Med. Assn., Dec. 16, 1916; Feb. 26, 1916, and March 19, 1921. *Quigley, J. K.*: Am. Jour. Obst., August, 1919. *Ochsner, E. H.*: Illinois Medical Journal, May 19, 1919, Surgery, Gynecology and Obstetrics, November 1920. *Galliatt, W., and Kennaway, E. L.*: Quart. Jour. Med., xii, Oct. 1911; Jan. 1919. *Lynch, F. W.*: Jour. Am. Med. Assn., August 16, 1919.

MARSH-STRONG BUILDING.

PRIMARY CARCINOMA OF THE FEMALE BLADDER, WITH REPORT OF A CASE*

By I. S. STONE, M.D., WASHINGTON, D. C.

THE object of this paper is to report a case in which early excision of a supposedly malignant bladder tumor, by combined vaginal and abdominal operation, has resulted in an apparent cure.

This subject appears to have been given rather scant attention in the literature. We find but little definite or specific description of the disease, its frequency, prognosis, or results of special operative treatment in female patients.

RELATIVE FREQUENCY IN MALE AND FEMALE PATIENTS

Albarran (footnote quoted by Watson and Cunningham) gives the proportion as 14 to 20 per cent in women and 80 to 86 per cent in men; while Winckel (quoted by Mundé) reported 37 cases, 33 of which were in women, or eight times as many as in men. These statistics are, of course, unreliable, having been published several years ago.

We have seen many cases of cancer of the bladder associated with cancer of the uterus, but only two of which were primary as far as we could discover. Allowance must be made for those cases seen in ward practice too late for accurate observation. By most of my associates cancer of the bladder has been considered hopeless from the start. My belief now is that this is wrong and that the present day efficiency in diagnosis and careful study will change this gloomy outlook to a more hopeful promise. One of the most disappointing features of case reports in the literature is the lack of a follow-up study of patients. Certainly there is no substantial progress possible until we know more than the immediate result of treatment.

CASE REPORT

Miss —, white, sixty-three, single and virgin, consulted me in February, 1920, on account of irritable bladder, with bloody urine. She had always been healthy since childhood, weighed 150 pounds, had the appearance of good circumstances and had no vices. At the time of her visit she was passing bloody urine every day, which she thought uninfluenced by exercise. After she came under observation we always found blood in specimens examined microscopically. She had not had any severe or alarming hemorrhage at any time. Blood examination showed 80 per cent hemoglobin and no constitutional disease, with blood pressure 130 systolic. Her urine was normal apart from the usual epithelium, shreds and elements from the growth in the bladder. Pelvic examination gave but little information. It was discovered that she always had residual urine in her bladder; generally two

*Read before the Southern Surgical Association, Pinehurst, N. C., December 13, 1921.

or three ounces. With a Kelly cystoscope a mass near the left ureteral orifice could be seen which had a ragged surface and was dark red in color, which easily accounted for the bloody urine and irritable bladder. She had not suffered severe pain but was obliged to empty her bladder at intervals of a few hours. This circumstance I now believe was partly due to the inability to completely empty the organ. (Incidentally, her bladder capacity was somewhat limited, being about ten ounces.) My colleague, Dr. G. Brown Miller, examined the patient at my request and gave an unqualified opinion that we had to deal with a malignant growth. He advised operative treatment.

The growth, as seen through the cystoscope, appeared to be about two centimeters vertically and not as wide as it was long. It was placed immediately adjoining the left ureteral orifice, being rather more above than below that point. The outline was in sharp contrast to the adjoining mucosa, being abruptly projected out from the bladder wall, which was practically of normal appearance. The growth was sessile and answers well to the description of papillomatous carcinoma.

Preliminary Treatment.—In order to sterilize the mucosa as well as possible a 2 per cent solution of protargol was injected in the bladder on alternate days for a time; the same treatment as that used in cystitis. It was seen that distention of the organ beyond a certain point always caused pain and increased bloody return. Operation, April 1920. The first steps of the operation were rather tedious; owing to the small size of the vagina. However, the anterior vaginal wall was opened in the median line and the bladder carefully and thoroughly separated from all attachments at its base, especially on the left of the median line and from the anterior surface of the uterus, an easy matter to those accustomed to the performance of vaginal hysterectomy or an interposition operation. The region about the ureter was thus investigated, the growth located, and its size estimated. Then the abdomen was opened and the operation completed from above. I wish particularly to call attention to the ease with which the operation was completed after the base of the bladder was freed. We could raise the organ considerably above its usual position and there was no special delay in the excision of the growth as the ureter was easily brought into view. In this case the ureter was displaced slightly, but not entirely separated from its lateral attachments, and was sutured in position as the wound was closed. A line of small plain catgut sutures closed the bladder and were tied on the inside. A second row of No. 2 catgut was added on the outside but under the peritoneal cover. A drain tube provided with fenestra was sutured to the anterior wall of the uterus and brought into the vagina to act in case of leakage, possible infection, or hemorrhage. As a matter of fact, there was need of this which we did not expect, for a small amount of urine escaped through it for more than a week. A selfretaining catheter was placed in the bladder. Although this catheter was doubtless retained within the bladder it is almost a certainty that its lumen was allowed to close and the leakage due to that mishap. However, there was at no time any serious delay in the patient's recovery. Complete and satisfactory wound closure proceeded rapidly and without infection. The bladder functionated satisfactorily in ten days.

The wound in the bladder extended from the apex to a point well below the left ureteral orifice and the growth excised with scissors, leaving a good margin of healthy tissue outside of the involved area. The pathologist of the hospital reported an "epithelioma" and I regret that the specimen has been lost. No treatment was required for cystitis, and although the patient has been kept under observation for nearly 20 months, no untoward symptom has occurred. The growth had involved the musculature of the bladder, but there was no evidence that the disease had extended outside. This, however, may have been due to the absence of lymphatics in the region of the ureteral orifice.

At my request, the patient came to my office December 5, 1921.* She reported herself well and we found her bladder in excellent condition, although she was still unable to completely empty it voluntarily before examination. She has gained in weight and feels confident that she is permanently cured. The urine is absolutely normal.

The description of operations for cancer upon the female bladder by the surgeons named below will prove interesting, the more so because they comprise about all of the special work of gynecologic operators in this field.

REFERENCES

Pawlik: Verhandl. d. X Internat. med. Cong., 1890, Berlin, 1891, 111, 8, Abst. 101-106, describes the first cystectomy upon a female patient for cancer of the bladder. He first sutured the ureters in the vagina and at a second operation a month later removed the bladder. The operation was performed in 1888. A year later, he says, the patient made a long journey to Berlin, spent the day in seeing the great city and was apparently enjoying life. *Munde, P. F.:* Am. Jour. Obst., New York, 1886, xix, 267, describes what appears to have been the first reported case in America. *Martin, F. H.:* Am. Obst. and Gyn. Jour., Chicago, 1900, May, xvi, 395. *Mann, M. D.:* Am. Jour. Obst., New York, 1906, p. 263. *Reynolds, E.:* Interstate Med. Jour., St. Louis, 1914, xxi, Extirpation by Way of Vagina. *Webster, J. C.:* Am. Jour. Obst., New York, 1905, lii, 873. *Boldt, H. J.:* Am. Jour. Obst., New York, 1906, p. 263.

In several reports of removal of uterus and resection of the bladder for cancer it would seem difficult to determine if these merit classification with the rest, as they were probably secondary rather than primary carcinomata.

STONELEIGH COURT.

---

*More than 18 months since operation.

HEMORRHAGE DURING THE EARLY MONTHS OF PREGNANCY*

BY ROBERT YOUNG SULLIVAN, M.D., F.A.C.S., WASHINGTON, D. C.

Associate Professor of Gynecology, Georgetown University; Attending Gynecologist to Columbia, Providence and Municipal Hospitals and Consulting Gynecologist, Government Hospital for the Insane, Washington, D. C.

A DISCUSSION on hemorrhage during the early months of pregnancy at once resolves itself into a consideration of the causes, diagnosis and treatment of the termination of pregnancy in the early months, both of the intrauterine and ectopic gestation. Inasmuch as the great majority of pregnancies are uterine and that the underlying causes of hemorrhage for both are for the greater part similar, ectopic pregnancy should be considered only in connection with the chief pathologic factors that cause bleeding. Abortion and miscarriage are terms that cover the hemorrhagic processes, the former, before the completion of the sixteenth week and the latter before the twenty-eighth week of gestation.

The frequency of hemorrhage during these periods is great, probably greater than we are able to truly estimate, since many are deliberately concealed and hospital statistics are faulty because only the more extreme types occur in clinics or in the hands of specialists who are interested in collecting statistics on this point. It is very frequent, however, being variously estimated from one in four to one in sixteen pregnancies. It is thought to be more frequent in multipara than primipara because of the greater number of the former and also because of the greater probability of pathologic conditions incident to the injuries of former pregnancy and the marital state. It is also greater among those who reside in the city and among the poorer class than those who live in the country and among the well to do. These conditions are possibly brought about by the stress of city life, the lack of healthful surroundings, conditions, and the nearness of the criminal abortionist.

The etiologic factors causing bleeding in early pregnancy have been classified as paternal, fetal and maternal. We may look upon it as the manifestation of some pathologic influence either without or within the uterus. Nearly all maternal causes are due to intrinsic uterine pathology. Returning for the moment to the first classification, paternal, fetal and maternal, we may say that frequently ova are fertilized with spermatozoa from such weakened and devitalized male individuals that the future development of the product lacks the impetus to attach itself and reach maturity. This is seen in

---

*Read before the Medical Society of the District of Columbia in a Symposium on Obstetrical Hemorrhage, February 23, 1921.

syphilis, lead poisoning, the alcoholic and even the excessive user of tobacco. It is closely allied with the problem of systemic or functional sterility of the male. The lack of continued impetus may be the cause of uncompleted development and hence, bleeding with expulsion.

Much more important and reasonable are the theories of primary fetal death. In this group we have a large list of active, reasonable causes acting either upon the fetus directly, as in acute and chronic infectious disease or in a secondary manner, upon the membranes and placenta, including high temperature and direct infection of the fetus as in influenza; hypercarbonization of the blood as in pneumonia or tuberculosis of the extreme type, as the effect of toxins in the placental site transferred from the circulation of the mother as in scarlet fever, smallpox and syphilis. It should be said at this point that in recent years the view concerning the force of syphilis has changed, the majority believing that this disease is a large factor in the hemorrhage of the latter half of pregnancy but not so prolific in the first half. There are many instances however, where abortion in the early weeks is due to syphilis and the influence is directly upon the fetus itself. Syphilis contracted at the time of conception usually results in fetal death and abortion. Syphilis contracted during pregnancy, both parents being healthy previous to the time of conception, results in fetal death and hemorrhage during the early months. Syphilis acquired in the latter months may result in the child escaping. The placenta here limits the excursion of toxins. Syphilis causes glandular hypertrophy of the endometrium with consequent hemorrhage usually in the latter half of pregnancy.

The product of conception succumbs from placental disease due to endarteritis, red and white infarcts, apoplectic tendencies, also the presence of hydatidiform degeneration. Endarteritis has definite relationship to both bacterial and syphilitic infection and the subsequent changes in the vessels. The effect of infarction is responsible for many abortions, the fetus dying because large sections of the placenta are improperly nourished. Similar effects occur from direct bleeding by rupture of vessels as in apoplexy. Many instances of fetal death and ultimate extrusion are the result of monstrosities. Specimens collected and examined closely seem to bear out the view that cases of hemorrhage and expulsion result because irregular development has occurred which forbids complete development or any further progress. Considerable importance seems to be attached to this and it is hoped that its better understanding at later dates may explain the misunderstood habitual abortion.

Other causes that should be mentioned as occurring in this group and affecting the fetus are acute polyhydramnion, oligohydramnion and amniotic adhesions restricting development, thereby causing fetal death.

In the maternal group there are numerous causes suggested. By far the largest number of active factors occur here. They should be classified first, as those factors outside the uterus and secondly, those having definite pathology within this organ. In the first instance occur some of the aforementioned systemic causes, high temperature, acute and chronic infectious disease, toxemias of the mother, as nephritis, the exanthemata and hypercarbonization. These influences seem to bring about irritation of the uterus and uterine contractions. This is evident in enteric fever, acute septicemia, as following acute appendicitis, periuterine infection usually of gonorrheal origin, the influence of pelvic and abdominal tumors, also traumatism, both at distant parts and near the uterus. It is believed that the effect of traumatism in its relationship to obstetrical hemorrhage is directly proportionate to the shock and ensuing sepsis, and may be better borne early rather than late in pregnancy. Hemorrhage following traumatism in general is thought to be secondary to some more potent cause as endometrial changes, nephritis, syphilis, etc.

Nephritis as a cause of hemorrhage is a positive factor. It is clear that a nephritis in existence before pregnancy ensues becomes a great problem for these reasons, first, the tendency to irritation of the uterine wall because of toxemia, secondly, because of reduced oxygenation of the blood, but particularly because of the tendency to cause the endometrium to become hemorrhagic. In the endometrium of the nephritic there are found many small hemorrhages, sclerosis of blood vessels and infarction; also destruction of the chronic villi due to toxemia. These factors lead to fetal death, hemorrhage and abortion.

By far the most active groups of hemorrhagic influences in pregnancy are those associated with pathologic change in the uterus itself, including faulty developmental defects, anteflexion, infantile uterus, double uterus, and general hypoplasia, all of which tend toward bringing about an irritable uterus. Again we have the presence of new growths, polypi, benign and malignant tumors, also injuries at previous confinements as laceration of the cervix and pelvic floor, retroversion and prolapse. These conditions all bear directly in changing the circulation and the endometrial lining, thus bringing about active or passive congestion which interferes with the proper attachment and maturity of the fertilized ovum.

The most prolific factor in hemorrhage is a disturbed endometrium, either the atrophic or hypertrophic type. From these causes there are many bleedings, probably more than all others. The influences that act from without, already mentioned, favor an originally developed anomaly here. There is present in many instances a condition independent of outside irritation, infections or tumors where there is increase in the glandular elements in the uterine mucosa which predisposes to hemorrhagic changes that separate the attachments of the product of conception. These conditions are accompanied by frequent hemorrhages into the endometrium which are inconsistent with the further course of pregnancy and with the doubtful exception of monstrosities probably constitutes the largest single cause of termination of pregnancy with early bleeding.

In ectopic pregnancy the same pathology is found. Usually the same conditions occur in the endometrium of the uterus as in the normal uterine pregnancy except that a thinner layer of fetal decidual cells is present. Hemorrhage occurs through the uterine mucosa because of fetal death in the tube. The etiologic factors outside of the endometrium need not be discussed in connection with this hemorrhage except to say that the bleeding is slight, dark and irregular. The hemorrhage which occurs within the tube in ruptured ectopic pregnancy is the most grave of all hemorrhages occurring in the early months. This is due to perforation of the tube wall and opening of large vessels by chorionic villi or by extrusion of the ovum into the pelvic cavity as in tubal abortion. In either case there is severe internal hemorrhage with attendant symptoms, collapse, rapid pulse, pallor, subnormal temperature, which of course demands immediate attention, operation and frequently transfusion.

The theories as to fetal death are: 1. Destruction of the fetus and formation of a foreign body. 2. Cessation of stimulation of the endometrium by the fetus, the alterations of this reflex bringing on abortion. 3. Destruction of the corpus luteum of pregnancy, thus depriving the uterus and ovum of this influence.

Missed abortion is described as that period from the point of fetal death to the time of extrusion of the product of conception. This introduces the matter of active hemorrhage and attempts, successful or not, toward emptying the uterus.

We are confronted with two types of aborting efforts, pathologic and traumatic, for convenience of description. In the former there is usually slight but continuous dark blood without typical uterine pain. The ectopic pregnancy belongs in this group up to the time of rupture. In traumatic abortion there is more often the bright red hemorrhage with definite labor contractions. The former is usually present in the first three months of pregnancy and is rather hopeless from the first. While it would seem at first that the contrary would be true, still this is reasonable when the pathology is considered that the satisfactory attachment and development of the fetus is impossible.

Traumatic abortion is much more hopeful of treatment if the uterus has not been entered. If entrance has occurred, abortion is almost inevitable. In either case a fair trial at arresting the process should be made by placing the patient in bed in care of a competent nurse and in favorable aseptic surroundings. Morphine in large doses should be administered hypodermically and opium and belladonna by suppository. When it is evident that abortion is inevitable the uterus should be emptied in the most conservative manner and at the first opportunity, but under the most careful aseptic surroundings, preferably in an obstetrical hospital. The product of conception should always be examined microscopically.

The technic of emptying the uterus is of considerable importance. When it is evident that expulsion of the fetus is probable and cannot be arrested by narcotics, the bleeding should be allowed to continue until the ovum is separated spontaneously. The uterus should then be emptied, preferably by the carefully sterilized finger with rubber glove covering. When this is impossible the product of conception or secundines should be removed with sponge forceps. Except in the rarest conditions curettage of any character is contraindicated. The same should be said regarding vaginal and intrauterine packing. As a rule such treatment is unnecessary, since rest, opium, pituitrin and ergot will usually control the hemorrhage. On the other hand, the risk of introducing packing in inevitable cases is attended with considerable danger of sepsis and as it is usually followed later by operative emptying of the uterus, it is therefore ill advised.

While the treatment of the bleeding is important for life and health, still the essential treatment of abortion and miscarriage is not obstetrical, but gynecological. The important treatment so far as the potential mortality and morbidity of early hemorrhage is concerned, is that which the patient should receive in the nonpregnant period. This may be outlined as follows: First, thorough investigation of the cause of disability after miscarriage, second, systematic correlation of the points learned by history and examination, third, appropriate treatment for systemic disease of acute or chronic nature, fourth, correction of all mechanical defects as lacerated pelvic floor and cervix, replacement of the uterus, removal of all foci and correction of all processes of inflammation, fifth, treatment of the endometrium by improving its circulation by the measures just mentioned. The sterilization of the uterine mucosa with iodine and cauterization of the cervix with iodine or the actual cautery should also be done.

Should these patients be subjected to routine curettage? Probably no greater surgical insult has been inflicted upon a larger class of patients than the women who have received routine curettage. The cure of the difficulties causing early bleeding cannot be brought about by scraping away the endometrium, but undoubtedly considerable harm is caused by increasing the already present irritation of the glandular areas in the uterine mucosa. Much more satisfactory results are brought about by directing our attention to the correction of systemic disease and definite local pathology.

Case Reports

COINCIDENT RUPTURED ECTOPIC GESTATION AND ACUTE SUPPURATIVE APPENDICITIS*

By Charles E. Ruth, M.D., F.A.C.S., Des Moines, Iowa

Cases such as this are rare enough to be well worth reporting, presenting difficulties too, in diagnosis, which makes them interesting. In over thirty years of dealing with these conditions I have never before seen them occur coincidently, so consider myself fortunate in making the diagnosis before operation.

The patient, Mrs. S., twenty-three years old, family history negative and general health good. She aborted in the summer of 1920, but recovered without incident. In October she menstruated normally but failed to menstruate at all in November. On December 7, she had an apparent attack of appendicitis accompanied by a slight menstrual flow, from which she recovered sufficiently to be about and at her work in three days.

Jan. 8 she was again taken suddenly ill. Her family physician, Dr. R. Fred Throckmorton, was called at two in the morning. She was in profound shock, pale, nearly pulseless, abdomen tender, rigid and distended with gas. Ordered to the hospital immediately, she did not arrive until late afternoon.

At ten in the evening of the same day her pulse, still weak, was markedly improved. She was no longer in severe shock. At this time her temperature was 101° F. Leucocytes 17,000. Pain, still severe, was more marked on the right side, as were also tenderness on pressure and muscular rigidity. Behind the uterus a mass filled the pelvic cavity.

Presumptive diagnosis of ruptured tubal pregnancy and acute appendicitis was made. Operation was postponed until morning, improvement from the shock seeming to indicate that hemorrhage had ceased and that further improvement was likely. Improvement did continue during the night so that she reached the operating room at eight o'clock in very fair condition.

Median incision below the umbilicus revealed the upper abdomen filled with pus, the lower abdomen and pelvis containing a large amount of partly coagulated blood. The right fallopian tube was found to be ruptured. It contained a placenta with attached cord and a three inch fetus. The tube was ligated, removed, and the stump covered with peritoneum. The pus in the upper abdomen came from a retrocecal appendix which was covered with a thin film of exudate. There seemed to be no attempt at limitation of the infection by adhesions of omentum or intestinal loops. The stump of the appendix was too thick and brittle to be ligated, but was inverted by suture. One large drainage tube was placed in the culdesac of Douglas and another behind the cecum.

The operation was concluded with as great speed and little exposure and trauma of tissue as possible. Postoperative condition fair. The patient was kept in a sitting position well inclined to the right. Proctoclysis was continuous. The wicking in the drainage tubes was removed at the end of twenty-four hours.

---

*Presented at the Thirty-Fourth Annual Meeting of the American Association of Obstetricians, Gynecologists, and Abdominal Surgeons, St. Louis, Mo., September 20-22, 1921.

Recovery was complete in four weeks at which time she was up and feeling well.

It is not always easy to decide in cases such as this, whether to operate immediately or wait until conditions are a little more favorable. I do not like to operate at night. I feel that I do better work in the day time. Except in cases where it is quite apparent that the progress of the case is backward and delay dangerous, I prefer to wait until morning.

In this case we did the proper thing for she rallied from the shock and came to the operation in better shape than she would have had the night before. And yet there was always the possibility that hemorrhage would recur or that she might have by morning absorbed enough of the toxins from the appendix to be beyond help. The latter danger we decreased by keeping her on her right side with the shoulders elevated, throughout the night. The danger from hemorrhage was lessened by limiting her movements with morphine and placing of an ice pack on the lower abdomen. The constant improvement during the night was not an absolute indication that we were safe. A hemorrhage might have occurred at any moment.

Twenty years ago suppurating appendicitis with diffuse peritonitis resulted in a mortality of about 90 per cent. Now 10 per cent is not expected, other complicating factors, such as we had in the case reported, being absent. The principal factors in reducing the former great mortality are, I think, five: (1) shorter time of operation; (2) continuous proctoclysis to supply the needed body fluid while the stomach is irritable; (3) Fowler position to aid drainage and prevent infection from gaining contact with the open mouthed lymphatics of the upper abdomen; (4) less trauma from atmospheric exposure, manual manipulation and contact of peritoneal surfaces with dry gauze; and (5) well placed, large drains.

415 IOWA BUILDING.   (*For discussion see p. 534.*)

DOUBLE UTERUS AND VAGINA*

By David Hadden, M.D., F.A.C.S., Oakland, California

IN December, 1919, Miss E. S., nineteen years old, consulted me because of indigestion and loss of weight following influenza. Her last menstrual period had occurred in May, though prior to that time she had menstruated regularly every 20 days since the beginning of her menstrual life at thirteen years. The only symptom referable to the pelvis was a heaviness in the lower abdomen.

External pelvic examination showed a normal introitus. On digital examination it was found that a cystic mass bulged from the right side into the vaginal canal. It began one inch from the hymen and extended to the right of the cervix and above its level. It was of sufficient size and tension to make examination of the cervix and uterus difficult. The uterus appeared to be of normal size; the cervix was normal but congested. The cystic mass was not tender.

A diagnosis of a probable cyst of the duct of Gärtner was made because of the normal outlet and the level at which the cyst had its origin.

Following a few local treatments and organotherapy, the menstrual function was established and continued regularly without distress of any kind.

In November of 1920 the girl was married. About Dec. 25, I was called to her home to find her suffering with acute peritoneal irritation and presenting the picture of pelvic abscess.

---

*Presented at the Thirty-Fourth Annual Meeting of the American Association of Obstetricians, Gynecologists, and Abdominal Surgeons, St. Louis, Mo., September 20-22, 1921.

Drainage of the culdesac, Dec. 28, produced large quantities of decomposed blood, and an opening into the cystic mass through the drainage incision, produced the same material. A diagnosis of double vagina and uterus with blind vaginal canal on the right side was made.

On Jan. 10, the acute symptoms having subsided, I did a laparotomy. The uterus was double, but the right side was connected at the internal os with the left, though the cervices and vaginae were independent. The right uterus was smaller. The tubes and ovaries were normal. The appendix was congested.

I removed the right uterus and tube and carefully closed the opening into the left uterus. I then made a permanent opening into the right vagina from below so as to care for any vaginal secretion, as a removal of that structure seemed inadvisable and unnecessary.

The woman has been normal since the operation and at the time of writing is probably six weeks' pregnant.

HERNIA OF THE ILEUM THROUGH A RENT IN THE MESENTERY

By F. H. Jackson, M.D., F.A.C.S., Houlton, Maine

UNDER the above title Darnall describes a case occurring in his practice.* He is able to find only one similar reported case in the literature and comments upon the rarity of the condition. Darnall's case was a woman of 46 who was operated upon by him for an uncomplicated uterine fibroid. The procedure employed was a supravaginal hysterectomy from which the patient made a prompt recovery. A month following her first operation she was taken with severe abdominal pain in the epigastrium accompanied by profuse vomiting. Twenty-four hours later the condition of the patient was much worse. Despite the fact that enemata brought away gas and feces a diagnosis of ileus was made and operation performed. The operative findings were as follows: Through an opening in the mesentery of the second convolution of the ileum there had slipped a loop of ileum belonging to the first convolution high up on the left under the spleen. The loop had undergone a twist, was gangrenous and perforated. In the left kidney pouch was an abscess and foci of pus in various locations in the upper abdomen. The whole abdominal cavity was filled with fluid and intestinal contents. A resection of the ileum by means of the Murphy button and drainage was employed. The patient died from shock five hours following operation. Commenting upon the pelvic findings Darnall states that there were no constricting bands or adhesions.

The following case came under observation in February, 1921, and while the hernia was through a rent in the mesentery it was situated in a different location. It is obvious that an exact diagnosis is impossible as to the cause of the obstruction in such a form of ileus. The fact that such a thing can and has occurred is worth bearing in mind when confronted with a patient presenting the more or less complete syndrome of a mechanical ileus.

L. W., age sixty-eight, F. M., was seen on February 21, 1921. Twenty years ago she had a complete supravaginal hysterectomy performed for a very large uterine fibroid complicated by very extensive adhesions. She informed me that the operation was a prolonged one, that the attending surgeon told her that her bladder was torn during the removal of the fibroid mass so that drainage was employed

---

*Wm. Edgar Darnall, Amer. Jour. Obst. and Gynec., 1921, i, No. 4.

and her recovery was tedious and prolonged. While able to live a fairly active life following her first operation, there has always been more or less abdominal pain. She had attacks of pain and distention which were overcome by enemata and cathartics. There has also been quite marked dysuria and frequency. She went on until sometime in the summer of 1920 when she had a very severe attack of general abdominal pain, accompanied by marked distention and vomiting. Relief was obtained by hot packs and enemata. Following this attack she claims never to have been entirely free from some abdominal discomfort but that it was very much less if she had a daily bowel movement. The attacks, however, became more frequent and increased in severity. On January 18th, 1921, the gall bladder was removed. She says that her symptoms immediately previous to the cholecystectomy were no different than in any of the previous attacks. A few days later she was seized with excruciating abdominal pain, accompanied by nausea, profuse vomiting, and distention. Her condition became critical, but relief was finally obtained after massive continuous hot packs to the abdomen and from enemata. A consultant who saw her during this attack stated that a diagnosis of ileus was made by him and that by rectal and vaginal examination he was able to make out a distinct mass in the pelvis. Following the relief of the very acute stage of her illness he was able to still make out the exquisitely tender mass in the same location.

The patient came under my care on the 21st of February and I was able to confirm the then attending physician's opinion. Operation was done on February 22, 1921. A median incision was made dissecting out the line of her previous lower abdominal incision. There was a bewildering mass of adherent intestines in the pelvis and a loop of ileum was found firmly adherent to the bladder. Even through the adherent intestines it was quite easy to make out the mass that was felt before operation. This was a loop of ileum of some ten inches in length that had slipped through a rent in the mesentery of the ileum in its lower part. The loop was partially twisted clockwise and was very adherent to the sigmoid. The rent in the ileum was an old one inasmuch as its surface was perfectly smooth. The ileum was removed from the bladder, the incarcerated loop released from the pelvis and the rent in the mesentery repaired. No attempt was made to interfere with the other adhesions as the condition of the patient was such that time was a marked factor in the case. Following the operation she had quite marked abdominal distention for a number of days but the response to massive hot packs and enemata was very gratifying. She was in the hospital about three weeks. When last seen (November, 1921,) the frequency and dysuria were quite bothersome but otherwise she was in very good condition.

FOUR CESAREAN OPERATIONS ON ONE PATIENT

By HERBERT THOMS, M.D., F.A.C.S., NEW HAVEN, CONN.

THE following report is interesting for two reasons: first, because of its bearing upon the question of the uterine scar, and, second, because of the performance of cesarean section for the fourth time upon the same patient.

Mrs. H. C., age twenty-seven, colored, admitted to the Obstetrical Service, Grace Hospital, Nov. 6, 1921. Patient had measles, mumps, pertussis and pneumonia as a child. History otherwise negative. Menstruation began at fourteen, always regular, 28-30 days, duration 4 days, moderate flow, no pain. Menstruated once or twice since last baby, does not know when, or when present pregnancy started. Thinks date of confinement is in early January.

Married four years, husband in good health, except for attacks of rheumatism. Two children alive and well, one child died of pneumonia at nine months. All pregnancies normal throughout, no history of vomiting, toxemia, etc.

First labor, May, 1918, delivered by cesarean section after 72 hours labor, in Waterbury Hospital, Waterbury, Conn. Baby 8¼ pounds. Convalescence normal.

Second labor, May, 1919, delivered by cesarean section after a trial of labor at St. Raphael's Hospital, New Haven. Baby 9½ pounds. Convalescence normal.

Third labor, Dec. 4, 1920. Entered Grace Hospital, New Haven at 8:30 P.M., membranes ruptured spontaneously shortly after admittance. At the time of her entrance she was having good contractions every three minutes and was seen at this time by Dr. T. V. Hynes, who ordered her prepared for immediate section. Operation was performed at this time by Dr. Hynes and myself. Upon opening the abdomen through a median incision the omentum was found densely adherent to the parietal peritoneum and anterior uterine wall and it was with considerable difficulty that the old uterine scar was exposed and the adhesions freed. Upon opening the uterine cavity the edge of the placenta protruded through the open wound, apparently having been implanted for a part at least over the uterine scar. This organ was pushed to one side and a live male child of 8½ pounds extracted. The uterus and abdomen were closed in the usual manner without drainage. The convalescence was normal and mother and child left the hospital in good condition 15 days after entrance. A Wassermann taken at this time was negative.

On October 25, 1921, the patient presented herself at the Prenatal Clinic of the Grace Hospital Dispensary. At that time the fundus was 8 cm. above the umbilicus. Abdomen showed old scar in midline about 15 cm. in length. No hernia, apparently well healed. The fetal and maternal hearts were normal. Urine negative. The measurements taken at this time were: spines, 22, crests 24.50, trochanters 29.00, extern. conj. 17.25.

On November 6, 1921, the patient was admitted to the Obstetrical Service having uterine contractions accompanied by some bloody discharge from the vagina. One hour after entrance she was seen by me and at this time it was apparent that labor had definitely started. Rectal examination revealed the cervix to be 4 cm. dilated and the membranes bulging. She was removed to the operating room and prepared for immediate operation. On incising the abdomen many adhesions were found as at previous operation, involving the peritoneum, omentum, intestine, and anterior surface of the uterus. These were freed and incision in uterus made in the midline. At the inception of this cut a large portion of the placenta protruded through the incision and it was evident that this organ was implanted upon the old scar. The uterine wall at this point was abnormally thin, not more than a millimeter or two in thickness, and it was apparent that labor could not have progressed much further without great danger of uterine rupture. The placenta was pushed to one side and a small live female baby delivered. The placenta and membranes were removed manually. The uterus contracted exceptionally well immediately and was closed in the usual manner. The patient was sterilized by the resection of a portion of both tubes and by the excision of a small wedge at each uterine cornu containing the uterine portion of each tube. The abdomen was closed without drainage in the usual manner. The convalescence of both mother and child was quite normal.

Comment.—The extreme thinness of the uterine wall at the site of the previous scar may have been due to (a) excavation due to poor union at previous operation, (b) thinning out due to intrauterine pressure at the time of labor, (c) syncytial erosion. It seems reasonable to suppose that all three processes may have shared in the condition.

Recent researches have taught us that the uterine wall underneath the placenta, even in normal pregnancy with normal implantation, is thinner at this point. It is also reasonable to suppose that the burrowing and penetrating properties of trophoblastic tissue and chorionic villi may invade the scar formation and thus weaken it. This is probably particularly true in instances such as the above where pregnancy has followed operation in such a short time. The history of this case well emphasizes the fact that the cesareanized woman needs extra medical supervision and during the last month of pregnancy such supervision should be constant. Because the puerperium following cesarean section is unattended by fever or other manifestations of infection, is it not assuming too much to claim that the scar in such instances is perfectly healed and will stand an equal amount of strain with any other portion of the uterine wall? The knowledge of the implantation of the placenta and of the condition of the scar would greatly strengthen our position in regard to our treatment of the cesareanized woman.

59 COLLEGE STREET.

Society Transactions

AMERICAN ASSOCIATION OF OBSTETRICIANS, GYNECOLOGISTS, AND ABDOMINAL SURGEONS. THIRTY-FOURTH ANNUAL MEETING HELD AT ST. LOUIS, MO., SEPTEMBER 20, 21, AND 22, 1921

(*Continued from the April issue.*)

DR. JAMES E. DAVIS, of Detroit, Mich., read a paper entitled **Neoplasia of the Kidney with Reports of Five Primary Cases.** (For original article see page 478.)

DISCUSSION

DR. GEORGE GELLHORN, ST. LOUIS, MISSOURI.—It seems a far cry between the adrenals and gynecology and yet, several years ago I published a case which shows that there may be a close connection between the two. The patient, a woman of sixty-four, was admitted to the hospital because of symptoms of mental confusion. She seemed to have pain in the left side of the abdomen, and on examination a large retroperitoneal tumor of obscure origin was found in that side. The next day when the nurse reported a suspicious vaginal discharge I was asked to examine the patient and found in the anterior vaginal wall just below the urethral swelling two small tumors the size and color of red raspberries, which could easily be shelled out with the finger nail. These were removed and when I examined them microscopically, I found adrenal structure. The large tumor, then, was diagnosed a hydronephroma. A few days later the woman died and on autopsy this diagnosis was confirmed.

Such vaginal metastases seem to be rather rare, because on careful search only nine other cases could be found in the literature. Whereas hydronephroma metastasizes quickly and extensively in other parts of the body, the genital system seems to be very rarely involved. However, I have a suspicion that many of the so-called primary sarcomata of the vagina, particularly in children, are in reality, secondary to undiscovered hydronephroma higher up. It might be wise, in the future, to think of the possibility of hydronephroma if one encounters such a vaginal tumor.

DR. DAVIS, (closing).—I desire to emphasize the age incidence of my cases. The first was fifty-one years of age, a female; the second was a patient fifty-six years of age, a female; the third was sixty years of age, a female; case four was a patient sixty-two years of age, a female; and case five, aged seven months, was a male.

DR. THOMAS B. NOBLE, of Indianapolis, Ind., presented a paper entitled **Transperitoneal Nephropexy.** (For original article see page 493.)

DISCUSSION

DR. ROLAND E. SKEEL, LOS ANGELES, CALIF.—In the discussion on radium yesterday the essayist observed that we were discussing something which would be obsolete in a few years; but he now has given us the technic of an operation which so rarely ought to be performed that it should have been obsolete for the past ten or fifteen years. Leaving aside the few patients with recurrent or persistent hydronephrosis, which we consider to be definitely surgical, why do a nephropexy on anyone?

Quadrupeds do not have movable or floating kidneys, but bipeds do; and the most beautiful illustration of useless surgery is that employed to fix a kidney in which the principal symptom is pain without evidence of retention of urine in the kidney pelvis. These patients are all physically inadequate and consequently neurasthenic and if one relieves the patient from a pain in one side, she develops pain in the other or in the back of her neck or elsewhere. Moreover, if consistent with life you might remove all the organs in the abdomen and the patient would still complain because the origin of her symptoms is in the central nervous system.

DR. K. ISADORE SANES, PITTSBURGH, PA.—Pyelography has demonstrated to us cases of prolapsed kidney that are pathological. We have seen cases of nephroptosis with such kinks and angulations, at times fixed by adhesions, that the flow of urine was greatly interfered with, causing a hydronephrosis and pyonephrosis. There is no question that there are cases which require surgical interference.

As to the operation suggested by the essayist, if I were to operate primarily for nephroptosis I would unquestionably choose the posterior route, but if, during an abdominal operation, with a sufficiently large incision, I had to do a nephropexy in addition, I think I would consider favorably the operation suggested by the author.

DR. C. W. MOOTS, TOLEDO, OHIO.—I would like to go a step further than Dr. Skeel and say that we should never operate for pain *per se*.

DR. MILES F. PORTER, FORT WAYNE, INDIANA.—''Never'' and ''always'' are very strong words. Never operate for pain? God forbid that I should ever find it necessary to consult that surgeon with a neuritis of the fifth nerve! Yes, we operate for pain!

DR. NOBLE, (closing).—The matter of displaced kidney is one that men have debated for years, as well as other visceroptoses, and because of the failure in many cases, discouragement has come to many, and certain operators have therefore quit working on the kidneys and allowed the patients to go on and suffer pain. They have approached the kidney through the back; which I believe is the wrong route.

Clinical progress and conversation with your confreres prove the statement that I make. This very day one of our Fellows told me of an experience which I am privileged to quote. Recently a patient was operated through the back for a floating kidney, followed by recurrence. Again operated in the back, and again followed by recurrence. This confrere then took the case, operated once more through the back, and again, recurrence. Then he operated through the abdomen to take the kidney out and found the patient had a pathological gall bladder to be taken care of. Another reason why we should go into the abdomen; we may find something else and thus make our patient well.

A few days ago, I saw a woman who had been cut in the back, with urinary drainage for months and months. There was a picture of renal stones in that kidney. She had been cut in the back but the renal fistulae continued and a subsequent picture showed a plugging of the ureter from another stone. I found her with a discouraged operator, and stone on the other side. She was turned over to me. But I said: if I do it I will do it my way. I will save the right kidney, if possible, and do with the left what I have to do. With a cut in front I found out (she was a fat woman and we could not make this discovery before) that she had a big, thick gall bladder plugged up with a stone exactly the size of the shadow on the right side. One would think at once, here is the solution of the trouble. I felt quite elated that I had gone in, for this was the pathological lesion. I removed the gall bladder and the stone. I was unable to palpate anything through the fat about her kidney and hoped I had removed the source of her trouble, but a photograph showed the same shadow. Four weeks later through the same incision, I removed the stone in the right kidney. She has yet to undergo a fourth operation for the trouble in the left side.

Among many of the cases, we find that to cure the patient we have to take care of the pyloric disease, of the accessory artery in the lower pole of the kidney, the head of the colon; we have to do with other pathology as well as that of the kidney, and through such an incision I maintain that I can do my patient more service than I can through the back.

DR. CHARLES W. MOOTS, of Toledo, Ohio, read a paper entitled **The Ice Bag in Appendicitis,—A Fetich.**

This article appears in full in the current volume (1921), of the Society's Transactions.

DISCUSSION

FREDERICK S. WETHERELL, SYRACUSE, N. Y.—Dr. Moots makes the statement that the ice bag on the abdomen has no effect on the growth of organisms in the appendix. He also makes the statement that the chance for gangrene is increased by interference with the circulation. I would like to have him explain how the cold gets down through the skin, the superficial fascia and muscles to the appendiceal branch of the ileocecal artery so as to change the circulation, without having any effect on the organisms.

DR. A. J. RONGY, NEW YORK CITY, N. Y.—In a series of experiments in cases with abdominal fistulae where the temperature was measured with ice bags on the top of the abdomen they had no effect on the internal viscera. What the ice bag does is to stop the pain by acting on the nerves of the skin. It does not change the temperature at all, and it cannot do it within the abdominal cavity.

DR. MOOTS, (closing).—In reply to Dr. Wetherell, I believe we agree entirely. I think it was bad rhetoric that permitted you to get the impression you did. I had in mind, when I wrote the sentence, to say that it did not do that much.

For twenty-six years I have been asked by many medical associations to take an active interest in legislation to protect the public from the so-called nonmedical cults. The object in writing this paper was to bring forcibly before you this fact, —that until our trained men will go home and do as well as they know, we have no right to ask legislation to protect the public.

DR. BENJAMIN R. MCCLELLAN, Xenia, O., reported two cases of **Torsion of Appendices Epiploicae.**

This article appears in full in the current volume (1921), of the Society's Transactions.

Dr. A. J. Rongy and Dr. S. S. Rosenfeld, of New York, presented a paper entitled **Transuterine Insufflation, a Diagnostic Aid in Sterility**. (For original article see page 496.)

DISCUSSION

Dr. James E. King, Buffalo, N. Y.—There is no question of the value of this method in determining the patency of the tubes. Dr. Rongy has described the dangers which arise from this procedure, and I think it should be emphasized that this method should be used only by the gynecologist or some one competent to determine whether there is an existing infection. I have in mind a case where a very severe and almost fatal pelvic infection resulted from the use of this procedure. The case was in the hands of a general practitioner. The patient applied to him because of her seven years' sterility and he, having read an article on this procedure, got into communication with an x-ray man, with the result that they found that at least one tube was patent. One day later the patient had a slight pain. Two days later she had very severe pain. I was asked to see her at this time and found her with a very rapidly spreading pelvic peritonitis. After four weeks of very serious illness she improved and I found upon examination before she left the hospital that her pelvis was practically wrecked. Her uterus was firmly fixed and her chances for pregnancy are gone unless great absorption takes place.

Dr. Rongy, (closing).—I never undertake the treatment of sterility unless the husband is examined and not only is the semen examined microscopically but we also try to determine how long the semen survives in the vaginal tract and we test it with many reagents in order to study their effects.

Dr. King is right—unless a man is sure of his pelvic pathology he should not undertake this work. One must ascertain by examination whether an infection exists in the pelvis. We never subject any woman to this examination when there is the slightest indication of any inflammation in or about the pelvis, which is of recent origin. It is in the clean cases that we use this method. To my mind this procedure is not only useful to determine the patency of the tubes but it also helps us to determine our procedure on the operating table.

The morning I left for St. Louis I operated on a woman who had a definite pathologic condition in the right tube, and while the woman was on the table and the abdomen open I made use of this method in order to determine whether the left tube was patent or not. Apparently the left tube seemed to be involved, but under pressure we succeeded in passing the gas through and therefore, left the tube in. I am sure that the gas introduced through the uterus under pressure will very often straighten kinks in the tubes and also expel the mucous plugs very often found in the outer portions of the tubes. We have often introduced the oxygen into the abdominal cavity under a pressure of 200 millimeters.

Dr. Budd Van Sweringen, Fort Wayne, Ind., read a paper on **Anomalous Location of the Duodenojejunal Junction**.

This article appears in full in the current volume (1921), of the Society's Transactions.

Dr. Charles E. Ruth, of Des Moines, Iowa, read a paper entitled **Coincident Ruptured Ectopic Gestation and Acute Suppurative Appendicitis**. (For original article see page 525.)

DISCUSSION

DR. STEPHEN E. TRACY, PHILADELPHIA, PENN.—Some years ago I saw a patient with a somewhat similar history, whom the family physician had treated for an acute attack of appendicitis. The patient had apparently recovered and the doctor had discharged himself. The following morning the patient was seized with violent abdominal pain. When the doctor arrived he found her in a state of collapse with marked tenderness over all the abdomen. She was sent to the hospital and the resident physician reported, that from the history, he thought she had a ruptured ectopic gestation. When I saw her later in the morning she had reacted and was in a fair condition, and an immediate operation was decided upon. The pelvis and lower abdomen contained a considerable quantity of liquid and clotted blood from a ruptured left tubal gestation. The appendix was retrocecal, acutely inflamed and filled with pus. The left fallopian tube and the appendix were removed and the patient had a normal convalescence.

DR. DAVID HADDEN, of Oakland, Calif., presented a paper entitled **Double Uterus and Vagina.** (For original article see page 526).

THE NEW YORK OBSTETRICAL SOCIETY

MEETING OF JANUARY 10, 1922.

DR. RALPH H. POMEROY IN THE CHAIR

DR. ELIOT BISHOP presented a report of two cases of **Myoma Causing Dysmenorrhea Cured by Operation.**

While fibromyomata are frequently operated on for other reasons, it is not common to find small ones causing dysmenorrhea, with operative cure demonstrating the etiologic relationship; so for this reason, I am briefly reporting the two following cases.

The first, a fourteen-year-old schoolgirl, whose family history, and past history are unimportant, except that she has never looked well-nourished. Her first period came in July, 1919, accompanied by severe emesis and syncope, but no pain. In September, pain began, and she had a heavy flow. Since then it has been a normal amount, but very painful, and during its duration of five to six days, she always vomits, and there is slight clotting toward the end of the flow. The pain is in the right iliac region, lancinating, paroxysmal and accompanied by right-sided backache. She is confined to bed during this time and has marked eructations. When seen first in June, 1920, she was not a particularly well-nourished girl, her heart and lungs were negative, with large tonsils whose removal had been advised, and in July, 1920, was done. There were no spinal lesions to account for the backache. Abdominal examination showed tenderness over the right kidney, and McBurney's point, and also deep in the right iliac region, but very slight on the left side, and no masses were demonstrable. Rectal examination showed a uterus normal in size, and position, and a mass in the right side five by four cm. which was presumed to be a cystic prolapsed right ovary, and operation was advised. However, it was postponed until the fall, and during the summer she had practically no dysmenorrhea, but had some attacks of vomiting, with right-sided pains, usually coming after a period. In one of these attacks, on November 3rd, I was called and she seemed so sick that a diagnosis of a twist of the pedicle of a cystic ovary was made, and she went to the hospital for observation. At the Brooklyn Hospital, on November 5, 1921, she had a temperature of 99.6° F. and a pulse of 100. Her urine was negative, a blood count showed 17,400 white cells, with 89 per cent polynuclears. A second count was done three hours later, which showed 19,800, with 98 per cent polynuclears. The patient looked sick. She was put in the knee-chest position for ten minutes in hope of untwisting a pedicle. After that she had an enema and received sixty grains of bromide by rectum, and a gastric lavage. Vomiting finally ceased, during the night, and after two days, as she had no fever, and the white cell count dropped to 9,400 with 60 per cent polynuclears, operation was decided upon, and the abdomen was opened on November 8, 1920. The mass felt by rectum was found to be intimately connected with the uterus, and a diagnosis of myoma was made. The right ovary was 1½ inches long and cystic; the right tube was occluded or obliterated for ¾ of an inch. The right adnexae were removed after Norris' method. The myoma was shelled out, and during this procedure, about an ounce and a half of black blood broke through from the center; the usual myomectomy technic was followed. The left adnexae were apparently normal. A sharply kinked appendix was removed, and the abdomen was closed in layers. The pathological report was "fibromyomatous tumor with hemorrhagic degeneration," but there was no mucosa in the cavity, thus demonstrating that it was not a uterine anomaly. She was seen in January, 1921, and again in January, 1922, and she reports no dysmenorrhea, or any symptoms at the periods, local or general, and no pelvic symptoms at any other time. Rectal examination shows the uterus in normal position, and the fornices negative.

The second case was a twenty-eight-year-old woman, who had had a hard labor with a stillbirth in 1914, with no other pregnancies. In 1916 her cervix was repaired at the Brooklyn Hospital, and since then she has had elsewhere, seven dilatations and curettements for her present trouble, and in 1919 she had her left ovary and appendix removed at the Norwegian Hospital. Her periods, which began at sixteen are regular and moderate, and until 1916 only moderately painful. She was first seen in May, 1921, complaining of pain in the left side for five years past, extending into the back, coming usually after, but occasionally with the periods; sometimes it would seem to be associated with alternating periods. The pain was unusually severe, and squeezing in character, and always accompanied by nausea. She showed a good pelvic floor, and the fundus was of good size and position, and, aside from resistance in the left fornix, the pelvis seemed to be negative. She was admitted on May 10 to the Brooklyn Hospital, for study, with a provisional diagnosis of varicosities of the broad ligament. The heart and lungs were negative, as was the urine; she had no fever, and her blood pressure was normal, the blood picture was also normal, and cystoscopy and pyelography demonstrated no lesion in the bladder, left ureter or kidney. The pelvic findings were so slight that consultation was requested and with the story of such prostration and onesided pain, exploration, was advised, and on May 14, the abdomen was opened. There was a difficult dissection through the old scar, but no intraperitoneal adhesions were found that needed freeing. The right adnexa showed a large, but free ovary, and an apparently normal tube. The left side showed that about one inch of the tube had been left, and was covered by an adhesion. About three quarters of an inch of the left tuboovarian ligament was found, and at the end there was possibly a slight portion of the left ovary. Just below the attachment of the left round ligament was found a fibromyoma, 2 by 1 cm. in the body of the uterus. The left side of the uterus and broad ligament was resected and peritonealized, and the abdomen closed in layers. We got no histological report on this tissue. The patient made an uneventful convalescence. She was seen a month after the operation, and had had one period, which was profuse and clotted, but painless. Examination showed slight tenderness, and a mass in the left, which was presumed to be an exudate. She was seen again, July 6th, having had a period June 15-22, premature, but painless, and examination showed a negative left fornix. She was seen in January, 1922, and reported that she has had no pain at any period since her operation, and examination showed her uterus in good position, and the left fornix was negative, and the right fornix showed apparently normal adnexa.

In the last few years, with more intensive case study, gynecological surgery has become more satisfactory in results, with the exception of surgery for dysmenorrhea, and the excellent result in these two cases gives me the excuse of reporting them. The first had a clear cut indication, but the lack of signs in the second shows us that we sometimes must take the chance of thorough exploration of the pelvis, even in a young woman.

DISCUSSION

DR. J. V. D. YOUNG.—I would like to report the case of a woman thirty-one years old, who was married and had borne no children. She came to me in June, 1920, with very severe dysmenorrhea of the character that Dr. Bishop has described, severe mental depression, and very pronounced backache. These symptoms had lasted ten years without relief. She had had no operation. She had a fibroid about 3 centimeters in diameter, which was felt in the left fornix. I advised removal of this fibroid, which was done by me in November, 1920. It was located in the uterine wall. Since its removal she has remained absolutely free from dysmenorrhea.

DR. OTTO H. SCHWARZ, St. Louis, Mo., presented (by invitation) a paper entitled **Diffuse Adenomyoma of the Uterus: Conditions Influencing Its Development.** (For original article see page 457.)

DISCUSSION

DR. W. P. HEALY.—Adenomyoma is a comparatively rare lesion in our experience. In five years up to January 1, 1920, we had only 14 cases of the diffuse type in the Roosevelt Hospital service. We had a number of ectopic adenomyomata occurring in other places, but of the diffuse type we had 14, and these three conditions to which our attention has been drawn as being associated with it, are quite common lesions in the uterus; that is, myomata, chronic metritis and hypertrophy. It would seem to me that if we were to assume that they are an underlying cause for the development of adenoma or adenomatous changes passing out into the corpus uteri from the endometrium, that we would meet with the lesion more frequently.

DR. J. O. POLAK.—The first thing that impresses one, in looking at the slides which were shown, is that adenomyoma is a distinct entity which has nothing whatsoever to do with the myomatous uterus. The second point which the doctor has brought out, and which is a point I think he makes clear, is the fact that the normal uterus is not subject to these invasions from the mucosa.

While the diffuse adenomyomata which the doctor describes and the cases he reports are relatively few, I feel certain that were we to make serial sections of our cases we would find them more frequently than we do. It has been surprising to find that where this has been done in cases which did not show definite evidence grossly of such lesions, microscopically the lesion was found.

Now, all adenomyomata do not occur as diffuse tumors. The class to which the doctor has called attention is easily explained by the invasion theory which was suggested by Cullen and which the doctor has shown so clearly in these cases of metritis, of subinvolution and of hypertrophy, where the fibers are actually spread and the uterus is relaxed to a greater or lesser extent. Again, we know that this invasion takes place along the blood vessels, particularly in cases associated with inflammatory lesions, and while it does not invade the blood vessels, you will find that these invasions of the mucosa and these causal rests are present in the bloodvessels. But there are several adenomyomas that are not explained, those of the rectogenital space, which Cullen has attempted to explain by an inversion of the peritoneum and that the peritoneal covering can take on the same characteristics as the cells lining the interior of the uterus. It seems at first hand that that is a rather improbable theory and still it is a fact that the large majority of the myomata which I have seen have been located in this region. The next most frequent location, in my experience, is at the cornu of the uterus, usually posterior; and whether the old theory that the wolffian duct and the müllerian (duct) crossing at that point, causing relaxation, has been the etiologic factor of the development (of the condition) at that point, or whether it is purely inflammatory and the result of an invasion and inclusion of the mucosa, as one expects to find at that point in chronic inflammations of the tubes, is the etiologic factor, it is difficult to say. Yet those are two very common locations in which we find adenomyomata. How can we explain on this invasion theory the adenomyomata that we find, for example, in the round ligament, in the broad ligament, and in a case that Dr. Pomeroy reported and one I reported of the umbilicus? It is hard to think of the invasion of the mucosa to such points as that.

This paper has been very illuminating, because, first, it has brought out so clearly that a healthy uterus seems to be protected; secondly, it is a distinct entity from fibroid of the uterus; and, thirdly, there is a relaxation, so to speak, and a broadening of the muscle fibers which allows of invasion of these mucosa rests.

DR. HERMANN GRAD.—In a study of a series of 100 uteri to find the cause of bleeding, I found that in only 3 of the cases had the pathologist reported penetrating uterine glands, and that was the only lesion that we found to account in some way for this bleeding, and in all there was this marked condition of subinvolution. In one of the 3 cases, in addition to the subinvolution, there was also what the pathologist, Dr. Strong called a myometritis.

DR. S. H. GEIST.—I have had the opportunity of looking at a great many uteri in the last ten or twelve years and have been struck with the comparative rarity of this condition. At Mount Sinai Hospital, where we have a fairly large service, we see not more than 6 to 10 cases of diffuse adenomyoma cases a year. We see more frequently adenomyoma, a distinct tumor, in which there are islands of uterine mucosa.

It is not my recollection that the lesions which Dr. Schwarz describes are always present. We have diffuse adenomyomata without any type of lesion, either fibroid, hypertrophy or the condition which he describes as subinvolution. The hypertrophied condition of the mucosa, I believe, is an entirely different problem. That is a condition which we find associated, as the doctor has stated, with fibroids, and particularly with the types of cases that are called "essential bleeding." I believe that the lesion in the mucosa has nothing to do with the process in the uterus, and that it is probably an expression of some other factor. However, I think that there is undoubtedly a great deal to be said in favor of the invasional theory, in view of the fact that in the presence of chronic irritation, whether because of subinvolution or the rare finding of a chronic metritis there is a stimulus to the normal uterine mucosa which has no submucosa to protect the uterine wall and allows this so-called invasion. I think invasion is a badly chosen term because it gives one the impression of a malignant tumor, and these conditions of adenomyomatosis are not malignant; they are benign and simply give rise to the local symptoms which we deal with in these cases.

I think that in the presence of an inflammatory process or some other irritative factor, we might have one possible etiology for the infiltration of the so-called normal mucosa into muscularis or fibrous tissue wall of the uterus.

DR. H. B. MATTHEWS.—It seems to me that this invasion of the endometrium might be looked upon as the precursor, as it were, of cancer. It seems strange that this tissue can migrate out of its normal habitat into the interstices of this muscle tissue without finally acquiring some characteristics of malignancy.

DR. W. S. STONE.—Apropos of the remarks of the last speaker regarding the development of cancer in such a tumor, I have seen two cases of uterine cancer in which such a sequence of lesions seemed probable. Both of them were operated upon under the diagnosis of fibromyoma with the probable complication of some tubal disease. At operation, in both cases, the uterine tumors were found densely adherent to all the surrounding structures and the removal of the tumor was extremely difficult. Instead of an inflammatory cause for these adhesions we found a diffuse infiltration of the uterine wall with a malignant neoplasm which extended directly to the peritoneal surface and perimetrial structures, differing in its mode of distribution entirely from that which we see in the ordinary adenocarcinoma of the uterine body, and illustrating nicely how the anatomy of cancer is determined by the type of lesion that has previously existed. In both of these instances it seemed most probable that the cancer had its origin in a diffuse adenomyoma. Its diffuse distribution and its extent was such that it could not be accounted for in any other way.

DR. R. L. DICKINSON.—The clinician would ask the writer of the paper to carry the study further, if his histories admit, to tie his pathology to his symptomatology and treatment, whether the pain, the dysmenorrhea, the intermenstrual pain, the bleeding can be grouped as definitely with his pathology, so that we can fit our treatment to them.

DR. OTTO H. SCHWARZ.—It appears from the discussion that others do not feel that the lesion is as frequent as I indicate. I think the frequency in which this lesion is found depends directly upon the interest one has in the specimen, whether it is the operator or the pathologist. It has been my experience that most general pathologists are not particularly interested in this special field, and a man who is particularly interested in this subject will give more accurate data as regards the frequency of this lesion.

Inflammation accompanying this lesion in my series was not at all striking; it was so slight that we made no table of the cases in which this lesion occurred. However, in the case of cornual or tubal lesions, inflammation is present in almost every instance.

The term "invasion" was used in this paper in a mechanical sense, merely a flowing in of the endometrium between the muscle bundles, and in no sense invasive as compared to the invasion of a malignant growth.

As subinvolution is very frequently present in large uteri removed at operation, one might also ask the question, "If this condition has anything to do with the causation of adenomyoma, why do we not find it more frequently?" I feel that this might be explained by the fact that frequently in subinvoluted uteri we have an endometrium which is rather atrophic and it might be expected that such an endometrium would have less tendency to invade these clefts than a normal or more active endometrium might have.

In regard to the clinical aspect considerable data are embodied in the paper which I neglected to mention. In our series there were only six nulliparous uteri; in Cullen's series there were fifteen.

Menorrhagia was found most frequently in those cases with hyperplasia of the endometrium, which occurred in about twenty-six cases of my series. In every instance where hyperplasia was very definite the menorrhagia was quite profuse. This was also true of the cases of hyperplasia in Cullen's series. In the cases of subinvolution in my series only one-half gave a history of increased bleeding. In the cases of myoma alone, both nulliparous and multiparous, there was no hemorrhage in several.

OBSTETRICAL SOCIETY OF PHILADELPHIA

STATED MEETING NOVEMBER 3, 1921

THE PRESIDENT, DR. JOHN A. McGLINN, IN THE CHAIR

DR. AUGUSTUS KORNDOERFFER read (by invitation) a paper entitled **Further Experiences with Pituitary Extracts in Obstetrics.**

After enumerating the clinical indications for the employment of pituitary preparations, Dr. Korndoerffer stated that an exhaustive search of the literature failed to disclose any references to the use of this substance for the control of after-pains. Without attempting to enter into a prolonged discussion of the etiology of this condition, Dr. Korndoerffer stated his belief that an altered endocrine function or disturbance existed as the basal cause of the same. He assumed that if ergot had a sphere of action in this condition, the pituitary preparations would possess a similar one and it is therefore logical to inquire whether any objection could be offered to the use of pituitrin for the control of after-pains. In his own experience a variety of remedies usually employed for this purpose had proved unsatisfactory or disappointing. Dr. Korndoerffer based his indications on a study of the physiological action of the drug obtained from the literature. A routine order was issued in the maternity department of the Children's Homeopathic Hospital of Philadelphia that all cases of after-pains be treated with pituitrin. It was given in one mg. doses and while some cases suffered a short temporary aggravation, all others were relieved. As for contraindications, Dr. Korndoerffer's experience included neither uncompensated heart lesions, threatened respiratory collapse, nor arteriosclerosis. It was also given in cases of high blood pressure without ill effects. In the latter case he based his indications on the statement made by Heaney, of Chicago, who showed that in healthy individuals there is no rise in blood pressure if the injection is made subcutaneously and that it only occurs if intramuscular or intravenous injections are employed. In cases of acute nephritis in pregnancy pituitrin was administered in 1 mg. doses without bad results. In no instance was any depression noted. Convalescence seemed to be uninfluenced during the employment of the drug and the essayist concluded that pituitrin was a most useful and practically harmless means of relieving troublesome after-pains.

DISCUSSION

DR. WILLIAM E. PARKE.—I have never given pituitrin with the distinct purpose of controlling the after-pain. I have given it for bleeding and, so far as I know, the nurse has given it practically always intramuscularly and not subcutaneously. The occasions on which I would give it would be after long, tedious labors when I feared postpartum hemorrhage, or when there was actually an excessive amount of bleeding without a distinct hemorrhage. I have not thought of it along this line enough to know whether it was a factor in controlling after-pains in these particular instances.

DR. DANIEL LONGAKER.—With reference to the use of pituitrin after delivery, during the last six months it has been my practice routinely to administer 1 c.c. of pituitrin intramuscularly immediately on the delivery of the baby. I do believe in the speaker's contention that there has been less after-pain than when not given.

DR. LIDA STEWART COGILL.—I would like to ask Dr. Korndoerffer how he explains the action of pituitrin in relieving the pain. He spoke of the pituitrin producing muscle contraction and yet not being followed by any expulsion of clots, of its making the uterus firm and causing involution to go on much more rapidly. In the Maternity at the Woman's Hospital, we have not used pituitrin for after-pains. In fact we have very few of our multiparae complaining of after-pain where we are sure the uterus is kept free of clots. We are using less and less after-pain medication of any kind.

DR. J. E. JAMES.—I think one can readily agree upon the dearth of material relative to any accurate data or consideration upon the subject of after-pains, which necessarily, therefore, makes the present consideration of the subject a most important one. Patients oftentimes will complain more bitterly of afterpains than of the actual suffering during the course of labor. I think we can all readily agree, likewise, that the usual agents recommended, namely, ergot and opium, prove failures in the constant control of this most annoying condition of the puerperium. In my own clinic we have been using pituitrin for the past year or two in place of the different preparations of ergot as administered by mouth and rectum, but, in more or less of a haphazard fashion. Our attention has recently been called to the possibilities of this therapeutic agent by Dr. Korndoerffer in varied dosage and type of administration. Acting upon his recommendation for its use, I have been very agreeably surprised in many instances in the almost immediate effect in the control of the after-pain. Like ergot, it has not proved to be a specific or a panacea, but in the majority of instances, it has either immediately controlled, or produced amelioration. In two very recent cases, for example, after the administration of pituitrin, there was noted an aggravation for a period of one hour, but subsequent to this time, the patients were absolutely comfortable and remained so. In another case, even though the pituitrin was repeated several times, there was absolutely no effect on the pains.

In a general way, in my own experience, it has seemed that pituitrin offers itself as a much more potent therapeutic agent under such circumstances than our former remedies. We naturally propose to continue its use in a series of cases in order to see comparative results.

DR. KOENDOERFFER (closing).—I am perfectly frank to say I cannot explain the action of pituitrin in this condition. I will say that where I have given ergot we have seen absolutely no blood clots come from the uterus following its administration. I think it is begging the question when obstetricians state that the after-pains are due to retention of minute clots. The fact remains that I have seen severe after-pains where no membrane was discharged at any time and it is that fact which makes me believe there is a deeper cause explaining the after-pains. It is my impression that these pains are due to altered condition of the posterior lobe and although we know it is the anterior lobe of the pituitary which most actively participates in the hypertrophy of pregnancy, I cannot but believe that the anterior is closely correlated to the posterior lobe. I believe there exists a condition of what may be described as hypopituitarism although I believe the word is poorly chosen and does not express the thought we wish to convey. I believe there is an altered pituitary secretion. Whether that is altered in quantity or quality I do not stand willing to say and I believe that that primarily is the way the after-pain is relieved.

A Symposium on the Treatment of Cancer of the Uterus with Radium

DR. WILLIAM L. CLARK.—When I first engaged in the study of electricity in relation to the treatment of malignant disease nearly fifteen years ago the only serious methods employed by gynecologists for the treatment of cancer of the uterus were the curette, cautery, and operative surgery. Radium at that time was not considered a potent agent in the treatment of malignant disease. The curette and cautery were extensively employed as a palliative agent to get rid of the gross diseased mass, to stop bleeding, to deodorize, and to inhibit the disease. This treatment was invariably followed by recurrence, since the superficial action of the curette and cautery was inadequate to remove all the disease, but the use of these measures was, however, amply justified as a palliative in the absence of any more potent remedial measure. The results obtained by radical operative surgery, even in the early cases were unsatisfactory except in a very small percentage, hence treatment of cancer of the uterus was in a chaotic state and any improvement of these cases by any means was considered pure gain.

My studies with the high frequency currents led me to believe that these could be used to advantage as a substitute for the curette and cautery as a palliative and possibly in selected cases, if seen early enough, could effect a cure. The reason for this belief was based upon the following observations:

1. The heat penetration and deep destruction of tissue could be accomplished by this means, whereas the effect of the ordinary cautery application was comparatively superficial.

2. That the gross mass of cancerous tissue could be coagulated to any depth quickly and thoroughly.

3. That this treatment was not accompanied by bleeding; indeed, that severe hemorrhage could be stopped immediately.

4. That blood and lymph channels could be sealed, thereby avoiding reinfection, and inhibiting extension of disease and metastasis.

5. Results of experiments seemed to indicate that the heat penetration beyond the area actually coagulated had an inhibitory or destructive effect upon cancerous cells in the broad ligaments and even in the pelvic glands. This belief was based upon the fact that cancer cells succumb to a lower degree of heat than normal cells with recovery of normal cells.

6. That, owing to thorough sterilization of the cancerous mass, it could be deodorized.

7. That the action of the current could be controlled with precision after studying the characteristics of the current and employing proper technic.

8. That since satisfactory results were obtained in malignant disease in other anatomical locations, it seemed feasible the same effect could be obtained when applied to the uterus.

A series of thirty-six cases of cancer of the uterus, varying from incipiency to advanced stages, were treated by the electrocoagulation method. The results justified the belief that the electrocoagulation method was superior to the curette and cautery, since in my experience a longer period elapsed in most cases before recurrence and in some of the early cases apparent cures were effected.

When radium came into use by gynecologists, after studying the reports of Dr. John G. Clark and others, I felt that perhaps a more potent agent than electrocoagulation had been found. Not then having radium at my personal disposal, I referred my uterine cancer cases for radium treatment. Sixteen cases in all were referred and the results of treatment followed with interest. My conclusions after studying facts were that the results obtained were not any better than those obtained by the electrocoagulation method combined with x-rays; in fact the results obtained by the electrocoagulation method combined with x-rays appeared to be even better. After studying the radium problem and comparing the results of various workers, I noted a discrepancy in the reports of gynecologists of equal attainments. Some were enthusiastic about the value of radium, others had not yet formed definite conclusions, while others condemned its use altogether. Laboratory studies undertaken by trained physicists working in collaboration with physiologists and pathologists in different parts of the world seemed to show that radium produced a definite lethal action upon malignant cells in varying depths depending upon the dosage, filtration, etc., The difference in clinical results by different men and the discrepancies in the laboratory and clinical results led to the conclusion that, with improved technic, better results could be obtained. It was found that most gynecologists and radiologists depended upon the radium capsule inserted into the cervical canal, or capsules in tandem inserted up as far as the fundus. Sometimes a radium capsule was placed against the cervix without insertion into the canal. It seemed obvious that under these conditions it was impossible to irradiate the tissues to a sufficient depth to influence malignant involvement of the broad ligaments and structures remote from the point of contact and that this was the reason for disappointment.

Having procured some radium in hollow, metallic needles, I tried combining the capsule or capsules in the cervix or body of the uterus, using standard filtration, with radium needles inserted at the extreme margin of the cancerous mass, care being taken to avoid the ureters, also not to insert the needles into the bladder, rectum, or peritoneal cavity. It would seem that the radium rays by this combined method of application would penetrate farther than when the capsule in the cervix was used alone and that, instead of having a large quantity of radium concentrated at one point, by means of the radium needles crossfire radiation from needle to needle would be accomplished, rendering the rays received by the tissues more homogeneous and equally divided. It appeared that this radium treatment might be powerfully supplemented by massive x-ray treatment according to standard technic with portals of entry suprapubically, laterally, through the back and through the perineum. This treatment was applied to thirty-one cases. Such astonishing results have been obtained by these combined methods during the past four years that I certainly recommend them as an improved technic of employing radium to cancer of the uterus.

In some cases where there were large necrotic masses, it seemed a good plan to destroy the mass first by the electrocoagulation method so that it would not be necessary to irradiate such a large area. This has been practiced in some cases to advantage. If the tissue is firm, however, radium needle, capsule, and x-ray treatment combined may be employed without electrocoagulation. With proper dosage and filtration there will be no slough, the malignant tissue will retrogress and entirely disappear leaving in its place pale fibrous tissue. I shall not at this time attempt a statistical study of results, but in the near future hope to present in proper form what has been accomplished.

It has been suggested by some gynecologists that it might be advisable to practice hysterectomy after converting the case into an operable one by the use of radium. The question of the advisability of this is still in abeyance. It was practiced in two cases and the gynecologist was astonished at the freedom from malignancy in the uterus, also at the ease with which the operation was performed, since, owing to the action of the radium upon the blood vessels, the operation was comparatively bloodless. It was found in one case, after opening the abdomen, that there was some malignant disease in the tissues anterior to the rectum, also of the bladder wall, which could not have been detected without laparotomy. Radium needles were therefore inserted into the growths through the abdominal opening and left in place twenty-four hours, when they were easily withdrawn. An exploratory incision after radium has done its work should be seriously considered for the purpose of performing a hysterectomy or panhysterectomy if, after examination of the parts, this seems advisable, and to inspect the whole pelvic cavity, that radium in needles might be applied if there was any disease that had hitherto escaped notice. I believe some lives could be saved if this were practiced, since it may be done with comparative safety and some disease might be found that could not be discovered by any other method of examination.

Notwithstanding the opinion of one of our distinguished colleagues who says that radium is of no value in the treatment of malignant disease, we can definitely state that he is mistaken. It has not by any means failed. The future with improved technic of application will undoubtedly show it to be of greater value than is realized at the present time and when we consider the little hope that could be offered by the older methods, radium is a welcome addition to our armamentarium.

DR. GEORGE E. PFAHLER.—I will begin where Dr. Clark left off. I have had, as Dr. Clark has had, some patients who were very much distressed by the newspaper reports that have been circulated during the past two weeks or ten days. I have had some discontinue treatment. I have had others say, "Well, if it had not been for radium I would not be alive." It is a pleasure to hear that and annoying to hear the others. There are a great many people who have been made unhappy and discouraged. Some of them have entirely given up any form of treatment as the result. We must bear in mind that this subject of radiology is only at its beginning. It is being investigated by a number of skilled and careful men, but we must understand by comparison, surgery is hundreds of years old and surgery can claim today the most brilliant minds probably in the whole profession. What does radiology have by comparison? A few men who have taken this work up enthusiastically, many of them well trained, but they have almost no experience to go by, there is no preceding teaching. What is more, surgery has hundreds of millions of dollars invested in hospitals which have gradually built up surgical experience and yet the surgeons have not cured cancers and are not curing a sufficient number to be satisfied, or we would not have this subject under discussion tonight.

Therefore, why make this comparison? Don't forget that practically all the development of radiology up to the present time has been upon the basis of surgical failures, patients that have either been cast aside as hopeless from surgery, or that have been operated upon and the disease has recurred and then they are turned away to the radiologist for treatment. That is not imagination, it is an everyday experience with everybody who is using either radium or the x-ray and of all the optimistic people in the world none perhaps can equal the surgeons who have operated on the disease in the beginning, have had it recur and then assure the patient he will get well under radium. Now anybody can go into any good radiological laboratory, and spend a day and I believe there is not one of these laboratories from which the visitor will go away unconvinced of the value of radiation in the treatment of malignancy. Some time during the day they will see a case in which there can be no question of the value of radium and what it has done.

Coming to the real subject for which we have met tonight: When we discuss this subject of carcinoma of the uterus we must classify our cases, namely, first, the operable class, in which the disease is confined to the uterus and can be operated upon with reasonable success. When the disease has spread from the uterus into the vagina, into the parametrium, into the lymphatic glands then at the very beginning, they may be classed as borderline. These later may be termed as inoperable. Then we have the recurrent cases, which, of course, belong to the inoperable group because they have invaded the surrounding tissues. And finally the hopeless cases that are so far advanced that there is no hope of reaching all the disease by any means. Now these are the five groups of cases that we must deal with. There is only one group of the whole five concerning which we need to make any comparison with regard to surgery. With regard to the other four groups, what are you going to do for them? Now it is not the radiologist, pure and simple, today that is most enthusiastic about the treatment of carcinoma of the uterus by radium. It is the surgeon and the gynecologist who have taken up radiation thoroughly and have had a large clinic to work with and have had a reasonable quantity of radium, who are today the most enthusiastic. Dr. John G. Clark, whose work and results no one will question, says that his operable group is becoming less and less. Others have claimed that none of them should be considered operable any more. It is the gynecologists who have had experience with operation and experience with radiation and have come to this conclusion and there are a number of these who are not operating on any carcinomata of the uterus. Now there are some of these operators, such as Schmidt and Bailey, and several others, who have taken up the question of doing operation after the radiation. Dr. Schmidt, of Chicago, who is in charge of the gynecological clinic of two of the largest hospitals in Chicago, told me last week, when I asked him "how soon should a patient be operated upon after the application of radium in operable cases?" He said "Why operate? Radium will cure the disease if it is still in the uterus, and if it is outside surgery won't cure the disease and there is where it ends all." I applied some radium for one of our leading gynecologists week before last and I telegraphed to two of our leading men who have had the most experience in this line of work because the gynecologist intends to operate shortly after this application of radium. I wanted to advise him when it would be best to operate. I was not opposed to operating. The word came back from Dr. Bailey, of New York, saying, "If you have applied 2,000 mgs. hours in a carcinoma of the cervical canal operate within a week; if you have applied 4,000 mgs. hours operate after four weeks."

In a certain group there is still a question whether you should operate or not. I think the surgeons and gynecologists who have had experience should operate.

It will help them to find out what is best to be done and give the woman the advantage of surgery and radiology. The borderline cases have a better chance from radium than from operation. We cannot lay down any rule as to the application of the rays, because every case differs somewhat, but in general I think in this group where the disease has extended to the walls of the vagina, or even into the parametrium, that it is wise to make an application of radium against the cervix and the diseased area and then introduce radium into the uterine canal. I should use 100 mg. for 24 hours in radium pack; with vaginal walls and bladder packed as far away to prevent irritation. The bladder for this purpose should be emptied, if practicable kept empty by means of the catheter. The rectum should be thoroughly cleansed preceding the application of the radium. If we are going to treat carcinoma of the uterus we count on using 5,000 to 7,000 mg. hours. This is about the total amount you can use without causing too much destruction or injury of other tissues, but in these advanced cases where the disease has extended into the parametrium, or lymph nodes of the pelvis, we should add x-ray treatment, because by this process we can carry a certain amount of radiation into these diseased areas through the abdominal wall and we will get more cases well.

Now there has been a great deal written, especially in Germany, about the high voltage current. These voltages are gradually increased. An investigation by Dr. Coolidge led him to conclude that they were using very little more voltage than we were, but they were measuring by a different process and that they were using about 140,000 volts in comparison with about 127,000 volts that we were using, providing we spoke in the same language. We, however, speak of that same current generally in America as 90,000 volts. There are being developed machines that will produce 200,000 and even 300,000 actual effective voltage. That gives us radiation that approximates, though does not equal the gamma rays of radium and gives it to us in much larger quantity than we can get from radium. I believe when our technic has been thoroughly developed for that high voltage that we will accomplish results such as we cannot possibly hope to accomplish today. I must say that I am afraid of the propaganda that has been developed concerning this high voltage. I am afraid that a lot of untrained and enthusiastic people may take this high voltage up without sufficient training and do harm. I am getting letters every day from hospital authorities asking what they shall do about this matter. I think within a year we will have something we can use and depend upon.

Now in regard to the recurrent cases and the hopeless cases. I will first illustrate one of these inoperable cases that I have just spoken about. About a year ago Dr. Laplace at the Misercordia Hospital turned over to me a woman who had an inoperable carcinoma involving the entire cervix, with enlargement of the whole uterus and with extension of the carcinoma around three-fourths of the upper portion of the vagina and extending downward about an inch. I applied 100 mgms. into the uterine canal, filtered through 1 mm. of platinum and 1 mm. of rubber. At the same time I placed against the cervix 100 mg. of radium in pack. I left it 24 hours. In three weeks I applied the x-ray through the walls of the pelvis anteriorly, posteriorly and laterally, giving all the skin would stand in a period of a month. So far as any of us could tell all of the disease had disappeared and she regained her health perfectly. When I examined her in July there was apparently none present. She may die ultimately of the disease, but if she does we will have prolonged her life. That is an illustration of what we get in some of these very advanced cases which are inoperable. It is not a question of comparing surgery with these cases.

The recurrent cases are to me very discouraging. You may have a comparatively small amount of disease in the recurrence, but you cannot make the same impression. You may get the disease to disappear temporarily, but it recurs very generally. In the recurrent disease if you can treat thoroughly with the x-rays and destroy the local disease by implantation of radium needles, it is probably the best procedure.

DR. BROOKE M. ANSPACH.—About nine years ago, Dr. John G. Clark and some of the members of his staff went to Baltimore to spend the day with Dr. Kelly, who was then starting his work with radium. He was very enthusiastic. We came back hopeful, but skeptical. It happened that I had a patient who had been operated upon three or four months previously, a woman of sixty-five, with an advanced cancer of the cervix, for which I could do no more than curette and cauterize. She had been given the usual treatment with acetone, and had rapidly failed. I had spoken of Dr. Kelly's ideas with one of my associates, who was related to this woman, and he wished to try the radium in her case. Through the courtesy of Dr. Kelly, I obtained some emanations and later, some of the radium salt. The patient at that time, was rather emaciated, she had lost 40 pounds, there was a marked degree of anemia, an irregular temperature, constant pain which required opiates, and the vaginal discharge was so offensive that the burning of deodorizing cones was required. Her family were very much opposed to any plan of treatment, one physician having advised that she be given opiates and allowed to die. It was only after explaining the simple plan of placing the radium in the carcinomatous crater that the consent of one of her daughters was obtained. To make a long story short, within six months this woman had regained her usual weight, her blood picture was normal, she had no pain, and she did her own housework. She had a small rectovaginal fistula, which gave her very little trouble. She lived for four years apparently in good health, and then died after an acute illness of four days. No autopsy was allowed, so that I am unable to state the cause of death.

No one will deny that if a cancer is entirely localized in a certain spot, surgery is the best method of treatment, the surgical procedure being a removal of the carcinomatous area with a wide circle of normal tissue.

In the case of cancer of the cervix, the operation is difficult even in the early stages, and one man in the course of his surgical work has a comparatively limited experience. So far as I know, the largest experience was that of Wertheim, who, four or five years ago, reported 250 cases which he had operated on and followed for a period of five years, and in them the percentage of absolute cure was less than 20. In other words, less than one-fifth of the cases of cancer of the cervix which applied for treatment in his clinic were cured, a very discouraging result, and especially so, in view of the fact that in the earlier operations his mortality was as high as 25 per cent. As his experience and technic improved, the mortality was lowered, and of the whole series, if I remember correctly, it was about 11 per cent. As these facts demonstrate, surgery has not done all that might have been expected of it for cancer of the cervix. Moreover, there are few cases of cancer of the cervix seen in such an early stage that a cure appears feasible by a wide removal of the diseased area. In the face of such a situation, the remarkable result following the use of radium in the case which I have described, encouraged me to make a further use of it. I have no statistics of my own, as my cases were grouped with those in the gynecological service of Dr. John G. Clark at the University Hospital. Dr. Clark and Dr. Keene have recently reported the results in the series. The report deals with 313 cases. These include carcinomata of the uterus, vagina and external genitalia. At the end of four years, 24 per cent were alive and free of recurrence. In 60 per cent, there was local healing, that is, there was no bleeding or discharge. In a considerable percentage there was relief of pain. In about 10 per cent, the radium seemed to increase the rapidity of the growth, and in about 10 per cent, the use of radium was followed by the development of fistulae. Fistula as the result of radium treatment was more frequent in the cases treated earlier in the series than in the late ones, because in the late ones knowing more about the dose, fistulae could be avoided. Early in the series, every case of carcinoma was exposed to a maximum dose. Later, the very bad cases, that is, those in which the disease greatly involved the vesicovaginal or the rectovaginal septum were not treated at all, or at least, not given a full dose. When a full dose is given under such circumstances, fistulae invariably follow, and this adds to the misery of the patient, while ultimately it does them no good. At the present time, a smaller dose of radium, say one-half the usual dose, helps the discharge and the bleeding, does not produce fistulae and probably is the best method of treatment. The dose of radium used in this series was usually 100 mg. for 24 hours, or 2400 mg. hours. At first, in most of the cases this was applied in capsule, but recently needles have been employed, at least in part. As a result of experience, it is wise to give a full dose at the time of the first application, and it is unusual to derive any more benefit from a second application. There are, of course, exceptions to this rule.

The explanation offered by Clark and Keene for this fact, is that after the first treatment with radium, the cancer cells which remain are rather closely imbedded in the fibrous tissue, and the fibrous tissue itself being subnormally vascularized, may be itself affected by the radium. Recurrent cases are not favorable ones for the use of radium on account of the scar tissue, in which the cancerous cells are more or less embedded.

The ideal surgical procedure in early cases of cancer of the cervix would seem to be panhysterectomy immediately following the application of radium. I have had only one case of cancer of the cervix during the past year in which the cancer appeared to be early enough to make operation the procedure of choice. This carcinoma was in a young woman of 31 who had had one pregnancy ending in miscarriage at the fifth month. It was of the glandular type, and in spite of the previous radiation with a 100 mg. of radium for 24 hours, and the removal of the vaginal cuff and of the cellular tissue at the base of the broad ligaments and a perfect surgical convalescence, the disease recurred within six months in the iliac glands and she died. Notwithstanding the unfortunate outcome, which may be explained on the grounds of an unusually rapid growth, I believe this is the procedure of choice in the early cases. In carrying out such a plan, one must be very careful that the radiation is confined to the carcinoma itself and does not affect the vaginal fornices; otherwise, sloughing may take place.

DR. JOHN A. McGLINN.—All during my teaching career I have emphasized early diagnosis in cancer but the plea for early diagnosis and for the treatment of the precancerous lesions, in this country, at least in my experience, has not borne results. I very seldom ever see a case of really precancerous cervix. Although the extent of operability as the result of Wertheim's operation has undoubtedly increased yet it is very seldom we see a really operable case in comparison with the inoperable type. Wertheim in his early cases had a tremendous operative mortality. Then after developing his operation his operative mortality decreased, the extent of operability increased and yet he was able to cure about 20 per cent of his cases and that result has never been attained as far as I know in any other clinic. The Wertheim operation is a very difficult operation. I have attempted it a number of times, I have never properly performed it. Very few men in this country would have the temerity to risk the tremendous operative mortality by doing the operation to perfect themselves in the operative technic. So that I think it is safe to say that in no clinic in this country have Wertheim's figures ever been approached and the best you can hope for in clinics of the United States is at least 10 per cent in all cases of cancer of the uterus. I personally, have two cases living and well over the five year period from operation. About two years ago a woman walked into my hospital and that woman two years afterwards from an absolutely inoperable condition was absolutely free from disease and that was by the use of radium. A case that Dr. Clark speaks about a year and a half ago, weighed 80 pounds, hemoglobin of 30 per cent; she was bed-ridden and I would not give her two weeks to live. I have examined her since the radium treatment and her uterus is freely movable and there is no sign of cancer anywhere in the woman's pelvis. I saw a woman recently who had a fibroid of the uterus about the size of a bucket, the whole cervix was absolutely destroyed by a cauliflower growth. I took her to the hospital and she had a terrific hemorrhage after the use of the radium but this was readily controlled by packing. Because she had this hemorrhage I felt dubious, but four weeks later the uterus was half the size and healed over with normal mucous membrane. I then sent her to Dr. Pfahler for intensive x-ray treatment. Even though she had extensive thickening in the base of the left broad ligament, she is as free from cancer as physical examination can determine. I am not saying she is cured of her cancer. I am satisfied she is cured of her fibroid. I had a case only recently, absolutely inoperable, whom I examined ten days after the application of radium and the cervix was normal size, covered over with mucous membrane and you could not tell that woman had ever had a child, everything was so absolutely normal so far as the cervix was concerned. There is no question that in the inoperable cancers of the cervix, radium is the only thing to use. The important thing to be decided, and it can only be after more experience, is whether we should discard surgery, whether we are justified to use surgery, if we are going to do the proper operation and assume the high operative risk, or use radium in the operative cases where there is practically no risk. The best review of the subject appeared in Taussig's article in THE AMERICAN JOURNAL OF OBSTETRICS AND GYNECOLOGY. Statistics show there is practically no difference between radium and operation in Wertheim's clinic, but even in five years the technic in the application of radium has developed and is going to develop still further; whereas the technic in the cases referred to surgery is almost a finished article. Personally, I feel that if I met with a case of cancer of the cervix, an early operable case, I would use radium on it and not surgery. I am perfectly convinced if I had a member of my own family with early cancer of the cervix, knowing what I do of the effect of the unoperated cases, that it would be radium and not surgery.

DR. STEPHEN E. TRACY.—Unfortunately carcinoma of the uterus is so far advanced before the patients seek medical aid that we cannot expect a large percentage of permanent results by any method of treatment. I quite agree with Dr. McGlinn that the main thing is to educate the public on the cancer question so that the dangers will be recognized and the patients come for treatment early. It is pretty generally agreed that carcinoma of the corpus uteri, if seen at all early, should be treated by surgery. The results from surgery in the treatment of carcinoma of the cervix uteri have been so thoroughly unsatisfactory in the vast majority of cases that any form of treatment which promises relief for these patients is worthy of consideration and serious investigation.

There is another factor to be considered and that is the type of cancer with which we are dealing. Some cases in which we expected good results, were most disappointing; while good results were secured in what seemed hopeless cases. One patient, who had an extensive carcinoma of the cervix uteri, on whom we did a radical operation, is alive and well over twelve years after operation. Another patient is alive and well more than eight years after operation. I have had several advanced cases of carcinoma of the cervix uteri, on whom extensive cautery operations were performed, and some lived three and four years, and one nearly five years after operation. Most cases of carcinoma of the cervix uteri are beyond the operative stage when seen. Dr. Pfahler is seeking information as to whether patients treated with radium, in whom there is a marked improvement, should subsequently be subjected to surgery. Few men are willing to do a really radical operation on these patients, and, if there is a marked improvement, or an apparent cure, it would seem wise to leave well enough alone. There is no doubt, as Dr. Pfahler stated, that the cases which have been sent to the radiotherapists for treatment were either the hopeless cases or the ones in which there had been a recurrence, and radiotherapy has certainly done something for a certain percentage of these patients.

DR. RICHARD C. NORRIS.—I have considered treatment by radium and x-ray too technical to attempt its use and refer my patients to those specially qualified by training and experience. The diagnosis is very important and must be demonstrable in reported results. I distrust radium for its absolute curative value in uterine carcinoma in the early stage. To report a few cases of extensive carcinoma which are brilliantly and wonderfully cured and say nothing about all the other cases of failure, especially early cases not benefited, is not convincing. Each man tells of the cases that have been benefited. Many of these cases make us have the hope that future development of radium and x-ray treatment will prove efficient in all cases. Until we know more about cancer, in fact until we know more about radium, we cannot appraise its true value. It has occurred to me, and clinical experience bears it out, that in supposed early cases if cancer cells are deposited in the broad ligaments or elsewhere beyond the reach of surgery, there will be recurrence; if they happen to be beyond the influence of radium, then recurrence will also follow radium treatment. It is impossible to know to what extent this involvement may have occurred. We preach the doctrine to the laity and to our profession of early diagnosis, but until we know more about the cause of cancer and have more reliable early clinical and laboratory means of diagnosis it will even be too late in many cases to cure either by radium or by surgery. After the appearance of the first suggestive symptom, in a patient previously well, the patient goes through treatment by surgery or radium and dies promptly from recurrence. Another perfectly analogous case goes through radium or surgery and is alive eight or ten years afterwards. Such cases make me believe that very often it is not given to us to detect the beginnings of cancer or the degree of involvement in time for surgery or radium to cure. When we know more about cancer and its cause the future may throw light on many of these dark problems and early diagnosis, perhaps through serological or other laboratory method may aid us, but as I see it now certainly anyone near and dear to me with a suspicious or accurately diagnosed carcinoma of the cervix, and certainly of the uterine body, in what we now call an early stage, I certainly would not trust to radium. I would send her to a surgeon and radiate her afterwards with the proper precautions against fistulae. I think Dr. Deaver meant what he said, that the actual curative value of radium is overestimated as a routine procedure and that there was growing up a class, or group of radium practitioners who were holding out the hope to the laity that in radium we had found a well recognized cure for cancer. I believe Dr. Deaver meant what he said when he said we had not found that cure and I think the public needs to know it, to be protected from these men who claim it is a cure.

We are in the stage of investigation; no man can make absolute statements; we only know the usual hopelessness of surgery, we are finding out more and more the all too frequent hopelesness of radium as a cure. Another plan must come. Let us teach the woman at the menopause to seek her doctor, let us teach the doctor to be on the lookout for carcinoma, but if both woman and doctor are ever so urgent to find out if there are evidences of beginning cancer, we will still have cancer as an elusive disease. We can help ourselves improve our results because we do know that some early cases do get well, but not enough to satisfy us. With our present scant knowledge I believe the result is dependent upon the degree of involvement, the patient's resistance to and the character of the invading agent. When you cut or radiate beyond the area of involvement and get it all the patient will recover and the fact that not more than 10 to 20 per cent of cures follow means that in only 10 to 20 per cent do we reach and destroy all invaded tissue. Clinical diagnosis cannot at the present time make that selection of cases. We are forced to stumble on in the darkness, but let us remember that radium has not proved itself a cure for cancer because it sometimes brilliantly helps some aggravated cases that we know the surgeon cannot help. Let us be skeptical, let us have the evidence, not partial evidence, not hopeful evidence, but actual scientifically determined evidence by the results of radium treatment all over the world. In the meantime we do not wish to decry the use of radium. We want these men who have invested large sums of money and many hours of labor to make more and more effort in their investigations. We are not in a position to say that surgery should be abandoned or that radium and x-rays should be our only hope. They go together and if there is any value in radium to destroy a cancer cell I cannot understand why, in early cases, after you remove all you can surgically, radium or intensified x-rays should not be of value to destroy any cancer areas left behind within the range of safe radiation. If it can search out and destroy involved areas that we know the knife cannot safely reach, it surely should be so used and the radiologist should work out a technic efficient for that purpose and freed from danger of fistula. I defy anyone to tell by any means of examination, that in a particular case beyond the reach of surgery radium will reach and destroy all of the disease. The results show that it very often fails. In the early case I should prefer the surgery first and the radium afterwards. In advanced cases our only hope is radium and the x-ray, and in most of these cases they only palliate but do not cure. Their palliative value is unquestioned.

DR. GEORGE W. OUTERBRIDGE.—There is one point in the technic in handling cases of carcinoma of the cervix concerning which I should like to have the opinion of the radiologists. This is the question of removing by cautery, purely as a preliminary measure before the application of radium, as much tissue as possible through the vagina. In my association with Dr. Nicholson, this has become practically our routine procedure in advanced carcinoma of the cervix, especially those cases with large friable, easily bleeding, cauliflower masses projecting into the vaginal vault. As we understand it, the penetrating power of radium is distinctly limited, and it would seem rational, therefore, to remove mechanically, as much as possible of the malignant tissue, so as to be able to apply the radium that much closer to the deeper tissue, if this can be done with no danger of excitation of the growth. For this purpose, we have been using the Percy cautery, not at all as Percy uses it, with an idea of cooking surrounding tissue, but as a hot cautery for actual cutting away and cauterizing, because it carries the heat so much better than the ordinary small cautery knife. The operation can be done under nitrous oxide anesthesia and takes but a few minutes. I understand that at the University of Pennsylvania the feeling is against using the cautery preliminary to radium; it may be that this procedure is absolutely of no value; it may be that it does actual harm.

I should like to have an expression of opinion on this subject from the radiologists present.

DR. CLARK (closing).—My experience has been that it is very unwise to remove cauliflower growths by cautery or other means. Unless you can destroy cancer by one sweep of cautery, you had better not attempt the use of heat. I have seen many cases stimulated by this means. I have had cases of so-called fulguration and these cases almost invariably grow like wild fire. Unless you can get it all it is better not to use the cautery. Of course if you use capsules alone it might be the lesser of two evils to remove the gross mass so that the radium might penetrate, but where needles and shanks are used, the mass can be penetrated to the desired points; so it is unnecessary to remove a portion of the mass and I would strongly advise against it according to my own experience.

NEW YORK ACADEMY OF MEDICINE
SECTION ON OBSTETRICS AND GYNECOLOGY
STATED MEETING, HELD DECEMBER 27, 1921

DR. WILLIAM P. HEALY IN THE CHAIR

DR. HARBECK HALSTED reported a case of **General Edema of the Fetus Associated with Osteogenesis Imperfecta.**

Osteogenesis imperfecta is used as a general term to cover all imperfections in the development of the bones, consequently in the aggregate it is quite a common condition while at the same time any single type may be very rare. Ballantyne, who has gone into the subject very extensively, divides fetal bone diseases into five types and, after careful consideration, I am unable to place this case into any one of his divisions. The main defects in this case seem to be in the long bones and the bones of the skull. The long bones are very short and friable and there are evidences in the x-ray pictures that fractures have occurred *in utero*, with subsequent healing, in one place making a marked angulation, and in other places just represented by callus. The skull bones are only represented by small plaques of bone.

The patient was white, born in the United States, of American parents, a primipara. She was delivered November 13, 1921, about the seventh month. The mother was toxic and edematous. There was no history of any monster in the family. The patient does not remember having had the ordinary diseases of childhood. She had frequent attacks of tonsillitis and her tonsils were removed when she was ten years of age. She had jaundice when fourteen years of age. She began menstruating at fourteen years, regular, moderate. The first six months of this pregnancy were absolutely uneventful. One month before admission her urine showed a trace of albumin. She was given a vegetable diet and the albumin soon disappeared. One week before her admission she began to develop edema and a little albumin, and the blood pressure began to rise. These symptoms grew progressively worse and she was admitted to Sloane Hospital, Nov. 12, 1921. At this time her blood pressure was 170 systolic, 110 diastolic. The urine was acid, specific gravity 1,020;

albumin 85 per cent by gravity; an occasional red blood cell; many pus cells and an occasional hyaline cast. The patient was put on a salt-free, protein-free diet, and given morphine. The next morning she was given a colon irrigation, castor oil and quinine. Labor soon set in. The presentation was breech, R. S. A. After a few hours the breech and both feet presented at the vulva. Gentle traction was made on the right foot; the foot and part of the leg just above the ankle pulled off. Gentle traction was then made in both groins and when the baby was born it was seen that both groins had been split nearly down to the bone. As soon as the baby was born the cord broke about two feet from the baby's body. The stump of the leg and both tears in the groin bled for a short time and then stopped spontaneously; the cord did not bleed. The child's heart was beating and it took several breaths but soon died. The placenta and membranes delivered spontaneously almost immediately after the birth of the baby. The baby was a premature male weighing 3 pounds 9 ounces and was 32 cm. in length. The tissues were edematous, very friable, and very little bony structure could be made out by palpation. The skin was thin and easily macerated. The feet, legs, arms, and hands were short, deformed and flattened. The placenta was large, jelly-like, and very friable.

The patient bled rather freely postpartum, so was given ergot and pituitrin, and these were repeated in one hour. She was also given morphine and this was repeated in three hours. One hour and thirty minutes after delivery she seemed to be in fair condition and was put to bed. Almost immediately she had a convulsion. In the following two hours she had two more convulsions of slightly longer duration. After this she gradually improved, her blood pressure dropped and the urine gradually returned to normal.

Sections of the placenta showed only a few small villi; the majority are covered with a thick layer of syncytium. The villi contained many small vessels but very few large and conspicuous ones. The impression was given of less vascularity than normal. In some of the villi the connective tissue fibres were moderately separated, as if by edema; many, however, were compact. Microscopic examination of the cord showed the fibres of Wharton's jelly markedly separated, suggesting edema. The intima of all the vessels in the cord was markedly and irregularly thickened.

DISCUSSION

DR. L. T. LEWALD.—I do not believe the bone lesions are specific, and I think the history of the case bears that out. One must differentiate osteogenesis imperfecta from achondroplasia which is a peculiar type of bony development and which is also not specific. Both these are sometimes confused with syphilitic conditions. I regret that the microscopic study of the bone has not been made, and hope that some light on the etiology of the condition may result from it. The radiogram showing the healing of fractures *in utero* with the production of callous formation is exceeding interesting, and is a condition I have not seen before.

DR. H. C. WILLIAMSON.—I have had a case somewhat comparable to this, a para iii, delivered at the eighth month. She showed general edema before delivery and had six convulsions postpartum. In this instance the neck of the fetus was broken and there was a fracture of one humerus, but no radiograms were taken. The postmortem examination revealed acute degeneration of the kidneys, liver and spleen. The Wassermann reaction was negative.

DR. ABRAHAM RONGY read a paper entitled **Primary Sterility: A Study Based on 400 Cases.**

Dr. Rongy believed that the reason we cure relatively few cases of sterility is because our entire conception of the etiology and treatment of primary as well as relative sterility is entirely erroneous. The mechanical theory of sterility is untenable, and a new, and for the time being, a very promising and almost fascinating discovery has been "sprung" on the profession. The organs of internal secretion have been held responsible for all the ills to which human flesh is heir. Every sterile woman has been given all sorts of combinations of organic extracts. We soon found, however, that they were falling far short of the claims made for them. I feel that if we blindly accept the theory that the organs of internal secretion are responsible for sterility, we shall again be led astray for another thirty years, and in the meantime out attention will be detracted from the true causes of sterility in the largest number of women.

During the last decade, man's share for the responsibility for the sterility has, in my experience, undergone a great change. In a paper published by me in 1911, I found that the husband was at fault in nearly 50 per cent of the cases, and this coincided with the experience of a number of observers at that time. In this series it is less than 11 per cent. I believe that the educational campaigns conducted by the medical profession and the various public health agencies are just now beginning to bear fruit. While we have thoroughly investigated the male aspect of the question, and interesting points have been brought out from the academic standpoint, I feel that they have no practical value. In the light of our present knowledge we must pronounce the men well, if the examination of a condom specimen shows fully formed and viable spermatozoa. A number of our patients were inseminated; the semen was lodged high in the uterine cavity, in the hope that ovulation might be helped in that way. Not one of these patients became pregnant. The failure of conception to take place in these cases seems to indicate that something is wrong somewhere "higher up," and I am sure that if the problem of sterility is to be solved at all, it will have to be investigated from a purely biological and chemical standpoint. A great many women who are sterile have practically the same developmental characteristics; they are short, fat, stocky, and give a history of menstruating very irregularly.

Anatomic defects in the bony pelvis, were not found with the x-rays. A group of women and their husbands were selected for the purpose of having their blood typed, in the hope that it would show a characteristic grouping, but no material difference was found in the grouping between the sterile couples and those who had one or more children. Other experiments were carried out which showed that diet had no direct relation to sterility. It is my experience that those patients who give a history of having developed sudden and severe pain during the second or third day of their menstruation three or four years after puberty, are more likely to be permanently sterile. Inquiry was also made into the possible relationship between the exanthematous diseases and sterility. It is my impression that there is a greater prevalence of sterility among the women, who during their infancy or childhood had troublesome throat infections, also that women who had had scarlet fever, complicated by severe kidney disturbances, were not so likely to be sterile as those women who had a simple uncomplicated scarlet fever. While this is highly speculative, I feel that something might have taken place during an attack of scarlet fever or diphtheria, which prevented the ovary from properly developing and possibly at the same time caused permanent structural changes.

It seems to me that as yet, the endocrine label is but roughly qualitative and crudely quantitative, nevertheless the analysis of this series of cases from the endocrinological standpoint brought forth the interesting point that in answer to the question, "Whom do you resemble, father or mother?", 221 patients said that in physique and features they resembled their father, and 85 patients said they resembled their mother. While this may be purely accidental in this series of cases, nevertheless it may have some bearing from the biological standpoint.

A number of women were selected showing no evidence of inflammatory changes in the pelvis; they were given no treatment whatever, except a placebo from time to time. All of them were married a year or longer. Of 36 of these patients 6 became pregnant, four being delivered of full term babies. This is the best illustration that sterility is very often temporary in nature and that in a certain number of women some readjustment takes place and pregnancy ensues. I believe that no marriage ought to be considered sterile until two years have passed.

I cannot help feeling that displacement of the cervix and uterus plays a very small rôle in the etiology of sterility. The only findings of more or less importance are: (1) The small infantile body of the uterus, which is narrow from side to side, is usually associated with a small conical cervix and is frequently found in fair women. (2) The large hard body of the uterus with a long hypertrophied cervix and a history of rather profuse menstruation, which is usually found in the tall, dark, masculine type of women. To me such findings indicate a most unfavorable prognosis. I am sure that if these patients were let alone, some of them would have a better chance to become pregnant, for the various operations performed on them often result in the closure of the fallopian tubes, causing permanent sterility. Patients in whom one finds a small, cord-like body of the uterus, retroverted and often adherent posteriorly, must be severely let alone. I have never seen one of these patients become pregnant whether they were treated or not. Plastic operations on the fallopian tubes, in my experience, hold out very little hope for the cure of sterility. It seems to me that those patients whose tubes become closed because of gonorrheal infection, very often have a better chance if they are not operated upon, for such exudates in time may be absorbed and the tube will become patent. The reactionary exudate which follows an operation is less likely to be absorbed. To my mind it is still a mooted question whether to operate on patients who have fibroid tumors. I removed the fibroid tumors in 9 patients; one became pregnant and was delivered of a normal child, another became pregnant and miscarried at the end of the third month; the others are still sterile. In patients who are sterile and suffering from fibroid tumor of the uterus, if by insufflation I find the tubes open I do not advise operative interference, unless acute symptoms develop, for it is a well-known clinical fact that women who suffer from fibroid tumors of the uterus are more likely to become pregnant between the ages of thirty and forty than they are between the ages of twenty and thirty, and something may be gained by waiting. If, however, I find the tubes closed, I advise operation, for there is nothing to be gained by delay. Fifty-two patients had dilatation of the cervix and the insertion of the stem pessary for the purpose of correcting and enlarging the cervical canal. Eight of these patients became pregnant, one while the stem pessary was in place; the others remained sterile. I never saw a permanent enlargement of the cervical canal after a stem pessary operation. There are many other objections to the stem pessary. In eight patients with unilateral ovarian cysts, the tumors were removed; the other ovary in each of these patients was enlarged and cystic. The menstrual history in these patients remained unchanged, but they all remained sterile. Ovarian tumors in women who are sterile should be removed as soon as possible, because the tumor may act as an irritant to the other ovary, and by an early operation we may be able to save a small portion of the ovary which is less involved and has not, as yet, been destroyed. Three patients suffered from persistent vaginismus. The classical Pozzi operation was performed and they became pregnant shortly after. The real problem that confronts us in the treatment of sterility is in that group of patients which practically presents no anomaly of the genital tract, except possibly a moderate degree of flexion or version.

Dr. Rubin's method of insufflation for the purpose of ascertaining the patency of the fallopian tubes has changed the entire status of sterility and its treatment. We are now able for practical purposes to classify all patients who suffer from primary as well as relative sterility into two general groups: (1) The "clean group'' or patients who suffer from sterility due to some constitutional disturbance. (2) The "unclean group" or those who are still suffering from an inflammatory condition in or about the pelvis. At the Lebanon Hospital, during the past twelve months, we have made 152 examinations by this method. In our series the average rise in the patent cases was 132 mm. and 182 mm. in the closed cases. If oxygen is used, not more than 300 c.c. should be introduced. If carbon dioxide is used, a greater quantity can be introduced. In this series of cases 9, or 59.2 per cent, were positive, that is, air appeared in the abdominal cavity; in 62, or 40.8 per cent, no air was present in the abdominal cavity. As a general proposition, it may be stated that, whenever the air passes into the abdominal cavity through the tubes, they may be considered patent from the standpoint of mechanical obstruction to the passage of traveling spermatozoa. The fallopian tubes may be plugged by some inflammatory exudate or some mucogelatinous substance and still permit the passage of gas under pressure, yet, without artificial distention of the tubes the plugging may act as a barrier to the passage of spermatozoa. The contraindications to this method of examination are acute infections of the vagina or pelvic organs; also it must not be used in the presence of chronic infections, if the patient complains of pain. It should not be performed when the menstrual period is about to appear. Patients who have heart disease should not be subjected to this examination. In this series of examinations the only complications were a case of severe syncope, a case of syncope of lesser degree, and in a patient previously operated on for appendicitis, and later for intestinal obstruction, who had adhesions in the left pelvis, the examination evidently caused sufficient irritation so that the patient developed an acute inflammation of the left fornix, which subsided under palliative treatment. This method of examination should be used in every case in which the sterility is of doubtful origin. Four of these patients did not menstruate after the insufflation and upon examination were found to be pregnant. We do not believe that the occurrence of pregnancy in these patients was purely accidental. We feel that the force of the gas either expelled some mucous plugs or straightened out any kink that might have been present. We are certain that in a short time this method of examination will become a routine in office practice, and no patient will be given a definite opinion as to the cause of her sterility, before the patency of the tubes has been established.

The treatment of sterility consists chiefly in the art of being able to select the patients who are likely to respond to treatment. Those patients in whom we find congenitally defective organs ought to be let alone. On the whole there seems to be a group of patients who are suffering from sterility, who are hopelessly incurable and remain sterile for the rest of their lives, and still wander from doctor to doctor in the hope of selecting a cure. The hope held out to such patients by physicians has a tendency to create a suspicion in the minds of these women as to the integrity and honesty of the medical profession. We must be able to discriminate and select for treatment only those patients in whom we think we can obtain a cure.

DISCUSSION

DR. HARRY ARANOW.—Sterility may be considered in two main groups, namely, those in which the cause is evident, such as dyspareunia, vaginismus, marked stenosis of the cervix and those in which the cause is difficult to ascertain or is found to consist of obstruction in the tubes, maldevelopment or chronic disease of the ovaries which interfere with ovulation without giving any palpable physical signs. I believe the reason we have failed to cure sterility is because we have failed to put our finger on the underlying cause.

Dr. Rongy said cases which had remained sterile for two years after marriage might be considered sterile. I do not think we can consider a patient sterile until three years after marriage. A great many women even without prevention will not conceive for two years after marriage. I think we should allow three years before deciding that a woman is sterile. Some cases with anteflexion of the cervix are cured by dilatation. I have the same feeling about retroversion if it is not caused by an inflammatory process. The cases in which the sterility is due to inflammatory process are rather hopeless, but those in which no inflammation is present are sometimes helped by reposition and operation. I have the same hopeful feeling about fibroids. A woman of over forty recently consulted me, not because of sterility, but for fibroids which were causing pain by pressure. At operation I found five or six fibroids, some intramural, and a small uterus. That woman became pregnant and was delivered without difficulty though four or five incisions had been made in her uterus. I feel that those cases of sterility that have evidence of being caused by retroversion, or ovarian cyst or fibrosis or stenosis ought to be given the benefit of operation, for some of them may be helped. Of course before operation they should be thoroughly investigated by Dr. Rubin's insufflation method. The examination may be made under the fluoroscope in the office, and then we can answer the question as to the patency of the tubes at once.

One of the most complicated questions we have to consider is sterility. We can examine the cervix and the uterus fairly well, but when it comes to the tubes and ovaries, it is more difficult, and the question of endocrine imbalance may have something to do with the sterility. I think this method of insufflation should be made a routine procedure just as we examine the husband every time before undertaking to operate on a case.

One point Dr. Rongy brought out should be emphasized and that is that the gas may go through places where a spermatozoon cannot pass through.

DR. HERMAN LORBER.—We are probably all of the opinion that prophylaxis has its field of usefulness in the cure of sterility. The general custom of the young graduate providing himself with a set of curettes as his first instruments and using them when and where infection is very likely may be a contributing factor to so many cases of acquired sterility.

The eugenic test of the male and the cured chronic conditions of the prostate would also help to eliminate future possible cases of sterility. In cases of undeveloped uteri much has been done with endocrines and Dr. Hirst had cited cases treated with the galvanic current in which the uterus has almost doubled in size following his treatment.

DR. WILLIAM P. HEALY.—Dr. Rongy has shown that we now have available a very important method of clearing up the question of the patency of the tubes by means of Dr. Rubin's method by the injection of oxygen, and by the method of Dr. Cary of Brooklyn with salt solution. As Dr. Aranow has said, if we have something in the individual case that is pathologic it is well worth while relieving it in order to place the patient in as nearly normal condition as possible before giving up.

In regard to the question of using the stem pessary which Dr. Rongy discouraged, I believe it is a valuable form of treatment in dysmenorrhea and stenosis of the cervical canal and in sterility, not only because it acts as a dilator but because the cervical canal remains dilated thereafter, and also because it helps in the development of the uterus. It acts as a foreign body; the uterus makes an effort to expel it, and in spite of the fact that the pessary may be sutured *in situ* you will find it exceedingly difficult to make the pessary remain in place because the uterus will tend to expel it. That means the uterus has been undergoing mechanical massage, which causes it to increase in size and it is better for the pessary having been there. Of course putting a stem pessary in an inflamed uterus is another thing. The cases must be properly selected. Cases of dysmenorrhea are sometimes permanently cured by the stem pessary.

As to myomectomy in cases of sterility, I have not had good results. Very few have been benefited so far as the sterility is concerned. Occasionally one patient will be cured, but they are so few that they may be ignored. It is better, however, to do a myomectomy no doubt.

Dr. Rongy's paper brings out the necessity of knowing the condition of the tubes before instituting an operation for sterility. He stated that 60 per cent of the cases examined had clean tubes and only 40 per cent showed pathologic lesions needing treatment. That has been our experience; in cases of sterility approximately 60 per cent will be apparently normal and the husband is also normal. It is only in a small proportion of the cases in which conditions exist that we can succeed in curing by operation.

DR. RONGY (closing).—Regarding stenosis in the 152 cases which we insufflated, we used a No. 6 Holtzman syringe.

Regarding retroversion of the congenital type, it is not the uterus but the ovaries that are defective, and you do not correct the function of the ovaries by correcting the retroversion. In 1911, I reported 27 cases in which I used the stem pessary. It is true the stem pessary irritates the uterus and the uterus will expel it, but the reason the woman does not become pregnant is not because the uterus is small; she does not become pregnant because of some other difficulty. You may find the tube one-half the size they should be, or the ovaries hard and full of small cysts. While the uterus may be increased in size by the irritation of the pessary, that does not affect the sterility.

As to myomectomy, my experience coincides with that of Dr. Healy. I can recollect few cases in which I have done a myomectomy which have become pregnant. In a woman who has fibroids, the tumor is of no consequence as a cause of the sterility; it is the disturbance that causes the tumor which is responsible. I had a patient, a doctor's wife who was sterile for three years. She had fibroids which Dr. Cragin said should be removed, and two or three were removed. I said at that time that she would have more fibroids. Last week she came into my office with a fibroid as large as a fist. Women are not sterile as the result of fibroids, but fibroids are the result of sterility.

I have had very little experience with electricity. At one time I spent a considerable sum on electrical apparatus and treated various gynecologic conditions with it, but obtained no results whatever. When you increase the size of the uterus by electrical treatment you do not cure the patient. You may find the tubes patent, the husband well, and the woman having a small uterus; that woman's sterility is not a local condition but a constitutional one, and while we are not prepared to say what the cause of the sterility is, it will be found that it is away from the pelvis, and the sooner we learn this the less operating will be done in patients whose sterility cannot be cured by surgical procedures, and the better it will be for the patient.

Department of Reviews and Abstracts

CONDUCTED BY HUGO EHRENFEST, M.D., ASSOCIATE EDITOR

Collective Review

Toxemia of Early Pregnancy: Etiology and Treatment*
Part II: Treatment

BY PAUL TITUS, M.D., F.A.C.S., PITTSBURGH, PA.

THERE are as many, if not more, methods of treatment recommended for nausea and vomiting of early pregnancy as there are ideas regarding the origin of the condition. In all probability this is the result of the very fact that the etiology of all toxemia during pregnancy is still surrounded by so much uncertainty that Zweifel has quite correctly termed it "die Krankheit der Theorien."

Work which would discover the actual cause of toxemia of pregnancy would naturally produce appropriate therapeutic measures with which to combat the condition. At the same time it is not unlikely that successful though empiric treatment offers many clues to the sources of the trouble. A review of the more important methods of treatment of toxemia has, therefore, the double object of reasoning "whys" and gathering together "wherefores."

GENERALLY ACCEPTED METHODS OF TREATMENT

The milder cases of nausea and vomiting are often controlled by simple attention to the bowels, the diet, (DeLee) proper exercise and amusement, as well as sufficient rest (Williams).

The most widely accepted general plan of treatment when the nausea and vomiting has become at all severe consists in the rational and common-sense practice of establishing rest in bed, isolation from friends and relatives, the employment of gastric lavage and purgation, the use of chloral and bromides as sedatives, rectal feedings, and therapeutic abortion as a last resort. With this as a starting point the individual variations in treatment are legion, ranging all the way from organotherapy to pure dietetics.

TREATMENT OF PREDISPOSING PATHOLOGIC CONDITIONS

Many authorities, among whom may be included Williams, DeLee, Hirst, Tweedy and Wrench, and others, are of the opinion that vomiting of pregnancy may originate reflexly from various pathologic disturbances such as retrodisplacements of the gravid uterus or cervical erosions, and base their supposition on the fact that patients have obtained relief from their toxemic symptoms soon after the institution

*See first part in February, 1922, issue.

of appropriate treatment for these definite conditions. They recommend therefore that such factors be searched for and treated by surgical or other means. While the advisability of correcting gross lesions is freely admitted, Williams asserts it is by no means certain that the psychical effect of such treatment is not responsible for a large part of the benefit derived. Granting also the advantages to be gained from the treatment of lesions such as pyorrhea, tonsil and middle-ear disease, as well as sinus infections, the same reservation is to be made regarding Talbot's idea that a focal infection can be found as the underlying cause of practically all toxemia of pregnancy. Kingman goes so far as to state that appropriate treatment of hyperemesis consists in putting the patient into the knee-chest position, inflating the vagina and then packing it with wool tampons for twenty-four to thirty-six hours, because vomiting is so often due to anteflexion of the uterus with varying degrees of descent upon the pelvic floor.

C. H. Davis regards these as predisposing rather than causative factors, and points out that a carefully taken history will usually reveal any previous gastrointestinal disturbance, nervous disorder or other physical conditions which might make a patient more sensitive to the disturbed metabolism of pregnancy. The physical examination will reveal any source of local irritation or infection and he believes that dental work, removal of infected tonsils, the correction of uterine displacements, or acute cervicitis, should be undertaken merely as an incidental matter in connection with the general handling of a patient.

DIFFERENTIATION BETWEEN VARIOUS TYPES OF VOMITING

It must be recognized that there are several degrees of severity of symptoms, and of these the mild, or so-called "morning sickness" is most commonly seen. Indeed many women, as well as many physicians, have come to look upon this merely as an indication of the existence of a pregnancy, and because they have come to expect it, pay little or no attention to it. Bumm warns us, *a propos* of this that the emesis seen so frequently in hysterical women may readily develop into uncontrollable vomiting. It should, in fact, be more generally known that such vomiting is not necessary during pregnancy, according to Williams, and that it can be controlled by suitable hygienic and dietetic measures.

Women may pass from the "first period" (DuBois) into the "second period" where their vomiting is most distressing, often going rapidly from this stage into the "third period" where marked emaciation, dehydration, jaundice, acidosis, "coffee-ground" vomitus, and prostration are prominent, and death may supervene in spite of any measures which may now be undertaken.

The very fact that bizarre methods of treatment such as dilatation of the cervix recommended by Copeman, the use of electrical batteries, blisters to the spine, the ice-bag of Chapman, and the use of leeches applied to the cervix, have effected cures in apparently hopeless cases, has brought forward the idea first suggested by Kaltenbach that vomiting of pregnancy may be an hysterical manifestation. Kaltenbach even went so far as to state that practically all patients could be controlled by suggestive treatment.

The confusion which resulted from this has undoubtedly been the cause of a certain number of deaths from pernicious vomiting, since it became the tendency to pursue a waiting policy in the hope that some sudden change for the better would occur. It has seemed quite impossible to distinguish between patients that were apparently equally ill and yet might suddenly begin to improve as compared to those in whom delay beyond a certain point proved fatal, even a therapeutic abortion then being useless.

As a primary essential in treatment, therefore, Williams has attempted by means of the ammonia coefficient to distinguish between toxic and neurotic vomiting, believing as he does that all vomiting of pregnancy may be thus typed. If he can be convinced that the vomiting is neurotic in origin or type, he treats the patient by isolation from sympathetic relatives and friends, gastric lavage and forced feeding, the injection of normal salt solution under the breast using "dull needles," and the constant reiteration to the patient that these unpleasant measures will have to be repeated if there is no improvement. On the other hand, if the ammonia coefficient remains high in spite of forced feeding, he classes the case as one of toxic vomiting and induces abortion without undue delay. In accepting this as proof that neurotic vomiting is a distinct entity it must be remembered that this "suggestive" treatment is not entirely useless in combating an intoxication, especially if it consists in part of rest in bed, glucose and soda by bowel, sedatives, purges, and forced feeding.

DeLee agrees it is more than possible that a neurotic element is the basal cause of vomiting in hysterical or neurotic women, pointing out that in the presence of demonstrable disease the treatment of a displaced uterus or a diseased cervix simply relieves the patient of the peripheral irritant, while the vomiting ceases because the nervous system comes again into equilibrium.

Even the Freudian theory has been dragged in by its long hair through the suggestion of Schwab that a woman with hyperemesis is usually one who unconsciously has no love for her husband, the vomiting in this instance being not a symptom of a disease, but the expression of undesire, unwillingness, aversion and nausea. Death from hyperemesis gravidarum, he says, is a form of suicide, a hunger strike, these women protesting secretly and translating "I will not" into "I cannot." DeLee in abstracting this original article for the 1921 Year Book of Obstetrics, characterizes such notions as absurd.

It is probable that in all toxemia there is an element of neurosis which should be accorded consideration. On the other hand, it is hardly possible that neurotic vomiting as such could exist without any vestige of toxemia. In a given case, however, it is often difficult to say whether the toxemia or the neurosis is uppermost, and it should not be forgotten that lines of treatment successful without any apparent cause and therefore classed as suggestive, may have a reasonable physiologic basis for their success. For example, Williams believes that frequent meals begun before the patient arises in the morning and continued at stated intervals during the day are of benefit largely because of the mental effect which these careful directions have upon the patient. Duncan and Harding, as well as Titus, Hoffmann, and Givens, have shown that the beneficial results from such feedings are to be attributed to the avoidance of any long periods of hunger, or as it might be termed, mild starvation. The former believe that a direct carbohydrate starvation is responsible for hyperemesis gravidarum, and Harding in a later work points out the similarity between the symptoms supervening before death from this condition and that due to a deprivation of carbohydrate foods in a diabetic. The latter writers maintain that it is due to a combination of an actual carbohydrate starvation plus an increased demand for glycogen on the part of the fetus. Both groups of workers agree that a glycogen deficiency in the maternal liver, whether from the one or both causes, is responsible for practically all toxemia of early pregnancy by lowering individual liver resistance to toxins of whatever origin. That morning sickness is most common follows from the fact that the longest period of fasting in the twenty-four hours is during the night. This is merely a physiologic explanation of the simple fact that frequent meals, by night as well as by day, especially if carbohydrates predominate, will relieve the average case of vomiting of pregnancy, and that the neurosis in this instance is merely incidental.

That a neurosis could be solely responsible for the occurrence of any considerable number of cases can be conclusively proved only by effecting "cures" through the use of placebos alone, being careful that the generally accepted methods of treatment for such toxemia have not been used in conjunction with the spectacular and apparently inexplicable thing which suddenly brings about the "cure." Otherwise the process is too much like that of the patient with pneumonia who had a high fever in spite of all the doctors could do for six long days, when the family dismissed the doctors and called in an osteopath. He gave the patient one treatment, whereupon the fever disappeared that very night and the patient's life was thus saved!

DIETETIC INFLUENCE ON TOXEMIA

In conjunction with the generally accepted methods of rest, isolation, sodium bromide per rectum, gastric lavage, starvation for twenty-four hours, etc., the question of nourishment for the patient is obviously important.

DeLee uses rectal feeding, then dry diet with carbohydrates predominating, during the first few days after the initial period of starvation; Mack advises a milk diet with sodium bromide to be followed by milk plus eggs and zwieback, suggesting a preponderance of carbohydrates for the subsequent days; Tweedy believes that free purgation is the fundamental factor in successfully treating vomiting and proceeds cautiously with food, beginning with peptonized milk, whey, and albumin water, and increasing the amount of food intake very slowly. Shears says that dietetic treatment is less important than one would suppose and permits the personal preference of the patient to have considerable weight in the choice of food.

Duncan and Harding, as well as Titus, Hoffmann, and Givens, believe that frequent feedings of a high carbohydrate content are almost essential in the treatment of vomiting of pregnancy and begin with liquids, whereas Lynch urges absolute restriction of sweets and fruits, giving a diet of proteins with a limited amount of fats in what he terms the hyperacidity group of cases. He urges a dry, solid diet, stating that sweets invariably nauseate, and supplies carbohydrates through the rectal introduction of glucose and soda solution. C. H. Davis urges a middle course by suggesting a dry diet high in carbohydrates and low in fats and proteins.

Practically all writers agree that there should be an initial period of starvation or rest for the stomach, and during this interval attempt to supply nutriment in various forms per rectum. Some are content with the mere use of glucose and soda solution for enteroclysis, while Van Schaick concluded from two successful cases in which he used enemata or the Murphy drip of saline solution that to supply water in large amounts so that it is rapidly absorbed through the intestine will enable the mother to carry the child to term. Dehydration is undoubtedly an important item, but Van Schaick's assumption from two cases is scarcely conclusive.

Bacon has gone into the question of nutrient enemata in detail. He says that in this way all essential food elements can be supplied—water, salts, glucose, amino-acids and vitamins, while the deficiency in nitrogenous foods can be made up in part by giving an excess of glucose, and by alcohol. The latter he considers of great importance, and he adds that a calcium salt should also be supplied. Rectal feedings are discontinued gradually as stomach feedings are increased. His caloric values have been painstakingly worked out, as well as the various elements in the proportions which he considers essential, so that reference to his original article is well worth while.

Adair also insists that the proper treatment for vomiting of pregnancy has as its prime object the furnishing of food and fluid. In order to reduce the demands to a minimum, it is necessary to have absolute rest for mind and body. Supplying food is much more difficult as a rule than the administration of fluid, but in the main it should consist of carbohydrates and fats with a small amount of proteins.

It is perfectly obvious, of course, that carbohydrate metabolism is much simpler than that of proteins, although the latter can be broken up within the body into energy producing elements by a comparatively intricate process. From the standpoint of body chemistry, therefore, this use of carbohydrates is more logical than to utilize proteins, although proteins are by no means entirely unserviceable.

As long ago as 1913 LeLornier recommended subcutaneous infusions of sugar solution in addition to the rectal infusions during the first few days of treatment.

Considerable discussion has arisen over the similarity between the clinical pictures of pernicious vomiting of pregnancy and prolonged starvation. Underhill and Rand, in discussing Williams' work on the significance of the ammonia coefficient, emphasized this resemblance. They claim that little change can be detected in the nitrogenous urinary constituents so long as the carbohydrate store is not depleted and that this does not happen as rapidly as has been assumed. As soon, however, as the protein of the body is drawn on to furnish carbohydrate, acidosis appears and the ammonia nitrogen suddenly increases. They advised, therefore, that the patient be supplied with carbohydrates.by rectal enemata, their recommendation thus being physiologic rather than empiric. Benefit was obtained in a number of cases and they reasoned that it was because dextrose had been supplied solely for the energy obtained in its combustion. Their argument is partly erroneous because the dextrose supplied under such circumstances is only partly burned while a large part of it is stored in the liver, engorging and enriching its depleted cells with sugar whereupon a reserve supply is established and the liver is thus enabled the better to function in its detoxicating capacity. They say that supplying carbohydrate to the body should not affect the ammonia output in the urine, if the ammonia content of the urine is an evidence that the liver is out of function from irremedial lesions. Since that time, however, experimental evidence has been adduced, as described in Part I of this review, to the effect that a glycogen depletion of the liver from starvation or other causes is the explanation of the pathological liver lesions to be seen in these cases, and that to supply carbohydrates will cause a histological restoration of the damaged liver lobules.

Titus and Givens have confirmed this experimental evidence by clinical investigations, and recommend intravenous injections of large quantities of glucose in solution for pernicious vomiting as well as for eclampsia. They show that after such treatment, liver sections from fatal cases of both acute yellow atrophy and eclampsia have been restored so far toward normal that from them alone a pathologist could not interpret the specimens as belonging to these distinct clinical conditions from which the patients had died.

FLUID ABSORPTION FROM THE BOWEL

Practically all authorities agree that dehydration is an important factor in the progress of toxemia, and most writers urge the use of various fluids administered per rectum. Plain tap water may be used, although many prefer normal salt solution. Ringer's solution has been repeatedly advised and LeLornier says that one may choose between glucose and soda solution and Ringer's solution with equally good results. The tidal stand of glucose and soda solution utilized by Polak in his post-operative work probably effects the greatest amount of absorption with a minimum of discomfort to the patient.

It is hardly necessary to repeat that bromides or other sedatives may be administered in the fluid introduced into the rectum.

SEROLOGICAL TREATMENT

Murray speaks of the results obtained by Mayer and Freund who have advocated the injection of serum from normal pregnant women. Austin has had beneficial results in hyperemesis from such use of serum, but he varies the suggestion made originally, according to Williams, by Fieux and Dantin, in that he is careful to obtain the serum from a nontoxic woman whose pregnancy is of the same duration as that of the patient. Melgar has had favorable results from these methods of treatment, but was disappointed in the use of normal horse serum. This latter treatment has been variously recommended and referred to recently by Hannah in discussing the work of Newman.

Mack advises a trial of serum therapy but inclines to the opinion that its psychic effect on the patient is its greatest influence.

ORGANOTHERAPY

Lange, as well as Nicholson, believing that the trouble results from a failure of the thyroid to enlarge, administers thyroid extract. This has been more recently suggested again by Siegmund.

Zulogoa, as well as Cerecedo, and also Rebaudi, have attributed hyperemesis to some fault on the part of the adrenal glands. They have therefore considered the administration of adrenalin appropriate.

Eugene Cary recommends the use of 10 to 15 grains of desiccated placenta daily.

J. C. Hirst has attracted considerable attention to the use of corpus luteum extract for pernicious vomiting and many clinicians have followed his example with widely varying results. For instance, in 1919 he reported 111 cases of nausea and vomiting, 99 of which were favorably influenced by hypodermic intramuscular injections of commercial corpus luteum extract. More recently he has advised the intravenous injection of the extract. He now prefers this method of administration but in this paper gives no figures from which one can observe his results. After Hirst's first and preliminary report of five cases, P. J. Carter gave the method a trial and was able to present 20 consecutive cases without a failure. He gave the extract by hypodermic injection, and was most enthusiastic about the treatment. Quigley treated a series of 17 patients with relief for 12, while in Hirschfield's series of 15 patients only one showed no improvement.

DeLee in commenting on these results in the 1921 Year Book of Obstetrics states that he has used corpus luteum for hyperemesis by mouth and hypodermatically with varying success. Only half of his patients were benefited and in the toxemic varieties it has thus far failed entirely. Davis has seen little or no benefit from its use. In general, opinions on its value are still given with considerable reserve.

THERAPEUTIC ABORTION

Practically every textbook of obstetrics advises therapeutic abortion as means of last resort in profound and uncontrollable vomiting of pregnancy. A study of series of cases reported from various well-conducted clinics shows how infrequently this extreme means is necessary, but many patients have undoubtedly been lost who could have been saved had the operation not been unduly delayed.

The greatest conservatism must be observed, both in deciding to operate and in the method chosen, because the condition of patients actually needing a therapeutic abortion is usually grave.

RESUME OF TREATMENT

A brief summary of the general lines of successful treatment for hyperemesis gravidarum embraces (1) the ruling out of any independent disease such as gastrointestinal disturbances either acute or chronic, gall bladder disease, or appendicitis; (2) the removal of focal infections in the teeth, or tonsils, or elsewhere, and the correction of pelvic abnormalities such as uterine displacements or cervical erosions; (3) as careful and accurate a classification of the condition as possible, so that the element of neurosis may be given attention, and that the "period" (DuBois), or degree of severity, of the hyperemesis may be properly appreciated. (4) Rest is important at any stage, since it conserves energy, and (5) isolation from visitors is a form of rest. (6) The use of bromides and chloral by mouth or by bowel is helpful in obtaining absolute relaxation, while (7) gastric lavage is of value because it clears away mucus and food residue, at the same time permitting (8) the introduction of saline purges through the stomach tube. A period of (9) abstinence from food and water by mouth should be given to rest the revolting stomach, during which time (10) rectal feeding should be resorted to in order to combat both starvation and dehydration. Water, saline, glucose and soda solution, or nutritive solutions may be injected either by the "Murphy drip" or the "tidal stand" methods. (11) Subcutaneous injections of salt solution, as well as glucose solution have been utilized, and (12) intravenous injection of glucose dissolved in distilled water is also recommended.

With the return of stomach tolerance and improvement of the patient, (13) mouth feeding is cautiously resumed and one proceeds to give either liquids, or solids, or to adopt a middle course combining the two according to experience and preference. Carbohydrates should predominate in these feedings from the standpoint of simple metabolism although proteins may be more "tasty" and acceptable to the nauseated patient, being well though less readily utilized.

It is necessary to exercise keen judgment over all patients who fail to show improvement because a waiting policy may be prolonged beyond the danger point. In the presence of jaundice, epigastric pain, marked acidosis, "coffee-ground" or bloody vomitus, delirium, coma, increased pulse rate, etc., it is customary to (14) induce therapeutic abortion, although as a general thing this should be done before the patient has reached this stage of the disease, else even the abortion may be too late to save her life.

Having arrived, with the help of consultants, at a decision to empty the uterus, this should be done in the most conservative manner possible, using scopolamine and morphine to aid in the anesthesia. In early cases the uterus may be dilated and emptied at one operation, or vaginal anterior hysterotomy may be chosen in preference if the cervix cannot be readily dilated or if haste is essential.

BIBLIOGRAPHY

Adair: Med. and Surg., 1918, ii, 719. *Austin:* Med. Record, 1914, lxx, 705. *Bacon:* Jour. Am. Med. Assn., 1918, lxx, 1750. *Bumm:* Grundriss zum Studium der Geburtshilfe, ed. 5, Bergmann, Wiesbaden, 1908, p. 308. *Cary:* Surg., Gynec. and Obst., 1917, xxv, 206. *Cerecedo:* Siglo Med., 1913, lx, 546. *Copeman:* Brit. Med. Jour., 1875, i, 637. *Davis, C. H.:* Wisc. State Med. Jour., 1920, xviii, 350. *DeLee:* Principles and Practice of Obstetrics, ed. 3, Philadelphia, 1918, W. B. Saunders Co., pp. 354-366. Year Book of Obstetrics, 1921, v, 195. Loc. cit., p. 199. *DuBois:* Bull. de l'Acad. de Med., 1852, xii, 219. *Duncan and Harding:* Canad. Med. Assn. Jour., 1918, vii, 1057. *Hannah:* Texas State Jour. Med., 1917, xi, 243. *Harding:* Lancet, London, 1921, cci, 327. *Hirschfield:* Jour. Oklahoma State Med. Assn., 1921, iii, 26. *Hirst, B. C.:* A Textbook of Obstetrics, ed. 8, Philadelphia, 1918, W. B. Saunders Co., pp. 362-366. *Hirst, J. C.:* Am. Jour. Obst., 1919, lxxix, 327. Jour. Am. Med. Assn., 1921, lxxvi, 772. *Kaltenbach:* Ztschr. f. Geburtsh. u. Gynäk., 1891, xxi, 200. *Kingman:* Am. Med., 1913, viii, 519. *Lange:* Ztschr. f. Geburtsh. u. Gynäk., 1899, xl, 44. *LeLornier:* Clinique Paris, 1913, viii, 631. *Lynch:* Jour. Am. Med. Assn., 1919, lxxiii, 488. *Mack:* Ztschr. f. Geburtsh. u. Gynäk., 1921, lxxxiii, 653. *Melgar:* Cronica Medica, xxxv, 65 (Quoted in Jour. Am. Med. Assn., June 29, 1918). *Murray:* Jour. Obst. and Gynec., Brit. Emp., 1913, xxiii, 87. *Nicholson:* Trans. Obst. Soc. Edinburgh, March, 1902, iv, 452. *Polak:* Personal demonstration. *Quigley:* New York State Med. Jour., 1919, xix, 306. *Rebaudi:* Gior. d. Osp., Maria Vittoria, Torino, 1919, ix, 246. *Schwab:* Zentralbl. f. Gynäk., 1921, xxiv, 23. *Shears:* Obstetrics, ed. 2, Philadelphia, 1917, J. B. Lippincott Co., pp. 273-280. *Siegmund:* Zentralbl. f. Gynäk., 1910, xxxiv, 1349. *Talbot:* Jour. Am. Med. Assn., 1920, lxxiv, 736. *Titus and Givens:* Jour. Am. Med. Assn., 1922, lxxviii, 92. *Titus, Hoffmann, and Givens:*

Jour. Am. Med. Assn., 1920, lxxiv, 777. *Tweedy and Wrench:* Practical Obstetrics, ed. 4, Oxford Univ. Press, London, 1919, pp. 162-168. *Underhill and Rand:* Arch. Int. Med., 1910, v, 61. *Van Schaick:* Med. Rec., 1921, xcix, 746. *Williams:* Jour. Obst. and Gynec., Brit. Emp., 1912, xxii, 245. *Williams:* Obstetrics, ed 4, New York, 1919, D. Appleton and Co., pp. 549-562. *Zulogoa:* Arch. mens. d'Obstét., et de Gynéc., 1914, iii, 443.

1015 HIGHLAND BLDG.

Selected Abstracts

The Cervix

Hollender: The Treatment of Cervicitis and Endocervicitis with Bismuth Paste Injections. Illinois Medical Journal, 1921, xl, 323.

The author draws his conclusions from a series of 600 cases of endocervicitis treated with bismuth paste according to Beck's method. The therapeutic basis is a local leucocytosis set up by the bismuth injections which destroys the bacteria and heals the inflamed area.

Cancer, tuberculosis and syphilis as etiological factors are first excluded in each case. Deep-seated endometritis, pregnancy, malpositions and tubal involvement contraindicate the injection of bismuth into the cavity of the uterus. The cervical canal is cleaned by the coagulation of its mucous and purulent contents with 40 per cent silver nitrate. Following this, about one dram of 10 per cent bismuth subnitrate is injected without force into the uterus with a glass (urethral tip) syringe. Only the gentlest force is used in the injection. Some of the paste is then packed about the cervix and held in place by a tampon. At the end of twelve hours the tampon is removed and the patient takes a hot saline douche. This treatment is continued at intervals of from two to four days.

About 80 per cent of the cases were quickly cured by this method. No mention is made of the dangers of this method in the acute stages of cervical gonorrhea.

H. W. SHUTTER.

Matthews: A Study of Chronic Endocervicitis. Surgery, Gynecology and Obstetrics, 1921, xxxii, 249.

Chronic endocervicitis is a very common and intractable disease which, Matthews thinks, has far greater possibilities in the production of pelvic disease than has heretofore been supposed. Since, in the majority of cases, palliative measures are futile, he advises removal of the infected area by a method similar to Sturmdorf's. The infected area is outlined with scalpel, the mucosa of the portio is dissected off for a distance of 3 to 4 cm., forming a circular cuff. The infected area up to the internal os is then coned out and the flap of mucosa sewed into place. While the infected mucosa and submucosa must be thoroughly removed, care is taken not to remove any more of the muscularis than is absolutely necessary.

Though it is conceded that this is not a perfect method, it has many advantages over a cervical amputation. The results obtained with it are at least as good. In a series of 200 cases treated by this method, 64 per cent were cured, 28 per cent improved and only 8 per cent remained unimproved. R. E. WOBUS.

Donay: Surgical Treatment of Endocervicitis. Gynécologie et Obstétrique, 1921, iv, 137.

The frequency of lack of union by primary intention and cicatrization following the Schroeder operation and its modifications is emphasized by the author. He then dwells upon the operation described by Matthews of Brooklyn, a method founded on the work of Sturmdorf of New York, and Curtis of Chicago, similar in aim to the operation of Pouëy brought out in 1901. It consists in a circular incision of the cervix with a loosening of the vaginal mucosa of the cervix for a distance of from 3 to 4 cm., to permit of the covering of the bed of the endocervical tissue. The diseased endocervical mucosa is removed in a cone-shaped mass having for its apex the internal os and extending down to the musculature of the cervix. The free edge of the vaginal mucosa of the cervix is then brought in apposition with the uterine mucosa at the internal os by two U sutures, one anterior and the other posterior, which penetrate the whole thickness of the cervix from within outward and are tied on the vaginal surface of the cervix. This maneuver places the vaginal mucosa in contact with the mucosa at the bottom of the cervical canal, covers the denuded area and substitutes healthy vaginal mucosa for infected endocervical mucosa. R. T. LA VAKE.

Magid: Obstetrical End Results of the Tracheloplastic Operation. New York Medical Journal, 1921, cxiv, 387.

The author compares the end results of the Sturmdorf tracheloplastic operation with those of trachelorrhaphy and of cervical amputation. Leonard's review of the Hopkins series demonstrated that trachelorrhaphy did not relieve the endocervicitis which was the cause of symptoms, while a curative amputation was followed in four fifths of the cases by sterility. Half of the patients who became pregnant failed to carry to term, the remainder suffered severe cervical dystocia. Sturmdorf's tracheloplasty, on the other hand, cures the endocervicitis by removing the infected cervical mucosa, yet does not interfere with the cervical musculature and, therefore, has no bad effect on the possibility of future conception, pregnancy or labor. This operation may be justifiably performed during the childbearing period. The author quotes nine personal cases and mentions numerous successful deliveries by colleagues to support his contentions. MARGARET SCHULZE.

Heineberg: Diseases of the Cervix Uteri. New York Medical Journal, 1920, cxii, 706.

The ease with which the cervix may be amputated has frequently led to its removal without due consideration of other possible means of restoring it to a healthy condition. To insure complete removal of the diseased cervical mucosa and eroded area in badly diseased cervices, the internal incision in the formation of the flaps must be made so high across the mucous membrane of the cervical canal that the canal or internal os may be impaired. The latter may be left in a state of wide dilatation, the former may be tightly constricted by a ring of cicatrix perpendicular to the long axis of the cervix formed at the edges of the apposed flaps. A permanently dilated internal os favors infection of the uterine cavity with production of a leucorrheal discharge which is more difficult to cure than that which resulted from the preexisting cervical disease. Both produce unfavorable conditions for the retention of the impregnated ovum in the uterine cavity. Leonard has reported abortion or premature labor in 55 per cent of the pregnancies in a series of cases following amputations of the cervix.

Stenosis of the cervical canal produced by a dense ring of scar tissue formed along the edges of the flaps may obstruct the flow of menstrual discharge and be the cause of dysmenorrhea. Such a cicatricial ring may produce a prolonged and exhausting labor and such a history of succeeding difficult labor was found in nearly 70 per cent of Leonard's cases.

To reduce the amount of cervical tissue which must be removed, the author advises preliminary treatment. The tenacious cervical discharge is first removed by a mild alkaline solution, the mucous membrane is then treated with 50 per cent silver nitrate solution applied every 3 to 4 days. If the cervix is large and boggy, the applications are supplemented with boroglycerid tampons until the cervix is reduced in size. The patient is given an alkaline douche. In from three to six months, the cervix is markedly reduced in size, the erosion gradually decreased in area, the discharge is lessened in amount and has resumed its clear mucoid character. In more than half the cases, medical treatment alone was sufficient to cure the existing cervical disease. In most of the others, either trachelorrhaphy or moderate amputation restored the cervix to a practically normal state. MARGARET SCHULZE.

Book Reviews

Gynecology.—BROOKE M. ANSPACH, M.D., Associate in Gynecology, University of Pennsylvania. With an introduction by JOHN G. CLARK, M.D. 526 illustrations. Philadelphia and London, J. B. Lippincott Company.

In beginning a belated notice of this most readable book, the writer begs leave to make the personal confession that it is a labor of love, which, as one of the "old guard" of gynecology he undertakes in a somewhat different spirit from the ordinary perfunctory reviewer. As one who has had the honor of reviewing Emmet, Thomas, and all the works of the "giants of those days", it is really stimulating to catch the pungent taste of a new American monograph and to recognize how old and well-known truths are revivified in passing through the mind of a modern teacher, truly characterized in Dr. Clark's admirable introduction, as "well-balanced." Whether it is better adapted to the student than to the general practitioner is a question to be determined by those who are more familiar with the advanced medical teaching of the present day. It is certainly difficult to find any subject, directly or remotely connected with pelvic disease, which has not been touched and freshened by the text and illustrations. To the writer it reflects perfectly the spirit of modern gynecology, as compared with the old, when the study of pelvic disease "smoked of the lamp" and dealt with theory more than with facts, and refutes the oft-repeated criticism of the general surgeon that gynecology is a "narrow specialty", crystallized and no longer progressive.

The arrangement of the subject matter after the classical introductory chapters on embryology, anatomy and physiology is certainly novel and, it must be confessed, a little confusing to one familiar with an old-fashioned table of contents. The author jumps around a bit, though he omits nothing. It may seem best to him in the next edition to condense somewhat by including under their natural headings subjects which now seem to bob up in unsuspected places, leading the inexperienced to think that they are "after-thoughts."

However the conservative may question the propriety of including under the caption "gynecology" diseases of the abdominal viscera and their operative treatment (the old and still active criticism of the general surgeon), the modern reader must recognize the fact that this is the essential element in the new and broader view of a specialty which has grown, and will continue to grow, since it has a solid foundation in pathology and long ago ceased to apologize for its *raison d'être*. The only criticism is,—is not such an extended review of abdominal diseases confusing to the student unless it is closely linked up with his studies in general surgery? The weak point in the old gynecology was that it was divorced from obstetrics, hence the outworn theories of traumatic lesions, which we recognized after they had occurred and not *when* and *how* were caused. The author shows this clearly in the chapter on physiology (p. 75-81).

Chapters VI to VIII deserve careful study, not only by the student but by all who teach. Chapter IX, on examination of the urinary organs, is most thorough and exhaustive,—too formidable for the student and general practitioner, one would think, who would do better to refer such cases to the urologist. Under the chapter on diseases of the external genitals the author struggles manfully with pruritus vulvae, the *bête noir* of the gynecologist, and, after enumerating the familiar list of "sure cures", wisely concludes that "in some cases pruritus cannot be ascribed to any demonstrable affection." Injuries of the perineum and their results (Chapter XIII) are well handled and illustrated. Personally we would be glad to see the term "perineum" eliminated in favor of "pelvic floor" and more attention paid to lesions of the fascia, rather than of the muscles, neither do we regard Hegar's and Emmet's operations as modern.

Notwithstanding the modern teaching of locking up the bowels for a week or more after operations for complete laceration we have seen too many failures in the best hands to favor this teaching, which dates back to the time of Emmet. It does not seem to be dictated by common sense, even if it is "scientific". Of the cystocele operations described we are not inclined to regard the Martin and Sänger operations as modern, neither do we regard Watkin's interposition operation as comparable with Goffe's, the modified Mayo's or, above all, the ingenious and rational overlapping of the fascia devised by Bissell. Doubtless there is room for all, but the routine follow-up of such cases proves that "by their fruits ye shall know them."

Under diseases of the cervix (Chapter XIV) we note with surprise the brief reference to the pathology and treatment of endocervicitis. Surely Sturmdorf's and Bonney's operations are preferable to amputation, or rather excision, even in obstinate cases. There is moreover no reference to these procedures in the bibliography. The sections on laceration of the cervix are equally disappointing; in this day we would not expect to read "except where the indications for operation are urgent (!) * * * it is a good plan to try palliative measures before resorting to operative treatment." We could wish that more stress had been laid upon the importance of laceration and erosion as a causal factor in the development of "cancer." Some of the last words that the reviewer heard from the lips of Dr. T. A. Emmet were that he believed that this was his most important contribution to gynecology and that he would advise letting a lacerated cervix alone, or else amputating it promptly. Under the section on trachelotomy (p. 234) we note the expression "high" as compared with "low" amputation, a difference that cannot be too strongly emphasized from the standpoint of the obstetrician, to whom the former procedure is anathema.

Chapter XV, on displacements of the uterus, is clear and instructive. We note with approval here, as elsewhere, the author's skepticism with reference to the frequency of "various reflex symptoms",—our old cloak of ignorance. The operations, especially Simpson's, are briefly, but clearly described and illustrated. In the operative treatment of complete procidentia the author inclines rather to fixation-methods and to disregard the restoration of the lower fascial supports. It is comforting to one of the old school to find that such a progressive teacher does not discard entirely the humble pessary, which has no place in the armamentarium of many gynecologists, who view their specialty as essentially surgical. The freshening influence of the author's mind is evident by the way in which he describes the simple operation of curettement (not "curetment" or "curetage") on page

289, and incidentally in the section on perforation of the uterus on page 287. After all is it not a good test of originality to be able to put an old theme in a new light?

Chapter XVII, on myomata of the uterus, is excellent and the accompanying illustrations are a joy to the eye. We note many interesting practical hints which we would quote if space permitted. "At the present time," says the author on page 310, "the weight of evidence is against the use of the Röntgen ray or radium as curative agents in cases of myoma uteri, except under certain conditions." "Hysteromyomectomy is the operation of necessity in bad (?) cases; myomectomy is the operation of choice in good operative risks with favorably situated tumors." (This statement on page 312 is a little ambiguous.) He favors supravaginal amputation over panhysterectomy,—unless there is an "evidence of malignant complications" after amputation. With regard to the treatment of the ovaries we must agree with the wise conclusion that an ovary should either be let alone (not reseceted), or removed entirely.

In the chapter on malignant tumors of the uterus we note the author's preference for the radical operation in early cases and his advocacy of the Percy method in the treatment of inoperable cases. It is only fair to mention that both procedures seem to be losing ground in the light of more extended experience.

Diseases of the tubes (including ectopic) and of the ovaries (Chapters XIX and XX) are modern in text and illustrations, though the pathology is somewhat condensed. We heartily agree with the author that so-called "chronic" oophoritis is to be regarded usually as an "end-result" rather than an inflammatory process *per se*. The old nomenclature was a stumbling block to the student, to whom connective tissue was an old friend until the pathologists made use of it to bolster up their theories of so-called "chronic inflammation." Among minor slips one notes the scant attention paid to prolapse of the ovary (page 409) and its treatment. We doubt the statement that "any of the operations for suspension of the uterus will correct a coincident displacement of the ovary." Chapter XXI, on pelvic inflammatory disease, shows how easily and naturally the author deals with a subject which has been so frequently mishandled and rendered confusing to the beginner. We recommend page 423 to any practitioner who still has doubts as to the proper treatment of intrauterine infection. "Intrauterine douching and curetting are meddlesome and dangerous."

Cellulitis (our old enemy) has been robbed of its terrors to the distracted student of Thomas and Emmet by modern pathology and we now know that old cicatrices, "localized indurations", etc., are not dangerous foci which "light up" possible acute inflammation. Chapters XXII to XXV deal with diseases of the urinary tract from the meatus to the kidney. (There is a curious little lost child sandwiched in between them—Chapter XXIV, on urinary fistula—and leaves nothing to be desired.) Thence we pass to an ambitious general survey (Chapter XXVI) of the abdominal viscera, from appendicitis through intestinal stasis and enteroptosis to diverticulitis, the aim being to give the student an idea of the varied extrapelvic conditions which are related to, or associated with, pelvic disorders. One cannot avoid the hope that in succeeding editions (we expect many) this chapter will be placed near the end of the book, as it interrupts the natural sequence in its present position.

The chapter on backache (XXVIII) deserves careful study by all who are familiar with the work of the writers mentioned in the bibliography, especially Dickinson and Reynolds, in our own department. There could be no more striking commentary on the fact that gynecology has traveled far since the time when backache and various so-called "reflex" symptoms were explained (to the satisfaction of the doctor, if not of the patient) by the presence of a lacerated cervix or retroverted uterus.

Chapters XXIX—XXXI, on gonorrhea, tuberculosis and syphilis of the generative organs, seem rather lonely in their present situation. Perhaps that is why they are grouped together, but why they are interposed between backache and disorders of menstruation is not clear. The latter subject is treated fully and judiciously, especially dysmenorrhea of the so-called "obstructive" type, usually dismissed with some dogmatic statement which does not appeal to the scientific mind. The sections on the menopause—normal and abnormal—are thoroughly modern. The difference in the action of radium in menorrhagia and metrorrhagia is properly accentuated. Endocrines are not overlooked. The succeeding chapter on sterility is full and satisfactory. The author adheres to the theory that the ovum is always impregnated in the tube—"usually in the outer third" (?) He believes that exploratory incision may be the ultimate resort in cases in which intrapelvic adhesions are suspected, with the consent of the patient and her husband. On the whole he is wisely conservative. It would be interesting to know how much more one will know about this obscure subject fifty years hence.

Chapters XXXV to XXXVIII deal with operative technic, pre- and postoperative treatment, and complications, and deserve careful study. They compare most favorably with similar chapters in recent works on gynecology. Chapter XXXIX is in some respects a repetition of former matter and might be introduced earlier in the book with advantage.

Radium and Röntgen ray therapy is new and illuminating. The indications and contraindications of radiation are clearly stated. In cancer of the uterus the author favors radiation just before operation. It is not the procedure of choice in the early and distinctly operable stage. In borderline cases radium only should be used. Its postoperative application he dismisses as "not very successful." More than half of the inoperable cases are benefited as regards the relief of pain, hemorrhage and foul discharge. In "benign" uterine hemorrhage the use of radium is nearly always beneficial.

In this cursory review of a work which has the essential qualities of a "best seller" (to use a common phrase, applicable to ephemeral literature) we may have seemed to be hypercritical with regard to its unusual scope and the unorthodox arrangement of the subject matter. Doubtless some of these criticisms may be considered in another edition, which we expect will appear not long after this belated notice. In concluding with our approval of the careful work shown in the preparation of the table of contents, the index and the bibliography, we voice our unqualified approval of the book as a whole and congratulate the author on the offspring of his brain, which is "eminently viable." H. C. COE, M.D.

ERRATA

In printing the paper of F. F. Snyder and G. W. Corner in the April number an error was made in the table of specimens, lines 4-6 on page 362. The table should read:

Nonpregnant: First to third day of cycle, 4 specimens; fourth to seventh day, 5; eighth to tenth day, 4; tenth to fifteenth day, 3; fifteenth to twentieth day, 2. Pregnant blastocysts in uterus, 1; embryos of 17-18 days, 2.

The American Journal of Obstetrics and Gynecology

Original Communications

PHYSIOLOGY THE BASIS OF FUTURE GYNECOLOGY*

BY GEORGE GRAY WARD, JR., M.D., NEW YORK CITY

MY earliest gynecological aspirations were the result of the stimulus received from one of our Founders, Alexander J. C. Skene. Among my earliest medical memories the American Gynecological Society stands forth indelibly stamped on my mind as the apotheosis and acme of scientific acumen in all that related to the functions and disorders peculiar to women. I can well remember the awe with which I heard narrated the details of the meeting of 1892 which was held in Brooklyn. I was deeply impressed with the lofty position and scientific attainments which were a "sine qua non" to Fellowship. I am frank to state, I was fired with an ambition that some day I might aspire to become one of that select company of savants. It seems a far cry from that time to the present, and how much lower the altitude, and how much humbler our attainments appear when viewed from this end.

To attain Fellowship in our beloved Society was indeed a cherished honor; to be entrusted with the responsible and arduous duties of the Secretaryship was a mark of your confidence and trust, and became a labor of love; to become your Presiding Officer is to receive the highest honor you can bestow, and my unworthiness and its unexpectedness only serve to accentuate my deep feelings of appreciation and thanks for this signal mark of your esteem.

*Presidential Address, American Gynecological Society, Forty-seventh Annual Meeting, Washington, D. C., May 1-3, 1922.

NOTE: The Editor accepts no responsibility for the views and statements of authors as published in their "Original Communications."

During the past year all of our Active Fellowship may still answer *"Adsum,"* but two of our Honorary Fellows have entered into

"that sweet sleep that medicines all pain."

On June 23, 1921, Seth Chase Gordon, a former President and a Fellow since 1888, and an Honorary Fellow since 1915, passed to his eternal rest at his home in Portland, Maine, in his ninety-first year; and Bennet Bernard Browne, elected to Fellowship in 1881, and an Honorary Fellow since 1912, died in Baltimore on March 10th, at the age of seventy-nine. They lived long lives of usefulness to womankind and they loved this Society which was honored by their membership. Their memories will remain as an inspiration to us.

This yearly toll that Nature exacts from our roll of elder Fellows serves but to remind us that the men who in the earlier years built the foundations of this Society on a bed rock of real scientific attainment, a spirit of research, and irreproachable personal character, are rapidly becoming but memories. Of the thirty-nine Founders but one is alive today. Our ranks are filling with younger generations and it behooves us to take care at this stage of our existence as a Society to carefully study the history of our earliest years in order that we may fully appreciate the wisdom of our Founders and the ideals and principles upon which this Society was launched. That their wisdom was sound is proved by the fact that we are approaching our fiftieth anniversary and are in a vigorous state of health despite the storms and gloomy prognostications we have often encountered.

At this time of general unrest when the tendencies are everywhere manifest to overturn the old order of things, to push conservatism to the wall and to lean towards socialism, I believe our Society is in danger of losing its prestige and the high position which its Fellowship implies, if those who are entrusted with its guidance fail to grasp the intent of its Founders and deviate from the compass directions they laid down.

Let us glance back and study the words that have been uttered by some of the Founders relating to this matter. At the inaugural meeting for the foundation of this Society held in New York on June 3d, 1876, Chadwick of Boston, to whose happy inspiration the Society owes its birth, said, "It has been generally conceded to be better for our Society to have a restricted membership and to require high qualification in the candidates for admission. By this means membership will come to be coveted and our discussions more profitable."

The distinguished first President of the Society, Fordyce Barker, in the first Presidential Address said, "Without insisting that our selection of members should depend solely, or even chiefly, on the literary quality of the candidate, we surely may demand that one who has acquired such a reputation as to make him a desirable member of the Society should furnish such written justification of that reputation as would merit a place in our Transactions * * * the status of this Society in the Scientific world will be determined by the character and value of the papers published in its Transactions and by the tone and ability of its discussions," and again, he warned the Fellows of the importance of care in the selection of only those who have won a right to Fellowship by a conceded personal and professional eminence, and not those who give promise as to the future,—"as they can afford to wait until time has demonstrated that the buds and blossoms of youth have developed the fruit which ripens in an established reputation with the profession at large. Honors cheapened by being made common are but slightly esteemed." He further says, "In a Society of this kind in which Fellowship is restricted to a small number, it is of vital importance that all should be active working members."

Skene in his Presidential Address reminded the Society that it was the design of the Founders that it should be devoted to the advancement of science and art and the cultivation of the higher social elements of life and he warned against the careless selection of Fellows.

Wilson, another Founder, believed that as it was by invitation that the Society was formed, * * * that it should be by invitation continued.

Our Founders in their wisdom considered that a thesis demonstrating the fitness of a candidate should be required for Fellowship. This was a requisite for forty years, until in 1916 this requirement was done away with for supposedly good and sufficient reasons. But while it may be admitted that this requisite was often unnecessary and superfluous, and even absurd in the case of men of acknowledged preeminence, it must be apparent that it leaves a dangerous gap in our breastworks through which unqualified men may slip in should the vigilance of our sentries be relaxed. As Secretary of the Society for the preceding five years, I am in a position to state that this is no phantom peril. The plan that the Council has recently adopted of inviting as guests men who are known to have accomplished creditable work in the gynecological or obstetrical field, to present papers before the Society in order that we may judge of their suitability for Fellowship, is admirable in my opinion and is in a way a substitute for the thesis. I believe that the Society would be wise to adopt this procedure as a requirement in all cases before receiving proposals for Fellowship.

Our Society has the distinction of being the pioneer national gynecological organization of the world and Fellowship is naturally regarded as the highest honor to which a rising man can attain, consequently without the thesis requirement we must be doubly careful in our scrutiny of the scientific and personal qualifications of candidates. How can we expect to carry on the spirit and high ideals of the Founders, and maintain the standard of our contributions if extraordinary care is not exercised in the selection of Fellows?

I do not agree with the idea that I have heard expressed that we should enlarge the Society and that it is our duty to lift up to higher levels the "weaker brother" by admitting him to Fellowship, and neither do I believe that it is wise to take in younger men of promise *before* they have proved themselves. As the Autocrat of the Breakfast Table well says, "Knowledge and timber shouldn't be much used until they are seasoned." I believe it is our duty to carry on the spirit of our Founders and to jealously guard our heritage against anything tending to lower the character of the Fellowship of the Society. As Polk told us we should be "ever loyal to our forefathers, we should look to them for inspiration and guidance and ever remember our obligations to their wisdom, their courage and their fidelity, and to the trust they have passed on to us."

They blazed the trail and set the standards and ideals of the Society on a high plane. In these days when it is so easy to drift away from the old paths it is our duty to see that we do not allow the quality of our Fellowship to fall below the plane that the Founders established, in order that we may maintain for American Gynecology the proud preeminence that has already been achieved.

In previous presidential addresses you have been told of the wonderful achievements of the Society with the scalpel and in the devising of new operations and treatments, so that it would be a work of supererogation for me to remind you of them, but I cannot refrain from calling your attention to the fact that this Society has also done and is doing its share in the broader field of the general advancement of public health and welfare. In 1912 a prominent feature of the scientific program was a symposium on cancer statistics and as a result of the interest awakened by the presentations and discussions, on the motion of Dr. Reuben Peterson a committee was formed to draw up a plan of action to arouse the public to a full appreciation of this terrible scourge, and the result was the formation of the American Society for the Control of Cancer, with whose efficient work you are all familiar. The benefits of this work to mankind are comparable only to the results obtained in the world wide propaganda on tuberculosis. The American Gynecological Society has rendered a signal service to humanity in thus instituting popular education on cancer which will be the means of saving many lives.

At the present time a committee of this Society under the Chairmanship of Dr. Adair is doing valuable constructive work in cooperation with the American Child Hygiene Association in perfecting a program of maternal welfare. This work assumes great importance since Congress has passed the Sheppard-Towner Bill.

I have little patience with those who harp on the passing of gynecology as a specialty. These pessimistic harpings are but the vaporings of narrow minds who can only see cutting and sewing of the pelvic organs as the sum total of our work. As I have said elsewhere the science of medicine has become so complex with the discovery of new truths and the requirements of modern diagnostic methods and treatments, that specialization is perforce an inevitable necessity. The sister specialties of obstetrics and gynecology are interdependent and neither can be obliterated, in spite of the wishes of the general surgeon. As long as women continue to bear children the specialty of obstetrics cannot die, and until we reach the Utopian Age of anatomical and physiological perfection we will have reconstructive surgery to do on the female genitalia as a result of child-bearing. As well advocate the abandonment of orthopedics or urology because both fields are invaded by the general surgeon. He cannot do all there is in surgery equally well, and I believe, as in Pope's apt lines, that

"One science only will one genius fit
So vast is art, so narrow human wit."

Those who imagine that the race of gynecology as a specialty is run, should realize that during its subversion to pure surgery it was under bonds that restrained its advance by suppressing the equally important nonsurgical aspects of gynecic science. Gynecology is today throwing off the fetters which bound it to pure surgery, to its great benefit, and it is entering into a new field of a broader gynecology, which studies woman in a larger way in all her economic relations to the public weal, and which is as yet scarcely begun.

Who is better prepared than the gynecologist and obstetrician to study and promote investigations relating to woman from the standpoint of the great field of state medicine in all that concerns her development, education, fitness for marriage and maternity, her evolution; and also her degeneracies as a criminal, as a pauper, or as a prostitute?

If anyone imagines that there is not sufficient work left for this Society to do in the future, let him remember that our constitution states that our objects are to promote *all* that relates to diseases of women, obstetrics and abdominal surgery. That means that in addition to the need of our studying disease and perfecting surgical technic and treatments, there is abundant work at hand waiting to be done in the perfecting of our hospital care of patients. One of the great pieces of work lying before us as a Society of leaders in surgical practice is to demand, and to show by our example, that a "surgical conscience" shall guide us in what we do for those who place their lives and future happiness in our hands. The awakening to the need for a "surgical conscience" was the result of Codman's stimulus to end result study, and the necessity has been made manifest by the nationwide movement for Hospital Standardization inaugurated by our Fellow Member and past President, Franklin H. Martin, of whose vision and achievements of organization we are justly proud. The honest auditing of our surgical results, just as our finances are audited, is the only way to make us realize our grave shortcomings in this important matter. At first thought we would all treat with indignation any doubt as to our not giving our best judgment and care to all our patients, whether ward or private. Yet I fear that too often we are at fault in not studying our cases with sufficient thoroughness before subjecting them to the serious risks incurred by sometimes unnecessary or ill-chosen operations. That "familiarity breeds contempt" is undoubtedly true in our often careless invasion of the human organism.

I would commend to your attention Simpson's pungent criticism of our careless care of our ward patients in many instances. Greater humanity should be manifested by providing recovery wards with expert nursing, secluded and quiet rooms for the dangerously sick or dying, and competent and sufficient nurses for night duty, in order to overcome the horror of hospitals still latent in many lay minds. Hospital Standardization leads to more perfect and efficient service to our patients.

The importance of the teaching function of the hospital should not be lost sight of. In order to facilitate this, it is our duty to see that a uniform nomenclature, uniform methods of compiling statistics, and that mortality and morbidity standards are established and adopted on the lines so ably planned by Dickinson.

PHYSIOLOGY THE BASIS OF FUTURE GYNECOLOGY

While I have thus called your attention to a few of the many problems of the broader gynecology that await your solution, I would not have it thought that the field of scientific investigation relating to our obstetrical and gynecological problems is becoming exhausted. On the contrary, there is a vast field relating to our specialty, the surface of which has been barely scratched. I speak of the science of physiology in its relation to obstetrics, gynecology and abdominal surgery. As Clark has pointed out to us, in practical achievements we need fear no other nation by comparison, but that in scientific research we have left much undone. Coe urged that we give more attention to the study of pathology and prophesied that the future gynecology would aim at something more than surgical technic; and Cullen, in a recent address, states that "If America is to lead the world in surgery in the near future, every surgeon must be trained in surgical pathology."

While there can be no dispute as to the necessity and importance of our training in surgical pathology, I believe that there is certainly an equal if not greater need for our future scientific progress, and that is our appreciation and study of that vital element, the relation of physiology to surgical practice. While the study of the dead tissues is of vast import in developing our knowledge of disease, we should not forget that we are daily dealing with live tissues, and I am convinced that the future development of our specialty lies in our increasing interest in physiology. E. P. Davis has well said, "A new cellular pathology is yet to be written from the standpoint of cellular metabolism." It is still true that the physiology of the female pelvic organs is so little known that all its essentials have yet to be studied. Our patients have had their pathology studied for years in the specimens removed from their bodies, but it is only in recent years that more attention is being paid to preoperative physiological conditions. We do not yet see, however, intraoperative and postoperative physiological studies made with sufficient frequency. We as yet know little or nothing about what is going on in this living biochemical laboratory during the time of operation, or during the actual processes of childbearing. Beyond recording the pulse and respirations, and perhaps the blood-pressure, we have been content to consider that we have all the knowledge necessary. The chemical and physical changes produced in the blood and its containers, in the great nerve centers, and in the ultimate cells, by anesthesia, trauma of operation, hemorrhages, liberation of toxins, etc., are waiting to be revealed. We simply put our patients to bed after operation and expect them to get well as a matter of course, and only record the temperature, pulse and excretions. If peritonitis or embolism develop we throw up our hands in our helplessness, for we have yet to find the cure for these great curses that still too frequently overshadow our surgery, and that often when we least expect it blast our successful results with the blight of death.

Our further understanding of our many unsolved problems lies in our acquiring biochemical knowledge as was so admirably called to our attention last year by Blair Bell. Bayliss, the great English physiologist, says, "As physiologists our task is to refer, as far as we can, all phenomena of life to the laws of physics and chemistry." Through experimental biology and biochemistry will be elucidated the laws of what is normal in our bodies, and how these laws may be disturbed or altered by anesthesia and operative procedures as well as by disease. We recognize today that the human body is a vast chemical factory in which complex chemical and physical reactions are constantly occurring. A disturbance from their normal functioning means disease. Invading microorganisms produce their destructive work by chemical agencies, their toxins poisoning the vital centers.

In the protoplasm of the ultimate cell, chemical reactions take place which determine health or disease. Haldane, the physiologist, states that, "There is a constant molecular interchange between the cell and its environment. Cell secretion, cell respiration, and cell nutrition are clearly only different aspects of the same whirl of molecular activity." The study of the blood and its circulation is a vast field that is of vital interest to us in its practical relation to our daily operative work. As socially it is asked how blue the blood is, so surgically it should be asked how red it is, for upon the state of the blood may largely depend the operative risk. This means not only the investigation as to the amount of hemoglobin and the number and proportion of the cells, but also its coagulability, viscosity, CO_2 combining power as a measure of possible acidosis, the state of the blood cells, and the tone of the vessels.

How many surgeons do we see studying blood pressure before and after operation as a routine? How many know what the expected fall in pressure should be after an operation of a certain severity, and what are the limits of safety? How many know how high a preliminary rise in blood pressure in the pre-operative excitement stage may be safe for a patient who already has a high blood pressure? What is the normal rise in leucocytes after a clean operation? The importance of Walters' recent studies in the Mayo Clinic relating to the coagulation time of the blood and the effect of calcium chloride in shortening the time is an example of a physiological study that directly interests us as surgeons. The effect of anesthesia on the blood and the introduction of various solutions and colloidal suspensions directly into the circulation opens up a large field for fruitful observations. Studies of blood chemistry should be made in peritonitis. Opie has already determined that carbohydrates act in a protective manner.

The elucidation of many obscure problems of surgery relating to diabetes, nephritis, acidosis, and the possibility of traumatic toxemia being a factor in surgical shock, must be solved by the physiologist and biochemist. He may also aid us in our studies on the mystery of thrombus formation, and the control of the formation of peritoneal adhesions. Williams pointed out to us that we had done nothing in the way of the biological or biochemical aspects of pregnancy, or of the normal metabolism of pregnancy and the puerperium or of involution. The causation of the onset of labor and the physiology of uterine contractions await us, as do the etiology of abortion and the toxemias of pregnancy. Indeed, the need of biochemical and physiological research in the obstetrical field is a reproach to us. Kosmak, in the Report to this Society of the "Special Committee on Research Work," in 1920, called our attention to our responsibilities as a national Society made up of leaders, in promoting obstetrical research and in taking our part in solving the more general sociological problems affecting the future welfare of mankind. How may we best accomplish this desirable end? I must admit that the task I have outlined presents many difficulties. First, there is the need of adequate laboratory facilities for making biochemical and physiological studies in close conjunction with our operating rooms and wards. Many of our hospital laboratories while equipped to make routine examinations are not prepared to carry out research work of the type required. Next and most difficult is to find biochemists and physiologists to aid us in this work. There are very few men so trained who are available and they are largely absorbed by the university laboratories.

What we need in our daily clinical research problems are the services of a physiological chemist available in our hospital laboratories, who will study these vital problems with us as they occur in our patients in the operating room as well as in the wards. We as clinicians are as necessary to them as they are to us in collaborating in this research if practical results are to be obtained. Erlanger, whose studies in postoperative shock and hemorrhage are familiar to us all, has lamented his inability to carry out certain researches on account of the lack of opportunity to apply his work clinically in our hospitals.

To provide the physiologists and the necessary laboratory facilities means a considerable expenditure of money, more than many hospital trustees may feel able to meet at the present time, but as they have been brought to see the necessity for a pathologist and an efficient laboratory as an essential part of every hospital today, so in the near future we may hope that they may be made to appreciate the need of a physiologist with biochemical equipment as a necessary part of the resources of every hospital which expects to further medical knowledge. At the Rockefeller Institute in New York and elsewhere such biochemical studies are being carried out at the present time largely on important medical problems, and the extent of their work must necessarily be limited by the number of available hospital beds at their disposal. Our many surgical hospitals have a vast material awaiting to be studied.

Here lies a great opportunity for the Rockefeller, Carnegie, and other Foundations that are interested in the advancement of medical knowledge, to make use of this vast clinical material in our surgical wards for biochemical study, by providing such research workers and the necessary equipment to hospitals that are desirous of carrying on scientific work of this kind. I know that I would be very glad to see the Woman's Hospital in New York make use of such an opportunity.

As the future of gynecology and obstetrics lies in the broad field of physiological research, what is more fitting than that this national Society of men pre-eminent in the specialty, should show the way?

What would more truly carry out the wish of the founders? They were early interested in physiological studies. At the first meeting in 1876 a letter was read from Dr. John C. Dalton, Professor of Physiology in the College of Physicians and Surgeons of New York, asking the cooperation of the Fellows in studies he was making of the corpus luteum, and at the second annual meeting he rendered an exhaustive report of the results of his observations, and he was made an Honorary Fellow.

Our fiftieth year is approaching and we must soon consider the means of an appropriate celebration of that auspicious event. Who shall dare say that the achievements of the past half century will not have more than justified our *raison d'etre?* Are we to weep like Alexander because we have no more worlds to conquer? We know that the first gleam of organized science in the world was due to Aristotle who anticipated the modern scientific movement in his realization of the importance of ordered knowledge, yet do we realize that it is only seventy generations to the time of Philip of Macedon when Aristotle lived, and that it is seven hundred generations to our cave men ancestors? The evolutionary processes move slowly and the ultimate perfection we may hope to attain is yet far off. Surely, we have done well in the short time of our existence as a Society, but we have scarce begun, and when we remember that great men in the past history of science have considered that they have spoken the last word on many problems which in the light of our present knowledge seems absurd, how dare we say that our work is finished?

The American Gynecological Society has a heritage of work accomplished to be proud of, its Fellows have explored the unbeaten paths in the past and shown the way to successful abdominal surgery. It is now time for them to still show the way in these new fields of exploration.

Truly our work is not yet finished, and as is so well expressed in the words of James Russell Lowell's beautiful hymn,—

"New occasions teach new duties;
Time makes ancient good uncouth;
They must upward still and onward
Who would keep abreast of Truth."

48 EAST FIFTY-SECOND STREET.

THE OVARIAN FUNCTION*

BY WILLIAM P. GRAVES, M.D., BOSTON, MASS.

CONSERVATION of the ovaries is a topic worn so threadbare by discussion that its very mention before a group of gynecologists almost demands an apology. In the minds of many of the profession and laity the ovary is firmly established as the supreme arbiter not only of the pelvic functions, but also of many of the general forces that control the physical and moral character of woman. The high estate that the ovary has attained in professional esteem has been greatly enhanced by its somewhat tardy initiation into the sacred association of the endocrine glands, and the general belief thus created of an important direct and indirect influence exerted on its more powerful and vital fellow organs. By the majority of surgeons the question of ovarian conservation has been regarded therefore as forever settled, and it has become a well-nigh universal canon that in the performance of radical pelvic surgery, ovarian tissue, even if it be only a minute vestigium, must whenever possible, be religiously preserved. Unhappily the serenity of this doctrine has recently been disturbed by the advent of radium in the treatment of fibroids and hemorrhagic myopathies involving as it does the frequent destruction of ovarian function, and the conservationist is now confronted from a new angle by the same old problem, which he had supposed to be so comfortably solved. Moreover there has existed a small minority of operators who have detected in the overenthusiastic preservation of ovarian tissue in certain radical pelvic operations a serious menace to the patient's health. They have suspected that the alleged influence of the ovary on the mature human organism may possibly be exaggerated, and they have recognized that a permanent absence of the ovarian function may in certain cases be less detrimental to the patient than an irritating impairment of function resulting from mutilated organs. These and other considerations have determined me to undertake this brief review of the subject.

The first step in such a review is to make a frank inquiry of what value the ovaries actually are to the human organism. In answering this it must first be realized that the glands of internal secretion possess different functional values at different periods of the individual's existence. An extreme example is the thymus gland, which though important during early life atrophies and becomes completely defunctionated after the age of puberty.

---

*Read before the Philadelphia Obstetrical Society, December 1, 1921.

The ovary is no exception to this law. During the developmental period it appears to act chiefly as an organ of internal secretion and is of great importance in the attainment of the normal growth and maturity of the entire organistic structure, including the brain. To the practical gynecologist the early phase of the ovaries is of little moment, for the occasions during this period for the necessity of interfering with the ovarian function are so rare and are of such an exclusively life-saving character that they need no special consideration. After the age of puberty the ovaries assume an entirely new rôle their chief function now being specifically devoted to the purposes of reproduction. Outside the office of reproduction the essentially internal secretory function is henceforth in abeyance, and is so equivocal that no one yet has defined exactly what it is nor what its manifestations may be. In fact it is entirely possible that so far as the general organism is concerned the ovarian secretion has little or no positive significance after full maturity and that it acts only negatively in the sense of a temporary balance check to other more powerful endocrine organs. In view of our present lack of knowledge of the chemistry of the ovary our chief means of information regarding the effects of the ovarian secretion of the human body is by the observation of castrated women. Operations requiring ablation of the ovaries are so common that it would seem to be a very simple matter to collect data showing whatever bodily changes take place. One would suppose too that observations so abundant and readily obtained would exhibit a general agreement among different investigators. Such, however, is not the case and there exists a very wide diversity of opinion as to the effect of castration in women among observers who are doing exactly similar operations and on similar types of patients. There is also unlimited opportunity to study the permanent effects of the absence of ovarian secretion in women after the menopause.

In what respects one may ask, does a women possessing normally functionating ovaries and uterus differ from one whose ovaries have been ablated by operation or defunctionated by the application of radium or atrophied by the natural menopause? The changes that occur may be classified as those that are permanent and those that are temporary. Of the permanent changes there are two, namely (1) cessation of menstruation, and (2) local atrophy of the external genitals. Of the temporary changes there are vasomotor disturbances, by no means constant, the only definite manifestations of which are represented by hot flushes. These three phenomena indicate the probable existence of an ovarian secretion, of either a positive or inhibitory character. Cessation of menstruation as a fact *per se* has no specific permanent effect on a woman's general organism. Mental disturbances referable to a contemplation of the absence of menstruation are the result of repressed sentimentalism or emotionalism induced by intervening external influences usually of a domestic nature. There is no definite nerve connection between the ovaries and the brain, the breaking of which may produce a psychotic change in the cerebrum. Atrophy of the external genitals is, on the other hand, a real tissue change, constant in occurrence and anatomically demonstrable. It has some definite relationship to the absence of ovarian activity, and is theoretically due to a direct local action on the part of other gland or glands previously held in check by the ovarian secretion. The ovarian conservationists have much to say of the dangers of genital atrophy, and it is necessary to pause a moment on this point. Genital atrophy appears quickly after castration and radium defunctionation. It comes on more slowly at the normal menopause, often appearing at a considerable period before the cessation of catamenia. Postoperative atrophy is confined exclusively to the genitals with a later, often unnoticeable, effect on the breasts. It is not accompanied by atrophic degeneration in other parts of the body either physical or mental, such as whitening of the hair, defects of the teeth, senility or other aspects of aging. Occasionally the local atrophy is extreme and causes distressing symptoms, and it is this outcome that the conservationalists have seized upon as one of their most potent arguments against the ablation of the ovaries during an operation of hysterectomy. It may be said, however, that abnormal postoperative atrophy is a rare occurrence, and is no more frequent after hystero-oophorectomy than after the natural menopause. Personal experience convinces me that in both cases the condition is due to a specific idiosyncrasy residing in the other glands of internal secretion, or possibly in the local tissues themselves. Patients of this type when not operated upon have an early menopause, and undergo a general premature senility. In other words artificial ablation or defunctionation of the ovaries in normally constituted individuals does not produce abnormal progressive genital atrophy even when performed in comparatively young women.

The vasomotor disturbances of the artificial menopause need only a passing notice. They are not an inevitable sequence of ablation, occurring in about 80 per cent of cases. They appear with equal frequency after castration and radiation. They are more frequent, but of shorter duration, in the artificial than in the natural menopause, and are somewhat more frequent after a hysterectomy where the ovaries have been ablated than after one where the ovaries have been left *in situ*. They are of temporary duration lasting for an average of three or four months. They may be persistent in women of unstable nervous equilibrium, or in association with long standing disquieting postoperative complications, and especially following improperly performed hysterectomies that result in pelvic adhesions, or sagging of the pelvic supporting structure. The thousand and one other nervous symptoms commonly ascribed to the influence of ablation are not in any sense definitely characteristic of the operation, occurring as they do with equal frequency after other surgical operations that do not entail a removal of the ovaries.

Consider now a woman whose ovarian function has been terminated either by surgery or by radium, and who has passed through the temporary disturbances of the menopause. Do we find in such a patient degenerative changes of an organic or functional nature that can be ascribed to the presence of ovarian activity? In our personal experience we do not, with the single exception of the genital atrophy which as we have pointed out is pathologically significant only in rare instances. Omitting the possible effects of unforeseen surgical complications, we find no impairment of any of the vital organs. Neither do we observe after close follow-up study of our cases extending over years any specifically detrimental influence on the general nervous organization. In fact in the majority of cases the reverse is true, for as a rule the condition for which the operation or treatment was initiated, has been the source of nerve irritation, and its removal has consequently served as a means of relief to the nervous system. This important phase of the subject I have discussed at length in other papers. .

The popular fallacies regarding bodily changes following loss of ovarian activity need something more than passing mention for even at the present day it is necessary frequently to discuss them with patients, when radical treatment for certain pelvic lesions is contemplated. One of the commonest and most extravagant of these superstitions is the fear of a reversion, or perhaps one might more correctly say a metaphysis to the masculine type, manifested by a deepening of the voice, appearance of facial hair and acquisition of male instincts and mental attributes. How so absurd a notion as this could ever have attained such wide credence it is difficult to imagine. It can only be explained by an unreasoning converse analogy to the high-pitched voices of eunuchs.

It is quite probable that after full maturity ovarian defunctionation causes little if any impairment of sexual sensibility if such has previously been normally established. Neither does it produce any diminution in intellectual energy and productivity, nor in the skill that is dependent on nicely balanced physical reflexes. We make this statement with confidence after the intimate observation of writers, artists, singers, players of musical instruments, etc., who for various causes have been subjected to a loss of ovarian function by means of surgery or radium.

A fear of the acquisition of abnormal fat after ovarian ablation is another popular superstition for which there is no foundation in experience when the operation has been performed *after full maturity*. Certain circulatory and chemical changes in the body have been noted after ablation, but these changes are inconstant and are of doubtful significance.

After a study of cases observed over many years we are confirmed in our belief that after complete constitutional maturity the chief province of the ovary is one of reproduction and that as an organ of internal secretion it is otherwise comparatively unimportant to the general human organism.

This conclusion, contrary as it is to generally accepted beliefs, is one of unusual importance at the present time for the advent of radium with its astonishing influence on the functions of the pelvic organs is introducing new possibilities for treating certain ailments in the presence of which we were formerly more or less helpless. In other words the question of the advisability of defunctionating ovarian activity in order to attain certain constitutional results is one that is confronting the gynecologist more and more frequently.

The bald statement of our views concerning the status of the ovary as an organ of internal secretion is peculiarly liable to misinterpretation, as the writer is well aware from previous experience. In order therefore to make our position as clear as possible, it is necessary to enumerate specific examples of the more important crises in which the question at issue is presented. The following is a brief recapitulation of our views based on personal experience.

During the period of infancy and childhood the ovaries are essential as glands of internal secretion in growth and development either by their own agency or in intimate association with other more powerful organs. Their preservation is therefore all-important. Pelvic surgery is at that time, however, so rarely necessary that it needs no discussion here.

After puberty the ovaries assume their rôle as reproductive organs, and probably continue in a gradually lessening degree to be of influence in development until the age of complete physical and mental maturity, the average of which may be set at about twenty-two years though it has wide individual variation. During this period the ovaries should be sacredly preserved, both for their reproductive and secretory value. Omitting such rare conditions as bilateral dermoids, sarcomata, etc., the chief dangers that beset the ovaries between puberty and full maturity are the destructive processes of pelvic peritonitis, and the intractable menorrhagias. If operation is required for the former, it should be as conservative as possible, and should not be deferred until the inflammatory processes have destroyed the ovarian tissue beyond all possibility of repair. The entire endometrial surface should be spared. As much ovarian tissue as possible in both ovaries should be preserved, even if it involves tedious dissection from beds of adhesions and careful piecing together of ragged shreds. If both tubes must be sacrificed auto-transplantation of ovarian tissue into the uterine cornua should be carried out to furnish at least a chance for future impregnation. The severe intractable menorrhagias which in former times occasionally required a radical pelvic operation are fortunately now entirely amenable to radium. Radium may be applied in these immature cases with practically no danger of terminating menstruation, or of causing permanent sterility. By judicious dosage the excessive flow may be modulated and the periods restored with more or less accuracy to a normal rhythm. In our earlier cases we were greatly apprehensive of establishing a complete menopause in these young girls, but our experience seems to prove that the younger the ovary the more difficult it is to stop the menses by radiation.

In the decade following the establishment of full maturity the integrity of the ovaries should be carefully guarded for this is the most important child-bearing epoch of the woman's life. Hence from this standpoint all that has been said regarding pelvic inflammation and menorrhagia of prematurity applies also to this period. In addition to these two affections, one must also take into consideration in the third decade the not infrequent appearance of bleeding or rapidly growing fibroids. These must be treated with the utmost regard to preserving the reproductive power. Unless there be some serious constitutional contraindication to surgical operation fibroids at this age should not be treated by radium since their growth can be inhibited only by a dosage of radium that will also terminate the menses, and produce sterility. Fibroids at this age should in all cases wherever physically possible be treated by myomectomy with a conscientious safeguarding of the endometrium and ovarian tissues. Even extensive dissections are permissible, but extreme care should be exercised in repairing the uterus thus mutilated, to prevent weak areas in the wall that may rupture in future pregnancies.

Inasmuch as the ovaries have fulfilled their chief function as organs of internal secretion in the early part of the third decade, and are thenceforward less necessary to the constitutional well-being of the patient, they demand *from that particular standpoint* correspondingly less consideration if the question arises of their ablation in order to attain a permanent cure.

In order to make this point clear, let us take a specific example. Assume that a woman of twenty-seven, married and with two living children, has been suffering from a chronic pelvic inflammation that requires operation. The patient is poor, and does her own work. She stipulates that she wishes never to have another operation. On opening the abdomen the adnexa are found extensively involved. It would be possible to leave only sufficient ovarian and endometrial tissue to maintain for a while a scanty menstruation. The possibility of restoring fertility is out of the question. In such a case in our personal practice, we should not hesitate to make a clean sweep of the pelvis by a supravaginal hysterectomy with removal of the adnexa. We should consider the incomplete preservation of the ovarian function as of little weight in comparison with the chance of reformation of adhesions, recurring invalidism and a future operation, or if such be not the case the liklihood of a premature, prolonged and disquieting menopause.

In this case we have made our decision of radicalism only after taking the patient's social condition into careful consideration. In ablating the ovaries we have done so with a clear conscience, confident that the absence of ovarian activity will do the patient no permanent harm, and that our operation has given the best assurance of freedom from future invalidism that might otherwise result from a recurrence of her pelvic disability, had extreme conservatism been carried out.

We may summarize by saying that during the third decade conservatism should be observed as far as possible but that if radicalism seems necessary for the patient's welfare, it may be practiced without fear of injury from the loss of ovarian function.

Complete defunctionation by radium is rarely necessary during this period.

During the fourth decade of life, occasions raising the question of ovarian preservation or ablation multiply rapidly. During the early thirties much the same conditions obtain as during the third decade and the same rules are in general to be observed.

As the years go on however and one enters the second half of this period, that is, the age from thirty-five to forty, women have in the majority of cases established their families or have become reconciled to a life of sterility or maidenhood. The question of safeguarding the reproductive function becomes gradually less poignant. The gynecologist is correspondingly better prepared to meet at this age the newer problems of treatment that are evolving from our increasing experience with radium. These problems appertain chiefly to the treatment of menstrual disorders, and embrace such conditions as menorrhagia from uterine insufficiency, menorrhagia from fibroids, severe menstrual headaches, uncontrollable dysmenorrhea, periodic psychoneuroses, and the various other ailments that depend for their existence on the presence of the menses. The value of radium in terminating ovarian and menstrual function in this class of cases is now firmly established.

After the age of forty there is a great increase in the number of pelvic diseases, the treatment of which both by surgery and radiation demands for the best interest of the patients' future health, an ablation or defunctionation of the ovaries. During this decade the importance of the ovary as an organ of internal secretion becomes less and less significant until by the middle of the period it need scarcely be regarded at all, except from a purely sentimental standpoint.

This decade of a woman's life is the age of hysterectomies and for the sake of completeness it is necessary to repeat here our personal views regarding the retention of ovaries in operations that require a removal of the uterus. These views have been expressed by me in the literature so frequently and discussed at such length that only the following brief statement is required: We do not believe in leaving the ovaries *in situ* in operations where a removal of the uterus is necessary. Our reasons for this belief may be summarized without further discussion by saying that experience has convinced us that ovaries left *in situ* though possibly diminishing to some extent the vasomotor disturbances of the artificial menopause are of no permanent benefit, but on the other hand may be the source of later serious complications.

We may add parenthetically that we also do not believe in those mutilating operations, such as are enthusiastically exploited by Blair Bell, of Liverpool, that seek to preserve minute portions of the ovaries and endometrium so as to maintain some semblance of the menstrual function. Such operations in our experience often lead to a premature, long-drawn out and distressing menopause, and may become associated with serious psychoneurotic states. If menstruation is to be preserved, enough tissue should be left to maintain full menstrual activity.

It remains now to discuss the ovary from the standpoint of glandular therapeutics.

Once more it is necessary to emphasize our estimate of the ovary as an organ of internal secretion. Be it remembered that we do not deny the existence of an ovarian secretion, but we do maintain that after the age of full maturity it is devoted chiefly to the function of reproduction, and is of comparatively little importance to the general organism in its other capacities. This theory seems to be substantiated by the therapeutic effects of ovarian extracts, for we find by experience that the influence exerted by ovarian substance is evident only in some relationship with the reproductive mechanism.

Thus we find that ovarian therapy is valuable in treating the hot flushes of the artificial and natural menopause. It has an uncertain but nevertheless unequivocal effect on certain dysmenorrheas. The same may be said of its influence in cases of amenorrhea, delayed menses, clotting, menstrual headaches, etc. We have in our experience an increasing number of cases which seem to prove that it may stimulate fertility. Even at its best the action of ovarian extract is uncertain and excepting in occasional brilliant instances rather feeble. Outside its specific relationship to the reproductive functions, the influence of ovarian substance on the rest of the bodily organism is slight.

244 MARLBOROUGH STREET. (*For discussion, see p. 663.*)

THE APPLICATION OF METABOLISM STUDIES TO THE FETAL AND NEONATAL PERIODS OF LIFE*

BY HAROLD BAILEY, M.D., NEW YORK, N. Y.

Associate Professor of Obstetrics and Gynecology, Cornell University

CONSIDERABLE attention by lay organizations and nursing bodies has been directed toward prenatal and postnatal care with the object of reducing infant mortality. Two-thirds of obstetric practice is in the hands of midwives and doctors untrained in this special branch of surgery and the maternity center organizations have done a great work in calling the attention of the public to the lack of scientific care in the treatment of the pregnant and parturient woman. Maternal mortality of pregnancy and labor has not been greatly reduced and the upward trend of other branches of modern surgery has left this subject behind. Infant mortality from stillbirths and deaths in the first month of life is as high as 8.3 per cent (Cragin)[1] under the best conditions as regards obstetric care. In 10,000 cases from the Johns Hopkins Clinic[2] there were 7 per cent of infant deaths from the seventh month of pregnancy to two weeks postpartum and at the Sloane in the cases collected by Holt and Babbitt[3] for the same period of pregnancy and infant life, it was 7.2 per cent. The stillbirths at the Manhattan Maternity Hospital were 3.6 per cent in 14,468 births but the figures for the mortality during the first month are not available.[4] Many of these stillbirths were due to accidents of labor (32 per cent at the Manhattan Maternity Hospital) or to syphilis or congenital anomalies but a considerable proportion were due to prematurity.

Of 389 cases collected by Cragin, of newborn infants dying from the hour of birth to the thirteenth day (series of 10,000, 3.89 per cent) 50.3 per cent were premature and 43.9 per cent had no other known abnormality than congenital weakness. Schwarz and Kohn,[5] found

---

*Read at a meeting of the Association for the Advancement of Science, Toronto, Ont., December 28, 1921.

from 2 to 5 per cent of all viable births result in children of low birth weight and that the mortality from this type of case is ten times that of the normal. In their total of 272 cases from the Berwind Maternity Clinic, there were 39 deaths during the first week of life or a mortality of 14 per cent for this group.

From these facts it is evident that we have to contend with a tremendous death rate during the first weeks of life due in a large part to prematurity and low birth weight. In addition there is a stillbirth incidence of very great moment from this same condition. A premature infant is not able to withstand long continued head pressure and trauma occurring in labor.

The diagnosis of prematurity is nearly always made on low birth weight. When the weight is under 2000 grams, this is a correct method. However, in considering children who are under weight one should make a careful measurement of the length in order to determine more accurately their status, for the mortality is always higher in the premature as compared with the full term infant that is under weight.

What are the causes of interruption of pregnancy before term? Toxemia must be placed foremost. Pregnancy kidney with associated changes in the liver and accompanying disturbances of the maternal metabolism lead not infrequently to death of the fetus or to its expulsion from the uterus. Syphilis also has a tendency to produce miscarriage and premature labor owing to degenerated processes in the placenta. These two conditions are controllable to a certain extent by properly conducted prenatal care. The toxemia of pregnancy may be combated in its early stages by a correction of the metabolic disturbances and by relieving the liver and kidneys of further strain, by placing the patient upon a carbohydrate diet. While it is perfectly true that a small proportion of cases of toxemia will require the induction of labor, considerable experience in private practice shows that under proper care this procedure is seldom necessary.

Syphilis may be treated effectively during pregnancy by injections of salvarsan and mercury and a recent report by A. C. Beck[6] indicates how successful this treatment is. In a group of 32 syphilitic mothers, he was able to treat thoroughly seventeen and these women gave birth to fourteen living and apparently nonsyphilitic children. These results demonstrate very conclusively the value of antenatal treatment.

There are a certain number of premature births due to anomalies of the fetus and a small proportion to faulty implantation of the placenta but in the light of our present knowledge they must be considered as an irreducible minimum.

Premature labor is sometimes brought about by poor maternal nutrition and by the manual exertions made necessary by the numerous duties of the household. At the Manhattan Maternity Hospital normal cases are admitted only as they go into labor and as a result many of the women spend the last four weeks of their pregnancy attending to their regular home duties and under a poor dietary regime. In a report in this paper of the birth weights in the feeding experiments at the Manhattan Maternity Hospital, the 200 babies were taken in consecutive order in sets of 50, excluding all prematures, and yet there were 66 children or 33 per cent that had a birth weight between six and seven pounds. Thirty-six of these babies were male. A birth weight below seven pounds is not the ordinary conception of the weight of a mature, newborn infant.

On the Bellevue service where there is a waiting ward, many of the women spend the last three weeks in the hospital where they have a plentiful food supply and no household cares or worries. It has been noticed that they generally go to term and not infrequently pass the day of expected labor.

It is proper here to consider the effectiveness of prenatal care as ordinarily furnished by maternity center organizations. All well regulated maternity hospitals have Social Service Departments with workers who follow up delinquent patients and urge them to return to the hospital for antenatal examinations. Now, however, the prenatal nurse partly assumes the duties of a doctor, taking the blood pressure, examining the urine and even prescribing to some limited extent. Her observations are believed to be quite satisfactory to all concerned and the patient's visits to the antenatal clinic at the hospital are less numerous than formerly.

As a matter of fact at one hospital with which I am connected, if the patient applies in the seventh month of her pregnancy, she is advised to come back in six weeks and again on the day of her expected labor. During the rest of this period, the most important time of her pregnancy, she is in the hands of maternity center nurses. At the time of her labor the nurse attends and is of great aid to the doctor. The doctor delivers the patient and does not visit her again until the tenth day, all the postpartum care resting with the nurse. If our object is to reduce maternal and infant mortality, this must be looked upon as a ridiculous procedure and a step backward toward the nonmedical control of the puerpera.

Returning to the consideration of prematurity, there is a very wide field for these maternity center organizations. The majority of patients during their last month of pregnancy must cook, scrub, wash and attend to the many household demands. These patients should be aided and the prenatal service should provide a woman of the practical nurse type to relieve them of the heavier portions of their work. Nursing supervision should be given as regards diet, rest and proper care of the eliminative functions. When possible the last two weeks of pregnancy should be spent in the waiting ward of a hospital. The welfare of the prospective mother should be the care of the State and where it is necessary a subsidy should be granted to release the patient from the arduous tasks during the last month of her pregnancy and the first month following her delivery.

CONSIDERATION OF THE FETAL METABOLISM

In mammals the transfer of food material from the mother to the fetus is largely by osmosis through the placenta. We have the studies of Slemons[7] and his associates of the chemical blood analysis of the mother and of the child at the moment of birth. The nitrogenous bodies are found to be in equilibrium or nearly so on each side of the placenta, with the exception of the amino acids, which are always slightly in excess on the fetal side. The figures are so close, however, that the conclusion is forced upon one that the placenta acts as a filter.

Carbohydrates were studied by the analysis of the blood sugar. In nineteen of twenty-four cases there were slightly higher values for the mother but in the remaining five, the values were identical. The average for the mother in twenty-four cases was 0.132 per cent and for the fetus, 0.115 per cent. Slemons had one case of double ovum twins and the average blood sugar of each fetus was determined. In one fetus it was 0.099 per cent and the other, 0.096 per cent. The maternal blood showed a figure of 0.12 per cent which would indicate that there is diffusion through these placentae from the higher concentration of the mother to the infants.

We have evidence that the fetus depends upon the supply of glucose for its nutrition to a large extent. The analysis of the blood of the umbilical vein and artery by Cohnstein and Zuntz[8] result in a respiratory quotient of 1.0 and 1.6 respectively in two cases, indicating that carbohydrate is the source of energy. Bohr[9] measured the total respiratory exchange of pregnant guinea pigs before and after clamping the umbilical cord and noted the differences which gave a respiratory quotient for the embryo in the neighborhood of unity (Murlin). In the human subject, respiratory quotients in the neighborhood of one were found in a number of instances where the newborn was examined within a few hours after birth and led to a conclusion that the source of energy at this time is the glycogen stored in the liver and tissues of the fetus.

Murlin and I[10] found the total fat in the fetal blood to be much lower than that of the maternal. However, there seems to be some definite relation between the two as a high maternal fat invariably leads to high fat percentage in the umbilical vein. Slemons found that neither neutral fat nor cholesterol esters pass the placental barrier.

Cholesterol, however, does pass through the placenta. Since this substance acts as a colloid it cannot pass by diffusion and if its origin is not in the tissues of the fetus, which seems unlikely, its passage suggests some selective activity of the placenta. Attempts by Hoffström and others to pass stained fat from the maternal to the fetal circulation were unsuccessful. We may conclude that the fat of the fetus does not come from the mother except as it is formed by the fetus from either carbohydrate or protein.

CONSIDERATION OF THE MATERNAL METABOLISM

Let us now turn to the metabolism of the mother. Hoffström[11] in one case and Wilson[12] in two cases, have shown that there is a very considerable retention of nitrogen during the last months of pregnancy. The requirements of the fetus are greatly exceeded and in Hoffström's case, the nitrogen retention was 209 grams. For one of Wilson's it was 210.9 and for the other, 284.5 grams. It would appear that the mother ends her pregnancy with a considerable gain in nitrogen. This is of great practical importance in arranging dietary schemes in the last month of pregnancy.

Furthermore, Zuntz,[13] Carpenter and Murlin,[14] and Hasselbalch[15] found an increase in the metabolism for pregnant women near term. While they make the suggestion that this may be an effort of the body to maintain the hydrogen-ion concentration of the blood, one may very reasonably come to another conclusion, namely that in late pregnancy there is extra heat production somewhat proportional to the weight of the fetus. Carpenter and Murlin were able to show this by the measurement of the metabolism in three pregnant women and later in the puerperal women with their children. The difference in metabolism did not vary by 1 per cent in two cases and 7 per cent in the third. It is apparent that the higher demands of the newborn just compensate for the loss of the oxidation processes in the placenta, membranes and cord.

There is no definite means of knowing exactly how much change there is in the metabolism of the infant from fetal to neonatal life but it is probably considerable. The difference in its heat dissipation is so great that it is reasonable to suppose that its metabolism is placed on a much higher level immediately after delivery. Reubner expresses the belief that the law of surface area applies to the embryo as well as to the newborn and he claims that the average metabolism per unit of weight of any newborn animal would be approximately twice that of the mother (Murlin).

We know that the mother in the latter part of her pregnancy has a considerable hyperglycemia, very likely for the purpose of supplying the infant with sufficient carbohydrate but as Benedict and Talbot[16] state, "the oxygen and food are obtained from the blood of the mother, and while the fetus, may be glycogen-rich, the liver of the mother is likewise glycogen-rich, and hence it may be unreasonable to expect a specific gaseous metabolism of the embryo in the prenatal state."

PRACTICAL APPLICATION

Experience shows that the fat of the newborn is laid on largely during the last month of pregnancy. A baby with a considerable fat layer has a metabolism perhaps even lower than the premature or the thin baby because the fat conserves the heat. At the same time it answers for the energy requirements until the milk supply of the mother is sufficient.

We must then find a way of providing the newborn child with the proper amount of fat. It happens that there has been experimental work dealing with this very problem but from another angle. In the treatment of pelvic deformity, an attempt has been made to cut down the weight of the fetus by limiting the carbohydrates of the mother and the Prochownik[17] diet does this. On a food supply consisting mainly of protein, the weight of the fetus is reduced because it is thinner. However, the bony growth remains the same and the idea is a failure as regards the treatment of pelvic deformity. We may, however, argue inversely, that a carbohydrate diet will increase the weight.

A carbohydrate diet during the last month of pregnancy for the mother has proved to be a satisfactory one in combating toxemia. It provides the patient with a proper food supply when a small amount of fat is added and there is no complaint of the absence of the proteins. We may conclude, therefore, that a carbohydrate diet with small amounts of fat is a sufficient one for the last four weeks of pregnancy. It will reduce the incidence of toxemia and at the same time provide the fetus with an ample supply of glucose which is its main energy requirement.

METABOLISM STUDIES OF THE NEWBORN

Hasselbalch[18] in 1904 conducted metabolism experiments in children in the first hours of life and came to some important conclusions. He believes that the metabolism of the normally well nourished fetus consists of the oxidation of carbohydrates and that the newborn child at term has a store of this substance in its organs which is spent in a few hours.

Murlin and I[19] made 28 observations on six infants from the age of six hours to twelve days and in five instances found the respiratory quotient above 0.90. We had for comparison as regards weight, two infants, a light baby (6 pounds) and a heavy one (10 pounds, 3 ounces) who were examined at the same age in hours during the first five days. We came to the conclusion that the energy requirements of the newborn could be placed between 1.7 to 2.0 calories per kg. per hour or 40 to 48 calories per kg. per twenty-four hours or 25 calories per hour per square meter of surface (Table I). (Meeh's Formula.)

TABLE I
SHOWING METABOLISM OF NEWBORN INFANTS (BAILEY AND MURLIN)

WEIGHT, KGM.	AGE HOURS	CAL. PER HOUR	CAL. PER KGM. AND HOUR	CAL. PER SQUARE METER AND HOUR (MEEH)
W. 2.9	6	5.649	1.94	23.67
B. 4.6	6	6.724	1.46	20.43
W. 2.82	31	6.255	1.94	26.54
B. 4.49	31	8.704	2.22	26.87
W. 2.75	80	5.972	2.18	25.57
B. 4.27	80	7.101	1.66	22.67
W. 2.75	104	5.252	1.83	21.85
B. 4.27	104	7.500	1.77	23.47
W. Average	...	5.782	2.04	24.43
B. Average	...	7.514	1.70	23.36

Benedict and Talbot found the respiratory quotient for 74 infants on the first day of life was 0.80. This would represent the combustion of one-third carbohydrate and two-thirds fat. On the third day they found the average respiratory quotient was 0.73, representing nearly a pure fat combustion, (62 infants examined) and on the sixth day there was a rise to 0.82 (22 infants examined). It is apparent from these results that the energy requirement of the newborn is not fulfilled during the first days of life. They placed the basal energy requirement for infants from one and one-half to six days old at 44 calories per kg. of body weight or 12.65 calories per square meter of body surface per unit of length.

PRACTICAL APPLICATION OF METABOLISM STUDIES TO THE NEONATAL PERIOD

The loss in weight during the first few days of life is partly due to the loss of water from the skin and lungs, partly to the passage of meconium and urine, but the larger part is due to the combustion of fat to provide the energy requirements. The colostrum that is present in the breasts for the first few days has a high caloric value, but there is very little of it until the third day. Von Ruess[20] in 25 cases found none on the first day, 54 grams on the second day, 173 grams on the third day and 263 grams of secretion on the fourth day, when true milk may be said to be present.

In 1912 on the Bellevue service we began efforts to reduce the early loss in weight by feeding a milk formula after every nursing during the first three days. This proceeding was moderately successful but entailed considerable extra work on the part of the nurses and was eventually discontinued.

AVERAGE OF FIFTY CONSECUTIVE CASES IN EACH GROUP. (EXCLUDING PREMATURES)

1. *Two-Hour Feedings:* Alternate breast and sugar solution every six hours, 1st, and 2nd days, then breast nursing every 2 hours. *Ten breast feedings.*
   Average Birth Weight..............3652.2 grams
   " Weight 4th day............3367.8 "   —Loss of 284.4 grams
   "   " 10th day............3574.2 "   — "   " 78.0 "

2. *Three-Hour Feedings:* Alternate breast and sugar solution 1st and 2nd days, then breast nursing every 3 hours. *Seven breast feedings.*
   Average Birth Weight..............3634.2 grams
   " Weight 4th day............3393.6 "   —Loss of 240.6 grams
   "   " 10th day............3450.0 "   — "   " 184.2 "

3. *Four-Hour Feedings:* Breast every 4 hours except night feeding. 2 A. M. feeding of 5 x 20 formula. *Five breast feedings.*
   Average Birth Weight..............3538.8 grams
   " Weight 4th day............3299.8 "   —Loss of 239.0 grams
   "   " 10th day............3361.8 "   — "   " 177.0 "

4. *Four-Hour Feeding and Formula for Three Days.*
   Average Birth Weight..............3511.8 grams
   " Weight 4th day............3322.2 "   —Loss of 189.6 grams
   "   " 10th day............3394.8 "   — "   " 117.0 "

5. *Three-Hour Feeding and Formula for Three Days.*
   (Former report from Bellevue Service)
   Average Loss on 4th day............ 159.0 grams
   "   "   " 8th day............ 98.0 "

Formerly feeding intervals were every two hours or ten breast feedings in twenty-four hours. Increasing the number of the feedings in twenty-four hours does not help the infant because the exposure leads to an increased heat production. Many hospitals adopted the three-hour feeding routine. This calls for seven feedings in the twenty-four-hour period. During the last two years the four-hour feeding has been given a trial. The regime at the Manhattan Maternity Hospital is to give five breast feedings and one 5 x 20 formula feeding at 2 A.M. The infants under the four-hour period of nursing have less exposure and there is decidedly less crying and exertion. The mothers are happier and gain an eight-hour rest. There is less nipple disturbance and breast inflammation. Feeding 5 × 20 formula, 1½ ounces supplementary feedings on the first three days with the three- and four-hour feedings, led to a smaller loss by the fourth day and a return to the neighborhood of 100 grams below birth weight by the tenth day.

A comparison of the figures and chart shows the relative value of these different methods.

In none of the cases was there any disturbance from the supplementary feedings. While fulfilling the requirements as regards the quantity of calories in the diet, there is still a loss on the fourth day of between 5 and 6 ounces and a tenth-day weight that is 3 to 4 ounces below the weight of birth. The figures show an improvement over the regular methods of feeding and it is my belief that the supplementary formula should be generally adopted. It is interesting to see how closely the figures of the three- and four-hour intervals of feeding parallel each other. The differences on any one day are so slight that they may be disregarded.

The energy requirement of premature infants should be close to that of the mature and Litzenberg[11] has presented a series of charts showing that long interval feeding is feasible. It is probable that the freedom from disturbances and exposure lowers the heat production and in this way counterbalances the gain that should follow two-hour nursings.

Benedict and Talbot cite the importance of conservation of the body heat immediately after birth and suggest that the baby be oiled on the first day and the bath dispensed with. This is a very important point. The custom in some maternities of immediately greasing the baby, thus leaving it exposed in a room of ordinary temperature, is a pernicious one for in these first moments the heat regulating mechanism of the body is imperfect. It would be far better to place each newborn in one of the open electric heaters such as are in use for prematures at the Manhattan and Bellevue Hospitals.

It is appropriate here to suggest again that in maternity hospitals the newborn be turned over to the pediatrician. Obstetricians have been carrying this appalling death rate in the neonatal period with little concerted effort toward its reduction and it is time that we relinquished it to men better trained in pediatrics.

CONCLUSIONS

In order to prevent premature births, the care of the prospective mother must include a reduction of her manual work during the last month of pregnancy and the insistence upon a dietary regime composed largely of carbohydrates. The high death rate in the neonatal period must be looked upon as preventable to a certain extent and provision of the energy requirement of the newborn is the first step in that direction.

REFERENCES

(1) *Cragin:* Obstetrics, Phila. 1916, pp. 837-839. (2 Jour. Am. Med. Assn., Jan. 9, 1915, lxiv, No. 2, p. 95. (3) Jour. Am. Med. Assn., Jan. 23, 1915, lxiv, No. 4. (4) New York State Med. Jour., Oct., 1918, xxiii, No. 10. (5) Am. Jour. Dis. Child., March, 1921, xxi, pp. 296-306. (6) AM. JOUR. OBST. AND GYNEC., October, 1921, ii, No. 4. (7) Am. Jour. Obst., 1919. (8) Pflüger's Arch., 1884, xxxiv, 173. Ibid., 1888, xlii, 342. (9) Skan. Arch. f.

Physiol., 1900, x, 413. (10) Am. Jour. Obst., June, 1917, lxxv, No. 6, pp. 913-953. (11) Skan. Arch. f. Physiol., 1910, xxiii, 326. (12) Bull. Johns Hopkins Hosp., 1916, xxvi, 121. (13) Arch. f. Gynäk., 1910, xc, 452. (14) Arch. Int. Med., 1911, vii, 184. (15) Skan. Arch. f. Physiol., 1912, xxvii, 1. (16) Carnegie Inst. Publication, 1915, No. 233. (17) Centralbl. f. Gynäk., 1889, No. 33. (18) Trans., Benedict & Talbot, Car. Inst. Pub., 1915, No. 233. (19) Am. Jour. Obst., 1915, lxxi, No. 3. (20) Die Krankheiten des Neugeborenen, 1914, 90. (21) Arch. Int. Med., Dec., 1912, iv, pp. 383-390.

22 EAST SIXTY-EIGHTH STREET.

TERATOMATA OF THE OVARY*

By Miles F. Porter, M.D., F.A.C.S., Fort Wayne, Ind.

THE word teratoma comes from *teras* meaning monster and *oma*, a termination meaning tumor. Some of the other names applied to tumors of this class are dermoid, teratoid, embryoid, morular. The term dermoid means "like skin" and, therefore, strictly speaking should be used to define only those tumors formed by skin inclusions and composed only of epiblastic tissue. As a matter of fact no tumor composed solely of epiblastic tissue has ever been described. Generally speaking, the word dermoid has been used to signify a rather large class of cystic ovarian tumors composed of the three embryonal layers which are rarely malignant. Bland-Sutton, Hertzler, and others, use the word teratoma to indicate a solid tumor made up of the same structures as the dermoids but composed of a larger proportion of embryonal cells and, for this reason, peculiarly prone to malignancy. Hurdon says "teratomata are solid embryomata and are malignant." The majority of authorities, I think, today accept the classification of Eden and Lockyear who divide teratomata of the ovary into two classes—cystic (usually called dermoids) and solid. This classification is also that suggested by Adami, Nicholls, and Ewing.

Concerning the origin of these tumors, Waldeyer and Wilms hold that they are ovigenic; Conheim, that they arise from early ectodermal inclusions. Krömer is satisfied that these tumors are of ovarian origin, the cystic element coming from the follicle and the tissue elements from the ovule. Douglas, on the other hand, says the whole question is hypothetical. We may take either of the positions indicated and be sure of being in good company. Certain it is that there are two forms of teratoma of the ovary; the one cystic, quite common and little prone to malignancy and commonly reported as dermoids; the other is rare, solid and frequently malignant.

It is well here to emphasize the fact that so-called dermoids of the

---

*Read at the Thirty-Fourth Annual Meeting of the American Association of Obstetricians, Gynecologists, and Abdominal Surgeons, St. Louis, Mo., September 20-22, 1921.

ovary are much more frequently malignant than was formerly supposed to be the case. Ewing puts the rate of malignancy at 3 per cent. Hoehne says malignancy is more frequent in bilateral dermoids. The moot question, as to whether these tumors are congenital or postnatal in origin, is not, perhaps, of great practical importance. The writer has met with no case of malignant cystic teratoma in an experience covering an hundred cases, or more; while he has had one sarcomatous teratoma of the solid variety in an experience covering less than a score of cases.

This specimen was removed from an 18 year old virgin; it was entirely solid, the size of an adult head, pedunculated, without adhesions, encapsulated, symptomless, save from its presence, and sprang from the right ovary. The operation was done thirty years ago and the specimen examined by Drs. McCaskey, McCullough, and myself. At first it was regarded as a fibroma, but upon further investigation the diagnosis of sarcoma was made and later confirmed in a foreign laboratory.

It is of interest to note that the patient, now the mother of a family, is still living and, at last account, in good health. The presence of granulation tissue containing foreign body cells in the cyst wall is evidence of the irritating nature of the semi-solid contents of the cysts often found in these tumors.

The frequency of occurrence of teratomata is placed all the way from 4 per cent (Olshausen) to 18 per cent (Martin) of ovarian tumors. It is beyond doubt true that many of these tumors have been, especially in the past, placed in the category of ordinary cysts of the ovary for the reason that frequently they partake largely of the character of simple cysts and careful examination is necessary to reveal their true nature.

Concerning the composition and structure of these tumors, it may be briefly stated that it varies much, from nails to eyelashes, including glands, organs of special sense, genital organs, nerve centers and nerves. The identification of rudimentary organs in these tumors, usually requires microscopic examination.

Teratomata, like adenomata, of the ovary are apt to affect both ovaries at once. If one bears this point in mind when a patient presents herself to the surgeon with double ovarian tumor, he will at once suspect the trouble to be either adenoma or teratoma. Teratoma frequently so distort the ovaries, that the true ovarian tissues may be unrecognizable to the naked eye; and yet, these organs be able to perform their full functions.

Usually, these tumors are of slow growth; but they may grow very rapidly. Sutton reports a case of a seventeen-year-old girl in whom a cyst, containing 78 liters of fluid, formed within three years. Unusual rapidity of growth suggests malignancy. Teratoma of the ovary may appear at any age, often in childhood, but most frequently between the ages of 30 and 40. The symptoms do not differ from those due to other forms of ovarian tumors.

Concerning the accidents likely to occur to teratomata, it may be said that they are more prone to torsion of the pedicle, because of their irregularity, asymmetry and size, smaller than ordinary cysts on the average, less liable to rupture because of their thicker walls, and more liable to malignant change because of the variety of tissue cells they contain and because of the irritating nature of the cyst contents.

It is held by some that teratomata are peculiarly offensive to the uterus. Their presence is apt to cause abortion and both before and after delivery there is said to be great danger of infection. Personally, I have seen no cases of abortion due to these tumors and but one probable case of twisted pedicle. The patient whose case is herewith reported gave birth to a dead child and suffered a mild infection in which the tumors may be fairly said to have played a contributory part. The "probable" case of twisted pedicle was from a girl ten years old upon whom I operated for a supposed appendicitis and found instead, a right ovarian cyst, the size of a small orange, with a twisted pedicle. The diagnosis of teratomata was based on the irregular contour and consistency of the cyst, its size, and the age of the patient. There was no minute examination made to determine its exact nature.

CASE REPORT.—Mrs. J. W. W., housewife, age thirty-five, married three years. Family history unimportant. Had never been seriously ill prior to present trouble. Menstrual history normal. She had noticed that her abdomen was large as long ago as ten years, but thought it was "natural." On May 5th she gave birth to a child which the attending physician stated had evidently been dead for some days. Before the birth the doctor diagnosed a right sided ovarian tumor of large dimensions. Both patient and the doctor thought that she had gone over her time about twenty days. After the labor there was a low grade fever, and she had vomited prior to coming to the hospital, so that the doctor suspected bowel obstruction.

On May 10, 5 days after labor, she was brought to the hospital. I found a rather tall, well-nourished woman, with an abdomen as large as it should be at term, but rather fat and flabby. Fluctuation could be made out over the whole abdomen, except the epigastrium and left iliac region. The fluctuating area was dull. Aside from the abdominal findings, the examination was negative. No bimanual examination was made. I thought I detected the uterus, as large as a cocoanut, to the left. The patient was having some "gas pains," the bowels were loose, no appetite, lochia normal, temperature 100° F. Diagnosis right ovarian cyst.

Operation 10 days after arrival at hospital. Through a midline incision a large cyst was uncovered, tapped, delivered, the pedicle tied in sections, and removed. Examination of the left side revealed another cyst, the size of a cocoanut, of the left ovary. This also was removed and the abdomen closed, without drainage, although many lymph splotches were noted on the peritoneum; there was a little fluid in the peritoneal cavity and both cysts were universally adherent by wet-paper adhesions. The patient's recovery was tedious and slow with a low grade fever, some tendency to gas pains and abdominal tenderness, especially in the gall bladder region. It should be remarked here that the cyst on the right side was plastered to the under surface of the liver. There was no tympany. Blood culture revealed a paratyphoid infection.

The patient was finally allowed to go home although she showed an evening rise in temperature at times as high as 100°. It should be stated here that the wound healed by first intention throughout; but at the end of three weeks, there were a few drops of whitish pus from the upper end of the incision. The bulk of the right cyst was a clear fluid although there was a considerable quantity of the usual emulsion. The fluid contents measured 9 quarts. The solid portion of the tumor consisted of teeth, hair, and skin. The left tumor was of the same general character as the right.

REMARKS

The operation was not done immediately on the patient's arrival at the hospital because she had not entirely recovered from a rather acute illness following her delivery, and because of the fear of an infection or other accident; and, it was also thought the tumor would interfere with involution. For these reasons it was thought wise to operate as above indicated. The outcome of the case to date is satisfactory. The question of a possible malignancy, however, leaves a fear in my mind that only time can either confirm or remove, for through carelessness the specimens were lost before a microscopic study of them had been made.

This case presents the following points which are of more than usual interest. The enormous size of the tumors without the patient's knowledge or suspicion that anything serious was wrong with her. Complete functioning of the ovaries, including pregnancy occurring in the presence of bilateral ovarian teratomata, child carried beyond term, born naturally but dead. The development of a paratyphoid infection during the puerperium. The time of operation for ovarian tumors during pregnancy and during the puerperium.

REFERENCES

Spalding: Am. Jour. Obst., 1919, lxxx, 401. *Hurdon, Kelly and Noble*: Gynecology and Abdominal Surgery, 1908, i, 198. *Adami and Nichols*: Principles of Pathology, 855. *Ewing*: Neoplastic Diseases, 1919, 593. *Douglas*: Surgical Diseases of the Abdomen, 1903, 780. *Bland-Sutton*: Tumors, Innocent and Malignant, 1908, ed. 4, p. 484. *Hertzler*: Treatise on Tumors, 1913, p. 623.

2326 FAIRFIELD AVENUE.

CONGENITAL MALFORMATION OF THE FEMALE GENITALIA

By Philip J. Reel, M.D., Columbus, Ohio

(*From the Department of Surgery and Gynecology, College of Medicine, Ohio State University.*)

REALDUS COLUMBUS in 1752 was first to record a case of congenital absence of the uterus and vagina. In 1777, Hill reported a case with absence of the uterus, tubes, ligaments, and vagina. Burrage was the first American author to write on this subject. In 1897 he found 360 cases of absent uterus recorded by 239 writers. The anatomical findings were presented in 35 cases, 24 of which were adults, 2 children, and the rest were monstrosities with various other malformations. Ovaries and tubes presenting a greater or lesser degree of development were found in all but six cases. In practically all the patients some pretense of vaginal formation was encountered, consisting in most instances of a blind sac. At the present time there are some 400 cases recorded.

The rarity alone would seem to be sufficient reason for recording the study of each case encountered.

Mrs. M. C., white, aged twenty-two, consulted me on June 9, 1921, complaining of amenorrhea and what she and her husband both stated as ''having very unsatisfactory sexual intercourse.'' She has never menstruated or experienced any form of vicarious bleeding. Since the age of fourteen years she has had periodic pain in the right lower abdomen lasting three or four days, associated with a sensitiveness of the breasts. During the past six months these pains have increased in severity. This patient experiences libido sexualis but complains because the introduction of the penis is obstructed about one and one-half inches from the vulvar orifice, causing pain.

Physical examination reveals a young woman of distinctly feminine type. The facial expression, hands, feet, hips, waist line, and bust are all decidedly characteristic of a well-developed young female. The mammary glands are well formed with protruding nipples. Pelvic examination shows the external genitalia to be normal in every respect. The pudendal hair is fine and ends abruptly in a transverse line across the lower abdomen. Vaginal examination reveals a small narrow blind pouch which admits two fingers with difficulty to the depth of about one and one-half inches. The membrane lining this sac is moist and sensitive. No cervix or fundus uteri can be palpated either by vaginal or rectal examination. Palpation in the tuboovarian regions causes some pain in the right side but no masses or irregularities are to be felt.

The patient was told that she had a congenital malformation which in all probability included an absence of the uterus. The periodic pain was attributed to a rudimentary misplaced tube which at times experienced the congestion of menstruation. Inasmuch as she was capable of libido sexualis we explained to her the operation advocated by Baldwin. After discussing the problem with her husband, she decided not to undergo the operation for formation of a new vagina, but requested an exploration for the purpose of determining and correcting if possible the cause of her attacks of periodic pain.

On June 22, 1921, under ether anesthesia the lower abdomen was opened and inspection revealed the pelvis to be clean and smooth, presenting a fold of peritoneum reflected from the bladder, with a free margin to either side, extending directly across to the lateral walls of the pelvis. Behind this the blind pouch of the vagina could easily be everted for one and one-half inches. The rectum was centrally placed, presenting no gross abnormalities. The sigmoid seemed to be more lateral than usual with but little mobility. On the left side at the brim of the pelvis was found a large elongated ovary firmly attached to the peritoneum. There was no evidence of a tube in this region. On the right side at the pelvic brim was found a second elongated and enlarged ovary held by a very firm and broad attachment to the parietal peritoneum. Behind and fastened to the under surface of the ovary was a very small rudimentary tube measuring 2 cm. in length. The fimbriated extremity was quite well developed. In front of the ovary, held by a fold of peritoneum, was a tumor mass 7 cm. in length and roughly pear-shaped in outline. The lower extremity faded gradually into the subperitoneal structures near the bladder. This mass and the rudimentary tube were removed. Both ovaries were allowed to remain. This possibility had been discussed prior to operation and she was advised that unless there were some definite indication for removal, it would be best to permit any ovarian tissues found to remain. Examination at the time of operation revealed nothing of note except that they both presented evidence of physiologic activity characterized by a recent mature graafian follicle in one and a rather large corpus luteum could be easily seen directly under the capsule of the other.

The cecum had practically no mobility, being held to the posterior abdominal wall by the parietal peritoneum. The appendix for 2 cm. at the cecal extremity was as wide as the normal ileum. The remainder was tubular and of the average dimensions. Several rather strong adhesive bands were present running from the appendix to the upper parietal wall of the pelvis. These were separated along with the routine appendectomy.

A general inspection of the remainder of the abdomen failed to reveal anything of note. The postoperative convalescence was uneventful and the patient reports herself at the present time (Jan. 1, 1922) as free from symptoms.

Gross section of the small tumor removed does not show any pretense of cavity formation. It resembles in the gross the structure of a typical fibroid. Under the microscope the same applies in that the structure comprises a dense connective tissue undergoing areas of hyaline degeneration associated with a very scant blood supply. In the outer third of a section of this fibrous tissue is found a very small tubular structure lined with mucous membrane. The cells are cuboid and columnar in type. There is no glandular arrangement found in the many sections studied. The presence of this rudimentary cavity lined with mucous membrane would seem to substantiate the opinion that this tumor was derived from the middle portion of the right müllerian duct. Microscopic section of the tube reveals nothing other than an atrophic development of all its coats.

The exact etiology of congenital maldevelopments of the female genitalia is still unsolved. Embryology can explain how the one differs from the normal in development but does not attempt a solution of why this occurs. Most authors agree with Kussmaul that the müllerian ducts in their middle and lower portions fuse to form the uterus and upper part of the vagina. The upper portions which remain unfused eventually become the fallopian tubes. The ovaries have their origin in the genital germinal parenchyma on either side of the wolffian bodies, on their vesical surfaces. The external genitalia arise from the urogenital sinus, the tubercle and the genital fold. Because of this it is possible, and in many instances the condition encountered, to find that the external development is normal, while the uterus and fallopian tubes or ovaries, or the uterus and the adnexa may be deformed. Such was the condition in the patient under discussion. The external genitalia were anatomically perfect while the vagina, uterus, and certain of the adnexa presented a marked deformity in development.

It would seem reasonable to interpret the findings as a total lack of development of the left müllerian duct inasmuch as there was no evidence on that side of its ever having been present. On the right side the condition varied in that a rudimentary tube and in addition a fibrous tumor mass closely associated to the tube and ovary was found which extended downward towards the vagina. This in all probability represents the efforts of the duct on this side to follow out its embryologic progression in the formation of a vagina and uterus. The fact that the upper portion of the müllerian duct does not fuse in the normal development but serves to form the fallopian tube would seem to substantiate the assumption that but one duct ever developed in this patient inasmuch as the right side only presented any evidence of its ever having been present.

SUMMARY

Congenital maldevelopments of the female genitalia are of sufficient rarity to warrant a study and report of each case encountered. The patient used as a basis for this discussion was a young woman presenting in every respect typical feminine characteristics in external physcial development while the internal genital tract revealed an absence of one tube, the uterus, and vagina. That the rudimentary structures on the right side at times endeavored to undergo some menstrual change seems logical since she has been entirely free from attacks of periodic pain in this region since their removal by operation. Embryology can explain why certain portions of the generative apparatus can develop into normal proportions but cannot offer at this time a solution of the problem concerning the primary etiologic factors entering into the causation of the maldevelopments.

BIBLIOGRAPHY

Barne, C.: Am. Jour. Insanity, April, 1895, li. 475. *Bins, F.*: Monatschr. Geburtsh. u. Gynäk., 1920, liii, 176. *Bridgeman, W. E.*: Med. Stand., 1896, xviii, 1904. *Burrage*: Am. Jour. Med. Sc., 1897, cxli, 310. *Chowdry, B. K. (India)*: New York Med. Jour., 1914, c, 471. *Coleman, M. A.*: Med. Stand., Aug., 1895, xvii, 254. *Cotterill, J. M.*: Brit. Med. Jour., April 7, 1900, p. 837. *Macnaughton*: Brit. Gynec. Jour., April, 1902. *Mundé, P. F.*: Am. Jour. Obst., Mar., 1899. *Parakh, F. R.*: Brit. Med. Jour., 1919, ii, 496. *Robertson, B. O.*: South. Med. Jour., 1920, xiii, 206. *Robinson, M. R.*: Surg. Gynec. and Obst., 1920, xxxi, No. 1, p. 51. *Thorell, M.*: Ann. de gynéc. et d'obst., 1918-19, xiv, 2nd. ser., p. 294.

A METHOD OF KEEPING FALLOPIAN TUBES OPEN

BY WILLIAM T. KENNEDY, M.D., NEW YORK, N. Y.

INTRODUCTION

THE insufflation of the fallopian tubes with CO_2 gas as done by Rubin[1] has led to the detection of obstructions which produce sterility. After the diagnosis of occluded tubes has been established and there is no evidence of acute or subacute salpingitis, a laparotomy is done, adhesions about the fimbriae of the tubes are separated, and a resection of either tube is done when necessary. Some material is now required to preserve the patency of the tubes. Huber[2] experimentally has observed the superiority of alcoholized tissue in nerve surgery. For some time I have used Cargile membrane hardened in alcohol for at least 48 hours, threading it through the fallopian tubes and the cavity of the uterus to keep these tubes open both into the uterine cavity and into the peritoneal cavity. The membrane is flexible and strong, nonirritating to the contact tissues and is slowly absorbed, giving all raw surfaces time to heal and allowing this part of the genital tract to remain patent.

TECHNIC

The accompanying diagram (Fig. 1) illustrates the apparatus used and the method of procedure.

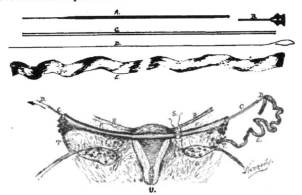

Fig. 1.—*A*, silver probe—length about 10 cm.; diameter .75 mm. to 1.00 mm., having a bristle about .45 mm. in diameter mounted in one end. *B*, cannula—to attach a Luer hypodermic syringe at one end and a hollow probe *C* at the other. *C*, hollow silver probe—length about 25 cm., diameter the same as *A*. *D*, strand of piano wire—about 3 cm. longer than *C*, looped at one end to serve as a membrane carrier. *E*, strip of Cargile membrane about 40 cm. long and 3 cm. wide. *F*, Fallopian tubes. *U*, uterus. *O*, ovary. *R*, round ligament. *T*, point of attachment of one end of the membrane. *S*, plastic sutures to anastomose the excised ends after a resection.

The Probe A is passed down the fallopian canal. The bristle enters first the isthmus of the tube, then the uterine cavity, directs the probe and makes the canal large enough to allow the passage of Probe C. Probe A is now removed and used to treat the other tube in the same manner. If there are any signs of an old inflammatory process each fallopian tube can be slowly irrigated from the fimbria into the uterine cavity with alcohol, using the Luer syringe attached to B and C. If for any reason the resection of a part of either tube is found necessary, that should now be done. Then thread Probe C through one fallopian tube, the cavity of the uterus, and the other fallopian tube as illustrated. Insert and tie all plastic sutures, S with C in position, to eliminate any possible obliteration of the canal. Now insert D into C and thread E on the wire loop, withdraw C, D and E together and leave the membrane through this part of the genital tract. Thread one end of the membrane on a round needle, pass it through the portion of the broad ligament at T and ligate it. Fasten the other end in the same manner to the other broad ligament at T. This will leave a loop of the membrane in the peritoneal cavity at each side to accommodate a possible pregnancy before the membrane becomes absorbed.

All cases diagnosed as acute or subacute salpingitis must wait at least six months and the treatment of any such cases not suspected on diagnosing, but so found by laparotomy, must be postponed. The procedure takes from 10 to 30 minutes. Accessory, malposition and other pathological conditions are treated when indicated.

REFERENCES

(1) Jour. Am. Med. Assn., lxxv, 661. Am. Jour. Roentgen., March, 1921, p. 120.
(2) Surg., Gynec. and Obst., May, 1920, p. 464.

163 EAST SIXTY-FIRST STREET.

IS CONSERVATIVE OBSTETRICS TO BE ABANDONED?

By W. C. Danforth, B.S., M.D., F.A.C.S., Evanston, Ill.

THE past three or four years have brought forth a number of new ideas in the way of routine delivery of normal or approximately normal cases. The parturient woman is entitled to and should receive all amelioration of suffering which may safely be given her, that is, without endangering her or her child. Efforts to diminish the duration and suffering of labor are commendable, provided they genuinely accomplish the objects sought for, and provided, also, that operative measures which are made use of in the effort to accomplish this end, are carried out by men of sufficient technical skill and of judgment sufficiently mature that the operation itself does not become a menace.

It may well be questioned whether the routine teaching of operative measures which are to be employed generally to classes of students is wise. Indeed it is a grave question whether the teaching of such methods to the profession as a whole is justified. In such teaching must be included the description of methods in widely circulated periodicals. Such publication must necessarily indicate the recommendation of the author for the procedure and the caution, often added, that certain operative procedures are for the experienced operator only, does but little good, for there are not wanting in every community of any size, men who do not hesitate to attempt any operative maneuver, obstetric or otherwise, with a minimum of preparation or with none whatever.

At a recent meeting, the able director of a well-known clinic in an eastern city presented some interesting statistics pertaining to a series of 1000 ward cases delivered in that clinic, demonstrating very well the results of an expectant plan of treatment, seconded, when definite indications existed, by expert operative intervention. The results, as indicated by fetal mortality, maternal mortality and morbidity, and showing a low incidence of operative intervention were excellent. The essayist, however, stated that in dealing with his private work the operative incidence ran higher. This, of course, is the experience of every obstetric specialist, as his practice tends to include a greater number of cases in which intervention of some sort is unavoidable.

It is with the desire of showing that, in a series of cases which includes a considerable number of private patients, expectant methods not only are possible, but will yield good results, that this series is reported.

It includes first my own private work composed of cases largely coming from a district containing probably as large a proportion of people of comfortable means as any residential section anywhere, and a very fair number of families, the female members of which have been accustomed to every luxury that ample means may procure, in short, the class of women among whom it is said that revolt against the normal processes of labor exists. Among the number, too, are a considerable number of cases who come, as they come to all men who specialize, because of trouble in a previous labor, or who are sent by their physicians because of anticipated pathology. A number of these had come long distances for some of the reasons named. It includes the cases of the junior attending man and also of a number of other members of the hospital staff who all follow our definitely established technic and who are usually prompt to call assistance in case of grave pathology. It includes also a modest number of ward cases which were delivered by internes under the supervision of the junior attending man. These were less than 20 per cent of the whole number.

The cases number 500,—multiparae 283 and primiparae 217. Our cases are drawn as indicated above from a neighborhood in which malnutrition is rare and the women are largely of native extraction, hence pelvic deformity is uncommon. There was one case of generally contracted and five of simple flat pevis.

Cephalic presentation occurred as follows: L. O. A. 330—66 per cent; R. O. P. 65—13 per cent; R. O. A. 40—8 per cent; L. O. P. 1.7 per cent; and Face 1—0.2 per cent.

Posterior positions were treated expectantly and the greater number of them rotated anteriorly without interference. The remainder were delivered by operative means.

Abnormal presentations included the following: Breech 28; Prolapse of arm 1; and Prolapse of cord 4.

The incidence of operative intervention included 12 high, 25 mid and 61 low forceps, a total of 98, or 19.6 per cent.

Version was done 9 times, breech extraction 18, cesarean section 8, induction of labor by bag 19; and the uterus packed 9 times.

The incidence of operation in this series is larger than in the report alluded to above, but a series containing a large proportion of private patients must contain more cases needing intervention of some sort than one composed purely of clinic cases. What I desire to bring out is, that private patients will go through normal labor without a demand for routine shortening of the normal processes of parturition by operative methods. The low forceps deliveries were done after a reasonable delay on the perineum, and in estimating what is reasonable, we are accustomed to give the mother the benefit of the doubt and to interfere after a short time if progress is not continuing. We auscultate the heart tones frequently as the head nears the perineum, using the head stethoscope of Hillis, interfering at once if notable slowing in the fetal heart rate is apparent. Cragin reported a series of 500 private cases in which the frequency of forceps was 22.6 per cent. This is about the same frequency as we note in this series. Cragin also reported an incidence of forceps of 12.3 per cent in 20,000 cases in the Sloane Hospital.

I am strongly in favor of episiotomy in primiparae, should laceration appear likely, and believe that spontaneous delivery will occur if it is used in some cases which without it would require application of forceps. I believe, also, that if this is done, it should be done before the perineum is greatly stretched in order to avoid damage to the perineal structures. It has seemed to me that a better ultimate result is obtained when one repairs a clean incision through structures, the integrity of which has not been impaired by too great stretching and possible submucous separation than by allowing either a laceration or submucous injury to occur. Inspection of a large number of these, six to eight weeks after labor has shown that satisfactory results are obtained.

Version has been used only on definite indication, in this series for prolapsed cord three times, placenta previa twice, and for a compound presentation, with one arm prolapsed, once.

While admitting the skill in the performance of version which is possessed by the foremost advocate of its elective use and admitting also the elaboration of its technic which has resulted from his work, we cannot agree with the indications for which he does this operation. Our own corrected fetal mortality in labor of 1.4 per cent with expectant methods supplemented by operative intervention when indicated, as compared with a rate of 7.5 per cent with routine elective version will speak for the correctness of this view. One of the followers of the originator of the method of elective version publishes fetal mortality rates of 8 per cent to 17.5 per cent. Surely this is too high a price to pay for a little shortening of the normal course of labor, particularly when the pain of the second stage can be so greatly mitigated as is possible today. Some of the cases in the report last referred to were delivered by beginners. A high degree of operative skill cannot be expected when that is the case. However, one may not unreasonably argue from that fact that operative work should be taught only to those who have attained proficiency in normal work.

Our use of the bag practically is limited to induction of labor for toxemia and for placenta previa. For induction of labor in cases other than these, castor oil and quinine with digital loosening of the membranes is used, and even in the milder degrees of toxemia, where need for haste is not so apparent, it is first tried. It is very rarely used for the treatment of contracted pelvis, and in this year's work, has not been so used at all.

My experience with the bag corresponds with that of some other observers. I have not found that it will always accomplish the result we desire. Many of us have introduced bags, only to find that after the expulsion of the bag labor ceases. I saw in consultation one case this year, a para 3, in which three bags had been used in a mild case of toxemia, labor ceasing on the expulsion of each bag. It was advised to let the woman alone as the toxemia was not alarming. Two days later she delivered herself precipitately. It must, of course, be admitted, that in reserving the bag for those cases which have proved refractory to less vigorous measures, causes it to be applied in those which are hardest to bring into labor, hence we have a larger proportion of unsatisfactory results than in services in which it is more routinely used. We cannot fail to recognize the danger of infection which accompanies the use of hydrostatic bags. Even though this, in well run institutions and with a proper technic, may be greatly reduced, still the introduction and retention of the bag within the uterus must carry with it some slight risk of infection. I have been asked to see two cases in which intrapartum rise of temperature had followed the introduction of in one case two, and in another, three bags.

Cesarean section was done more frequently than would be the case in a series composed of clinic cases exclusively. This is because of the number of women coming in with the history of a former disastrous labor, or who were sent by their physicians because of fear of possible complications. The indications shown in Table I were present in our series.

TABLE I

Flat pelvis,—previous child lost—test of labor	2
Primiparity at 43 with toxemia—rigid cervix	2
Flat pelvis, (prior section in Europe)	1
Flat pelvis,—primipara,—test of labor	1
Flat pelvis,—transverse position,—primipara—no test of labor	1
Generally contracted pelvis,—previous pubiotomy	1

We have tried to limit abdominal section to those cases in which reasonable indication existed. It was adopted in the cases of the elderly primiparae because it seemed likely that labor would be difficult, and because the mothers were extremely desirous of saving the babies, as they represented probably their only chances for children. The indication is, of course, relative, but, I believe, fair. The constantly widening indications which are being invoked for the employment of this operation should be carefully scrutinized, even though we admit the great value of the operation in properly selected cases. In the lesser degrees of pelvic contraction, the high percentage of cases in which spontaneous delivery occurs, or in which delivery may finally be accomplished by simple low forceps, has caused us to be slow to adopt this mode of delivery without a preliminary trial of labor, which often demonstrates the lack of need of section. In addition to the cases of flat pelvis shown in Table I as sectioned after a trial of labor there were a larger number in whom the possibility of operation was considered, but which delivered either spontaneously or with the aid of forceps. In one case, in which the possibility of section was considered, labor was allowed to proceed with the idea of terminating if necessary after a thorough trial of labor by a low section. The head however after some time engaged and the labor was ended by forceps. The child did not do well and died in 48 hours. Autopsy showed no cranial injury whatever but that atelectasis was the cause of death. It is a question whether, had early section been done, the child would not have been lost from the same cause. We employ section but rarely in placenta previa and have not treated a case by section in the past four or five years. It is not excluded and would be considered in a perfectly clean case, with undilated cervix, with a central previa and preferably in a primipara. Such cases are, however, rare.

Complications of pregnancy included: toxemia 11; cardiac disease 1; placenta previa 5; placenta ablata 2; hydramnion 8; and prolapse of cord 6.

Excluding 5 premature babies and considering those delivered at or near term the fetal mortality is as follows: dead at delivery 10; dead after delivery 8; hemorrhage 2; malformation 3 including one each of anencephalus, spina bifida, and cleft palate harelip.

The smallest child which we were successful in saving weighed just over three pounds at birth, the weight declining to two pounds, fourteen ounces. For co-operation in cases of this sort, in case of hemorrhage of the newborn, and in fact in all matters pertaining to the babies, I am under obligation to the attending pediatrician and his associates, who assume entire charge of them.

The difference in mortality rate between that which I have just given and those obtained by elective version are sufficiently striking. Let me emphasize again that immediate intervention in the second stage is done when auscultation indicates any fetal danger. Furthermore, the mother is never allowed indefinitely to exhaust herself at this time in the absence of definite progress.

Complications affecting the mothers. Rupture of uterus, 1; postpartum hemorrhage, 11; suppurative mastitis, 1; infection, 1; embolism, 1; deaths, 2.

Of the two deaths, that charged to embolism was unavoidable. The woman bled moderately severely, the uterus was packed at once by the junior attending man who was her attendant, but she became promptly cyanotic although the pulse rate did not go over 100. She died in an hour. In reviewing this case later I could not see that anything had been overlooked which should have been done. There was no autopsy. The other death followed a version done in a case of placenta previa by an interne before the arrival of the junior attending man. The rupture was not detected by an intrauterine revision of the field after the operation and its presence was not suspected until too late. Autopsy showed a tear upward on the right side in the region of the broad ligament with retroperitoneal bleeding. It is fair to ask ourselves whether this case should not have been saved.

Our mortality from all causes up to the end of labor was 2 per cent. Of children born dead at term there were 10. Of these one was a case of toxemia in which the child was dead at the onset of labor and one was the child of a woman with a flat pelvis, admitted after many hours of labor, with the cord and one arm prolapsed and the child already dead. This case was treated by craniotomy. Eight, therefore, were living at the onset of labor and died during or immediately after labor. One of these was an anencephalus; one died immediately after delivery in a case of placenta previa treated by metreurysis and version, one of asphyxiation caused by the cord being around the neck and one arm, one following a high forceps delivery and three were breech cases, two complicated by prolapse of the cord. Two of these were service cases and three were patients of physicians not especially interested in obstetrics. Concerning three of these cases, the high forceps and the breech cases not complicated by cord prolapse and the baby lost by asphyxiation due to the cord being around the neck and arm, we may inquire whether better obstetrics might not have saved one or two of the babies.

There were eleven premature babies, reckoning all born before the beginning of the ninth month as premature. Of these four were saved and the remainder lost. Five of the seven which were lost were less than seven months.

Of babies born alive but dying before the mother's discharge, there were eight. One of these was the smaller one of a pair of twins, the other twin surviving. One was a child referred to above which died of atelectasis as shown by autopsy. Another died of atelectasis two days after delivery, no autopsy. One was a spina bifida which lived one day. Another was a child which lived thirty-six hours after a normal delivery, but was constantly cyanotic. Autopsy showed an unusually large opening in the interventricular septum which had failed to close. Another was a child delivered by breech extraction in a primiparous labor. This child lived 24 hours and died, probably of cerebral injury. No autopsy was obtained.

The total number of deaths, therefore, was 18. This includes all deaths up to the time of the mother's discharge and gives a total infant mortality of 3.06 per cent. Obviously we cannot be charged with the loss of the child which was dead at the time its parturient mother was admitted nor with the loss of the anencephalic child as neither of these was lost as a result of our obstetric errors. Allowing for these gives a corrected fetal mortality in labor of 1.4 per cent. We may ask ourselves whether some of these could not have been saved.

Of those dying before the mother's discharge, it seems fair to assume that neither the spina bifida nor the loss of the tiny twin could be ascribed to technical errors. The loss of the child with the patent ductus botalli could also not be ascribed to lack of skill on the part of the physician. The corrected mortality for this group would be 1 per cent, or a total corrected mortality previous to discharge of 2.4 per cent. In estimating these mortalities I have not included premature babies, as the loss of these infants is as a rule not fairly chargeable against obstetric errors.

The results of a series of 167 cases under my own care, almost all of which form part of the large series discussed already, are as follows: L. O. A., 122; R. O. P., 28; O. D. A., 2; L. O. P., 4; breech, 3. Operative incidence in this series is as follows: Low forceps, 33; mid forceps, 7; high forceps, 5; version, 1; cesarean section, 6.

There were four premature deliveries counting those prior to the end of the eighth month as premature. Of these three were less than seven months and were lost. Two of these were dead on admission, one on account of a severe toxemia and another following a separation of the placenta in a woman who had a chronic nephritis. The fourth one was a baby of a little over seven months which lived.

There were no maternal deaths. Of fetal deaths during or immediately following labor at term there were two, one due to asphyxia caused by the cord being around the neck and one arm, and one case in which the child died about half an hour after delivery in a case of placenta previa treated by version. This was a referred case, considerable bleeding having occurred before the case arrived in the hospital.

One death occurred forty-eight hours after labor, this being the one alluded to before in which death was the result of atalectasis as shown by autopsy, the child having been delivered by forceps in a case of flat pelvis.

The total fetal mortality at term from all causes in this series is 3, a percentage of 1.79 per cent from all causes up to the time of discharge. This of course represents results attained by rigid prenatal observation with immediate meeting of any indication disclosed by observation and immediate admission to the hospital and constant observation after the onset of labor. Forceps incidence in this series is 26.9 per cent, considerably higher than the percentage for the entire year's work in the maternity, but this smaller series contains a very much larger number of women who had had previous difficult labors or who were referred because of complications present or feared.

It has been interesting to note, as indicating the comparative results of hospital obstetrics as compared with that carried out in homes, the difference in the fetal mortality in the large series reported in this paper and that reported for the Municipality of Evanston. The latter was almost 50 per cent greater. When one considers that this district contains only a very small number of midwives, that the general average of the medical practitioners is above that found in most areas of Chicago or indeed any large city which would correspond in size to the district considered here, and finally that the figures above considered as well as all deaths reported from a neighboring hospital within the town are reckoned into the report of mortality from the whole town, it would seem a striking argument in favor of the safety of carefully conducted institutional work.

This comparison becomes more striking if one considers that our hospital series contains many cases from the northern part of Chicago and elsewhere, a considerable portion of which had come because of former abnormality or fear of complications.

The safety of institutional methods, however, it seems fair to conclude, depends very largely upon the judgment and skill of those who determine them. We believe that a watchful conservatism, allowing the forces of Nature to accomplish delivery if possible, with careful operative interference at once upon proper indication, still remains the safest standard of obstetric practice.

800 DAVIS STREET.

A DEVICE FOR ASEPTIC INTRAUTERINE MANIPULATIONS*

By F. C. Hendrickson, M.D., Cincinnati, Ohio

THE maintenance of asepsis during intravaginal or intrauterine manipulations in the pregnant woman has always been difficult, if not impossible, and many methods and devices[1] have been designed to maintain asepsis. The writer has developed an apparatus and a method which he believes makes possible an almost perfect asepsis in performing any of the ordinary obstetrical manipulations except the cutting operations. This means that when the writer's device is used there need be no fear of infecting a parturient woman such as by a manual removal of adherent placenta, even though the woman should have a suppurating bartholinitis.

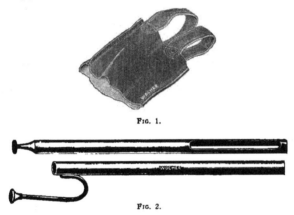

Fig. 1.

Fig. 2.

The fact that the device really works and is convenient to use in practice was demonstrated by its use in fifty obstetrical cases in the Cincinnati General Hospital. Besides the routine vaginal examination, some of the operations in which the device has been used are as follows: high forceps delivery, insertion of the Braun bag into the vagina, inspection and repair of the lacerated cervix following delivery, podalic version and extraction, manual dilatation of the cervix, and digital removal of products of conception following incomplete abortion.

The apparatus consists of two parts, namely, a "vulvar shield" (Fig. 1) which is a cylinder of cambric rubber sheeting with loops attached, and a "shield

---
[1]Kuhn: Am. J. Obst. & Gyn., 1921, 721.
*Received for publication, January 25, 1922.

everter'' (Fig. 2) made of two pieces of nickel-plated brass tubing with thumb pieces.

The technic for using the device is as follows: sterilization is first accomplished by autoclaving the shield and by boiling the shield everter. The parts are then ready to be assembled by the nurse, who works with sterile gloves. The rubber

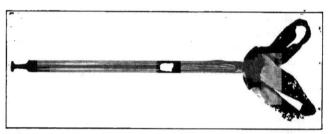

FIG. 3.

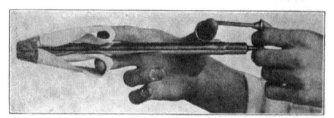

FIG. 4.

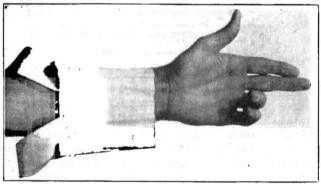

FIG. 5.

side of the shield is turned outward and is lubricated with a sterilized solution made up with soft soap (U. S. P.) 2 ounces, in 4 ounces of water. The shield is then tightly folded and inserted into the inner tube as illustrated in Fig. 3. The outer tube is now slipped over the inner tube so that the two tubes occupy the relative positions shown in Fig. 4.

When ready to examine the patient the accoucheur should take the device as assembled and proceed as follows: the barrel of the shield everter is lubricated with the soap emulsion. The cuff of the protruding shield is turned down over the end of the shield everter and the loops and handles are grasped as shown in Fig. 4. The cuff of the shield is inserted just into the introitus of the vagina. About three pounds steady traction are applied on the loops of the shield and at the same time an in-and-out piston-like motion is imparted to the inner tube, the excursions of which should be about ½ inch. With each excursion of the inner tube the shield is pushed a little way into the vagina.

It will be seen that the shield is fed into the vagina in such a way that there is no sliding motion along the walls of the vagina, but that the shield rolls from within outward and therefore absolutely avoids the transference of bacteria from the vaginal walls up to the uterus. Herein lies the fundamental idea of the device. Each part of the shield is protected in its upward passage until it is everted out against the vaginal wall where it is to stay permanently, neither sliding up nor down. The instrument is now withdrawn, leaving the shield in the vagina.

After thorough lubrication with the soap solution the hand, or any instrument, may be easily introduced through the shield into the uterus without having come in contact with the external genitalia or with the walls of the vagina. This absolutely rules out the possibility of transference of any infectious material that might come from the genital tract lying below the cervix. The examining fingers pass safely up through the shield regardless of the number of bacteria on the external genitalia.

If it is desired merely to examine the woman digitally, the two fingers are introduced through the shield up to the cervix uteri and then the shield is drawn out of the vagina up over the forearm (Fig. 5) leaving the examining fingers unhampered in their manipulations. It is to be noted that in cases of manual removal of placenta or in podalic version and extraction that the shield is removed before the extraction of the placenta or the baby. After the application of the blades in a forceps operation, the shield is withdrawn over the handles of the forceps and laid aside. In the same manner the shield may be removed after the aseptic application of a sterile speculum.

In every instance where the device has been used it has worked perfectly just as described. It is not adapted to low forceps operations though it works well with high forceps. Neither is it adapted to any of the cutting operations such as vaginal hysterotomy, curettage, etc. Strangely enough it has been found that the shield facilitates passing the hand into a small vagina. The reason for this is that the labia are prevented from rolling inward by traction on the loops of the shield.

It is the writer's belief that the device should be used routinely in practically all obstetrical manipulations, and especially in the manual removal of placenta and in the routine vaginal examination. It is a safe and convenient expedient in preliminary vaginal examinations where the pubic hair has not been shaved and in cases of suppurative bartholinitis. Furthermore, it would seem that the practice of vaginal examination through the shield should to a large extent supplant the practice of rectal touch as used so commonly at the present time.

CINCINNATI GENERAL HOSPITAL.

TREATMENT OF CARDIAC FAILURE DURING PREGNANCY*

By Harold E. B. Pardee, M.D., New York, N. Y.

I DESIRE at the outset to make a distinction between the importance of cardiac disease during pregnancy and of cardiac failure during pregnancy and to explain exactly what I wish to have understood by the term cardiac failure. Evident cardiac disease with loud murmurs may be present without any sign of cardiac failure. Mitral regurgitation, or mitral stenosis, or aortic regurgitation or combinations of these may exist and yet the patient may not be conscious even after ordinary exercise of any abnormality of the heart. Such a person has cardiac disease but not cardiac failure. On the other hand even a normal person will suffer from breathlessness or palpitation after exercise, if only the exercise is sufficiently strenuous or prolonged. This breathlessness is due to a cardiac failure which might be called physiologic. Pathologic failure is present when these symptoms make their appearance after exertions which the person was formerly able to undertake without causing them, and it is this degree of cardiac failure which concerns us at present.

One will realize readily that there will be many grades of cardiac failure. The mildest sort is shown by the patient who complains of an unusual breathlessness after climbing two or more flights of stairs, and the most severe sort by a patient in whom even the exertion of turning over in bed causes palpitation and shortness of breath.

When considering cardiac failure during pregnancy we must bear in mind that a normal woman who becomes pregnant will find her ability to exercise without causing dyspnea and palpitation is less than it was in her nonpregnant state. Such a degree of cardiac failure during pregnancy is physiologic and not abnormal. There are also many women otherwise normal, who develop more or less edema of the legs during pregnancy because of pressure upon the veins by the pregnant uterus, so that if a patient with heart disease shows a slight limitation of her ability to exercise during pregnancy, and perhaps also a certain amount of edema of the legs we must not feel that these signs are a cause of alarm.

There is a long standing tradition in medicine, supported by even so high an authority as Sir James Mackenzie,[1] that mitral stenosis is

---
*Read before the Section on Obstetrics and Gynecology of the New York Academy of Medicine, January 24, 1922.

The observations upon which these statements are based were made at the New York Lying-In Hospital through the kindness of Dr. Asa B. Davis. The author wishes to thank Dr. Davis and the others of the attending staff for their cooperation and their interest in the work.

a most serious lesion for the pregnant woman. This has not been my experience at all, for though some patients with mitral stenosis have been the cause of much trouble and anxiety, yet others have gone through with no untoward event, their hearts behaving quite as if there were no cardiac disease at all. I believe that the reason for this impression of the seriousness of mitral stenosis is, that there are twice as many patients with mitral stenosis as with aortic disease. It would be reasonable then to have twice as much trouble from the former patients as from the latter if the lesions were of equal gravity. As a matter of fact 4 of the 8 uncomplicated aortic cases which I have observed have had serious heart failure, while only 4 of 17 uncomplicated mitral stenosis cases had serious heart failure. Certainly from this experience mitral stenosis does not seem to be as dangerous as aortic regurgitation.

When a pregnant woman presents herself with evident signs of cardiac disease, we are less concerned with the nature of the disease than with the finding of symptoms or signs of cardiac failure, and with a determination of the severity of these symptoms or signs. This question of the fitness for pregnancy is a difficult one of itself and is being dealt with elsewhere. The subject I wish to emphasize at present is the treatment of those patients who show signs or symptoms of cardiac failure.

Two factors are of prime importance in the treatment of such a woman, and their importance is almost equal though in a quite different way. One is the degree or the relative severity of the patient's cardiac failure, while the other is whether we first see the patient before or after labor has set in.

SEVERE FAILURE DURING LABOR

The most dangerous situation is that of severe cardiac failure which has come on during labor. The patient may have had much shortness of breath on exertion during her pregnancy or she may have had but little. The important thing is that during labor it has been noticed and has become steadily more severe. The pulse is rapid, 120 or more per minute, and there may be a marked sense of suffocation with cyanosis and the coughing up of a pinkish frothy mucus. The patient is unable to lie down because of the dyspnea. The lungs show diffuse râles and the veins of the neck are much distended. This is the extreme picture of severe decompensation with edema of the lungs and shows that the heart has been severely overtaxed by the strain of labor. It is an acute decompensation or at least an acute exacerbation of one of lesser grade, and since the strain of labor was the provocation, the indication for treatment is an imperative one to do away with this strain and at the same time to treat the acute cardiac failure.

A hypodermic of morphine sulphate ¼ grain along with atropine sulphate $\frac{1}{50}$ grain helps these patients greatly, so does phlebotomy, if the neck veins are markedly distended, withdrawing enough blood to relieve the distention. From 6 to 8 or 10 ounces will usually suffice. If the patient has not had digitalis previously she should receive digitoxin intravenously in a single dose of $\frac{1}{60}$ of a grain, which should not be repeated as it is half of the average therapeutic dose. If digitalis has been given previously we cannot give an intravenous dose without knowing exactly how much the patient has received.

If the morphine stops the labor temporarily so much the better,—for the patient and the patient's heart will have a temporary rest. Operative interference at such a juncture is a very bad risk, but if labor continues, or starts up again and there is no indication that the treatment has helped the heart to regain control of the circulation, then the uterus should be emptied as quickly and with as little manipulation of the mother as possible. I feel that abdominal section is the best method if the head is high and a forceps extraction if it is in a low position. Do not move the patient from her home to a hospital without bearing in mind that the strain of the removal on a heart in this precarious state of compensation may be the deciding factor against her recovery. I would object to version because of the shock which accompanies intrauterine manipulations, and to vaginal section because it is a slower process and accompanied by more trauma to the patient than is the abdominal operation. It seems to me necessary to consider the effect of operative manipulations on the mother.

I believe that ether preceded by a small amount of chloroform is a better anesthetic than gas and oxygen because of the strain on the heart. I have seen an attack of acute decompensation brought on by the giving of gas to lance an infected finger, the patient being in the sixth month at the time and later going through a labor which was accelerated by version and rapid extraction of the child, without showing signs of more than slight embarrassment of the heart.

SEVERE FAILURE DURING PREGNANCY

Patients may have a severe acute decompensation during pregnancy at any time after the second or third month, because of excessive physical activity, either prolonged or of an acute nature. I have known sexual intercourse to cause this in several cases. Treatment of these patients is in no respect different from that described above except that if other measures fail to diminish the cyanosis, inhalations of oxygen are indicated. The reduction of cyanosis must be of great benefit to the heart muscle, for this likewise suffers from lack of oxygen.² The heart can often be observed to slow down when the cyanosis is diminished. Oxygen must be given from a closed inhaler or by nasal tube for at least 10- or 15-minute periods or more to be sure of producing its full effect. The pulmonary edema makes it difficult to get the gas into contact with the pulmonary capillaries. The objection to giving it to a case in labor is that it may, by preventing sleep, keep the morphine from checking the labor and giving the heart a much needed rest.

Operative interference of any sort is extremely dangerous when the heart is severely decompensated even when the patient is not in labor and therefore should not be undertaken unless there are indications that the compensation will fail still further, and that the patient is not reacting to treatment. If it is considered imperative for either of these reasons, then I feel that abdominal section is the operation of choice for the reasons which have been already mentioned.

When the patient has regained her compensation—and it is our experience that they always have done so from the first attack, though not always from a later one—then it is advisable to consider very carefully whether the pregnancy should be allowed to proceed to term. The question to be faced is how much chance we shall take with the mother's life in order that this child shall be borne. How important is it that she should have this child?

In some cases pregnancy will proceed successfully and uneventfully even after a severe decompensation, while in other cases it does not. It is beyond our present knowledge to determine with exactness whether a given woman will or will not have trouble during labor. Difficult labor will be more likely in a primipara with a large child however, and so cardiac failure will be more likely under these circumstances than if a multipara should have a precipitate delivery of a seven or eight months' child.

If we are willing to take a certain chance, I believe that even a woman who has had an acute decompensation during pregnancy can be safely carried along with proper medical supervision as will be detailed later. If she should have a second acute attack, the uterus should be emptied as soon as compensation is sufficiently regained, but with proper care a second acute attack will but rarely occur. Such a patient should never be allowed to go longer than the fortieth week of gestation, for a large child will be an added strain at delivery. To be safe on this point, if we think that the pelvis is small or if the woman is a primipara, it might be better to induce labor before this time. Opinions differ as to whether induced labor at the eighth month is easier than at term. The features of the individual case will often be decisive on this point.

When labor starts we must watch very carefully for the first indication that the heart is not standing the strain, and be ready to perform an abdominal section, unless the head should be in a position for a quick forceps delivery. Here again the shock of a version seems to contraindicate this procedure, and a high forceps operation or a vaginal section is too slow a method for the emergency of a failing heart. We must do away with the strain of the labor, with as little trauma to the patient as possible.

The indications of heart failure during labor which should point to prompt interference are a quickening of the pulse to over 95 per minute, or of the respiration to over 25 per minute, or the appearance of any sensation of distress such as dyspnea, or cough, or precordial discomfort. The more of these signs or symptoms that appear the more urgent the state of the patient. We should never wait for marked dyspnea and a pulse of 120 or more, for the strain of operation at that time will almost surely be too much for the already overtaxed heart. Watch the patient from the beginning of labor, and if the pulse or respiration is increasing I believe it is safer for both mother and child to operate at once, than to wait in the hope that delivery will take place before the strain has resulted fatally for the mother. We should operate when the decompensation is slight or moderate, in order to avoid having to operate when it is severe.

LESSER GRADES OF FAILURE

In regard to patients with lesser grades of heart failure it is difficult to make general statements which will apply equally to every case. There is, besides the variation in the degree of cardiac insufficiency from one patient to another, a variation in the same patient from time to time. Some patients grow worse during the course of their pregnancy, while others improve surprisingly in their cardiac power. Moreover there is the greatest variety in the activities which different women pursue during pregnancy, and the more active woman is naturally more liable to overstrain her heart.

I would never advise abortion or premature delivery before the eighth month unless it had first been demonstrated that with proper treatment by rest and digitalis, the signs and symptoms of cardiac failure were persistently increasing.

At the outset of treatment the patient should be kept in bed. This applies not only to the severe cases, but also to the mild cases of decompensation, and they should be kept there as long as any noteworthy increase in the pulse or respiration results from such efforts as sitting up or turning over in bed. They will usually be more comfortable in bed with a backrest on account of the dyspnea. When the patient is able to move about freely in bed without any discomfort from her heart she should be allowed to try the effect of sitting in a chair. If this causes no fatigue or dyspnea or palpitation, she may, after being in the chair a few hours each day for from seven to ten days, be allowed to walk a few steps. If this does not cause discomfort she may gradually be up more and more, always keeping short of any exertion which is followed by palpitation or a sense of shortness of breath or any other discomfort. As long as she keeps this principle in mind she will not harm her heart by overstrain.

When the patient is allowed to be up the pulse rate should be taken twice daily and she should be carefully questioned from time to time as to what she is doing and what abnormal sensations, if any, may arise. If she is of the type who persist in doing more than they should, then she must be kept in her room or in the house or even in bed if necessary to prevent this overdoing. Similar patients when not pregnant feel better and do better when they are allowed a certain degree of freedom and activity than when kept closely confined, and though my experience with such patients during pregnancy is more limited than with uncomplicated cardiac failure of the same degree, yet I have seen nothing to make me feel that the treatment should be any different in principle merely because of the abdominal tumor and the increased vascularity of the uterus, though it is plain enough that the same degree of activity is more strain during pregnancy than before.

If a patient who is allowed up does not continue her improvement, or if the pulse tends to remain above 85 per minute, then it is likely that a further period of two or three weeks' rest in bed or sitting about her room will be helpful in improving her compensation. Her heart was evidently having too frequent demands upon it and rest is needed to allow it to recover from its state of chronic fatigue. Some patients, while keeping short of a severe overstrain, will continually throughout the day, push the demands upon their heart so near to its limit that it can just hold its own. A little extra rest will enable it to gain an ability which may be more than adequate for the former demands.

The diet is of but secondary importance in these patients unless the cardiac failure is severe, and then should be restricted as to fluids and salt according to the well-recognized principles for the treatment of such patients.

At the outset of treatment digitalis should be used. If a preliminary intravenous dose of digitoxin has been given because of the urgency of the symptoms, it should be followed in two or three hours by the oral administration of 30 minims of the tincture well diluted with water so that the nauseous taste will not cause vomiting as it often does with the congested stomach present with severe failure. The less severe cases who do not need the intravenous dose may be started at once with the tincture or the powdered leaf, the dosage depending upon the urgency for obtaining an effect. At the outset at least as much as 60 minims of the tincture should be given per day, or 6 grains of the powdered leaf. Digitalis is best given at intervals of at least twelve hours, following the initial doses which may be given at smaller intervals, so that 30 minims or 3 grains night and morning would be a proper dose with which to continue the medication, or even for starting it if there was no urgency for obtaining digitalis effects. With this dosage we must watch the patient carefully for the early signs of full digitalization, for they will appear at some time between the third and the seventh or eighth day. Stop the drug promptly at the first sign of its activity and resume after a two or three day intermission with 10 minims of the tincture or 1 grain of the leaf night and morning. The further course of digitalis treatment must be carefully individualized for each patient, so that enough is given to maintain the effect and yet not so much that severe toxic symptoms will make their appearance.

The question of how long digitalis should be continued is also one that will have to be determined for each case. It should be kept up as long as the patient continues to improve and for a week or ten days thereafter. It should be resumed if there is any sign of a relapse on stopping the drug, continued for another month and then stopped again to see whether it has not become superfluous. Possibly it might be well during the month preceding the expected labor, to thoroughly digitalize all patients who have shown any signs of failure during pregnancy, considering it as a sort of prophylactic against a serious break in compensation at that time.

SUMMARY

The important feature of a patient with heart disease during pregnancy is the degree of cardiac failure. If this is slight the disease is of little importance.

Even with a moderate degree of failure it will be possible for the child to be born if the mother is allowed to take a risk which is not so great as sometimes stated.

The first attack of severe decompensation can usually be recovered from with proper treatment, unless the attack should occur during labor.

With proper observation and prompt operation severe decompensation should not occur during labor.

Abdominal section is the operation of choice in the emergency, provided a low forceps cannot be done. Ether anesthesia started by chloroform is a better anesthetic for these patients than gas-oxygen.

Oxygen inhalations from a mask are helpful to clear up a persistent cyanosis.

Without severe cardiac failure or after recovery from it, most patients can be carried through to term or to an induced labor during the eighth month.

During labor, watch for a pulse over 95 or respiration over 25 per minute, precordial discomfort, dyspnea, cough, and do not let these little signs become big before putting an end to the labor.

In treating lesser grades of failure during pregnancy, the patient must rest enough to spare the heart from overstrain, but this may not necessitate rest in bed for more than a short time.

Digitalis should be given in doses sufficient to insure an effect.

With this treatment I feel sure it will be possible to diminish the present mortality of about 25 per cent for severe cases and 10 per cent for all cases to a figure which is less disquieting.

REFERENCES

(1) Heart Disease and Pregnancy, Oxford University Press, London, 1921. (2) Jour. Am. Med. Assn., 1922, xxviii, 1188. (3) *Baruch, A. L.,* and *Wordwell, M. N.:* Arch. Int. Med., 1921, xxviii, 367.

74 WEST FORTY-EIGHTH STREET. *(For discussion, see p.* 649.)

A NEW HYDROSTATIC BAG FOR THE INDUCTION OF LABOR

By Geo. H. Lee, M.D., Galveston, Texas

THE recent attention which the postmature child has been receiving in certain clinics, the very carefully developed methods of measurement by which the size of the child, the weight, the diameters of the head and the month of gestation can be determined, and the very accurate results in expert hands which these systems of measurement have given, serve to emphasize the importance of the induction of labor at term and to direct attention to the means available for that purpose. In addition, the various toxemias of pregnancy, as well as certain cases of dystocia, frequently render the induction of labor necessary.

The hydrostatic rubber bag is assuredly the safest and most certain instrument for this purpose. It can be sterilized and can be introduced without becoming contaminated, which is often not true of gauze and other agents sometimes employed. It can be folded upon itself in the grasp of a uterine dressing forceps so as to be sufficiently small to pass into a very slightly dilated cervical canal and when distended becomes a very efficient foreign body in exciting uterine contractions.

The bags which are most used in the present time belong to two classes. The one is represented by the Barnes fiddle-shaped bag which is designed to dilate the cervical canal, and is not bulky at the point which is within the uterus when the bag is in place.

The other group is typified by the Champetier de Ribes and Voorhees bags. These are designed to be distended within the lower uterine zone where the bag acts as a foreign body and this action can be intensified by hanging a weight to the protruding tube of the bag. These bags are not designed to distend or stretch the cervical ring or canal.

Each type of bag has certain good features. And to each there are some points which are objectionable.

The Barnes bag (even the larger size) is too small. When distended it loses its fiddle shape, and as it has no expanded portion on the end which should be within the internal os, it readily slips out of the cervix before it has produced satisfactory dilatation of the cervix or brought about satisfactory uterine contractions. Moreover, the material of which these bags are made is a rubber which is really too light to give service.

The Champetier de Ribes bag is bulky. It is constructed of silk covered with rubber and in order to introduce an ordinarily satisfactory size the cervix must be dilated 2.5 to 3 cms. Then the bag is designed to rest entirely within the lower zone of the uterus, either intra- or extraovularly and no provision is made for *elastic* dilatation of the cervical canal. Moreover, the shape of the tube from the bag is such that the tube distends the vulva—being at that point from 4 to 5 cms. in diameter—and in this manner must increase the opportunity for the introduction of infection.

The Voorhees bag is cone-shaped like the Champetier de Ribes and thus is designed to be placed entirely within the lower zone of the uterus with no provision for elastic dilatation of the cervix. The tube from the bag is small, but the material is light and will not permit the attachment of a weight to drag the bag against the cervix.

The bag* illustrated in Fig. 1 has been designed to combine the good features of both these types of bags, and to eliminate the objectionable points. The tube A is 1 cm. in diameter and joins B, a swelling which is designed to rest in the vagina just outside the cervix. At the point C the bag has a constriction which fits into the cervical canal and

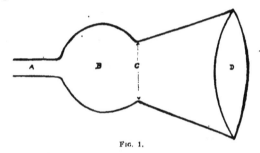

Fig. 1.

when the bag is distended will dilate the cervix, thus adding to the irritation produced by the foreign body, the enlarged portion of the bag D which is placed within the lower uterine zone. This bag combines the two desirable features of the Barnes bags and of the Champetier de Ribes and Voorhees bags; i.e., dilating the cervical canal and supplying an efficient foreign body within the lower zone of the uterus to excite uterine contraction. The extracervical enlarged portion B is small enough to rest well within the vagina and nothing protrudes from the vulva except the rubber tube 1 cm. in diameter. These bags are made in two sizes, the diameters of each at the points indicated being as follows:

Larger: A, 1 cm. B, 7.5 cms. C, 5 cms. D, 10 cms.
Smaller: A, 1 cm. B, 6 cms. C, 4 cms. D, 7.5 cms.

It will be noted that the diameter of the base of the larger bag is

---
*These bags can be had from The Kny-Scheerer Corporntion, at No. 56 West 23rd Street, New York City.

10 cms., which will be extruded through the os uteri when the cervix is practically fully dilated.

These bags are made of a fairly heavy, good quality of soft rubber and can be folded within the grasp of a uterine dressing forceps, so that the bag can be introduced through a cervix which will admit the index finger. The quality of the rubber will permit of the attachment of a weight to the extending tube in appropriate cases.

AN UNUSUAL CASE OF EXTRAUTERINE PREGNANCY

By John W. Riley, M.D., F.A.C.S., Oklahoma City, Okla.

EXTRAUTERINE gestation is such a common condition or disease, that, ordinarily, one might feel like apologizing for presenting this report. However, I feel that this case is so unusual and so atypical, that it is worthy of record.

This patient had the usual signs of pregnancy and felt the fetal movements. These, without the usual evidence that accompanies tubal rupture, suddenly ceased between seven and one-half and eight months of the pregnancy. Outside of the presence of an abdominal tumor, she enjoyed good health, and one year subsequently, gave birth to a full term, living child. Her pregnancy and labor were normal in every way.

She subsequently gave birth to four children, two of whom were born dead. There was no history of any abnormality during these pregnancies or labors.

On admission to the hospital, she complained of frequent urination and the presence of an abdominal tumor. Her menses began when she was thirteen years of age, and had been regular except during her pregnancies. She was married August 9, 1909.

In January, 1912, she had an attack of nausea and vomiting associated with a noticeable weakness. When her family physician arrived, he noticed that she was pulseless and appeared to be in a very weakened condition. A few hours after this, she noticed pain, which radiated to the shoulder, in the left upper abdomen. She was in bed for two months following this experience. She was troubled with cramping pains after eating and felt weak, but recovered from this attack gradually and appeared as well as ever. Her periods up to this time had been perfectly normal in every way. Did the tubal rupture occur at this time?

In February, 1912, she noticed a partial cessation of the menses, the flow at this time being very scant. Experiencing no morning sickness, she thought that she had a normal pregnancy and felt fetal movements in May, 1912. During May, she experienced a rather severe pain in the left upper abdomen. This pain radiated to the shoulder. She thought that she had miscarried, although there had been no flow and no evidence of abortion. Her physician assured her that was not the case, as there were no symptoms of this condition.

These symptoms ceased and the pregnancy proceeded without any complication until August, 1912, when she failed to feel the movements of the child. There were no pains or unusual symptoms at this time. She had observed that the abdomen had increased in size as it would in a normal pregnancy. After the cessation of the fetal movements, she thought that the child would be born and waited for its birth.

In September, 1912, having been examined by her physician who noted that there were no movements, no fetal heart sounds, no dilatation of the cervix, and thinking she might have a tubal pregnancy, he advised operation, but she did not follow this advice.

She continued to feel well and had no untoward symptoms of any kind. The abdomen did not increase in size to any noticeable extent, and after a year it began to decrease. She experienced some pain in the right lower quadrant, which was more noticeable when she was lying on the right side.

The bowels and urination were normal, except for a slight urinary frequency which she had experienced throughout her life. The abdominal mass was about the size of a double fist, and seemed to be in the right lower quadrant, near the midline.

On August 12, 1913, she gave birth to a normal, living child, weighing six pounds. The labor lasted for two hours and was easy and normal. The pregnancy had been normal with no complications of any kind. There was no laceration. The child was delivered alive and is living at the present time. She was in bed for two weeks following her labor, had no chills or fever, and made an uneventful recovery.

A second living child was born sixteen months later. There was no complication throughout the pregnancy and the labor was normal, lasting three hours. There were no complications, chills or fever following delivery.

Following this, she had one miscarriage at three months with no untoward symptoms.

The third labor was in June, 1919. The child was stillborn at eight months. The mother ceased to feel life two months prior to delivery. The labor was easy, spontaneous, and without laceration. The child appeared normal and the puerperium was normal. She miscarried again at three months.

The fourth child was born in January, 1920, an eight months' baby, born dead. It appeared normal. Life had been felt up to one week prior to delivery. At this labor she experienced more pain than she had in the previous ones. The labor lasted three hours and there was a slight laceration. She had no chills or fever following. She has not been pregnant since.

Her weight at marriage in 1909 was 130 pounds, and in 1919, she weighed 160 pounds. At the time of her examination, October 3, 1921, she weighed 100¾ pounds.

On admission, the patient gave a history of having frequent, painful urination for the past six months, and at the time of the examination, she was urinating every two hours during the day and night. She had noticed no blood or pus in the urine. For the last three or four months she had noticed that every time she voided, the bowels would move, or there would be considerable straining. There were no bloody or abnormal stools and they varied in amount from a small to a normal quantity.

She complained of what she thought was a slight prolapsus of the uterus. One year ago she had a colic-like attack of abdominal pain which subsided after a few days. There was a moderate amount of whitish vaginal discharge which was non-irritating. She had belching and bloating at times, lumbar backache was noticeable in the morning, and pain in the right lower quadrant, which was variable in severity, but never agonizing. She thought there was an obstruction in the rectum, as it troubled her when her bowels moved. She had lost fifty pounds in the last year and a half. She felt weak, but otherwise, the history was negative.

The examination showed a poorly nourished woman with a small amount of subcutaneous fat. The height five feet and six inches, pulse 116, temperature 99.6° F. blood pressure 110-68. The abdomen was distended, the muscle tone increased on the right, no hernia, tympany in both flanks. There was a distinct suprapubic mass, the superior surface of the mass being on a level about midway between the navel and the symphysis. The perineum was relaxed, the vaginal mucous membrane pale, the uterus in anterior position and deviated to the right.

A firm, croquet-ball sized tumor was firmly attached to the left of the uterus, causing considerable pain upon examination. It was fixed and immovable. It was rather irregular and hard like a myoma. No crepitus was elicited. Rectal examination was very painful and the mass felt irregular to the examining finger.

The husband inquired if this tumor could be an extrauterine fetus. I felt that it was not possible for a woman to give birth to four full term children without trouble and have an extrauterine fetus as large as this mass appeared to be, and I believed the tumor to be a myoma. The tubes and ovaries could not be palpated.

The blood Wassermann test was negative, white blood cells, 8,750, polynuclears 82, lymphocytes, 18, urine, negative.

A median suprapubic incision was made, about eight inches long. On opening the abdomen, the peritoneum in front of the bladder and uterus was pulled up and attached to a mass of loops of small bowel and the sigmoid colon. The intraperitoneal space in front of the bladder and uterus was obliterated. At the point where the peritoneum, mass and coils of bowel met, there was a stellate scar appearance, which made one feel as if he might be dealing with a carcinoma of the large bowel. It was possible to introduce the hand behind the uterus and broad ligament on the right side. The culdesac was not obliterated. The right tube and ovary were normal. On the left side, however, the mass and intestines blocked the way for any entrance into the culdesac. The uterus was about the size of a Bartlett pear, and was pushed to the right and backward by the mass in the left broad ligament.

On attempting to dissect the bladder from the mass, it was opened. A finger was introduced and the bladder dissected loose and then sutured. My dissection had opened a cavity from which a very foul odor emanated. I found the cranial bones of a fetus buried slightly below the surface of the capsule of the mass. The abdominal cavity had been completely walled off and the opening into the sac was enlarged and it was found to contain the bones of the fetus and a large amount (several ounces) of foul smelling, milky colored fluid.

The fluid was evacuated, the bones removed and the sac swabbed out with pure phenol followed by alcohol. Several of the bones were embedded in the walls of the sac and had to be dug out. Although there was no evidence of intestinal perforation at this time, this subsequently, appeared to have occurred. The cavity was about the size of a large grape fruit.

On account of the dense adhesions of the bowels and the structures of the pelvis, and the probable presence of infection, the peritoneal cavity was closed above the sac and the cavity of the sac was packed with iodoform gauze and a rubber drainage tube inserted. This brought the packing and whatever discharge might occur, extraperitoneally. At the close of the operation, a catheter was passed into the bladder and the urine was slightly blood streaked.

The patient showed no evidence of shock and was returned to her room in good condition. She was then given one pint of 5 per cent glucose and 5 per cent sodium bicarbonate solutions per rectum.

On removing the iodoform packing, about thirty-six hours after the operation, fecal matter was observed coming from the cavity. This did not cause any particular trouble, gradually becoming less and less. She had some trouble in emptying her bladder for a few days. She was catheterized and irrigated with one to two-thousand silver nitrate solution, and this condition rapidly improved.

A small sinus discharging fecal matter persisted, and on January 14, 1922, the abdomen was reopened and the sinus carefully dissected down to the sac of the previous operation. The sac had contracted to about the size of a lemon. It was thick walled and attached to the bladder, lateral pelvis and the pelvic colon. There were no adhesions except those immediately about the sac. A small opening was

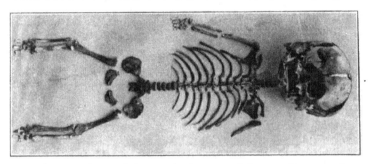

Fig. 1.—Photograph of skeletonized extrauterine fetus, removed nine years after rupture of sac.

found extending from the upper part of the sac into the pelvic colon. This was closed with silk and the abdomen closed with drainage down to the peritoneum. She made a very nice recovery. A recent report shows that she is perfectly well.

The bones of the fetus were entirely clean of all tissue. My colleague, Dr. Kernodle, has made a rather remarkable assembly of them as the accompanying photograph (Fig. 1) will readily show. It measures seventeen inches in height, and apparently represents the size of a fetus at seven and one-half to eight months' pregnancy.

119 WEST FIFTH STREET.

PELVIC HEMATOCELE FROM CAUSES OTHER THAN ECTOPIC PREGNANCY

By J. Wesley Bovée, M.D., F.A.C.S., Washington, D. C.

FROM its derivation it is not difficult to appreciate that "hematocele" means escape of blood into the peritoneal cavity and that pelvic hematocele denotes the escape of blood into the pelvic portion of the peritoneal cavity.

While the source of hematocele may be any blood vessel next to the peritoneum or organ projecting into it, the accumulation of blood in the pelvis from structures in the upper abdomen is rare and will not be considered here. The same may be said of hemorrhage from traumatism of the anterior abdominal wall or more remote structures. The limitation, then excludes consideration of malignant or other tumors, ulcers, and traumatisms situated in the abdomen except those originating in the pelvis. Nor will I concern myself with such conditions reported by Sauter,[53] Freund and others, as endocarditis, adhesive pericarditis, emphysema, endarteritis, nephritis and pneumonia. They have reported well authenticated cases of pelvic hematocele from these various causes and were I to stress treatment of pelvic hematocele in this paper I would have to consider these admittedly very rare conditions as related to accumulations of blood in the pelvic peritoneum.

That ectopic pregnancy is preeminently the most common cause of pelvic hematocele will scarcely be disputed.

That fact has led to carelessness in diagnosis of causes of such hemorrhages and to haphazard conclusion without routine careful investigation of tissues. It has led to unreliable statistics of ectopic pregnancy, pelvic hematocele and of other causes of the latter. It has led no doubt to arraignment of the chastity of girls, widows and other women.

H. P. Newman,[42] by the aid of microscopic study, was able to dissipate such suggestion in a case of a widow above reproach in which an operative diagnosis of ectopic pregnancy was made. Ellsworth[10] reports the case of a girl of eighteen years in which a lacerated fallopian tube was removed. There was no history of traumatism available. A careful microscopic examination was made and not the slightest indication of pregnancy was found.

The dictum of Henry Formad,[15] coroner's physician of Philadelphia, "I may state that I now class hematoceles of the tubes as ectopic pregnancies even if no fetus is discovered," has been as a two-edged sword. His report was based upon thirty-five cases of ectopic pregnancy he had found in thirty-eight hundred autopsies made in women dying suddenly. Another notable feature of his report was regarding the presence of the fetus. In one-third of the cases none was found; in two they popped out of the abdomen with escaping fluid and in the remainder the fetuses were *located quite remotely from the gestation sac*. It may be interesting to add that all his cases were in women from twenty to forty years of age and no pregnancy had advanced longer than four months.

While Formad's[15] paper did very much in a timely way to crystallize due appreciation of the danger and frequency of ruptured ectopic pregnancy and the necessity for prompt surgical care, it intimated that, given a hemorrhagic inundation of the peritoneal cavity of a woman in the procreative age, an immediate diagnosis of ruptured ectopic pregnancy was to be made.

In every case a uterine decidua or very plain remnants of one was found, microscopically, which was regarded only as confirmatory evidence.

Add to this the declaration of Horrocks,[27] that in many cases it is virtually impossible to distinguish microscopically between chorionic villi and altered blood clot, and we can appreciate the tendency to reliance upon Formad's dictum. McMurtry[41] in discussing Primrose's[47] paper said that in his operative experience covering several hundred cases of hemorrhage into the peritoneum presenting similar findings to those described in the paper, in every instance the condition proved to be ectopic pregnancy.

However, pelvic hematocele was found by careful observers, under conditions that eliminated probability or even the possibility of pregnancy.

It was found at puberty (Fordyce,[14] Hortolomey,[28] Jayle[31]) and even as late in life as "long past the menopause," as reported by Richard H. Harte.[22] Moreover, many surgeons found that routine microscopical examination of tissues and blood clots removed from the pelvis in cases of suspected early ectopic pregnancy in which fetuses were not found, revealed not only the absence of pregnancy but the presence of pathologic lesions which could be declared as positively the causes of the hemorrhages. Hundreds of papers illustrative of this fact have been added to medical literature during the past twenty-five years. In 1897, my experience having convinced me that the attention of the profession should be directed to this subject, I published a paper, entitled: "Tubal and ovarian hemorrhages resembling ectopic pregnancy."

In discussing that paper Crofford[4] said, "I am satisfied now that I have had one case that was not extrauterine pregnancy which I thought was at the time, although I said nothing about it." This is only one of the many instances in which a lack of careful microscopic study of tissue has permitted erroneous diagnosis.

A perusal, even a very casual one, of the literature on hematosalpinx and pelvic hematocele will find many authors making the sweeping statement that such conditions are invariably the result of ectopic pregnancy.

We have unlearned many ideas given us by Formad. One is that only retroperitoneal ruptures afforded successful operations. Another is that perhaps more than half the cases of ectopic pregnancy recover without operation, even though expelled into the peritoneal cavity and nearly all the graver ones are saved by operation, instead of having tragically fatal ending as stated by him. We have also learned that the microscope must decide for or against pregnancy in those doubtful conditions devoid of macroscopic proof. In fact the gloomy Formad picture of ectopic pregnancy has received a complete covering in cheerful color.

We may well inquire what conditions other than ectopic pregnancy are productive of pelvic hematocele.

Gordon Taylor[61] reports a case of twins in a gestation sac of right tubal origin that had ruptured into the right broad ligament and then into the peritoneal cavity. In a clot in the broad ligament he found a complete embryo and the head and shoulders of another, thus illustrating that pelvic hematocele can be produced by ruptures into the peritoneal cavity.

Tuboovarian varicocele is a term used considerably in the literature as rupture of it causes severe intraperitoneal hemorrhage. Hirst[26] reports a case of this kind upon which he successfully operated under a preliminary diagnosis of ectopic pregnancy.

The rupture of proliferous cysts in the pelvis and producing pelvic hematocele is reported by Reynes,[40] Finsterer[12] and Jacoulet.[29]

Hortolomey reports the case of a ruptured uterus in a girl of thirteen years from falling against a writing desk, receiving the blow in the hypogastrium. Three months later he operated for a rapidly growing abdominal tumor. At the time of operation she was very weak and had had a metrostasis for three weeks. The tumor was found to be a pelvic hematocele extending up into the abdomen and its source was from a ruptured uterus.

Sauter[53] and several others have reported cases from pelvic hyperemia and some of them stress this cause.

Hemorrhage from uterine fibroids is reported by a large number of writers, including Bégouin,[1] Lemoine,[36] Perrier,[44] Clarke,[3] Jaschka,[30] Pollosson,[46] Tédenat,[62] Wallace,[66] Turner,[64] Laroyenne[34] and Lilienthal.[37] Some of the tumors were interstitial. In some of the cases, reported by Littler,[38] Vanverts,[65] Steinbuchel,[57] Stein,[56] Martin,[40] and

Turner,[64] the hemorrhage was from rupture of the pedicle of subserous fibroids. In the cases of Littler[38] and Turner[64] a fall had been the exciting cause. Torsion of the pedicle had occurred in some of the reported cases.

Hartmann,[23] reports one case caused by a hypernephroma in the uterus. A considerable number were found to be fibroids and hematosalpinx. Ferguson,[11] Fortin,[16] McNaughton Jones[33] and Perrier,[44] report very tragic cases, many of them fatal.

Some authors are impressed with the older view of Puech[48] that menstruation occurs in some people from the mucosa of the fallopian tubes as well as from that of the uterine body and I must confess I am inclined to the same belief. In all events hematosalpinx of the nongestational variety is commonly seen. The following case of mine serves as an example:

Case of Double Hematosalpinx.—Miss Frances C.—white, twenty-two years of age, clerk. Menses, 14, 5, 28, rarely has cramps or backache. In 1917, had a slow fever and menstruated every two weeks over a period of three months. Then had curettage and "straightening of womb." The result was good until December, 1919, when she had an attack of influenza to be followed by menstruation every two weeks and lasting 7-8 days and from June 1st, 1920, to July 2nd, 1920, had been constantly flowing. On the latter date I first saw her. Then she stated the above and that she worked steadily but has become very nervous. An examination revealed a very short anterior vaginal wall that was attached to the cervix near the external os and pulled that orifice to very near the pubic arch. The body of uterus well down in Douglas' pouch. The slightly enlarged ovaries were under it, uterosacral ligaments not felt. No excessive tenderness in pelvis. She was given bromide of sodium and ergot and an Albert Smith pessary was fitted. Operation was advised and performed July 10, 1920, as follows: The anterior vaginal wall was transplanted on cervix to opposite internal os; the uterosacral ligaments triplicated and the anterior surface of the broad ligaments were plicated. The uterus was found to be slightly undersized. The fallopian tubes were each about five inches in length and in their outer two-thirds, about double normal size. They were nonadherent with open fimbriated ends and each contained about four drams of fluid blood.

The ovaries were about double normal size but apparently normal, free from adhesions and lying in Douglas' pouch. Neither of them contained a true corpus luteum but were surrounded by fluid blood.

The hematosalpinx with hematocele was attributed to the influenza infection and the congenital displacement as a complication. A recent letter from her does not allude to her health and I am inclined to think she is well.

Doran[7] reported a case in which no evidence of pathology existed. Tartanson[59] cites many such in his splendid thesis. Galabin,[19] Tédenat,[62] Richardson,[50] Townsend,[63] Freund,[18] Strawn,[58] Pilliet,[45] Croom,[5] Bloodgood,[2] and others have writtten voluminously on the subject or reported cases and in most instances an existing inflammation, usually of a chronic form, has been considered the exciting cause. Freeman[17] reported the case of an athletic young woman who, in vaulting over a fence, experienced a violent pain in the lower abdomen and went into collapse. The abdomen was opened and a fallopian tube found torn near its middle. The uterus and appendages were otherwise normal with no evidence of pregnancy. I have already referred to the case reported by Eliot Ellsworth,[10] in which in operating for appendicitis in a girl of eighteen years, he found the appendix normal but the pelvis completely filled with blood that had escaped from a small laceration of the right fallopian tube, about one inch from its fimbriated end, which was still bleeding. Morris Richardson[50] stated: "A hematosalpinx that is not associated with pregnancy may give rise to as rapid and as fatal symptoms as a ruptured extrauterine fetal sac." Puech[45] stated they may be rapidly fatal or so slight as to give only trifling symptoms.

Fogt[15] found in his case an anomalous condition existed in that the tube was connected with the bicornate uterus only through the means of a thin membranous structure 2 cm. in length. He collected fifty-five cases of bicornate uterus, seen clinically by reporters, (1876 to 1919), thirteen of which were associated with voluminous hematosalpinges. Freund[18] and others are bold enough to use the term "hemorrhagic salpingitis" in this connection.

The gynecologic surgeon is quite accustomed to dealing with hematosalpinx on one or both sides and usually there is not much blood in the peritoneal cavity. But he cannot understand why there is not more. Often he finds much more.

The late Robert P. Harris collected about a dozen cases of cesarean section by violence in which some, or most of them, were caused by goring of bulls. One was that of a squaw gored by a bison bull.

Malignant growths in the pelvic organs cannot be ignored in their causative relation to pelvic hematocele as one needs little imagination to realize malignant growth of the ovary, parovarium, fallopian tube or uterus may give rise to free intraperitoneal hemorrhage. Such an one is that reported by Harte[22] occurring in an old woman whom he opened for appendicitis with emphatic symptoms to find only severe hemorrhage from a rupture of an angiosarcoma of the ovary.

We now come to consider the ovary, an organ which is more frequently the seat of hemorrhage than any other organ of the body. This organ seems to be the principal one concerned in the production of nongravid pelvic hematocele, and, therefore, your attention is specially directed to hemorrhages from and in it.

Ovarian hemorrhage arises from (1) the graafian follicle; (2) the atretic follicle; (3) the corpus luteum; (4) the stroma, and (5) ovarian tumors.

Ovarian tumors may, by revolving on their pedicles, produce laceration of the pedicles with resulting hemorrhage into the peritoneal cavity primarily or, more often, hemorrhage into the cyst. In several cases reported a secondary rupture into peritoneal cavity has occurred. These were in the larger sized cysts. Hemorrhage of both characters may also occur with solid tumors of the ovary. Lee,[35] Douglas,[9] Hedley,[24] Lockyear,[39] Giles,[20] Herman,[25] Doran,[8] Depage,[6] Jones,[32] Taylor,[61] Jayle,[31] DeRouville[62] and hosts of others have reported cases and discussed the subject of ovarian cyst hemorrhage as related to pelvic hematocele. Such growths have been found in one and in both ovaries. In many instances the cysts were very small,—simply follicular cysts or corpus luteum cysts.

Probably of greater account are the many papers comprising the literature on ovarian hematomata and ovarian hemorrhage other than from cysts,—at least cysts other than microcysts.

Perhaps the most frequent form of ovarian hemorrhage is that of the atretic follicle though the stromal variety likely occurs about as often. Authors differ as to the relative frequency of the latter.

The graafian follicle variety is probably least frequent and the corpus luteum kind the most striking in gross appearance of the organ.

While it has been found before birth (Tate,[60] Schultze,[55] Riedel,[51]) and in very advanced age (Harte,[22]) it seems to occur frequently at puberty and most often during the procreative period of the life of women.

Causes.—It is presumable that in most cases a local abnormality is at least a contributory factor.

These may be classed as: (1) menstrual, excessive congestion; (2) nonmenstrual, (a) active hyperemia from infections or their results; (b) passive hyperemia, thrombosis, prolapse, varicosities, torsions, adhesions; (c) new growths.

But there are often remote or general causes activating or promoting. Among them are, (1) acute or chronic poisoning; (2) various diseases already mentioned which embarrass the circulation, causing passive hyperemia; (3) various general infectious diseases; (4) hemophilia; (5) burns and ulcers; (6) diseases producing marked blood changes.

It is not necessary to mention the possible various combinations of these causes.

The amount of blood loss may be trivial, or so great as to produce rapid death, or be between these extremes. The danger of grave hemorrhage is practically limited to the pelvic hematocele, the ovarian hematomata being usually circumscribed and therefore permitting less blood loss. While the atretic follicular, follicular and stromal types are usually small, they may coalesce, thus forming one large hematoma that may in turn rupture, thus permitting uncontrolled hemorrhage into the pelvic cavity. The corpus luteal variety seems prone to provide a grave type of hemorrhage with its associated phenomena. Both ovaries may coincidently be affected or one after the other.

Symptoms.—The symptoms of free hemorrhage from the ovary are so little understood that a mistaken diagnosis is usually made. They vary with the amount of blood loss probably more consistently than when the lost blood is contained in the ovary. Probably the greater proportion of cases having ovarian hemorrhage, or even tubal, into the peritoneum have symptoms so slight that they are ignored, or attributed to menstruation which they commonly accompany. Those of the grave forms may be of an overwhelming character such as are noted in profuse and rapid intraperitoneal hemorrhage from any cause. Usually the attack is ushered in by sudden and severe localized pain with collapse and metrostasis. In many instances the attack promptly follows some physical exertion such as moving heavy furniture (Primrose,[47]) or hanging up clothing in a wardrobe. Accidents have been noted as exciting causes. Menstruation is frequently found to be present or appearing shortly afterward. In those from the corpus luteum Novak[43] has found menstruation has usually ceased several days in advance. If local disease be a predisposing cause manifestations of its existence, such as localized pain, painful or habitually delayed menstruation will be present. If the process be a slow but practically continuous one the uterine bleeding is apt to continue, and a feature stressed by Savariaud[54] is the peculiar yellowish color of the blanched skin and conjunctivæ. Acute infections have their characteristic phenomena. Physical examination, especially at the onset would reveal hypogastric and pelvic hypersensitiveness and perhaps abdominal distention and the usual evidence of concealed hemorrhage. After the blood has attempted organization the mass may be recognized by vaginoabdominal or rectoabdominal examination. After a few weeks in a moderate case a tender pelvic mass may be outlined in one or both sides of the pelvis. Of course rectal and vesical symptoms may be expected from the presence of such masses.

Diagnosis.—The diagnosis of pelvic hematocele in mild cases is a matter of extreme difficulty. In fact it is practically never made before operation. As already mentioned it is probable that often the condition is regarded as a stormy menstrual period or straining of the uterine supports, indigestion, very mild appendicitis, or ovarian congestion. If a history of previous pelvic infection, overexertion, pelvic injuries incident to parturition or becoming chilled at or just preceding a menstrual period exists, then such conditions by means of their sequelæ are regarded as the sum total of the actual conditions present.

When the condition is pronounced, as in the case of rupture of a tube or a large rupture of an ovary accompanied with a rapid and profuse hemorrhage, or profuse hemorrhage from or into a tumor in the pelvis, then the two cardinal symptoms of hemorrhage and pain point to either a hematoma or usually, a hematocele in the pelvis. During the child-bearing age the question of ectopic pregnancy must be settled. Usually the nonpregnant condition occurs at a menstrual period except in the corpus luteal hemorrhage when the attack is apt to occur ten to fifteen days subsequent to menstruation and has less indication of ectopic pregnancy. But when the tissue injury and pain are moderate in degree the condition has to be differentiated from acute appendicitis, ruptured ectopic pregnancy, torsion of the pedicle of a pelvic tumor,—such as a pediculated uterine fibroid or an ovarian tumor, and threatened or incomplete abortion in a uterine pregnancy. In the moderate and severe forms, the hemorrhage may be detected by study of the blood and perhaps by the usual symptoms of profuse, concealed hemorrhage. The leucocyte, especially, and the red cell count, as well as the hemoglobin percentage should be higher in acute appendicitis than in pelvic hematocele. Physical exertion at or just preceding the onset is a feature in pelvic hematocele and not in acute appendicitis.

Burns, ulcers and trauma are likewise productive of hematocele rather than appendicitis. After several days or weeks have followed the onset without surgical intervention, prolonged metrostasis and localized pain may easily lead to suspicion of early tubal or ovarian pregnancy or incomplete abortion as well as pelvic hematocele. The presence or expulsion of a uterine decidua would not occur in nongravid pelvic hematocele. But the history of regular menstruation, long continued metrostasis and the presence of a tender mass lateral to the uterus in either or both sides, without enlargement or material softening of the uterus together with the history of onset and progress point to pelvic hematocele. A boggy mass felt in the culdesac of Douglas would be confirmatory.

The following case history illustrates this class:

Case of Ovarian Hematoma.—Mrs. Hyman G. referred to me by Dr. Mary Holmes for examination and opinion November 11, 1918. She was twenty-seven years of age, had a good family history except that her mother, fourteen years before, had been subjected to nephrectomy for a twelve pound tumor.

This patient had become frail just after puberty. Her menses had appeared first at the age of thirteen years, occurring semimonthly the first year, becoming normal, only that the duration was 7 to 8 days, scanty, and for the first two or three days painful. She was married at twenty-two and ten months later gave birth to a baby, after forceps, with laceration, (July, 1914). Two years later had an abortion of a two months' pregnancy, attributed to laceration of cervix, and was operated upon for lacerations and appendicitis in February, 1917. Was much improved by it except frequent and painful micturition and constipation persisted. The following June she was operated upon for hemorrhoids. In July, 1918, had pain throughout menstrual period and also in each period since, the last continuing October 5 to today,—forty-four days. She suffers with sacralgia, groinache, abdominal distension, headache, insomnia and nervousness.

Patient's weight, 113 pounds, blood pressure, 134-40; perineum relaxed; a scar in the base of each broad ligament, extending out from the uterus; the uterus had a good position, size and density, but to its left side is felt a pulpy, globular mass two inches in diameter that was very sensitive to touch and thought to be an ovarian hematoma. The next day, November 19, 1918, I wrote Dr. Holmes "I believe an ovarian hemorrhage with blood accumulated in the ovary constitutes a mass intimately connected with the uterus near the middle of its left side and has been the cause of her prolonged metrostasis, I would recommend an operation for its removal.''

The operation.—Left salpingooophorectomy, was done December 6, 1918. The right appendage seemed normal and left tube and ovary were adherent. The ovary enlarged about 100 per cent, showed a brown discoloration and contained a hemorrhagic cyst. The tube was adherent to it. The appendage was examined microscopically and pronounced nongestational.

October 6, 1919, she was again referred by Dr. Holmes, complaining of pain in the right side of the pelvis. Her last two menstrual periods were five weeks apart. Her right ovary was found doubled in size and hypersensitive but otherwise normal to touch. November 17, 1920, Dr. Holmes informed me the patient has a child fourteen months of age, and is in fine health.

This case was interesting from another standpoint,—that of preoperational diagnosis, a very rare occurrence as shown in another part of this paper.

Prognosis.—It is conjectured the majority of cases of pelvic hematocele are never recognized and recover with or without treatment.

It is common knowledge that very frequently blood is found in the culdesac when the peritoneal cavity has been opened for recognized pathology accountable for the symptoms. But like ectopic pregnancy and appendicitis nongravid hemorrhage into the pelvic peritoneum may be of very grave import. A large number of fatalities have occurred from it either with or without operation. Many were discovered by autopsy following sudden death.

Then it appears that a certain (quite large) percentage die before proper aid is secured and many are promptly operated upon successfully.

In this respect the result parallels ruptured tubal pregnancy, it being a question of the amount and rapidity of the blood loss and the reaction of the patient to such loss.

Treatment.—As may be inferred, the mild variety will respond favorably to rest in bed, with or without morphia, and perhaps icebags applied locally and resort to means to lessen the blood supply to the pelvic structures.

In the tragic variety nicety of judgment must decide whether prompt invasion of the peritoneal cavity should be made. If such invasion is done it should be after conclusion that the hemorrhage continues or will likely resume at any moment to a fatal degree and that it must be made with due guarding at the patient's vitality and primarily to end the blood loss.

Removal of pathologic structures should be of secondary consideration. Here, again, good surgical judgment is needed, for the removal of an ovarian tumor with a twisted pedicle or, having ruptured, has caused the hemorrhage or of a bleeding subperitoneal uterine fibroid may be required to check the blood loss.

The various methods of combating the results of blood loss, such as transfusion, are of very great importance, but their employment before the bleeding vessels have been secured may cause further blood loss and be therefore, rendered futile.

REFERENCES

(1) Bull. Soc. d'Anat. et Physiol. de Bordeaux, 1892, xiii, 51. (2) Tr. Am. Surg. Assoc., 1912, xxx, 617-625. (3) Lancet, London, 1907, i, 8. (4) Trans. S. Surg. and Gyn. Assn., 1897, x, 57. (5) Med. Press and Circ., London, 1891, N. S., li, 189. (6) Anjou Méd. Angers, 1898, v, 89-91. (7) Tr. Obst. Soc., London, (1898) 1899, xl, 180-188. (8) Proc. Roy. Soc. of Med., London, 1909, part 2, Obst. and Gyn. Sect., p. 88. (9) Trans. South. Surg. and Gynaec. Assn., 1897, x, 57. (10) Tr. Am. Surg. Assn., 1912, xxx, 617-625. (11) Am. Jour. Obst., New York, 1895, xxxi, 879. (12) Wien. Klin. Wchnschr., 1912, xxv, 1959. (13) Ann. de gyn. et d'obst., Paris, 1918-19, xiii, 531-561. (14) New York Med. Jour., 1889, xlix, 180. (15) Tr. Path. Soc., Philadelphia, 1889-91, xv, 349-353. (16) Normandie méd. Rouen, 1905, xx, 511. (17) Tr. Am. Surg. Assn., 1912, xxx, 617-625. (18) Centralbl. f. Gynäk., 1903, xxvii, p. 853. (19) Brit. Med. Jour., 1892, ii, 291. (20) Proc. Roy. Soc. Med., London, 1910, iii, pt. 2, Obst. and Gyn. Sect. (21) Am. Jour. Obst., New York, 1904, l, 119. (22) Tr. Am. Surg. Assn., 1912, xxx, 617-625. (23) Bull. Acad. de Méd., Paris, 1920, lxxxiii, 90. (24) Proc. Roy. Soc. of Med., London, 1908, pt. 2. Obst. and Gyn. Sect., pg. 6. (25) Diseases of Women, ed. 3, New York, 1907, p. 292. (26) Univ. Penn. Med. Bull., 1909-10, xxii, 260. (27) Discussion on Paper of J. B. Sutton, Brit. Med. Jour. 1892, ii. (28) Bull. et Mém. de la Soc. des Médecins et Naturalistes de Jassy, 1916, xxx (year), 42-46. (29) Prog. Méd., Paris, 1911, xxvii, 55-60. (30) Centralbl. f. Gynäk., 1910, xxxiv, 625-28. (31) Rev. de Gynec. et de Chir. Abdom., 1909, xiii, 185-222. (32) Surg. Gynec. and Obst., 1913, xvi, 63-74. (33) Proc. Royal Soc. of Med., London, 1907-8, i, Obst. and Gynec. Sect., 122-124. (34) Lyon Méd., 1882, xl, 13-14. (35) Brooklyn Med. Jour., 1905, xix, 209. (36) Hématome Intraperit. an Cours Fibrom-Uteri Thèse de Montpellier, 1906-7. (37) Tr. Am. Surg. Assn., 1912, xxx, 617-625. (38) Jour. Obst. and Gynaec., Brit. Emp., 1910, xvii, 423-5. (39) Proc. Roy. Soc. of Med., London, 1901, iii, part 2, Obst. and Gynec. Sect., 206. (40) Normandie Méd., Rouen, 1897, xii, 360-65. (41) Tr. Am. Surg. Assn., 1912, xxx, 617-625. (42) Am. Jour. Obst., 1893, xxvii, 271. (43) Jour. Am. Med. Assn., 1917, lxviii, 1160. (44) Des hémorragies intrapéritonéales dans les cas de fibromes utérins. Lyon, 1904, 52 p. 8. (45) Ann. de Gynec. et d'Obst., Paris, 1893, xl, 366-371. (46) Lyon Méd., 1904, ciii, 280-282. (47) Tr. Am. Surg. Assn., 1912, xxx, 599-607. (48) De l'hématocèle périutérine et des sources .8°, Montpellier, 1858. (49) Marseilles Méd., 1920, lvii, 369. (50) Ann. Surg., 1894, xx, 705-730. (51) Ein Fall von Haematoma Ovarii bei einem Neugeborenen., Dissertat., Halle, 1896. (52) Ann. de Gynec. et d'Obst., Paris, 1908, 2nd Ser., v, 222-7. (53) Ztschr. f. Heilk., (abth. f. path. anat.) Wien. u., Leipz., 1900, xxi, 187-199. (54) Gaz. de Gynäk., 1913, xxviii, 81-82. (55) Quoted by Riedel, Wm. A. (56) Monatschr. f. Geburtsh. u. Gynäk., Berlin, 1905, xxii, 637-42. (57) Wien. klin. Wchnschr., 1905, xviii, 945-947. (58) Jour. Am. Inst. Homeop., Chicago, 1919-20, xii, 45-48. (59) Les Hémorrhagies et L'Hématoceles Pelviennes Sans Grossesse Ectopique, Thèse de Lyon, 1909. (60) Tr. South. Surg. and Gynaec. Assn., 1904, xvii, 335-347. (61) Practitioner, London, 1918, ci, 37-39. (62) Bull. Soc. d'Obst. et de Gynéc. de Paris, 1920, ix, 81-85. (63) Boston Med. and Surg. Jour., 1893 cxxix, 438-440. (64) Med. Press, London, 1920, N. S., cix, 483. (65) Bull. Soc. Anat. de Paris, 1896, lxxi, 753-757. (66) Jour. Obst. and Gynec., Brit. Emp., London, 1910, xviii, 357-367.

Society Transactions

NEW YORK ACADEMY OF MEDICINE
SECTION ON OBSTETRICS AND GYNECOLOGY
STATED MEETING, HELD JANUARY 24, 1922

DR. WILLIAM P. HEALY IN THE CHAIR

DR. H. DAWSON FURNISS reported **Two Cases of Supernumerary Ureters Emptying Extravesically.**

Supernumerary ureters are fairly numerous, but those with extravesical openings rare. Of 20 personally observed cases presenting three ureters, only two have been of the latter type. When he reported his first case he could find records of only 19 others. Since then Judd of the Mayo Clinic has recorded two and Tovey has personally communicated one.

The first patient was a girl of nineteen, who came on account of incessant dribbling urine since birth, although able to void naturally. This history pointed clearly to some congenital anomaly, one in which urine was discharged distal to the urethra. With this in mind she was cystoscoped after intravenous injection of indigo-carmine. The dye was eliminated promptly through normally situated right and left ureters. The vagina and vestibule were packed with cotton. After a wait of ten minutes it was found that the cotton just below the urethral meatus was stained. A careful search revealed a minute opening, into which a ureteral catheter could be introduced four inches. Vaginal palpation showed this to run to the left side.

Operution—After catheterizing the ureter an attempt was made to dissect it out, and turn it into the bladder. A thin fusiform sac, intimately adherent was found. This was opened accidentally. After this an incision was made into the bladder through the opposite wall of the sac, and the vesical and ureteral mucosa united with catgut. The distal end of the ureter was closed, the accidental wound sutured and the vagina brought over it with chromic catgut. A retention catheter was placed in the bladder. Seven days later the old ureteral leakage returned. After three weeks the ureter was exposed through the vagina, and it was then found to be twice the normal thickness on the kidney side of the fusiform sac. After mobilizing three-fourths of an inch of the ureter, a sound was placed in the bladder, depressing the bladder just in front of the ureter. A hole was cut at this point, a suture placed through the ureter and tied to the sound. On withdrawing the sound the ureter was pulled into the bladder, where it was sutured with chromic catgut and the vaginal wound closed. The incontinence was cured. After operation the new opening was shown to function by the appearance of indigo-carmine elimination. After six months this ceased. Attempts to catheterize this ureter were vain.

The second patient was a woman of thirty-eight, with a similar history, incessant dribbling and normal micturition. Cystoscopy showed two normally placed ureters, both eliminating indigo-carmine promptly, but an opening of an extravesical ureter could not be found. Cotton pledgets were placed after indigo-carmine administration to detect any extra-vesical discharge, but none was found. On vaginal examination the urethra appeared more full and prominent than usual. A metal catheter was placed in the bladder and the urethra again palpated without detecting any swelling underneath.

The patient had a fibroid uterus the size of a grapefruit, and because of three weekly profuse bleedings Dr. Furniss did a supravaginal hysterectomy. On the right side of the pelvis was found a soft elastic swelling extraperitoneal, about three-quarters to an inch in diameter, running from below upwards, over the brim of the pelvis. The history, together with the knowledge of two normally placed ureters, each promptly eliminating indigo-carmine, gave the clue to the diagnosis. Palpation of the right kidney showed a mass the size of a hickory nut on the superior pole.

Not trusting the efficiency of simple ligation of the ureter, an upper right rectus incision was made through the peritoneum, on the outer side of the colon, which was displaced inwards, exposing the kidney. At the pelvic brim the dilated ureter covered the other so that it was not to be seen. The ureter was freed three inches from the pelvis, double clamped and cut. The lower end was ligated with chromic catgut and dropped. The renal end was freed up to the vessels going to the lower part of the kidney and then passed above them. It normally ran posteriorly to the vessels. The kidney was normal in shape with the part attached to the extra ureter perched on top. Two small arteries ran to it,— the veins could not be seen. This part of the kidney was represented by a sac, three-quarters of an inch in diameter, with a small layer of kidney tissue attached to the kidney, the whole being enclosed in a fibrous capsule. It was resected without difficulty and without bleeding. A stab wound was made in the flank, through which a cigarette drain was placed; the posterior peritoneal incision, the anterior peritoneal incision, and the abdominal wall were closed. There was only slight bloody drainage. The drain was removed on the second day. Recovery was uneventful with complete relief of urinary drainage.

DISCUSSION

DR. DAVID TOVEY.—I should like to report a case which I am interested in observing at the present time, a young woman, twenty-six years of age, who all her life has wet her underclothes. Since becoming a nurse she is in the habit of tamponing her vagina, but if the tampon is in place for a long time and becomes saturated the urine runs out. I have injected indigo-carmine and find she has two normal ureters. I waited a half hour to find where the supernumerary ureter emptied but was unable to locate the opening. There was indigo-carmine in the bladder but none at all in the vagina. This patient tells me that after she went home she found the cotton tampon stained with blue colored urine. I have not had her back to finish making observations and to find the extra ureter. It is often difficult to find the opening of these supernumerary ureters. The second patient of mine of whom Dr. Furniss spoke was operated upon three or four times, had the vesical sphincter shortened and an interposition operation done, thinking that would make pressure on the neck of the bladder and cure the incontinence of urine. After all these procedures, a ureteral opening was found beneath the urethra. This demonstrates the difficulty of locating the opening in some instances.

DR. FURNISS.—I think the radical operation as performed in the second case is easier than the plastic procedure used in the first case. There is no reason why one has to go through the peritoneum; it can be done extraperitoneally. It is difficult to transplant a greatly distended ureter. Should infection occur in it such infection is prone to persist on account of urinary stasis. As to Dr. Tovey's case in which he has not found the opening of the supernumerary ureter, there is so little functioning tissue drained by such a ureter that it takes a great deal of time for the injected indigo-carmine to show itself. As to the operative procedure, I think I prefer resection, for we must remember that the vessels in the kidney are terminal vessels and that makes resection easy. If the amount of kidney tissue drained by the supernumerary ureter is large, the ureter not greatly dilated, and infection absent, a ureterovesical anastomosis is preferable.

DR. WILLIAM H. W. KNIPE reported a case of **Vaginal Caesarean for Eclampsia.**

This patient, twenty-nine years of age, a Roumanian, para iii, 7 months' pregnant was admitted to Gouverneur Hospital with complaints of headache, and disturbed vision, followed by convulsions. The patient's general health had always been excellent; no diseases of childhood were remembered by the patient; she had two previous uncomplicated pregnancies and labors; no miscarriages.

Patient was seven months pregnant and for the last 2 months had considerable edema of both lower extremities. She had recently called in a physician who took her blood pressure and examined the urine. On the day before admission to the hospital, she had severe headache with restlessness and disturbed vision; during that night she had three convulsions at home; on the next morning the ambulance was called and immediately after entering the hospital another convulsion lasting 5 minutes took place. Upon admission the patient's blood pressure was 240 systolic, 144 diastolic, temperature normal, pulse 72. The eyelids were edematous, pupils contracted and regular, and did not react to light. The heart and lungs were normal; there was marked edema of the lower extremities, and the reflexes were hyperactive. The cervix was firm and unyielding and the external os admitted one finger. The urine was very dark colored, was loaded with albumin and showed many casts of all varieties. There was a vertex presentation of the child and the fetal heart was 160.

Upon admission to the hospital the patient was given morphine gr. ¼ and fl. ext. veratrum viride m. x by hypo; the veratrum was repeated in one hour and a hot colon irrigation of 3 gallons was given and the patient was then taken to the operating room where a vaginal cesarean section was done, using a filled No. 4 Voorhees bag as a tractor, and the patient delivered of a living child with the aid of forceps. The convalescence from the operative procedure was in no way different from a normal labor, and there was no abdominal disturbance.

One hour after delivery patient had a slight convulsion, and afterwards was treated with veratrum viride and morphine, alkaline carthartics, colon irrigations of soda bicarbonate 5 per cent solution; Murphy drip of glucose or soda bicarbonate, hot packs, imperial drink, diuretin, carbohydrate diet.

The patient was blind for several days and the blood pressure went down to 138 systolic, which after delivery rose again to 188 and remained higher than normal for two weeks. The urine also remained distinctly abnormal for some time but at the end of sixteen days patient was discharged in fairly good condition as regards her severe kidney lesion, with a cervix that had healed by primary union, but with a retroversion of the uterus for which a pessary was inserted. The baby was also thriving at this time.

It seems a reasonable proposition to state that a woman with eclampsia should be delivered by that method which will subject the patient to the least shock and the method adopted must depend upon the different factors present in the individual case, depending upon the size of the pelvis, upon the rigidity and dilating possibilities of the cervix, upon the size and viability of the child and upon the condition of the mother. With a normal sized pelvis, with a small or premature child and where the only obstacle to a speedy delivery is a hard rigid and undilating cervix, the performance of a vaginal cesarean operation offers the simplest, quickest and least harmful method of facilitating delivery of the child. It should not be used however if the child is large.

DR. KNIPE also reported a case of **Ectopic Gestation and Ovarian Abscess.**

This patient entered the hospital because she had been bleeding vaginally to a slight degree for a period of two weeks. She was thirty years of age, a Russian, and had always been well except for the discomfort incident to hemorrhoids; she had two children, one 6 years and one 3 years and no miscarriages; her menstrual history had been normal in all respects up to the present trouble.

Six weeks before entering the hospital the patient had a normal menstruation; when the next menstruation was due, she had some cramps in the lower abdomen and began to bleed slightly. She visited one of the dispensaries in this city, where she was informed that she had aborted and was advised to stay in bed at home for a few days, which advice was followed. Upon resuming her household duties she continued to bleed slightly and felt feverish; at this time she also complained of burning and difficult micturition.

Examination upon admission showed a well developed woman with a normal temperature and pulse, who had a slight bloody vaginal discharge, somewhat dark in color. The abdomen was soft, with no rigidity but with marked tenderness on slight pressure upon the left lower quadrant of the abdomen. Upon vaginal examination, the uterus was found to be very slightly enlarged, the right tube and ovary seemed normal but the left appendage was felt as a mass about the size of a large walnut—which upon light pressure elicited signs of moderate tenderness.

Two days after admission to the hospital the patient's temperature took an abrupt rise to 103° F. and ranged between 100° F. and 104° F. thereafter. The pulse rate ranged between 88 and 110. At the same time the small mass in the left pelvis grew gradually until the fifth day when it was the size of a large orange. The leucocyte count at this time was 22,000 with 93 per cent of polymorphonuclear cells, hemoglobin 90 per cent, red cells 4,900,000. A diagnosis of ectopic gestation was made with the additional probability of an infected hematocele and it was determined that a laparotomy was necessary.

Upon opening the abdomen the peritoneum showed an acute infection added to an old process as shown by the presence of new gelatinous exudate mixed with old, dense adhesions which were difficult to separate. The left fallopian tube showed an unruptured ectopic gestation of six weeks' duration situated at the uterine half of the tube. About two ounces of foul smelling light brownish pus surrounded the left ovary and the ovary itself was a pus sac. The fallopian tube and ovarian wall were extremely friable. Dense adhesions and the condition of the tissues made the operation difficult. The tube and ovary were removed and two large cigarette drains were inserted to the bottom of the pelvic cavity and the abdomen closed.

The patient improved considerably for three days; then became weaker and upon the fifth day died, evidently from a general peritonitis.

This case illustrates the difficulty in making a differential diagnosis between ectopic and inflammatory pelvic conditions especially when both are present in the same case; it also shows the difficulty of treatment in a patient with two pathologic conditions requiring diametrically opposite lines of attack—the ectopic, I believe all will agree, should be operated upon as soon as it is diagnosed—the inflammatory condition as shown by the gelatinous exudate, was operated upon too soon,—if there had been no ectopic present the best course of treatment would have been to wait longer before operating.

DISCUSSION

DR. CHARLES G. CHILD, JR.—I believe Dr. Knipe is right in thinking that the vaginal cesarean operation when indicated offers the simplest, quickest and least harmful method of immediate delivery. Of course we should use the least serious operative procedure when we believe that immediate delivery is needed in a case of eclampsia. In the last case in which I did a vaginal cesarean section, I was not as fortunate as Dr. Knipe. My patient rapidly succumbed to her eclampsia and I do not think the cesarean section hastened or retarded in any way her demise, nor do I feel that in a serious case of eclampsia immediate delivery is an advantage. I believe those cases are better treated by attempts to establish proper elimination than by operative measures.

In the second case it would be interesting to know why the acute inflammation started up after the patient was brought to the hospital. I feel that the fatal result was produced by the rupture of the abscess. The walls of such abscesses are often very friable, as in Dr. Knipe's case, and I can readily understand how an examination could easily cause a rupture. I say this not in the way of criticism, but if one has any idea that he is examining a case in which there is an ovarian abscess he should be most gentle in his manipulations.

DR. HERMAN LORBER.—About fifteen years ago I did my first vaginal cesarean section for a marginal placenta previa. This patient made an uneventful recovery. Last year I had two cases in which I was not so fortunate. Both cases came into the hospital in coma and both ended fatally. One woman had been in coma for twelve hours and it was a question whether to let her alone or to operate. It was finally decided to do a vaginal cesarean section without an anesthetic. This was done and the woman died as a result of her eclampsia. The other patient also died as a result of the eclampsia. I think vaginal cesarean section has a decided field in eclampsia if one believes that evacuation of the uterus is one way of treating eclampsia and there is no dilatation, but most of us feel that the administration of morphine, etc., and waiting, is the better way of dealing with such cases.

As to Dr. Knipe's second case, while we believe that ectopic pregnancy should be operated upon early, I think that in the presence of an acute inflammation one would be justified in waiting until this had subsided. A high temperature may be considered almost an indication for waiting. In fact in many cases even without inflammation it is better to wait until the shock is over and then to go ahead with the operation.

DR. W. H. HEALY.—The second case was so complicated that I doubt whether any one could have handled it in any better way. The clinical history indicated an ectopic gestation so the diagnosis was not obscure at the time of admission to the hospital. The development of the acute ovarian abscess as a complication changed the picture entirely. You cannot delay operating on an ovarian abscess. An ovarian abscess is always a great responsibility for if it ruptures it leads to peritonitis. Dr. Knipe really had no choice in the matter for an acute ovarian abscess cannot be handled like an acute pyosalpinx. An acute pyosalpinx can be kept waiting with much greater advantage than if operated on immediately.

DR. KNIPE, (closing).—It was not my intention to take up the treatment of eclampsia except insofar as one would choose the operative procedure which would add least to the burden the patient was already bearing.

As to the treatment in the second case, if I had known as much at that time as I know now, I do not think I could have treated the case any better. I have delayed with an ovarian abscess until it almost filled the abdomen and then had a bad case with which to deal, a peritonitis. In this case my diagnosis was ectopic gestation with a possible secondary infection. It is sometimes exceedingly difficult to differentiate between an ectopic gestation and an inflammatory condition.

DR. HAROLD E. B. PARDEE read a paper entitled **Treatment of Cardiac Failure During Pregnancy.** (For original article, see p. 620.)

DISCUSSION

DR. KNIPE.—I should like to ask what percentage of patients with chronic valvular disease give trouble before or during labor. Some years ago I used to be very much afraid of cases with mitral stenosis. I did not so much mind those with regurgitation but I felt that it was very dangerous to allow those with mitral stenosis to go to labor. But I have found that the cases with mitral stenosis have no trouble. It is rare to have an acute loss of compensation in these cases, so I am not as much alarmed by them as I used to be. Dr. Pardee mentions having recourse to cesarean section in cases of acute decompensation. Personally, a cesarean section would be the last thing I would want to do under those circumstances, because I would fear that the sudden release of pressure, when the child is delivered within ten seconds from the beginning of the incision, might cause further embarrassment to the heart. It would seem to me that the more gradual emptying of the uterus would be better for the heart; I would prefer a low or medium forceps operation, or a version.

DR. CHILD.—The literature is unsatisfactory in regard to the study of cardiac cases during pregnancy, and especially during labor. I believe the functional efficiency of the heart, one of the most important things to consider during pregnancy and labor, has been much neglected. It is a subject which often requires the combined attention of the internist, the cardiologist and the obstetrician. As obstetricians we have not given the internist sufficient material of this kind to work with. I am glad to hear that the Lying-in-Hospital is participating in an effort to study the heart in pregnancy and labor.

The mere occurrence of abnormal heart sounds need not alarm us as much as formerly, now that we have a better understanding of the heart in pregnancy, but it alarms the family and makes them very anxious if the obstetrician does not show what they consider to be a proper amount of apprehension for these patients. Many times inefficient hearts are no different during pregnancy than under any other condition. In patients with cardiac lesions labor should always be so conducted as not to bring undue strain on the heart. Therefore there are times when cesarean section should be chosen. I do not think the sudden delivery of the child causes any additional danger for cases occur with sudden rupture of the membranes in hydramnios without any serious heart changes. In fact the sudden change of pressure, in my experience seems to help rather than interfere with the heart or the ultimate outcome. Functional efficiency is the keynote to successful treatment in all cases of cardiac failure in the pregnant woman, and the first duty of the physician is to determine as soon as possible the degree of efficiency, and to recognize danger signals early.

We cannot judge cardiac inefficiency by the presence of abnormal signs alone, as these give no indication of the degree of functional efficiency or inefficiency. As a rule there may be little apprehension felt if the functional efficiency is not impaired to a greater extent than would exist with a normal pregnancy. In the presence of mitral stenosis the pregnancy should be allowed to continue only under the closest and most careful observation, and then only so long as no marked signs of failure make their appearance. When dyspnea is present exercise should be prohibited. When, in addition there is cyanosis and edema of the lungs the patient should be confined to bed and all activities restricted to the minimum. When the signs of failure threaten life, then the pregnancy should be shortened by the induction of a miscarriage or premature labor. Medicinal treatment, has not, in my hands, ever been quite satisfactory in cases of mitral stenosis, but where marked auricular fibrillation is present, tincture of digitalis in fifteen to twenty drop doses three times a day until the pulse rate drops below 70 has been of help.

If the symptoms of heart failure can be satisfactorily kept in check then as a rule the pregnancy may be allowed to proceed, and in many such cases labor starts early, and is not necessarily complicated by any great strain on the heart. When decompensation develops during labor delivery should generally be facilitated by the early use of forceps if possible, and the administration of ether to avoid undue straining on the part of the patient. The general management of these cases is of the utmost importance, and the patient's life should be regulated so as to avoid, if possible, even the slightest strain. Digestive disturbances, insomnia and worry should receive proper recognition.

While many a bad heart will go through a pregnancy and labor without decompensating, serious signs of failure, such as dropsy, enlargement of the liver, edema and crepitation at the base of the lungs, and cyanosis, should always be watched for. The systolic murmurs need cause little anxiety in pregnancy where there are no other signs, and where the patient responds to physical tests satisfactorily.

Mitral stenosis is undoubtedly a most serious heart complication of pregnancy and labor, and a prognosis should never be favorable except after the most exhaustive functional tests have been carried out.

Aortic regurgitation, when the heart is otherwise normal, and functional tests favorable, is not a contraindication to pregnancy, unless there is marked hypertrophy of the ventricle present.

Great alarm is often caused in pregnancy, and many a pregnancy forbidden or interrupted, because of failure to understand and estimate at their proper significance heart murmurs and disturbance of rhythm. In this connection it might be well to emphasize the fact that the purely neurotic heart should never be taken as a contraindication to pregnancy.

I think Dr. Pardee knows so much about his subject that I should like to take this opportunity to ask his advice on a patient I saw in consultation last week. This woman is thirty-six years of age and has been delivered of four children who are all alive and well today. With each pregnancy she has had signs of cardiac failure. The first pregnancy terminated in spontaneous delivery with slight symptoms of dilatation of the heart, requiring no special treatment. In the second pregnancy signs of decompensation appeared during the middle part of the pregnancy, she then improved and went to term without further difficulty. Three years later she was again delivered spontaneously with slight dypsnea, and some edema of the lungs and extremities. In 1912 she was delivered spontaneously at term with a great deal of cardiac distress. She was attended by a general practitioner at this time. She suffered with dyspnea, cyanosis, and edema of the extremities throughout her pregnancy but with general medical care, she came through. In 1915, her last pregnancy, she developed symptoms of decompensation early and these were more severe than in former pregnancies. At the third month she was taken to Baltimore and the pregnancy terminated at the fourth month. From this she had an uneventful recovery. With these four children there would appear little reason for her to run any further risk. However, she was now married a second time and very anxious to have a child by the second husband. She is now six months pregnant with only slight symptoms. She has a mitral stenosis and a slightly dilated heart, has been in bed two weeks and says she feels as well as in any preceding pregnancy. I would like to know what Dr. Pardee would advise in this case.

DR. SAMUEL J. SCADRON.—I would like to say a word with regard to the cases of cardiac decompensation during pregnancy that have improved under appropriate treatment. I think it is not advisable to permit those patients to continue their pregnancies to full term and induce labor on them at about the thirty-sixth or thirty-seventh week of gestation. It is of paramount importance in all cardiac cases to diminish the physical and mental strain during labor. I found that with the use of morphine sulphate, ¼ grain, at the onset of active labor, and small doses of scopolamine, $\frac{1}{400}$ of a grain, repeated at regular intervals as labor advances, we can greatly alleviate the strain of labor. Fortunately cardiac cases progress in labor very rapidly, and nature seems to be very kind to them as their cervices are usually soft and dilatable. I think therefore that with the analgesic effect of morphine and scopolamine we can practically terminate labor with the minimum shock to the patients.

I must agree with the previous speaker in regard to performing cesarean section in cardiac cases with failure of compensation. I felt that the sudden decrease of intraabdominal pressure would be of serious detriment to the patient.

During my prenatal work I found a large percentage of normal cases develop functional murmurs in the pulmonic area. I would like to ask Dr. Pardee if he considers these murmurs of any significance; they are audible for a long period after labor.

DR. PARDEE, (closing).—In reply to Dr. Knipe's question, out of 2500 labors we have had 33 patients with heart disease, in eight of whom the condition was serious enough to give trouble. There were three deaths, a mortality of 40 per cent among the serious cases and 10 per cent of all cardiac cases.

In doing this work at the Lying-in Hospital my attitude has been that the obstetricians should know more about it than I did owing to their large experience. However, I have seen enough to be able to draw some conclusions as to bettering the treatment in vogue. I have not urged much, I have mostly watched and said very little, but I have had the cooperation of the attending staff who have been very good in following the suggestions that I have made. I did not make any suggestions as I did not feel sure of my ground at first. I did not know just how much the condition of pregnancy changed the ordinary principles of the treatment of heart conditions. The great thing we have done is the work in the prenatal clinic. We have seen these women early in their pregnancy and have saved some of them from severe decompensation and that is well worth while. It is also important to follow them after delivery. The case Dr. Child has told of gives me the impression that she should be allowed to continue this pregnancy as long as she is as well as described at present. A a rule however, the seriousness of cardiac disease is greater in multiparae than in primiparae. In this case she apparently will have an easy delivery. Why she had the difficult time in 1915 is hard to say. There may have been reasons why she did badly at that time. She may have had an infection or she may have been doing a great deal of housework. So long as the signs and symptoms are stationary it is no harm to let her continue.

As to cesarean section, I am interested to have the question discussed because we must reach a definite conclusion as to its effect upon the mother. We do not know whether or not rapid diminution of intraabdominal pressure does harm, but it does increase the amount of blood in the abdominal veins and that is in effect like a phlebotomy, a desirable form of treatment when the heart is overtaxed. The obeservation that the discharge of a large amount of fluid improved the condition of the cardiac patient was of interest. I have as yet no experience with cesarean section used in this way. Version and extraction have been done and also high forceps, but both of these seem to be a very severe operation to impose upon a cardiac patient. It may be advisable to induce labor in an interval when cardiac syptoms are more or less quiescent but that is a problem to be decided for each individual case.

It has been observed that blood pressure rises during labor and mental strain can be an important factor in causing this. That may be why scopolamine is helpful inasmuch as it diminishes mental activity.

DR. LORBER.—Is it possible by means of the electrocardiogram or by other means to determine what the heart will stand?

DR. PARDEE.—We do not think the electrocardiogram provides a method of determining the fitness of the heart but only gives information with reference to the structural integrity. A heart may be much impaired and yet be quite fit, or it may be little diseased and be quite unfit. We must determine fitness by the reaction to a test exercise.

DR. SCADRON.—During your antenatal work did you find any functional murmurs in the pulmonic area?

DR. PARDEE.—Yes, and we have seen them persist after delivery, but, as you know, many of those murmurs are found in men, so they probably are not caused by pregnancy.

NEW YORK ACADEMY OF MEDICINE
SECTION ON OBSTETRICS AND GYNECOLOGY
STATED MEETING, HELD FEBRUARY 28, 1922

DR. WILLIAM E. CALDWELL IN THE CHAIR

DR. HENRY C. COWLES presented a case of **Pregnancy Following Cesarean Section with Subtotal Hysterectomy in a Case of Unrecognized Uterus Duplex.**

Double uterus with double vagina of equal size developed to the extent of functioning successfully, is sufficiently infrequent to warrant recording. Furthermore each case seems to present certain features which are individual both from the standpoint of antepartum diagnosis and of obstetrical management.

CASE REPORT.—Mrs. X, age twenty-three, married four years, family history negative. She was particularly healthy and active as a child, and had no illness except diphtheria when 12 years old. Menses appeared during thirteenth year, were regular, 28-day type, seven days' duration with slight crampy pains just prior to the flow. She was married four years ago and became pregnant in August, 1919. This pregnancy was uneventful and near the appointed time in 1920 she went into labor. The pains were light and intermittent for forty-eight hours, the membranes then ruptured and the pains became more severe. After forty-eight hours more of labor without progress the physician who then had her in charge decided upon delivery by cesarean section. At this stage it was recognized that the patient had a double vagina. The left side apparently ended in a culdesac. The right connected with the pregnant uterus, being very narrow and fibrous in the upper portion and apparently slightly dilated. On account of the membranes having been ruptured forty-eight hours and a number of examinations having been made, the operator reasoned that hysterectomy after removal of the child would obviate potential infection. This was done. The right ovary and tube were not disturbed. The operator states that he found but one broad ligament and one ovary. The patient was advised that further conception would not occur. The child, a boy, was normal save for a slight deformity of the left hand, the terminal phalanges of all fingers and thumb being absent. Convalescence of the mother was normal.

One month after delivery she menstruated normally and continued regular until March 6, 1921, when amenorrhea became established and was considered a natural sequence of the hysterectomy. But during May there was a characteristic gastric disturbance with enlargement and soreness of the breasts, and on July 1 she felt life. I examined the patient first August 17, 1921, and noted: an abdomen enlarged, presenting the scar of a previous cesarean section around the umbilicus one-half above, one-half below. The breasts were pigmented and scant secretion was present. An abdominal tumor the size of a five months' pregnancy, showed fetal movements and fetal heart sounds. The introitus was markedly discolored and separation of the labia revealed two distinct openings, the septum between which was about a quarter of an inch thick and continuous to the vaginal vault. In the vault of the right vagina a small firm cervix could be felt. In the vault of the left vagina there was presented a cervix typical of pregnancy in consistency, though smaller than normal. Ballottement was obtained, yet the uterine sac seemed tense and thin. Pelvic measurements were ample. From the foregoing a diagnosis of pregnancy in the left half of what had been a completely double uterus was made, though due consideration was given to the fact that this part of the generative tract might be little more than a tube connected with a rudimentary cervix. However, as the pregnant organ had developed to this stage without symptoms of rupture it was decided to carry the patient to term if possible and to deliver her again by cesarean section.

The pregnancy developed normally, though at each observation the sense of thinness and tenseness of the uterine wall was evident.

Delivery by cesarean section was done December 10, 1921, and when the abdomen was opened the uterus which presented seemed normal in shape but tense. When emptied of its contents, however, and contracted the wall was seen to be thinner than usual and there was a distinct flattening of the right side, the side originally juxtaposed to its mate previously removed. This right side was devoid of tube, ovary and ligaments. The left side was normal in all respects. The pelvis was then explored and the ovary and tube of the ablated right uterus was found and seemed to be normal. This child which was a female weighing 6 pounds 12 ounces presented a slight deformity, a readily remediable left talipes calcaneovalgus which probably was due to intrauterine pressure.

DISCUSSION

DR. H. N. VINEBERG.—I have seen several of these cases. The first was a woman who had had numerous pregnancies, several resulting in miscarriages. She was then pregnant in the left uterus and aborted at the fourth month. The vaginal septum was rather distinct and extended only about two-thirds the length of the vaginal canal. Both cervices were lacerated, making it evident that both uteri had been pregnant. Probably one uterus was pregnant one time and the other the next time. That woman showed the typical characteristics of uterus didelphys, she had a rather wide pelvis. I have had a patient in my private practice who, when she first came to me, had two distinct vaginae and two cervices. Pregnancy occurred in the left side and the right uterus enlarged. During the puerperium there was slight rise in temperature, and I found that by pressing upon the right uterus I was able to expel some tissue, evidently decidua. Following this the temperature dropped and the patient had no futher fever. In her second pregnancy, and this occurred in the same uterus, the puerperium was afebrile the whole time.

Only last week a patient came into my office who was thirty-one years of age and had had three children. She began to bleed two weeks after her last menstruation and kept on bleeding. Upon examination, I detected two uteri with a vaginal septum and pregnancy had evidently occurred in both uteri at different times. She had never been told that she had this condition and was not at all aware of it. The bleeding came from the right cervix and as the cervix was rather patulous I was able to curette it gently and to remove some tissue. At her next visit there was bleeding from her left side and none from the right uterus. Most authorities deny that true uterus didelphys is met with excepting in newly born babies, for it is always attended with so many other vital deformities that life is not possible. They think the so-called didelphic uteri are merely instances of extreme uterus bicornus. Pfannenstiel, however, did not accept this view, for he reported twelve cases in adult life.

DR. A. J. RONGY.—I do not think that uterus didelphys is so infrequent. I saw one case, of a woman miscarried in the fourth month, and five months later she gave birth to a full term child. In another case the pregnancy occurred in the right uterus; the left uterus enlarged and caused obstruction to the passage of the child. The child was delivered by cesarean section and the empty uterus was removed at the same time.

I do not think the Porro operation was indicated in this case. In these patients, in whom many vaginal examinations have been made or who have been in labor for some time, and in whom infection is presupposed, I usually pack the uterus with iodoform gauze; that, to my mind prevents a great deal of intrauterine decomposition and, at the same time, causes the uterus to contract, and the chances of infection are therefore lessened.

It is a question whether, in view of the history, the second cesarean section was indicated, and the mere fact that the patient demanded it is certainly no indication.

DR. W. E. CALDWELL.—It strikes me that where a hysterectomy was done on one side in this case of uterus didelphys, one would probably find distortion and atresia of the cervix on the opposite side. Did the condition of soft parts make the second cesarean section necessary?

DR. COWLES (closing).—So far as defending the hysterectomy is concerned, I am not defending it. I did not do the hysterectomy. That was done in another city. I think the cesarean section was indicated but I think there was no indication for the hysterectomy. So far as the second cesarean section was concerned, the uterus felt as though it would rupture. The tension was great and the wall thin. Furthermore she had four days of labor with the first baby with no progress whatsoever. In the vault of that vagina there was a distinct sense of fibrosis. I feared rupture and did not want to take the risk of the amount of effort that would be required to dilate that cervix.

DR. GEORGE L. BRODHEAD reported a case of **Hydatiform Mole.**

This case is of an exceptional interest, because of the fact that in addition to the typical vesicular mass, a perfect fœtus was found. Edgar in his textbook states that he had seen hydatiform mole four times in 15,000 cases of labor observed in hospital and private practice and that the condition tends to recur. In a personal communication Edgar also states that he has never seen a fetus with hydatiform mole.

In the discussion of our case we would be glad to learn of cases of recurrence for in our experience we have no record of any. The condition is very rare and cases are still more infrequent where a fetus is found. As DeLee states in his work, the rule is that the fetus dies very early in pregnancy and is absorbed. This opinion coincides with our experience, for at the Harlem Hospital in the last eight years, during which time we have had about 11,000 labors and abortions, we have found hydatiform mole in only six cases, in only one of which a fetus was present. The symptoms calling our attention to the condition are atypical hemorrhage, soft boggy uterus, enlargement of the uterus, in some cases beyond the known or supposed period of gestation and the appearance in the vaginal discharge of typical diseased chorionic villi.

Our patient, a white primipara, aged twenty-four, came into the hospital bleeding profusely. The uterus was enlarged to about the size of a four months' pregnancy. No fetal heart could be heard neither was it possible to map out a fetus. The patient was put under ether, one c.c. of pituitary extract was given and a large vesicular mole was removed together with a well-formed four months' fetus. Her temperature on admission was 100° F. For several days there was a moderate rise of temperature, but the patient left the hospital in good condition on the eleventh day. The subsequent history was unobtainable as the woman could not be located.

DISCUSSION

DR. H. N. VINEBERG.—What is surprising to me is the small number of cases of hydatiform mole in so large a number of deliveries. The reason I assume maternity clinics see comparatively so few cases is due to the fact that they have a tendency to miscarry early and the patients are more likely to go to the gynecologic clinic where they are treated for early abortion. I have been particularly interested in hydatiform moles because of their tendency to be followed by chorioepithelioma. This makes it almost a necessity in every case of hydatiform mole to do a vaginal hysterotomy. This may not always be necessary, but one should palpate the entire interior of the uterus to see that there are no growths remaining. It seems to me that in some cases of chorioepithelioma the growth is present at the time the mole is removed. In these cases, bleeding recurs and the uterus is curetted three or four times perhaps and finally when the correct diagnosis is made the patient is too far gone to be saved. In every case of hydatidiform mole one should see that all the vesicles are removed and that there is not present a chorioepithelioma growth.

DR. HOLDEN.—The reason the fetus was present was that this was a twin pregnancy. I have never seen a fetus with a hydatiform mole in a single pregnancy. Very likely this was a twin pregnancy with the degeneration of one fetus and the implantation of the mole. The statement has been made that 50 per cent of hydatiform moles are followed by chorioepithelioma. Dr. Symmers tells me that at Bellevue they have had 18 hydatiform moles in five years and not a single case of chorioepithelioma.

DR. MILTON A. SHLENKER.—Within the past two years I have presented to this section three or four specimens of hydatidiform mole. I do not consider their occurrence as infrequent as quoted by Dr. Brodhead. I think that the most recent compilation of statistics on this subject show that they occur as often as 1 in 2500 cases.

As to the occurrence of the fetus with the mole, I am of the same opinion as the previous speaker, that this fetus is one of a twin pregnancy which had not undergone an absorption. This is the usual etiology of cases where a fetus is found with chorionic degeneration.

DR. VINEBERG.—The statistics show that 50 per cent of chorioepitheliomata are preceded by hydatiform moles. Now as to what number of hydatiform moles are followed by chorioepithelioma; that is stated variously, sometimes as high as 16 per cent and even higher, while others give it lower. In my nine personal cases of chorioepithelioma four were preceded by hydatiform moles.

DR. BRODHEAD.—Dr. Vineberg is perfectly correct. I think the figures show that 50 per cent of chorioepitheliomas are preceded by hydatiform mole, but hydatiform moles are rarely followed by chorioepithelioma.

Reference was made to twin pregnancy. If it had been a twin pregnancy one would think that we might have found a perfectly normal placenta while the other placenta would have been degenerated.

DR. EDWIN C. LANGROCK reported a case of **Rupture of the Uterus Following Pituitrin.**

This case is reported to bring out the fact that even after the uterus has been completely emptied, the administration of pituitrin is not without risk, and that when used after the completion of the third stage, the dosage should be small.

The patient, Mrs. M. G., twenty-seven years of age, was at term in her second pregnancy. During the week prior to her delivery, Feb. 4, 1919, she sent for me twice thinking she was in labor. On account of these two false calls, when she was awakened at 6 A. M. on the above date, with a slight cramp in her abdomen, she refused to allow her nurse to call me. Against the wishes of the patient the nurse called me on the telephone. While she was talking to me the patient had a few very mild labor pains, and the baby, weighing 8 1/2 pounds, was born. I arrived at the house twenty-five minutes later, and found the patient in satisfactory condition. The placenta was delivered easily by the Credé method. Immediately after the birth of the placenta, the patient received 1 c.c. of "infundin." Fifteen minutes later the woman complained of a very severe pain in the left lower quadrant of her abdomen. Her general condition remained good, and I paid no particular attention to her complaint. The pain persisted, however, and shortly became very much more severe. The pain was constant, radiated to the left side of her back, and caused her to cry out. Her pulse rate had risen to 120, and she appeared anxious. I gave her 1/4 grain of morphine, and 1/150 grain of atropine, hypodermically. Thirty minutes thereafter, with but slight relief of the pain, her pulse had risen to 140, but the quality of the pulse remained good. She was not pallid but appeared dusky. Her features were pinched; marked tenderness developed over the whole left abdomen. Another dose of morphine was administered. This relieved her pain, and her general condition improved somewhat. During this time there was no abnormal bleeding.

About 2 P. M. of the same day, that is, about seven hours after her delivery, the patient appeared seriously ill. Her pulse was still 140; her facial expression was unchanged. Her pain had disappeared but tenderness remained. There was slight muscular rigidity, especially on deep pressure, in her left lower abdomen. An area of dullness on percussion had developed, which extended to the left flank, almost up to the margin of the ribs on the left side. Bleeding was normal.

The diagnosis was made either of a rupture of the uterus, or rupture of a vein in the left broad ligament, giving rise to a large retroperitoneal hematoma.

At 4 P. M., Dr. Brodhead saw the patient in consultation with me. The clinical picture was unchanged and the above diagnosis was considered as probably correct. For the next six hours her condition remained practically the same.

At 10 P. M., the patient was seen by Dr. Berg, who made a vaginal examination, and felt a rent in the lower uterine segment, extending out to the left broad ligament. She was treated conservatively with opiates for her pain and given general obstetrical care.

Four days later she had a hemorrhage which was moderately profuse, but was quickly checked by a vaginal pack of iodoform gauze. A similar hemorrhage occurred two and a half weeks later, and another one eight weeks later. Each time the bleeding was so free that vaginal packing was required.

Catheterization was necessary from the time of her delivery until she was discharged fourteen weeks later. During this time the pelvic hematoma became infected, as was evidenced by a variable fever, lasting for ten weeks. The pelvic abscess ruptured spontaneously and drained through the rent in the uterus into the vagina.

The patient was discharged fourteen weeks after her delivery as cured.

The interesting features of this case are the easy normal delivery without violent uterine contractions, the onset of the condition described, following the administration of 1 c.c. of pituitrin, the uterine rupture with the formation of a large retroperitoneal hematoma, the infection of the hematoma, and the spontaneous rupture of the abscess effecting the cure of the patient.

In closing, I wish to emphasize the point that at *all* times, and even when the uterus is empty, pituitrin should be used with caution, and the dose should be small.

DISCUSSION

DR. H. N. VINEBERG.—The statement that a small dose of pituitrin can cause the rupture of an empty uterus is a very serious matter. We give pituitrin so often and so freely postpartum that we shall have to analyze this case very carefully before we accept it as it has been given. Is it not more likely that the head came down abruptly and ruptured the lower segment? The child came very quickly and it is likely that the head tore the cervix into the base of the broad ligament and it took some time before sufficient blood was effused to cause symptoms. The dose of pituitrin would simply be a coincidence.

DR. BONGY.—It is unfortunate that neither Dr. Brodhead nor Dr. Langrock examined this patient. Pituitrin does not produce a tear, as described by Dr. Langrock. Rupture of the uterus, due to pituitrin, usually takes place in the body of the uterus, or if the uterus violently contracts, when the baby is still in the uterus, it many tear itself away from its vaginal insertion, but it does not tear from below upwards into the culdesac.

Mechanically it is impossible for the uterus to rupture when it is empty, and in this case the pituitrin was administered after the baby was born. The tear in this patient was caused by rapid labor; the child lacerated the cervix, and the tear extended into the broad ligaments.

DR. BRODHEAD.—I have nothing particular to say except that the facts are exactly as Dr. Langrock has given them. There was a mass running up into the left lumbar region. We felt that it would be better to let the woman alone and that vaginal examination was unnecessary. Dr. Berg came up and examined the patient and found the rupture of the uterus, above the cervix. Pituitrin, if given at all, at any stage of labor, must be given in small doses. I rarely use more than 2 minims. I usually start with 1 minim. With doses as small as these we have seen no harmful results.

DR. HERVEY C. WILLIAMSON.—I think Dr. Vineberg is probably correct. At Bellevue we had a case delivered by operative means, a difficult craniotomy. Both Dr. Gravelle and myself introduced our hands into the uterus and were satisfied that there was a rupture of the lower segment. There was not as much bleeding as in a normal delivery. No pituitrin was given. On the following day the patient had a temperature of 104° and a mass in the right iliac region. This subsided but it later became infected. I examined her and in putting my finger into the opening pus escaped. She then made an uneventful recovery.

I believe that Dr. Langrock's case would have had the same course postpartum with or without the pituitrins.

DR. LANGROCK.—I do not think that either Dr. Brodhead or myself saw any occasion to make a vaginal examination. The patient had either a rupture of the uterus or a bleeding vessel and there was nothing to do but what we did do. If we had made a vaginal examination nothing would have been found but the tear going up into the broad ligament. The general surgeon did what we would not do, and I did not feel that he was justified in making a vaginal examination. Dr. Berg is quite capable of making a diagnosis and he diagnosed a rent into the broad ligament. The bleeding was absolutely normal throughout the whole affair. It seems possible that the tear might have been due to a precipitate delivery, and this baby weighed more than the former one and the mother had very hard contractions at the time of delivery. Forty minutes later when I arrived she was in perfectly good condition. She was given the dose of pituitrin and within ten minutes she complained of pelvic pains. She very quickly had contractions and my feeling is that the uterus probably ruptured as a result of these severe contractions.

DR. ARTHUR STEIN presented a paper, which was read by Dr. Langrock, entitled **Treatment of Tuberculous Peritonitis by Oxygen Inflation of the Abdominal Cavity, Artificial Pneumoperitoneum,** of which the following is an abstract:

During the course of my studies of artificial pneumoperitoneum as an aid to roentgen-ray diagnosis, the idea occurred to me that oxygen inflations of the abdominal cavity might be utilized therapeutically for the treatment of tuberculous peritonitis. Clinical observation had shown marked improvement in several children with peritonitis after the performance of one oxygen inflation prior to roentgen examination.

The patient, Mrs. T. M., thirty-two years of age, was referred to me with the complaint of constant pain in the back and was seen for the first time on Oct. 26, 1920. She had had one confinement several years previously and gave a history of irregular and always painful menstruation. Urination was frequent by night as well as by day.

A general examination at the time revealed the heart, lungs, and abdomen to be normal. Deep pressure over McBurney's point elicited slight pain. The patient seemed in excellent health and weighed 156 pounds.

Vaginal examination showed the vulva and vagina to be normal, the cervix pointing toward the symphysis. The body of the uterus was retroflexed and fixed. The posterior parametrium exhibited marked tenderness upon effort to push the uterus back into position. The patient was advised to have the uterus replaced in the normal position, and an operation was performed by me at the end of October, 1920. At this time the appendix was removed. At the time of operation there was not the slightest evidence of tuberculosis of the parietal or visceral peritoneum, of the omentum or of either adnexa.

I did not see the patient again until March, 1921, about three months after her discharge from the hospital. At that time she complained of marked pains in the right lower abdomen and a sensation of fullness in the abdomen, which amounted to acute discomfort after eating. She did not look so well as formerly. She was given tonics and kept under observation. The abdominal pains became more severe, her abdomen increased in size and night sweats made their appearance.

On the evening of March 1, 1921, I was called to see the patient. Her temperature at that time was 105°, pulse 120. There was extreme distention of the abdomen accompanied by marked pain. Examination revealed the presence of free fluid in the abdomen, and a diagnosis of acute exudative tuberculous peritonitis was made. On the following day the patient was removed to the Lenox Hill Hospital and an x-ray picture taken following artificial pneumoperitoneum. Dr. Stewart reported that roentgenographically the case presented a tuberculous peritonitis. On the following day an x-ray picture of the lungs was taken, but no evidence of pulmonary tuberculosis was found.

The oxygen injected at the time of the x-ray examination was not withdrawn. Thirty-six hours later there was still some oxygen present. The whole procedure did not cause the patient the slightest discomfort and the improvement in her general condition after this single inflation was most marked. By April her temperature had dropped to about 100°. She was therefore given another therapeutic oxygen inflation. About 4 liters of oxygen were used. On April 5 and 11 two more oxygen inflations were given. The patient was discharged from the hospital on April 12 and from that time her temperature remained normal. Her condition continued to appear normal during April and she promptly began to take on weight.

Not long after, while visiting relatives in Baltimore, she had another attack. She was persuaded to remain in that city and to consult Dr. Maurice Lazenby, who later wrote Dr. Stein that he had made a diagnosis of papilloadenocystoma of the ovary with probable malignancy. He was unable to get into the abdomen through a median incision and then made a high right rectus incision. A large quantity of blood-tinged serous fluid with numerous flakes was found. The omentum was fastened firmly to the anterior wall of the abdomen. Upon exploring the upper part of the abdomen he came in contact with a nodule 2 cm. in diameter in the omentum. This was excised. Upon further exploration numerous nodules were found over the under surface of the liver and as far as the finger could reach on the peritoneum. There were numerous loops of gut adherent to the abdominal wall. The abdomen was then closed. Examination of the specimen showed numerous caseating tubercles.

The patient had had no other attacks and at the present time weighed 152 pounds stripped, whereas at the time of her illness in March, 1921, she weighed 124 pounds.

It is clear that the pneumoperitoneal method of oxygen inflation offers a tremendous advantage over laparotomy as a therapeutic measure. The pneumoperitoneal method may be employed as often as indicated, ten, twelve or fifteen times, while a laparotomy with its accompanying shock, may at the utmost be resorted to only twice. The patients experience little or no discomfort from the inflations, and realizing the immediate benefit, look forward cheerfully and contentedly to the next administration.

Recently a child of eleven years with a markedly distended abdomen was admitted to the Harlem Hospital. A diagnosis of exudative tuberculous peritonitis was made. Thus far the child has been inflated ten times with results that are simply amazing.

In passing it might be mentioned that it is advisable to remove the ascitic fluid. It will also be found that these ascitic patients can tolerate more inflation (up to 5 or 6 liters of oxygen) due to the distention of the abdominal walls by the ascitic fluid.

Dr. Stein believes that this is the first case to be reported in the United States of an apparent cure of tuberculous peritonitis of the exudative type by the sole means of pneumoperitoneum.

Since completing the above report, Dr. Max Einhorn of this city had referred to him for examination a young Greek girl, twenty-four years of age, who was suffering with a marked abdominal distention. Clinical as well as pneumoperitoneal x-ray examination revealed general tuberculous exudative peritonitis. So far this patient had received two oxygen inflations with very marked improvement in the abdominal condition.

DISCUSSION

DR. EDWIN A. RIESENFELD.—My experience with the treatment of exudative tuberculous peritonitis is limited to one case, which Dr. Stein mentions in his paper. This child was admitted to the Pediatric Department of the Harlem Hospital in October, 1921, and at Dr. Stein's suggestion this method of treatment was tried.

The family and previous history of this case has no bearing on the present condition. The present illness began in July, 1921, with elevation of temperature, cough and vague abdominal pains. The patient complained also of drowsiness and extreme weakness. After admission the diagnosis of tuberculosis was confirmed by x-ray examination which showed peribronchial gland thickening. While the patient was in the hospital the abdomen was distended but no fluid was obtained. The distention quickly disappeared and the child was taken from the hospital on request of the parents. Subsequently the abdomen again became distended. The child complained of severe intermittent cramp-like pains in the abdomen. The child's mother has noticed that the child had fever at night. Emaciation, anorexia and constipation were continually present and a cough which occurred each night when the child assumed the recumbent position.

Examination revealed a child with the most marked degree of emaciation I have ever seen. The heart was pushed upward, the apex beat being in the third interspace; the heart was otherwise normal. The lungs were negative. The abdomen was tremendously enlarged. Organs could not possibly be palpated due to the distention. By x-ray the peribronchial glands were seen to be thickened and the abdomen showed the presence of fluid. Examination of the latter negative for tuberculosis. The proportion of lymphocytes to polymorphonuclears was 6 to 1.

Inasmuch as pneumoperitoneum seemed to be a rational mode of treatment, it seemed advisable to give the method a trial. As Dr. Stein has stated in his paper, some ten or twelve treatments were given and the results were little short of marvellous.

In a study of the literature of the treatment of tuberculous peritonitis one is struck by the great number of methods of handling this condition, and one is forced to the conclusion that the reason of this is that no one method has been found successful. Laparotomy or operative interference should not be undertaken too lightly. One can perform one or two laparotomies on a case and then he is in the dilemma of what to do next. Some cases recover without any treatment whatever. Recently Rollier has treated some of these cases successfully by heliotherapy, but we have not the facilities for carrying out that form of treatment in this country. When the oxygen treatment is given the patient complains of no pain and no discomfort. The injection of oxygen may be repeated many times without harm to the patient. I cannot believe that the phlebitis from which the child suffered had anything to do with the first operation. The child's temperature became normal after about 50 days. I have recently seen the child's father and he tells me that she is out and continues to improve.

DR. L. T. LEWALD.--We have produced artificial pneumoperitoneum in several instances and there are records of thousands of cases in which the procedure has been employed during the last three or four years. Four fatal cases have been reported, two of which occurred in one hospital. One of these fatalities was due to air embolism and the cause of the other was unexplained, but possibly it was due to air embolism. Of two other accidents, one was the result of perforation of the small intestine which was adherent to the anterior abdominal wall. In another instance there was a puncture of the bowel. Both of these patients recovered. So, though the procedure of introducing air or gas into the peritoneal cavity by puncture is a relatively safe procedure, it is not devoid of all danger. Carelli demonstrated here recently the method used in 750 consecutive cases without a single accident. He also did a large number of air injections in the kidney region without accident and then had two accidents. In one case the fatality was due to air embolism. The needle was introduced from behind and was accidentally introduced into a vein. The heart removed at autopsy showed distinct air embolism. Dr. Keyes told me he had punctured the kidney in one instance, but there was very little damage from that, as he removed the kidney a few days later. Thus one has to think of the possible accidents in employing these methods, but I think the benefits outweigh the slight accidental injuries that may occur.

We had one case of tuberculosis of the mesenteric lymph nodes in which we were called upon to make an x-ray examination in order to demonstrate whether or not there was an intussusception. At operation the lymph nodes were demonstrated greatly enlarged, but they subsided afterwards. It was a little far fetched to think that tuberculous lymph nodes could be cured by air injection, but this case certainly was greatly benefited as a result of the laparotomy.

DR. RONGY.—I want to sound a note of warning that insufflation with oxygen or any other gas is not without danger. I performed a large number of intrauterine insufflations for the purpose of testing the patency of the tubes. In one case I introduced 300 c.c. of oxygen, which is not at all a large amount, and as soon as the patient assumed the erect position, the gas evidently pushed up the diaphragm, embarrassing the heart action, and she went into collapse. For a few moments it appeared that death was imminent.

We must be very careful with this method of treatment, especially in patients who are obese; some of these patients do not seem to bear this method of treatment as well as the patients who are normal weight or underweight.

DR. F. J. HOLDEN.—In our interview with the patient we have elicited the information that only a few weeks elapsed between the time of the original injection and the operation in Baltimore. It was a matter of eight months after the operation until Dr. Stein saw the patient again, during which time she became almost entirely well. There was an eight months' interval between the operation in Baltimore and the final injection of oxygen. Was the patient cured by the operation or the oxygen inflation? I believe this method which Dr. Stein has described has a great deal of value, but the facts as they have been given place the credit of the cure to the operative procedure rather than to the oxygen inflation.

DR. E. W. HOLLADAY.—I shall have to agree with Dr. Holden that the operative procedure is what effected the cure in this case and not the oxygen insufflation.

DR. LEROY BROUN.—As the reader of the paper has said, this is not a new method but one that has been tried out for several years. Dr. Shively, a specialist on tuberculosis, some six or eight years ago, showed a patient as cured by this treatment of transperitoneal oxygen inflation. Dr. Shively stated at the time that the patient was free from any evidence of tuberculosis at the time of his presenting her. He stated that the treatment was being tried out at tuberculosis sanitoria with hopes of proving its value. There were two classes of tuberculous peritonitis, namely, those in which a plastic form of the disease predominates and there is little fluid. In that class of cases oxygen inflation would be of doubtful benefit since in using oxygen in such a case there is a possibility of injuring the intestines on account of the fixation due to adhesions. But in the other group where the abdomen was much distended and one had reason to think the intestines were pushed back and the fluid was on top, I think this is a safe procedure and well worth trying. Repeated injections would depend on the amount of recurring fluid.

DR. REED.—Was there any way of knowing whether this was the bovine or the human form of tuberculosis? In Edinburgh, surgeons open the abdomen and resect portions of the bowel and cecum for tuberculosis, while in London they will not attempt to open the abdomen. The reason is because in London it is the human tubercle, while in Edinburgh it is the bovine. Is there any reason for saying whether this was human or bovine tuberculosis?

DR. RIESENFELD.—Intestinal tuberculosis in this country is usually of the bovine type. Unfortunately a bacteriologic examination was not made in this case.

The case which I presented was treated by tapping and injections of oxygen through a needle. It is quite true that a great number of these cases get well themselves. In the plastic type of the disease operation should not be attempted. If the bowel is torn and a fistula results, this is certainly worse than the original condition. In our case the number of injections was governed by the temperature as we had nothing else to guide us. The child stood the inflation well, and when the temperature fell to normal and the abdomen became flaccid and normal we ceased giving the inflations. The improvement in this child in ten weeks was amazing. From a wretched, emaciated child with no appetite she was changed to an almost normal child with a hearty appetite, and gaining in weight.

OBSTETRICAL SOCIETY OF PHILADELPHIA

MEETING OF DECEMBER 1, 1921.

DR. WILLIAM P. GRAVES, of Boston, by invitation, addressed the Society on **The Ovarian Function.** (For original article, see p. 583.)

DISCUSSION

DR. BARTON COOKE HIRST.—It is interesting to contrast the views of Dr. Graves with those of Dr. Bell and of Dr. Polak, I have long believed that we strove to retain ovarian tissue when it had better been removed. In my early career I first sacrificed ovaries too inconsiderately and then went to the other extreme to save ovarian tissue. I have been obliged to reopen the abdomen of a number of women after my own previous operations and after operations by other surgeons, to remove degenerated ovaries and I have now come fairly close to the opinion that I understand Dr. Graves holds, but we should remember Dr. Bell's experience with transplanted ovaries and Polak's advocacy of preserving the circulation of the broad ligaments.

I agree with Polak that if one can preserve the circulation of the broad ligament intact, ovarian tissue may be left with impunity. If the incision in the broad ligament is made so there is no interference with uterine and ovarian anastomosis, there is little likelihood of subsequent degeneration of the ovary. So if practicable it should be done. It is easy enough to take the ovaries out, but not so easy to put them back again.

Dr. Blair Bell's technic should receive wider trial than it has. His observations have extended over five years of cases in which he buried a segment of the interior of an ovary in the rectus muscle without exciting hemorrhage. In the great majority of these cases he has preserved the menstrual function. It is often important to do so from the psychological point of view. I know of three private patients who are in insane asylums in consequence of an operative menopause, which accentuates to the patient's mind the fact that she has been mutilated and unsexed. For this reason it may be important to conserve menstrual function by Polak's plan or if that is not practicable, by Bell's. Take another instance: I recall a young girl on whom I operated quite early in life, before she married, removing both tubes for gonorrheal infection but leaving both ovaries. She made a perfect recovery, married happily and ten years later consulted me as to the possibility of conception, stating that she was now reconciled to the thought of sterility but had she been aware at first that she had been mutilated and rendered incapable of bearing children, it would have prevented her marriage and spoiled her whole life. These psychologic considerations, therefore, deserve attention as well as the physical results of the operation. I was particularly interested in the statements about the physiological activity of the cells in the ovarian residue. I have always believed that the corpus luteum was the source of the internal secretion of the ovary, but from what Dr. Graves has said, we must evidently pay more attention in our endocrine treatment, to the product of the whole ovary.

DR. JOHN G. CLARK.—Dr. Graves' very interesting address, in which he lays much stress, and properly so, upon the embryological derivations of the ovaries, brings to my mind a series of injection experiments which were carried out by me under Dr. Mall and later under Professor His, on the circulation of the ovary. By tracing back the embryo to the earliest period when it could be successfully injected, at the time when the germinal hillock was well defined on the wolffian body, I found the circulation of the ovary and testicle diametrically opposite. In other words, at the earliest priod in fetal life, the sex of the embryo could invariably be ascertained with absolute precision by the way in which the arteries were distributed. The ovarian circulation enters the germinal hillock at its base, penetrates the mass of epithelium and branches fan-like, dividing and subdividing the ovary into its final primitive follicles, leaving the terminal capillary branches in the tunica albuginea, or fibrous covering of the ovary. Quite to the contrary is the circulation of the testicle. The spermatic artery courses over the dorsum of the testicle and surrounds the organ with rib or hoop-like laterals, which send their twigs into the depths of the organ and terminate as capillaries in the very center. I do not dissent from Dr. Graves' theories, but I must say that I cannot make these observations coincide with them. In other words, Phlüger's theory was similar to that reviewed by Dr. Graves, namely, that the follicles are formed from egg cords or tubes which penetrate the mass of germinal epithelium whereas Waldeyer believed that the egg cells were divided first into fan-like compartments by the inthrust of blood vessels and connective tissue into the general hillock, thence further subdivided into the primordial follicles. My observations in the development of the ovarian circulation were very convincingly in favor of the latter, hence, I would like to be convinced as to Dr. Graves' interpretation of the origin of the follicles and the interstitial cells. Dr. Graves quite properly says that Dr. Charles C. Norris and I will be difficult to convince that the conserved ovary in a young woman in the absence of the uterus is of no value. We have studied a comparative set of cases, comprising over a hundred, and we feel certain that a conserved healthy ovary is of vital import. But, in full justice to Dr. Graves' viewpoint, we find as a result of our comparative statistics in women of equal decades that the temperamental equation is more important than the age factor in this estimation. Our statistics seem to show that the menopause in its mildness or severity is not so intimately associated with the age factor. In other words, we feel, that given equal ages, women upon whom a hysterectomy is done and yet possess a conserved ovary will in the aggregate, suffer far less than those in whom a total ablation has been performed, but there are interesting temperamental variations which are not dependent upon the age factor. Thus, a highly strung woman of the nervous type may go through an exaggerated menopause at forty-eight years of age, whereas a woman of thirty years of the well poised type may suffer only fleeting symptoms of the change of life. We consider the atrophy of the vagina which almost invariably occurs in young women who have not borne children of very serious portent if she is married, rendering her sexual life a burden or making it impossible. By our own experience, we must be guided, and while I concede to Dr. Graves his viewpoint, because I know that he is a careful observer, I cannot accept it fully, and yet he has so carefully qualified it and hedged it about with qualifying conditions that after all, we are really not so far apart as would appear if both of us spoke without these limitations. As we have reached our conclusions after a clinical retrospect of our comparative statistics, we are confirmed in our belief in the value of the conservation of normal ovaries, but, to reiterate, we do not rest our views upon the age factor so much as upon the temperament of the patient. The woman of the highly wrought type should have the benefits of ovarian conservation even at some pathologic hazard.

DR. RICHARD C. NORRIS.—I shall have no remarks to make on the embryological, since I wish to discuss the clinical side. What Dr. Hirst has said is true, but it does not bear directly on Dr. Graves' paper. The technic of Polak or the method of Bell would be applied to the cases which Dr. Graves brought out as cases in which we should preserve ovarian function and is not the question at issue. The question at issue is what shall we do practically in women with inflammatory conditions, on the one hand, and fibroids on the other, in regard to conservation of their ovarian function? Should procreative or endocrine value of the ovary dominate our action? Does the endocrine value cease after a certain age? I have had to gather my knowledge individually, working it out for myself, as we all do and I must say, in retrospect, that as I have seen my cases, studying them in detail, they have been true as to what Dr. Graves has said. My attempts at conservative surgery of the ovary have been based on the reproductive rather than the endocrine value of the ovary. In younger women it has always been my aim to save the ovary not only for its reproductive power, but also for its endocrine value. I am very glad to hear Dr. Graves present and defend his opinions. I have had some fortunate and unfortunate results in the attempt to conserve the ovary. The method of Polak and the method of Bell will help us in that group in which we preserve ovarian function primarily for its endocrine value. Dr. Clark and Dr. Charles Norris and Dr. Graves have analyzed series of cases and have had their opinions verified. Statistical studies of after results will be prejudiced by what you want to find by your studies, however scientifically they may be carried out. This applies to Dr. Graves as well as Dr. Clark and Dr. Norris. If they want to prove that the saving of ovaries is of sentimental value only, they will prove it. If they want to disprove it, as Dr. Clark has done, they will disprove it. The real crux of the matter is what shall we do in pelvic inflammatory cases? What shall we do in fibroid cases? It is a great satisfaction to me to feel in the presence of a serious inflammatory lesion in a mature woman that I can remove the ovaries and not do the patient harm, since I believe it is wise to remove an infected uterus and by that removal I destroy reproductive function. It is a great satisfaction to have Dr. Graves' dictum that I may remove the ovaries in a woman past thirty and not do her any endocrinal harm because I know I will do her a great deal of good in curing the pain and other distressing symptoms that follow leaving partly diseased ovaries. On the other hand, if it is a fibroid to be removed, this communication of Dr. Graves strongly favors myomectomies, and it stimulates me to do more myomectomies. The more I do myomectomy the more I am satisfied with it even on pregnant women. In those cases in which the uterus is studded with fibroids and we know we must remove the uterus, the surgical problem will be more simplified by what Dr. Graves teaches than by what Dr. Clark teaches. If we can feel that after the woman is mature, her ovaries only have a reproductive value, it certainly simplifies our treatment and I trust further investigation will maintain Dr. Graves' theory. It is a great satisfaction to me; it has confirmed my opinion of the unsatisfactory results of resection. Even with technic which preserves ovarian circulation, the tendency is to atrophy; it is a great satisfaction to hear Dr. Graves' paper and realize we have not done these women injury by removing their ovaries. As to the sentimental side of this, and the views of the laity, we are partially to blame, if with uncertain knowledge, as in the past, we permit the layman and rank and file of the profession, to state that a woman is wrecked and whiskers will grow on her face whenever her ovaries are removed. If we let such doctrines go forth the majority will feel that way. If Dr. Graves is correct, and we can say with authority, that after a certain time a woman may lose her ovaries and the only penalty she pays is that she cannot procreate, a great many women with or without children will be blessed both in mind and body. The crux of the matter is, are the ovaries valuable to the woman when she is mature, in any respect other than reproduction? Dr. Graves' study tends to prove that after that period she is not damaged by the removal. That is a great consolation to me because in such cases I take them out. When they are not mature women or the uterus is preserved, I have done the conservative operations of resection and I must say sometimes pregnancy has occurred, but more often the other story is told and she comes back with pains and aches requiring further operation. If we feel we can remove ovaries and do no harm, except take away reproduction, in our pelvic inflammatory cases at least, Dr. Graves has fortified my belief and I shall go forward in my work in the future more determined than ever and say to the patient, "Disease has taken from you your power of reproduction, what I shall do will relieve you from pain and suffering and enable you to do your work." I welcome his address and think it one of the best things heard here in a long time. It helps to clarify my ideas which means in the future I shall do more and more of what I have done in the past, with more assurance that the reproductive function of the ovary, in a physiologically mature woman, is its dominant function.

DR. G. BETTON MASSEY.—I have been trying to make up my mind whether Dr. Norris was Pickwickian in his remarks or not. I agree, on the contrary with what Dr. Hirst had to say on the subject of removal of ovaries, for this is not the first time this question has been discussed in this Society. I can recall an occasion about twenty-five years ago when the late Dr. Goodell took part in a discussion on the result to the woman of the removal of her ovaries. Dr. Goodell was an older man at that time than the reader of the paper, and he repeated three cycles of his own personal opinion, which had either been printed in his book, or uttered on the floor of this body. As I recall it the first was that there was little or no effect upon a woman due to the removal of her ovaries. He referred this opinion back to his early operative career, and as you all know Dr. Goodell was a very active operator. He probably had not operated many times when he announced that opinion. His second opinion, quoted at this time as having been announced later, was that there was considerable influence upon a woman. Then he gave his final opinion—the man who did the greatest number of operations of this character in the city of Philadelphia at that time—that it had a most profound influence upon a woman's nature in every characteristic. He did not say that she grew whiskers or anything like that. In fact that is something new to me. But I have seen a number of women who have gone to the insane asylum as the result of the removal of the ovaries, one, unfortunately, at my own advice. I have been physician to a number who did not go to the insane asylums but whose condition mentally and physically and nervously was most deplorable. I feel very strongly on this point, and it is accentuated by another remark of the reader of the paper, that the only way to treat hemorrhages of the uterus in the absence of fibroid tumors is by hysterectomy or radium. For thirty years I have been demonstrating in a very quiet way, after getting somewhat tired of talking before this body, that that can be done by the Apostoli treatment. I fear the reader of the paper never heard of that treatment, now supplemented by deep x-ray therapy. It was simply the intrauterine anodic direct current, given with no destructive but constructive, ideas for the cure of disease. I dispute the correctness of the statement made by some one that it was not possible to remove the disease without removal of the ovaries.

DR. GRAVES (closing).—The occurrence of insanity after hysterectomy has in my experience been infrequent. I have encountered only two such cases. Both patients became insane immediately after operation as the result of shock, but both had histories of mental unbalance at previous periods in their lives. Both recovered completely. Regarding patients who become nervously upset by the contemplation of the loss of their organs, I intimated in my paper that this outcome is usually due to domestic influence. Dr. Hirst's case is an excellent illustration of this point. A husband sometimes employs the fact of a radical operation performed on his wife as an excuse for personal abuse or as grounds for divorce. A nervous and mental reaction on the part of the wife is under such conditions inevitable. The sentimental or domestic situation must always be taken into careful consideration by the surgeon, and is often a great weight in determining the proper procedure during an operation.

I am very glad to defer to Dr. Clark's observations regarding the embryonic blood supply of the sex glands and their sex differentiation. Dr. Clark by his excellent early investigations on this subject is an authority, his work having had world wide recognition. To what he says however with reference to Waldeyer's theory of the invasion of the sex gland by the mesonephric tubules I am unable to agree. The statement that I made has the authority of many of the later writers. In my own study of early human embryos I have been unable to detect any suggestion of such an invasion. In other words it seems to be generally accepted at the present day that the vestigia found at the hylus of the ovary, are not wolffian rests but are in reality relics of the early cordlike invasion of the germinal epithelium. This of course has a most important bearing on the question of the histogenesis of ovarian tumors.

I was extremely interested in Dr. Norris' remarks and am especially grateful to him for so forcibly supporting my contentions regarding ovarian conservation.

Department of Reviews and Abstracts

CONDUCTED BY HUGO EHRENFEST, M.D., ASSOCIATE EDITOR

Selected Abstracts

The Physiology of Pregnancy

Biedl, Peters and Hofstatter: Studies on Implantation and the Further Development of the Ovum in the Uterus. Zeitschrift für Geburtshülfe und Gynäkologie, 1921, lxxxiv, 58.

The experiments of the authors were made upon rabbits and sought to determine the influence of the ovary and particularly the corpus luteum upon the implantation and further development of fertilized ova. In this animal follicle rupture and the consequent development of a corpus luteum follows only upon coitus. Fertilized ova from one animal transplanted therefore into virginal animals or into those which had not recently had intercourse, were entirely removed from the influence of the corpus luteum. In the earlier experiments, attempts were made to transfer by forceps or other instruments, fertilized ova from the tube of one animal to that of the other, but this involved too much trauma and none of these ova developed. Soon it was found that at a slightly later period, when the ovum had descended into the uterine cornu, but had not yet been firmly implanted, it could be easily obtained by gently washing the cavity with normal salt solution and could then be placed directly into the uterine cavity of the second animal through a hysterotomy incision. The experiments on virginal animals were uniformly unsuccessful, possibly because the uterine mucosa of these animals was not sufficiently developed. In animals which had borne young but had not recently been pregnant, the results were in most cases unsuccessful. However, in one case further development to a considerable stage seemed to take place, when later, death of the ovum occurred. The authors conclude from this case that a fresh corpus luteum is not absolutely essential to implantation of the fertilized ovum. They suggest that possibly the presence of the fertilized ovum may lead to a reactivation of the corpus luteum of an earlier pregnancy; which might then exert its usual influence.

Other experiments were made with implantation of fertilized ova into uteri of puerperal animals which had been castrated immediately after delivery, or at the time of transplantation; into animals with ovaries damaged by x-ray, and into animals already pregnant, either retaining or destroying the animal's ovary, developing ova. In one puerperal animal the implanted ovum developed into a fetus which was born—this animal's ovaries showed no active corpora lutea. Others developed to a certain stage and then regressed or formed the so-called placentoma. The authors believe that the fertilized ovum itself may exert a very similar stimulus, possibly not purely hormonal in character, to that usually ascribed to the corpus luteum, which may in a certain sense be considered a function of the ovum.

Attempts to stimulate a decidual reaction in the uterus by trauma, they found with Leo Loeb, were successful only in the presence of corpora lutea. Transplanted fetal or placental tissue, however, caused decidual reaction, not only at the site of its implantation, but also elsewhere in the uterus. In certain of these cases, however, there seemed to be a reactivation of old corpora lutea by the presence of this tissue.

The authors give data on fertilization and migration of the ovum in rabbits which they feel may be of value to others who wish to undertake further experimental investigation.
MARGARET SCHULZE.

MacKenzie, W. R.: The Re ation of the Corpus Luteum to Menstruation and Pregnancy. British Medical Journal, March 4, 1922, p. 343.

The author reports several cases from which he draws the following conclusions: (1) Injury to either a true or false corpus luteum will simulate a ruptured extrauterine gestation; (2) Injury to a true corpus luteum will bring on an abortion, and (3) Rupture of a false corpus luteum will bring on menstruation and its accompanying ovulation.
F. L. ADAIR.

Oliver: Human Gestation and Our Embryological and Morphological Data. Edinburgh Medical Journal, 1921, xxvi, 245.

The author emphasizes that fertilization and the onset of gestation are not coetaneous phenomena. Fertilization we now know may take place at any time from the cessation of one period up to two days before the onset of the next. Gestation does not begin at the end of the last full period. In the two days preceding a period the uterus is in a condition to receive the fertilized ovum. Gestation begins, therefore, at this time and the period is held in abeyance. We are in the habit of reckoning the period of gestation from the last menstruation only because we make allowance for the time up to two days before the first missed period. If the woman is not of the 24 to 28-day type our method of figuring is of no value. The old practice is unscientific and the author criticizes its use by embryologists and physicians.
H. W. SHUTTER.

Frank and Nothmann: The Value of Renal Glycosuria of Pregnancy in the Early Diagnosis of Pregnancy. Münchener medizinische Wochenschrift, 1920, lxvii, 1433.

Pregnancy being frequently accompanied by an absolute renal glycosuria, i.e., sugar found in urine, but blood sugar normal, the authors attempted to produce a glycosuria in women in early pregnancy whose blood sugar and urine were normal. The method employed was first to examine the blood sugar and urine to see that they were normal. The bladder was catheterized, 100 grams of grape-sugar in 350-500 c.c. of tea were given by mouth, and after thirty minutes the urine was examined at 15 minute intervals for sugar.

The reaction was positive in 30 cases in the first trimester, negative in three cases of suspected pregnancy which later were found to be not pregnant. The reaction is positive in the first week of pregnancy. In two cases clinically diagnosed tubal pregnancy, the diagnosis was confirmed in one by means of this test, (later at operation found to be correct), and diagnosis held in reserve in the second (operation showed bilateral cyst).

The authors conclude: (1) An alimentary glycosuria was without exception produced in 30 pregnant women in the first trimester. (2) The renal glycosuria may be employed in the early diagnosis of pregnancy immediately following the cessation of menstruation, when the clinical signs are as yet insufficient for positive diagnosis. (3) Starch will give the same results in about 60 per cent of cases. (4) The experimental alimentary glycosuria also points the way to an early diagnosis of ectopic pregnancy.
S. B. SOLHAUG.

Kamnitzer and Joseph: Biologic Diagnosis of Pregnancy. Therapie der Gegenwart, 1921, lxii, 321-24.

Frank has found that in pregnancy the ingestion of 100 grams of glucose suffices to produce glycosuria, and with Nothmann he has applied this phenomenon as a means of diagnosing pregnancy earlier than it can be detected by physical findings.

Following Frank's lead, Kamnitzer and Joseph devised an acceptable test meal of 75 grams raw weight of rice, 100 grams of cane sugar, with tea *ad lib*, and produced glycosuria in 20 cases of pregnancy, of which 5 were in the first month and one was confirmed as a tubal pregnancy. In 30 nonpregnant females, no glycosuria resulted. When only 75 grams of cane sugar were used, results were not consistent. In half of 20 cases the blood sugar exceeded Frank's limit of 0.19 per cent, the maximum being 0.26 per cent.

They then experimented with phloridzin. "While the majority of healthy persons excrete no sugar after injection of 2.5 mg. of phloridzin, the injection of this amount into the pregnant apparently regularly produces a definite glycosuria within half an hour." This amount produced no response in 10 men, and a response in only 7 of 70 nonpregnant women; and in most of these 7 cases the response was delayed until an hour to 1½ hours after injection. Of 30 pregnant women, most of them in the first month of pregnancy, all responded within half an hour. In 9 cases of abortion the test became negative within 10 days. In the cases tested during menstruation, no glycosuria resulted.

The authors conclude that a positive test is therefore a strongly presumptive but not infallible sign of pregnancy, while a lack of response within two hours excludes pregnancy. The test is made with 2.5 c.c. of a fresh 1 per cent solution of phloridzin prepared with the aid of heat. The substance precipitates in the cold. The injection is intramuscular and evokes at most a transitory smarting.

RAMSAY SPILLMAN.

Nürnberger: Utilizing Renal Glycosuria in the Early Diagnosis of Pregnancy. Deutsche medizinische Wochenschrift, 1921, xlvii, 1124.

Frank and Nothmann first called attention to a low sugar tolerance in the first months of pregnancy and, in a certain proportion of patients, also in the later months. Since a low sugar tolerance exists also in other diseases, such as dysfunction of the liver, thyrotoxicosis, latent diabetes and, at times, in neurasthenia, it is, in itself, not pathognomonic. However, in these conditions there is an accompanying increase in the blood sugar which does not exist in pregnancy. This work has been substantiated and amplified by other observers of which Nürnberger is one. He sums up the matter as follows: If 100 gm. of glucose are given to a woman and thereupon sugar appears in her urine, a test for blood sugar should be made under the same conditions. If her blood contains less than 0.19 per cent of sugar, she is certainly pregnant. If it contains more, she is suffering from one of the other conditions. During the second and third months, normal sugar tolerance would exclude pregnancy.

Nürnberger found that after abortions in the second and third months the test was positive as long as the greater part of the placenta remained attached to the uterine wall. After the placenta was removed, the normal tolerance returned after a day or two. In extrauterine pregnancy the test was found positive in those cases where a considerable portion of the functionating placenta remained attached, or within a short time after its destruction. In two cases of eclampsia the sugar tolerance was found to be very low.

R. E. WOBUS.

Seitz and Jess: **Renal Glycosuria of Pregnancy in the Diagnosis of Pregnancy,** Münchener medizinische Wochenschrift, 1922, lxix, 6.

In following up the work of Frank and Nothmann (experimental glycosuria in diagnosis of pregnancy) the authors find: In about half the cases of pregnancy the administration of one hundred grams of grape sugar gives rise to a glycosuria without an abnormal increase of the blood sugar; the test is not constant in the early months of pregnancy, and almost always fails in the last two or three months; the test can only be considered a probable sign in the diagnosis and differential diagnosis of pregnancy. S. B. SOLHAUG.

Kast, L., Wardell, E. L. and Myers, V. C.: **The Significance of Small Amounts of Sugar in the Urine.** American Journal of the Medical Sciences, 1920, clx, 877.

Clinical interpretation placed upon glycosuria has progressed during the past few years.

With a delicate quantitative test for sugar, developed by Benedict and Osterberg, hourly variations of sugar output are detected in normal individuals. Such tests show increased output two or three hours following ingestion of food. In diabetics the relative increase in excretion of sugar is much greater at these times.

Conclusions: Sudden new appearance of sugar is rare. Occasional careful quantitative estimations of sugar output in 24 hour specimens are more valuable than daily routine qualitative estimations in treatment of diabetics. Routine qualitative estimations on morning specimens or specimens taken at random may be quite misleading. J. WARREN BELL.

Bartholomew, Sale and Calloway: **Diagnosis of Pregnancy by the Roentgen Ray.** Journal American Medical Association, 1921, lxxvi, 912.

Centers of ossification develop in the clavicles of the human fetus in the sixth or seventh month and, soon thereafter, in other bones. This fact, which is quite constant, has led to the attempt to diagnose pregnancy by means of the Roentgen ray. While Edling has succeeded in demonstrating parts of the fetal skeleton *in utero* as early as the end of the fourth month, the authors were unable, even in the most favorable cases, to demonstrate pregnancy by this method before the fifth month, and then only in one-third of the cases examined. During the sixth month, one-half of the cases examined were positive. R. E. WOBUS.

Corner: **Internal Migration of the Ovum.** Johns Hopkins Hospital Bulletin, 1921, xxxii, 78.

Corner says that with the rarest exceptions all human cases of migration of the ovum are explained by the external route (where the ovum passes from the ovary into the abdominal cavity and thence into the opposite tube). He cites the case of Andrews (1912) as the most satisfactory instance of internal migration where one of twin embryos was interstitial in the right side and one normally implanted in the uterine cavity, in a woman whose right tube and ovary were absent. In his work on the pregnant sow, he found (1915) that one or more ova migrate in at least one third of all cases. In the pig the number of corpora lutea probably represents accurately the number of eggs which are discharged into the Fallopian tubes at the ovulation which gave rise to the pregnancy. In examining the ovaries and uteri of 545 pigs he found that internal migration (where the ova pass through the homolateral tube into the uterus thence to be implanted in the opposite uterine cornu or tube) was the rule. He offers the hypothesis that internal migration in the sow is under physiologic regulation for useful ends, which hypothesis was fulfilled in 84 out of 113 cases with 29 trivial deviations. He thinks the embryos are shifted by the peristaltic action of the uterine musculature. Clinically, he states, the internal migration of the human ovum is to be regarded as occasionally possible, more especially perhaps in multiple gestation.　　　　　　　　　C. O. MALAND.

Litzenberg: Blood Pressure in Pregnancy. International Clinics, 1917, iv, Series 27.

Based upon the results obtained in a study of 528 cases, Litzenberg urges the taking of the blood pressure in every pregnant woman. He advises beginning early in pregnancy, since a gradual rise is of more importance than a relatively high blood pressure by itself. He has frequently found a rise in pressure to precede the appearance of albumin, in fact, an increasing hypertension was not always followed by an albuminuria. In this connection it is noted that eclampsia can occur without albuminuria or hypertension; however, this is rather infrequent.

Of patients with a systolic pressure of from 130 to 140, 3 per cent had other symptoms of toxemia; of those between 140 and 150, 9 per cent were toxemic; of those between 150 and 160, one-third were toxic. This ratio steadily increases and it is assumed that all classes showing a systolic pressure over 180 are definitely toxic.

Litzenberg does not find the diastolic pressure of any diagnostic value. The pulse pressure, he thinks, may be of prognostic value as well as a guide to proper treatment in cases of actual eclampsia. Low blood pressure indicates asthenia, the cause of which should be looked for and remedied on general principles. It is also not to be forgotten that hypertension may be due to other causes, such as chronic nephritis, which should be looked for.　　　　　　　　　R. E. WOBUS.

Didier and Philippe: Hemolytic Reaction in Normal Pregnancy. Presse Médicale, 1921, xxix, 473.

In this work the authors followed out the method advocated by Widal. They studied leucopenia in 26 women following the administration of 200 grams of milk. As a result of these observations they concluded that 35 per cent of the women showed some insufficiency in the capacity for protein assimilation. They also studied arterial tension and found that in two-thirds of the cases the arterial tension was lowered. In six cases out of eight there seemed to be a parallelism between the lowering of arterial tension and the modifications of the leucocytic formula. They were not able in nine instances to establish any relationship between the presence of urobilin, biliary salts of urine, the coefficient of Millard, and the hemolytic reaction. With their experiments on the administration of glucose they found that pregnant women react somewhat similar to diabetics and they concluded that their experiments confirmed the idea of hepatic insufficiency in a certain number of pregnant women. This insufficiency may or may not be parallel with insufficiency in assimilating proteins.　　　　　　　　　F. L. ADAIR.

Reynals: Intrauterine Anaphylaxis; Relation of Anaphylaxis to Pregnancy. Revista Española d' Obstetricia y Ginecologia, 1920, v, 458.

Brief review of literature: anaphylactic heredity, or transmission of anaphylactic hypersensitization from mother to progeny said to have been demonstrated first by Belin (C.-rend. Soc. de Biol., 1910). Report of animal (guinea-pigs, dogs) experiments with claim that said experiments proved maternal anaphylactic desensitization in the puerperal state; or in other words, after parturition the previously sensitized mother shows no, or very slight, anaphylactic shock on the second introduction of the antigen into her organism, but the newborn perish with rapid fatal anaphylaxis on injection of antigen. Desensitization of pregnant mother can take place in short time (2-4 days); Scaffidi (Archives Italiennes de Biologie, 1914) quoted. It is claimed also that the hereditary transmission of the anaphylactic state exists also when the mother has been sensitized before gestation. An attempt is made to explain a theory of anaphylactic transmission by gestation. Very little space is given to the actual experimental work. The author's conclusions are: (a) The sensitized mother can transmit this state to her young, whether the sensitization has been done before or during pregnancy; (b) the mother herself is desensitized by the pregnancy; (c) this desensitization is the more intense according as the pregnancy and the sensitization have coexisted a longer time; if the maternal sensitization has been done before gestation, it is effected with more difficulty; (d) the period of fetal sensitization is appreciably shorter than in the adult.

P. GRAFFAGNINO.

Berman: Auscultation of One Fetal Heart in a Twin Pregnancy Complicated by Hydramnios. Progrès Médicale, 1920, No. 45, p. 489.

Berman, in reporting a case of twin pregnancy complicated by hydramnios, points out the value of the auscultatory quality of the fetal heart as a great aid in the diagnosis of the existing condition. He claims that when the size of the abdomen indicates the existence of hydramnios, the fact that a fetal heart of marked intensity may be heard at a definite point on the abdominal wall, furnishes sufficient evidence to establish the diagnosis of a twin pregnancy. He bases this claim on the fact that the fetal heart of a single fetus in hydramnios is always weak and indistinct due to the fluid intervening between the fetus and the ear of the examiner. The foregoing complex he calls the sign of Professor Enrique a Boero.

THEODORE W. ADAMS.

Radasch: Superfetation or Superfecundation. Surgery Gynecology and Obstetrics, 1921, xxxii, 339.

After reviewing the literature, Radasch describes the product of a spontaneous abortion which contained, in a fused sac, one fetus 11.6 cm. from crown to coccyx or 16-17 weeks' development, and another 18 mm. or about 40 days' development. He considers this a case of superfetation.

R. E. WOBUS.

Ingram-Johnson, R. E.: Superfetation. British Medical Journal, July 23, 1921, p. 116.

The author reports a case of a woman who on March 2 was delivered of a five months' fetus and on March 4 had a second abortion in which she passed a sac containing a fetus of about six weeks' gestation. F. L. ADAIR.

Wijsenbeek: Observations on Uterine Movements. Nederlandsch Tijdschrift voor Geneeskunde, 1922, i, 1263.

This observer makes use of the method first used by Katsch and Borchers for observing peristaltic movements of the intestines. Under anesthesia and appropriate aseptic precautions, a piece of celluloid is sewn into an opening in the abdominal wall. With this window *in situ*, he has kept rabbits alive as long as 87 days. In guinea pigs the method was not successful, as they always succumbed after a few days, while the uterus of a cat is so far removed from the ventral wall that it cannot be observed. To exclude the by-effects of anesthetic and shock, observations were never recorded within three days after operation.

Wijsenbeek noticed several distinct peristaltic waves in the uterus. He compares the phenomenon to the turning of a rain worm. The main peristaltic wave travels at intervals from the end of the horn to the cervix. Occasionally it occurred in the opposite direction. An even more pronounced wave was observed in the vagina. Lesser peristaltic waves were observed traveling in an oblique direction from the round ligaments in spiral fashion towards the cervix.

In the pregnant organ the contractions become somewhat more irregular and occur at longer intervals. In the later stages of pregnancy there is a tendency towards longer periods of contraction of the entire organ, followed by longer periods of complete relaxation. In no case did he observe the so-called pendulum movements mentioned by other observers who removed the uterus partly from the organism.

After the injection of pituitrin, he observed very active contractions with deep transverse furrows. These contractions were of about one minute's duration and were followed by longer periods of rest, during which the uterus appeared cyanotic. These contractions were as severe and of the same duration 4 hours after injection of the pituitrin as at the beginning. R. E. WOBUS.

Naujoks, Hans: **The Influence of Anatomic Changes in the Membranes upon the Time of Their Rupture.** Zeitschrift für Geburtshülfe und Gynäkologie, 1921, lxxxiv, 304.

The author made histologic examinations of the membranes in a number of cases of labor to determine whether there were any anatomic changes to which premature or delayed rupture might be ascribed. In all cases of premature rupture for which no definite mechanical factors could be held accountable, he found two in which the structure was entirely normal; in 5 degenerative phenomena were more or less pronounced, usually affecting the chorionic epithelium; amniotic epithelium and membrana intermedia were at times affected. The most varied types of degenerations were observed, disintegration of the nucleus, pyknosis, vacuolization of the protoplasm, hyaline degeneration of the connective tissues as well as marked deposition of pigment in one case. Inflammatory changes were found in 3 cases; in 2 combined with degenerations, in 1 alone. The fact that the inflammatory changes were far more marked in the decidua and chorion than in the amnion indicates that they probably spread from the uterine cavity to the membranes rather than the reverse as a secondary result of premature rupture. Delicacy of certain layers, especially the two connective tissue layers and the absence of the membrana intermedia occurred in other cases, alone or combined with degenerations.

Out of 5 cases of delayed rupture he found definite anatomic changes in 4. These consisted in increased thickness and density of the connective tissue layers, or in an increase in the smooth muscle cells in the amniotic or chorionic connective tissue.

MARGARET SCHULZE.

Lorenzen: **The Body Weight of Pregnant Women and the Influence of Impending Labor upon It.** Zeitschrift für Geburtshülfe und Gynäkologie, 1921, lxxxiv, 426.

The author calls attention to Zangemeister's conclusions concerning the weight of pregnant women: The body weight of the pregnant woman increases almost uniformly after the 27th week; after the 36th week there is a slight increase in the amount of gain. From the third day before labor until the time of birth there is a sudden decrease in weight—in these two days the pregnant woman loses on an average 1 kg. In following daily the weight of 78 pregnant women, Lorenzen was unable to confirm Zangemeister's conclusions. He found that the factors of daily variation were so great that it was impossible to follow the general tendency of the weight curve except by averages of several days or a week, and impossible to prophesy impending labor merely because of the loss of a few hundred grams in weight. In analyzing Zangemeister's conclusions he found that a number of his cases had already begun to have pain at the last weighing; here the factor of decreased nutrition due to pain must be considered.

The author's conclusions are that the body weight of the pregnant woman increases uninterruptedly from the 31st week until labor; that there is no terminal drop in weight. The average total is 4.82 kg. The increase in weight is due not alone to the developing ovum, but in far greater measure to an increase in the body of the pregnant woman. This increase tends to be greater in younger women, in multiparae, and in those above the average weight. MARGARET SCHULZE.

Items

Professor John Willoughby Miller, engaged in pathological research at the University of Tübingen, Germany, is writing for an extensive medical handbook soon to be published, the section devoted to the diseases of the ovary. He desires to give accurate and complete references, but only those papers can be taken cognizance of which are available in unabridged form. Those authors who wish to have their contributions of recent years considered, are invited to forward reprints to Professor J. M. Miller, Hoelderlin Str. 19, Tübingen, Germany.

At the Annual Meeting of the American Gynecological Society held at Washington, D. C., May 1st, 2nd and 3rd, 1922, the following new officers were elected for the ensuing year: Pres.: Dr. John A. Sampson, Albany, N. Y. 1st Vice-Pres.: Dr. Brooke M. Anspach, Philadelphia, Pa. 2nd Vice-Pres.: Dr. Frank W. Lynch, San Francisco, Cal. Secretary: Dr. Arthur H. Curtis, Chicago, Ill. Treasurer: Dr. Charles C. Norris, Philadelphia, Pa. Other members of the Council: Dr. George Gray Ward, Jr., New York, Dr. Walter W. Chipman, Montreal, Dr. Robert L. Dickinson, New York, Dr. Franklin H. Martin, Chicago, Dr. R. R. Huggins, Pittsburgh, Pa. Dr. Le Roy Broun, New York.

Books Received

Acknowledgment is made of the receipt of the following books, selected reviews of which will appear in early numbers:

DISEASES OF THE GENITAL ORGANS OF ANIMALS. By W. L. WILLIAMS, Ithaca, N. Y., 1921, published by the author.

A MANUAL OF OBSTETRICAL NURSING, By NANCY E. CADMUS, New York, 1922, G. P. Putnam's Sons.

THE HEALTHY CHILD FROM TWO TO SEVEN. By DR. FRANCIS HAMILTON MACCARTHY, New York, 1922, The Macmillan Company.

PRENATAL CARE IN CHICAGO, A SURVEY. By THE CHICAGO COMMUNITY TRUST, Chicago, Ill., 1922, The Chicago Community Trust.

OBSTETRICAL NURSING. By CAROLYN CONANT VAN BLARCOM, New York, 1922, The Macmillan Company.

GYNECOLOGICAL AND OBSTETRICAL MONOGRAPHS, New York, 1922, D. Appleton Co.

BIRTH INJURIES OF THE CHILD. By DR. HUGO EHRENFEST.

PELVIC NEOPLASMS. DR. FRANK WORTHINGTON LYNCH.

GYNECOLOGICAL AND OBSTETRICAL PATHOLOGY. DR. ROBERT TILDEN FRANK.

TOXEMIAS OF PREGNANCY. DR. GEORGE WILLIAM KOSMAK.

STERILITY AND CONCEPTION. DR. CHARLES GARDNER CHILD.

INDEX

A

Abdominal drainage, Waldo, R., 436
Abortion, legal aspect of, Oakley, E. P., 37
Abortion, treatment of, Yates, H. W., 42
Adenomyoma, diffuse, of the uterus—conditions influencing its development, Schwarz, O. H., and McNally, F. P., 457
Adler, Meno- and metrorrhagia, (Abst.), 223
Adler, The treatment of cancer of the uterus, (Abst.), 337
Amenorrhea, a contribution to the clinical and pathological anatomy of, Novak and Graff, (Abst.), 223
Amenorrhea, in war, regressive gland changes of the endometrium, Graff and Novak, (Abst.), 222
American Association of Obstetricians, Gynecologists, and Abdominal Surgeons, Transactions of Thirty-Fourth Annual Meeting, 77, 188, 312, 431, 531
Anaphylaxis, intrauterine: Relation of anaphylaxis to pregnancy, Reynals, (Abst.), 672
Andrews, C. J., End results in obstetrics, 502
Antenatal factors of life and death, the —genetic, toxigenetic, gestational and obstetrical, Salesby, (Abst.), 449
Antenatal syphilis, the effect of legislature control on the incidence of, Cumpson, (Abst.), 450
Antenatal syphilitic environment, the dangers and treatment of, Sequiera, (Abst.), 450
Appendicitis in early life, the gynecologic significance of, Graves, (Abst.), 110
Appendicitis, the ice bag in,—a fetich, Moots, C. W., 533
Arnold, A brief review of recent obstetrical progress, (Abst.), 451

B

Bailey, H., Application of metabolism studies to the fetal and neonatal periods of life, 591
Report of a case of hemimelus or so-called congenital amputation, 72
Use of radium in cancer of the female generative organs, 117
Bainbridge, W. S., Oxygen in the peritoneal cavity, with report of cases, 419

Bandler, The "higher up" theory of sterility and its relation to the endocrines, (Abst.), 113
Bartholomew (with Sale and Calloway), Diagnosis of pregnancy by the Roentgen ray, (Abst.), 671
Bell, J. N., Diabetes in pregnancy, 20
Bell, W. Blair, Some common, but often unrecognized, obstetrical difficulties, (Abst.), 451
The prevention and treatment of puerperal infections, (Abst.), 454
Berman, Auscultation of one fetal heart in a twin pregnancy complicated by hydramnios, (Abst.), 673
Berreitter, The question of the frequency of malignancy in myomata, (Abst.), 330
Biedl, (with Peters and Hofstatter), Studies on implantation and the further development of the ovum in the uterus, (Abst.), 668
Bill, A. H., The choice of methods for making labor easy, 65
Bishop, E., Myoma causing dysmenorrhea cured by operation, 535
Blood pressure in pregnancy, Litzenberg, (Abst.), 672
Boggs, The treatment of carcinoma of the cervix and uterus by radium, supplemented by deep roentgen therapy, (Abst.), 339
Bonifield, C. L., Carcinoma uteri, 250
Bonney, The radical abdominal operation for carcinoma of the cervix, (Abst.), 336
Book Reviews: Gynecology, Anspach, B. M., 569
Diagnostische und therapeutische Irrtümer und deren Verhütung in der Frauenheilkunde, Schwalbe, J., 456
Les Hémorrhagies Méningées Sous-Dure-Mériennes Traumatiques du Nouveau-Né, Lantuéjoul, P., 456
Heart Disease and Pregnancy, MacKenzie, J., 456
Pneumoperitoneal Roentgen Ray Diagnosis (A Monograph with Atlas), Stein, A., and Stewart, W. H., 341
The Problem of Abortion from the Medical and Legal Standpoints, Kisch, F., 343
Die Prophylaxe und Therapie der Enteroptose, Knapp, L., 344
Bourne, The causation and prevention of puerperal sepsis, (Abst.), 454
Bovée, J. W., Pelvic hematocele from causes other than ectopic pregnancy, 634

Bram, Israel, Exophthalmic goiter and pregnancy, 352
Breast physiologically and pathologically considered with relation to bleeding from nipple, the, Dickinson, G. K., 31
Brodhead, G. L., (with Langrock, E. G.), A study of pituitary extract at the beginning of the third stage of labor. Its use in 100 cases, 170
Hydatidiforme mole. 655
Brown, G. Van A., Valuable methods used to extend operability in advanced cancer of the cervix, 263
Browne, Stillbirth: Its causes, pathology and prevention, (Abst.), 453
Burrows, The treatment of advanced carcinoma of the cervix of the uterus by radium, (Abst.), 340

C

Calloway, (with Bartholomew and Sale), Diagnosis of pregnancy by the roentgen ray, (Abst.), 671
Cancer infection, Ochsner, (Abst.), 329
of the female generative organs, the use of radium in, Bailey, H., and Quimby, Edith, 117
of the cervix, present status of the treatment of operable, Graves, (Abst.), 339
of the cervix, some phases in the evolution of the diagnosis and treatment of, Skeel, R. E., 252
of the cervix, valuable methods used to extend operability in advanced, Brown, G. Van A., 263
of uterus, increasing inoperability and its remedy, Winter, (Abst.), 332
of the uterus, the significance of early symptoms in the management of, Zweifel, (Abst.), 331
of the uterus, treatment of with radium, a symposium on the, 542
of the uterus, the treatment of, Adler, (Abst.), 337
of the uterus, the treatment of, Schmitz, (Abst.), 338
of the vagina, primary, Engelkens, (Abst.), 331
the control of the mortality of abdominal operations for, Crile, G. W., 272
the importance of early diagnosis of uterine, Highsmith, (Abst.), 333
Cancerous rectum, excision of, through vaginal section, Drueck, (Abst.), 340
Carcinoma, attempts to decrease the mortality of operation for uterine, Schweitzer, (Abst.), 335
of the cervix and uterus by radium, the treatment of, supplemented by deep roentgen therapy, Boggs, (Abst.), 339

Carcinoma—Cont'd.
of the cervix, early squamous-cell, Cullen, (Abst.), 335
of the cervix of the uterus, the treatment of advanced, by radium, Burrows, (Abst.), 340
of the cervix, prophylaxis in, Smiley, (Abst.), 334
of the cervix, the differential diagnosis of chancre and, Warthin and Noland, (Abst.), 333
of the cervix, the present position of the treatment of, Shaw, (Abst.), 340
of the cervix, the radical abdominal operation for, Bonney, (Abst.), 336
of the cervix, the technic of vaginal hysterectomy for, Cuneo and Picot, (Abst.), 336
of the uterus, early diagnosis of, Frankl, (Abst.), 333
of the white mouse, an organism associated with a transplantable, Nuzum, (Abst.), 329
of the female bladder, (case report), Stone, I. S., 517
treatment and dosage, Seitz, (Abst.), 338
uteri, Bonifield, C. L., 250
Cardiac failure during pregnancy, treatment of, Pardee, H. E. R., 620
Cervix and trachelorrhaphy, end results of amputation of the, Rawls, R. M., 1
Cervix uteri, diseases of the, Heineberg, (Abst.), 568
Cervicitis and endocervicitis, the treatment of, with bismuth paste injections, Hollender, (Abst.), 567
Cesarean operation, four, on one patient, Thoms, Herbert, 529
Cesarean section, vaginal, for eclampsia, Knipe, W. H. W., 646
Cesarean section with subtotal hysterectomy, pregnancy following, in a case of unrecognized uterus duplex, Cowles, H. C., 652
Chorioepithelioma, the diagnosis and treatment of, Geist, (Abst.), 334
Chorionepithelioma after the birth of viable children, early diagnosis of, Fink, (Abst.), 334
Ciliated epithelium in the pig, observations on the distribution and function of the uterine, with reference to certain clinical hypotheses, Snyder, F. F., and Corner, G. W., 358
Circumcision, Fagge, (Abst.), 455
Clow, Menstruation during school life, (Abst.), 220
Cord stump, indication for the management of, Willson, P., 506
Coffey, T., Use of lutein for the control of nausea and vomiting of pregnancy, 513

INDEX

Collective Reviews: Fear of the fetus; an ancient cause for the cesarean section, Ela, Alfred, 445
 Toxemia of early pregnancy, etiology and treatment, Titus, Paul, 209, 559
 The views of primitive people concerning the care of the parturient, Wright, J., 104
Cord, death of a fetus in twin pregnancy due to twists in the, Shlenker, M. A., 443
Corner, Internal migration of the ovum, (Abst.), 671
Corner, G. W., (with Snyder, F. F.), Observation on the distribution and function of the uterine ciliated epithelium in the pig, with reference to certain clinical hypotheses, 358
Corpus luteum and placenta on uterine hemorrhages, the menstrual cycle and menopause symptoms; the influence of lipoids from, Hermann, (Abst.), 224
Corpus luteum of menstruation and pregnancy, the, Morley, (Abst.), 217
Corpus luteum, the relation of, to menstruation and pregnancy, MacKenzie, W. R., (Abst.), 669
Couvelaire: A dispensary for syphilis as part of a maternity service, (Abst.), 450
Sterility in the female, (Abst.), 110
Cowles, H. C., Pregnancy following cesarean section with subtotal hysterectomy in a case of unrecognized uterus duplex, 652
Cron, R. S., Indications and contraindications for the use of pituitary extract in obstetrics, 300
Cullen, Early squamous-cell carcinoma of the cervix, (Abst.), 335
Cumpson, The effect of legislature control on the incidence of antenatal syphilis, (Abst.), 450
Cuneo, The technic of vaginal hysterectomy for carcinoma of the cervix, (Abst.), 336

D

Danforth, W. C., Is conservative obstetrics to be abandoned? 609
D'Aunoy, Rigney, (with King, E. L.), Lithopedion formation in extrauterine fetal masses, 377
Davis, J. E., Neoplasia of the kidney, 478
Delivery in normal cases, a method of, Tate, M. A., 61
Dice, W. G., Heart disease in pregnancy, 24
Dickinson, G. K., The breast physiologically and pathologically considered with relation to bleeding from the nipple, 31 .

Didier, (with Philippe), Hemolytic reaction in normal pregnancy, (Abst.), 672
Dittler, Parenteral injection of semen, (Abst.), 109
Donay, Surgical treatment of endocervicitis, (Abst.), 567
Doorenbos, parturition in Javenese women, (Abst.), 449
Dorman, F. A., Primary sarcomatous tumor of the umbilicus, 93
Drueck, Excision of cancerous rectum through vaginal section, (Abst.), 340
Duncan, Uterine cancer, (Abst.), 340
Dysmenorrhea, myoma causing, cured by operation, Bishop, E., 535
Dysmenorrhea, the results of operative treatment of, Forssner, (Abst.), 225

E

Ecbolics, the action of the commoner, in the first stage of labor, Rucker, P., 134
Eclampsia, treatment of, then and now, Moran, J. F., 155
Ectopic gestation, coincident ruptured, and acute suppurative appendicitis, Ruth, C. E., 525
Ectopic gestation and ovarian abscess, Knipe, W. H. W.. 647
Ectopic pregnancy, a study of the origin of bleeding in, Polak, J. O., and Welton, T. S., 164
Ectopic pregnancy, intraligamentous, Pfeiffer, W., 101
Ela, A., Fear of the fetus, an ancient cause for cesarean section, Collective review), 445
Electric waves, rhythmic, in gynecology, Massey, G. B., 426
Emetine hydrochloride, the action of, upon the uterus, Martin, Paul. 241
Endocervicitis, a study of chronic, Matthews. (Abst.), 567
Endocervicitis, surgical treatment of, Donay, (Abst.), 567
End results in obstetrics, Andrews, C. J., 502
Engelkens, Primary cancer of the vagina, (Abst.), 331
Exophthalmic goiter and pregnancy, Bram, Israel, 352
Extrauterine pregnancy, an unusual case of, Riley, J. W., 630
Evans, Malignant myomata and related tumors of the uterus, (Abst.), 329

F

Fallopian tubes, the nonoperative determination of patency of the, Rubin, (Abst.), 112
Fagge, Circumcision, (Abst.), 455

Farr, R. E., Gynecological operations under local anesthesia, 400, 431

Flatau, Sterilization by knotting the tubes, (Abst.), 115

Fetal and neonatal periods, the application of metabolism studies to, Bailey, H., 591

Fetus, general edema of the, associated with osteogenesis imperfecta, Halsted, H., 552

Findley, P., The slaughter of the innocents, 35

Fink, Early diagnosis of chorionepithelioma after the birth of viable children, (Abst.), 334

Forssner, The results of operative treatment of dysmenorrhea, (Abst.), 225

Frank, (with Nothman), The value of renal glycosuria of pregnancy in the early diagnosis of pregnancy, (Abst.), 669

Frankl, Early diagnosis of carcinoma of the uterus, (Abst.), 333

X-ray and radium treatment in gynecology, (Abst.), 338

Furniss, H. D., Supernumerary ureter emptying extravesically, 644

G

Garling, On the leucocytic blood picture during menstruation, (Abst.), 222

Geist, S. H., A contribution to the histogenesis of ovarian tumors, 231

The diagnosis and treatment of chorioepithelioma, (Abst.) 334

Gellhorn, G., The new trend in gynecological therapy, 275

Gestation, human, and our embryological and morphological data, Oliver, (Abst.), 669

Glycosuria in the early diagnosis of pregnancy, utilizing renal, Nürnberg, (Abst.), 670

Glycosuria, renal, of pregnancy, in the diagnosis of pregnancy, Seitz and Jess, (Abst.), 671

Glycosuria, renal, of pregnancy, the value of, in the early diagnosis of pregnancy, Frank and Nothman, (Abst.), 669

Gynecological operations under local anesthesia, Farr, R. E., 431

Gordon, O. A., Uterine torsion in pregnancy with fatal results, 197

Graff, A contribution to the clinical and pathological anatomy of amenorrhea, (Abst.), 223

Regressive gland changes of the endometrium in war amenorrhea, (Abst.), 222

Graves, W. P., Ovarian function, 583

The gynecologic significance of appendicitis in early life, (Abst.), 110

Graves, W. P.—Cont'd.

Present status of the treatment of operable cancer of the cervix, (Abst.), 339

Gynecologic operations under local anesthesia, Farr, R. E., 400

Gynecological therapy, the new trend in, Gellhorn, G., 275

H

Hadden, David, Double uterus and vagina, 526

Halsted, H., General edema of the fetus associated with osteogenesis imperfecta, 552

Haskell, The dangers of pituitary extract: Some clinical and experimental observations, (Abst.), 452

Healy, W. P., Recovery after postoperative tetany treated with calcium lactate, 99

Sudden death during the preoperative treatment of procidentia uteri, 99

Heineberg, Diseases of the cervix uteri, (Abst.), 568

Hellendall, A new method of tubal sterilization, (Abst.), 116

Pregnancy after ligation of both tubes, (Abst.), 116

Hemimelus or so-called congenital amputation, report of a case of, Bailey, H., 72

Hemolytic reaction in normal pregnancy, Didier and Philippe, (Abst.), 672

Hemorrhage during the early months of pregnancy, Sullivan, R. Y., 520

Hemorrhage, the treatment of uterine, not associated with pregnancy, Phillipe, (Abst.), 224

Hendrickson, F. C., A device for aseptic intrauterine manipulations, 617

Hermann, The influence of lipoids from corpus luteum and placenta on uterine hemorrhages, the menstrual cycle and menopause symptoms, (Abst.), 224

Hernia of the ileum through a rent in the mesentery, Jackson, F. H., 527

Highsmith, The importance of early diagnosis of uterine cancer, (Abst.), 333

Hoehne, The physiology of conception, (Abst.), 110

Hofstatter, (with Biedl and Peters), Studies on implantation and the further development of the ovum in the uterus, (Abst.), 668

Holden, F. C., Are the operations for absence of the vagina justifiable? 439

Hollender, The treatment of cervicitis and endocervicitis with bismuth paste injections, (Abst.), 567

Huggins, R. R., The indications for and the dangers in the use of spinal anesthesia in obstetrics, gynecology and abdominal surgery, 412

Hühner, Max, Methods of examining for spermatozoa in the diagnosis of sterility, (Abst.), 111

Humpstone, O. P., A case of rupture of the uterus in a placenta previa, 94

Hydatidiform mole, Shlenker, M. A., 441

Hydramnios, twin pregnancy complicated by, auscultation of one fetal heart in a, Berman, (Abst.), 673

I

Induction of labor, a new hydrostatic bag for, Lee, G. H., 628

Ingram-Johnson. Superfetation, (Abst.), 673

Insufflation, transuterine, a diagnostic aid in sterility, Rongy, A. J., and Rosenfeld, S. S., 496

Intrauterine manipulations, a device for aseptic, Hendrickson, F. C., 617

J

Jackson, F. H., Hernia of the ileum through a rent in the mesentery, 527

Janney, J. C., Report of three cases of a rare ovarian anomaly, 173

Jess, (with Seitz), Renal glycosuria of pregnancy in the diagnosis of pregnancy, (Abst.), 671

Joseph, (with Kamnitzer), Biologic diagnosis of pregnancy, (Abst.), 670

K

Kammerer, The relation of climate to puberty, (Abst.), 219

Kamnitzer, (with Joseph) Biologic diagnosis of pregnancy, (Abst.), 670

Kast, L. (with Wardell, E. L., and Myers, V. C.), The significance of small amounts of sugar in the urine, (Abst.), 671

Kellogg, F. S., The relationship between toxemia of pregnancy and uterine sepsis, a study of 400 toxemia cases, 366

Kennedy, W. T., Keeping fallopian tubes open, 607

Keukenschriever, Parturition in Javanese women, (Abst.), 449

Kidney, neoplasia of, (case reports), Davis, James E., 478

King, E. L. (with D'Aunoy R.), Lithopedion formation in extrauterine fetal masses, 377

King, J. E., Atresia and stricture of the vagina, 290

Korndoerffer, A., Further experiences with pituitary extracts in obstetrics, 540

Knipe, W. H. W., Vaginal cesarean section for eclampsia, 646
Ectopic gestation and ovarian abscess, 647

L

Labor, the choice of methods for making, easy, Bill, A. H., 65

Langrock, E. C., Rupture of uterus following pituitrin, 656

Langrock, E. C., (with Brodhead, G. L.), A study of pituitary extract at the beginning of the third stage of labor. Its use in 100 cases, 170

Lee, G. H., A new hydrostatic bag for the induction of labor, 628

Ley, The difficulties encountered in pregnancy, labor, and lactation in working class mothers and those of the educated class (Abst.), 449

Lithopedion formation in extrauterine fetal masses, D'Aunoy, Rigney, and King, E. L., 377

Litzenberg, Blood pressure in pregnancy, (Abst.), 672

Loeb, Effect of undernourishment on mammalian ovary and the sexual cycle, (Abst.), 219

Lorenzen, The body weight of pregnant women and the influence of impending labor, (Abst.), 674

Lutein solution for the control of nausea and vomiting of pregnancy, Coffey, T., 513

M

Macomber, Diagnosis in sterility, (Abst.), 111

Magid, Obstetrical end results of the tracheloplastic operation, (Abst.), 568

Malformation, congenital, of the female genitalia, Reel, P. J., 604

Martin, Paul, The action of emetine hydrochloride upon the uterus, 241

Massey, G. B., Rhythmic electric waves in gynecology, 426

Matthews, H. B., Pregnancy after nephrectomy, 327
Report of a case of B. Welchii blood stream infection of uterine origin, 307
A study of chronic endocervicitis, (Abst.), 567

MacKenzie, W. R., The relation of the corpus luteum to menstruation and pregnancy, (Abst.), 669

McKeown, Present day obstetrics, (Abst.), 452

McLean, S., Sarcoma of uterus in infant, 322

McNally, F. P. (with Schwarz, O. H.), Diffuse adenomyoma of the uterus, 457

Mendenhall, A. M., Teaching undergraduates obstetrics, 53

Medlener, Answer to Flatau's paper on sterilization, (Abst.), 116

Membranes, the influence of anatomic changes in, upon the time of their rupture, Naujoks, Hans, (Abst.), 674
Meno-and metrorrhagia, Adler, (Abst.), 223
Menstrual blood, the, Stickel and Zoudek, (Abst.), 221
Menstrual poison, Schick, (Abst.), 221
Menstruation, basal metabolism in, Wiltshire, (Abst.), 220
Menstruation during school life, Clow, (Abst.), 220
Menstruation, on the leucocytic blood picture during, Garling, (Abst.), 222
Menstruation, influence of, on the food tolerance in diabetes mellitus, Rosenbloom, (Abst.), 221
Moots, C. W., The ice bag in appendicitis—a fetich, 533
Moran, J. F., Treatment of eclampsia, 155
Morley, The corpus luteum of menstruation and pregnancy, (Abst.), 217
Mosher, G. C., Ten years of painless childbirth, 142
Myers, V. C., (with Kast, E. L. and Wardell, E. L.), The significance of small amounts of sugar in the urine, (Abst.), 671
Myomata, malignant, and related tumors of the uterus, Evans, (Abst.), 329
Myomata, the question of the frequency of malignancy in, Berreitter, (Abst.), 330

N

Nassauer, Treatment of sterility, (Abst.), 113
Naujoks, Hans, The influence of anatomic changes in the membranes upon the time of their rupture, (Abst.), 674
Nausea and vomiting of pregnancy, use of lutein solution hypodermatically for the control of, Coffey, T., 513
Nephropexy, transperitoneal, Noble, T. B., 493
New York Academy of Medicine, Section on Obstetrics and Gynecology, Transactions, 322, 441, 552, 644, 652
New York Obstetrical Society, Transactions, 93, 197, 436, 535
Nitrous oxide and oxygen continuous analgesia and anesthesia with rebreathing, in obstetrics. Technic of administration and summary of results, Rives, A. E., 296
Noble, T. B., Transperitoneal nephropexy, 493
Noland, The differential diagnosis of chancre and carcinoma of the cervix, (Abst.), 333
Nothman, (with Frank), The value of renal glycosuria of pregnancy in the early diagnosis of pregnancy, (Abst.), 669
Novak, A contribution to the clinical and pathological anatomy of amenorrhea, (Abst.), 223
Regressive gland changes of the endometrium in war amenorrhea (Abst.), 222
Nürnberger, Utilizing renal glycosuria in the early diagnosis of pregnancy, (Abst.), 670
Nuzum, An organism associated with a transplantable carcinoma of the white mouse, (Abst.), 329

O

Oakley, E. F., Legal aspect of abortion, 37
Obstetrical difficulties, some common, but often unrecognized, Bell, W. Blair, (Abst.), 451
Obstetrical Society of Philadelphia, Transactions, 540, 663
Obstetrical progress, a brief review of recent, Arnold, (Abst.), 451
Obstetric armamentarium, additions to our, Ziegler, C. E., 46
Obstetrics, is conservative, to be abandoned? Danforth, W. C., 609
Obstetrics, present day, McKeown, (Abst.), 452
Obstetric teaching, the defects in our, Polak, (Abst.), 453
Ochsner, cancer infection, (Abst.), 329
Oliver, Human gestation and our embryological and morphological data, Abst.), 669
Ovarian anomaly, report of three cases of a rare, Janney, J. C., 173
Ovarian function, studies on, Schickle, G., (Abst.), 218
Ovarian tumors, a contribution to the histogenesis of, Geist, S. H., 231
Ovary, mammalian, and the sexual cycle, effect of undernourishment on, Loeb, (Abst.), 219
Ovary, function, Graves, W. P., 583
Ovary, teratomata of the, Porter, M. F., 600
Ovulation, corpus luteum and menstruation, Tschirdewahn, (Abst.), 218
Ovum, internal migration of, Corner, (Abst.), 671
Ovum studies on implantation and the further development of, in the uterus, Biedl, Peters and Hofstatter, (Abst.), 668
Oxygen in the peritoneal cavity, with report of cases, Bainbridge, W. S., 424

P

Painless childbirth, ten years of, Mosher, G. C., 142
Pardee, G. E. B., Treatment of cardiac failure during pregnancy, 620, 649
Parturition in Javanese women, Keukenschriever and Doorenbos, (Abst.), 449
Pelves, the conduct of labor in contracted, Schmitt, (Abst.), 452
Pelvis, normal variations in type of the female, and their obstetrical significance, Williams, John T., 345
Peters, (with Biedl and Hofstatter) Studies on implantation and the further development of the ovum in the uterus, (Abst.), 668
Pfeiffer, W., Intraligamentous ectopic pregnancy, 101
Philippe, (with Didier), Hemolytic reaction in normal pregnancy, (Abst.), 672
Phillips, The treatment of uterine hemorrhage not associated with pregnancy, (Abst.), 224
Physiology the basis of future gynecology,—presidential address, Ward, G. G., Jr., 573
Picot, The technic of vaginal hysterectomy for carcinoma of the cervix, (Abst.), 336
Pituitary extract, the dangers of; Some clinical and experimental observations, Rucker and Haskell, (Abst.), 452
Pituitary extract in obstetrics, indications and contraindications for the use of, Cron, R. S., 300
Pituitary extract at the beginning of the third stage of labor, a study of, Brodhead, G. L., and Langrock, E. G., 170
Pituitary extract in obstetrics, further experiences with, Korndoerffer A., 540
Placenta, the premature separation of the normally implanted, Williamson, A. C., 385
Placenta previa, a case of rupture of the uterus in a, Humpstone, O. P., 94
Pneumoperitoneum, artificial, treatment of tuberculous peritonitis by, Stein, A., 658
Polak, J. O., The defects in our obstetric teaching, (Abst.), 453
(with Welton, T. S.) A study of the origin of bleeding in ectopic pregnancy, 164
Porter, M. F., Teratomata of the ovary, 600
Potter version, an analysis of the, Speidel, E., 150

Pregnancy after ligation of both tubes, Hellendall, (Abst.), 116
Pregnancy after nephrectomy, Matthews, H. B., 327
Pregnancy, biologic, diagnosis of, Kamnitzer and Joseph, (Abst.), 670
Pregnancy, diabetes in, Bell, J. N., 20
Pregnancy, diagnosis of, by the roentgen ray, Bartholomew, Sale, Calloway, (Abst.), 671
Pregnancy, exophthalmic goitre in, Bram, Israel, 352
Pregnancy, heart disease in, Dice, W. G., 24
Pregnancy, labor, and lactation, difficulties encountered in, in working class mothers and those of the educated class, Ley, (Abst.), 449
Pregnancy, uterine torsion in, with fatal results, Gordon, O. A., 197
Pregnant women, the body weight of, and the influence of impending labor, Lorenzen, (Abst.), 674
Prenatal and obstetric care, Taylor, (Abst.), 450
Procidentia uteri, sudden death during the preoperative treatment of, Healy, W. P., 99
Puberty, the relation of climate to, Steinach and Kammerer, (Abst.), 219
Puerperal fever, the prevention of, Schmitt, (Abst.), 454
Puerperal infections, the prevention and treatment of, Bell, W. Blair, (Abst.), 454
Pyelitis, double, complicating pregnancy at sixth month, Smith, W. S., 201

Q

Quimby, Edith, (with Bailey, H.), The use of radium in cancer of the female generative organs, 117

R

Radasch, Superfetation or superfecundation, (Abst.), 673
Rawls, R. M., End results of amputation of the cervix and trachelorrhaphy, 1
Reel, P. J., Congenital malformation of the female genitalia, 604
Reynolds, Diagnosis in sterility, (Abst.), 111
Reynals, Intrauterine anaphylaxis: Relation of anaphylaxis to pregnancy, (Abst.), 672
Riley, J. W., An unusual case of extrauterine pregnancy, 630
Rives, A. E., Nitrous oxide and oxygen continuous analgesia and anesthesia with rebreathing in obstetrics. Technic of administration and summary of results, 296

Rongy, A. J., (with Rosenfeld, S. S.), Transuterine insufflation, a diagnostic aid in sterility, 496
Rosenbloom, Influence of menstruation on the food tolerance in diabetes mellitus, (Abst.), 221
Rosenfeld, S. S., (with Rongy, A. J.), transuterine insufflation, a diagnostic aid in sterility, 496
Rubin, The nonoperative determination of patency of the fallopian tubes, (Abst.), 112
Rucker, P., The action of the commoner ecbolics in the first stage of labor, 134
The dangers of pituitary extract: Some clinical and experimental observations, (Abst.), 452
Ruth, Charles E., coincident ectopic gestation and acute suppurative appendicitis, 525

S

Sale, (with Bartholomew and Calloway), Diagnosis of pregnancy by the roentgen ray, (Abst.), 671
Salesby, The antenatal factors of life and death—genetic, toxigenetic, gestational and obstetrical, (Abst.), 449
Sancs, K. I., Ureteral obstructions, 405
Schick, Menstrual poison, (Abst.), 221
Schickle, G., Studies on ovarian function, (Abst.), 218
Schiffmann, The question of sterilization by means of ligation of the tubes, (Abst.), 114
Shlenker, M. A., Death of a fetus in twin pregnancy due to twists in the cord, 443
Schmitz, The treatment of cancer of the uterus, (Abst.), 338
Schmitt, The conduct of labor in contracted pelves, (Abst.), 452
The prevention of puerperal fever, (Abst.), 454
Schwarz, O. H., (with McNally, F. P.), Diffuse adenomyoma of the uterus, 457
Schweitzer, Attempts to decrease the mortality of operation for uterine carcinoma, (Abst.), 335
Seitz, Carcinoma treatment and dosage, (Abst.), 338
(with Jess), Renal glycosuria of pregnancy in the diagnosis of pregnancy, (Abst.), 671
Semen, parenteral injection of, (Abst.), Dittler, 109
Sepsis, the causation and prevention of puerperal, Bourne, (Abst.), 454
Sequiera, The dangers and treatment of antenatal syphilitic environment, (Abst.), 450

Shaw, The present position of the treatment of carcinoma of the cervix, (Abst.), 340
Shlenker, M. A., Hydatidiform mole, 441
Skeel, R. E., Some phases in the evolution of the diagnosis and treatment of cancer of the cervix, 252
Smiley, Prophylaxis in carcinoma of the cervix, (Abst.), 334
Smith, W. S., Double pyelitis complicating pregnancy at sixth month, 201
Snyder, F. F., (with Corner, G. W.), Observations on the distribution and function of the uterine ciliated epithelium in the pig, with reference to certain clinical hypotheses, 358
Speidel, E., An analysis of the Potter version, 150
Spencer, H. R., William Harvey, Obstetric physician and gynecologist, (Abst.), 448
Spermatozoa in the diagnosis and treatment of sterility, methods of examining for, Max Hühner, (Abst.), 111
Spinal anesthesia, the indications for and the dangers in the use of, in obstetrics, gynecology and abdominal surgery, Huggins, R. R., 412
Stein, A., Treatment of tuberculous peritonitis by oxygen inflation of the abdominal cavity, 658
Steinach, The relation of climate to puberty, (Abst.), 219
Sterility in the female, frigidity and, Talmey, (Abst.), 112
Sterility, diagnosis in, Reynolds and Macomber, (Abst.), 111
Sterility in the female, Couvelaire, (Abst.), 110
Sterility, treatment of, Nassauer, (Abst.), 113
Sterilization, a new method of temporary, Wessel, (Abst.), 114
Sterilization, a new method of tubal, Hellendall, (Abst.), 116
Sterilization, answer to Flatau's paper on, Medlener, (Abst.), 116
Sterilization by knotting the tubes, Flatau, (Abst.), 115
Sterility, the "higher-up" theory of, and its relation to the endocrines, Bandler, (Abst.), 113
Sterilization, the question of, Van der Velde, (Abst.), 115
Sterilization by means of ligation of the tubes, the question of, Schiffmann, (Abst.), 114
Stickel, The menstrual blood, (Abst.), 221
Stillbirth, Its causes, pathology and prevention, Browne, (Abst.), 453

Stone, I. S., Primary carcinoma of the female bladder, case report, 517
Sugar in the urine, the significance of small amounts of, Kast, L., Wardell, E. L., and Myers, V. C. (Abst.), 671
Sullivan, R. Y., Hemorrhage during the early months of pregnancy, 520
Superfetation, Ingram-Johnson, (Abst.), 673
Superfetation or superfecundation, Radasch, (Abst.), 673
Syphilis, a dispensary for, as part of a maternity service, (Abst.), 450

T

Talmey, Frigidity and sterility in the female, (Abst.), 112
Tate, M. A., A method of delivery in normal cases, 61
Taussig, F. J., The hypertrophiculcerative form of chronic vulvitis. (Elephantiasis, esthiomene, syphiloma), 281
Taylor, Prenatal and obstetric care, (Abst.), 450
Teaching undergraduates obstetrics, Mendenhall, A. M., 53
Tetany treated with calcium lactate, recovery after postoperative, Healy, W. P., 99
The slaughter of the innocents, Findley, P., 35
Thoms, Herbert, Four cesarean operations on one patient, 529
Titus, Paul, Toxemia of early pregnancy (Collective Review), 209
Toxemia of pregnancy and uterine sepsis, the relationship between, a study of 400 toxemia cases, Kellogg, F. S., 366
Tracheloplastic operation, obstetrical end results of the, Magid, (Abst.), 568
Tschirdewahn: Ovulation, corpus luteum and menstruation, (Abst.), 218

U

Umbilicus, primary sarcomatous tumor of the, Dorman, F. A., 93
Uterine cancer, Duncan, (Abst.), 340
Uterine movements, observations, on Wijsenbeek, (Abst.), 673
Uterus, double, and vagina, Hadden, David, 526
Uterus, rupture of, following pituitrin, Langrock, E. C., 656
Uterus, sarcoma of, in infant, McLean, S., 322
Ureter, supernumerary, emptying extravesically, Furniss, H. D., 644
Ureteral obstructions, Sanes, K. I., 405

V

Vagina, absence of, are the operations justifiable for? Holden, F. C., 439

Vagina, atresia and stricture of the, King, J. E., 290
Van der Velde, The question of sterilization, (Abst.), 115
Vulvitis, the hypertrophic-ulcerative form of chronic. (elephantiasis, esthiomene, syphiloma), Taussig, F. J., 281

W

Waldo, R., Abdominal drainage, 436
Ward, G. G., Jr., Presidential address, Amer. Gyn. Soc.—Forty-seventh annual meeting, 573
Wardell, E. L., (with Kast, L., and Myers, V. C.), The significance of small amounts of sugar in the urine, (Abst.), 671
Warthin, The differential diagnosis of chancre and carcinoma of the cervix, (Abst.), 333
Welchii, B., blood stream infection of uterine origin, report of a case of, Matthews, H. B., 307
Welton, T. S., (with Polak, J. O.), A study of the origin of bleeding in ectopic pregnancy, 164
Wessel, A new method of temporary sterilization, (Abst.), 114
Wijsenbeek, Observations on uterine movements, (Abst.), 673
William Harvey, obstetric physician and gynecologist, Spencer, H. R. (Abst.), 448
Williams, John T., Normal variations in type of the female genitalia and their obstetrical significance, 345
Williamson, A. C., The premature separation of the normally implanted placenta, 385
Willson, P., Indications for the management of the cord stump, 506
Wiltshire, Basal metabolism in menstruation, (Abst.), 220
Winter, Increasing inoperability of uterus cancer and its remedy, (Abst.), 332
Wright, T., Views of primitive people concerning the care of the parturient, (Collective Review), 104

X

X-ray and radium treatment in gynecology, Frankl, (Abst.), 338

Y

Yates, H. W., Treatment of abortion, 42

Z

Ziegler, C. E., Additions to our obstetric armamentarium, 46
Zoudek, The menstrual blood, (Abst.), 221
Zweifel, The significance of early symptoms in the management of cancer of the uterus, (Abst.), 331

The American Journal of Obstetrics and Gynecology

GEORGE W. KOSMAK, M.D., Editor   HUGO EHRENFEST, M.D., Associate Editor

Published by THE C. V. MOSBY COMPANY, 508 North Grand Ave., St. Louis, Mo.

Published Monthly. Subscriptions may begin at any time.

Editorial Communications

Original Contributions.—Contributions, letters, books for review, and all other communications relating to the editorial management of the Journal should be sent to Dr. George W. Kosmak, 23 East 93d Street, New York.

All articles published in this Journal must be contributed to it exclusively. If subsequently printed elsewhere (except in a volume of Society Transactions) due credit shall be given for original publication. The editor relies on all contributors conforming strictly to this rule.

Neither the editor nor the publisher accepts responsibility for the views and statements of authors as published in their "Original Communications."

Translations.—The Journal will be pleased to receive, and to translate contributions by Continental authors if on examination they prove desirable.

Illustrations.—A reasonable number of halftone illustrations will be reproduced free of cost to the author, but special arrangements must be made with the editor for color plates, elaborate tables or extra illustrations. Copy for zinc cuts (such as pen drawings and charts) should be drawn and lettered only in India ink, or black typewriter ribbon (when the typewriter is used), as ordinary blue ink or colors will not reproduce. Only good photographic prints or drawings should be supplied for halftone work.

Exchanges.—Contributions, letters, exchanges, reprints, and all other communications relating to the Abstract Department of the Journal should be sent to Dr. Hugo Ehrenfest, 713 Metropolitan Building, St. Louis, Mo. Writers on gynecological subjects are requested to place this address on their regular mailing list for reprints.

Reprints.—Reprints of articles published among "Original Communications," may be ordered specifically, in a separate communication to the Publishers, The C. V. Mosby Co., 508 North Grand Ave., St. Louis, U. S. A., who will send their schedule of prices.

Review of Books.—Publishers and Authors are informed that the space of the Journal is so fully occupied by matter pertaining to the branches to which it is devoted, that only works treating of these subjects can be noticed. Books and monographs, native and foreign, on Obstetrics, Gynecology and Abdominal Surgery will be reviewed according to their merits, and space at disposal. Send books to Dr. George W. Kosmak, 23 East 93rd Street, New York.

Business Communications

Business Communications.—All communications in regard to advertising, subscriptions, change of address, etc., should be addressed to the publishers, The C. V. Mosby Company, 508 North Grand Ave., St. Louis, Mo.

Subscription Rates.—Single copies, 75c. To anywhere in United States, Cuba, Porto Rico, Canal Zone, Mexico, Hawaii and Philippine Islands, $6.00 per year in advance. To Canada and under foreign postage, $6.40. Includes two volumes a year, January and July.

Remittances.—Remittances for subscriptions should be made by check, draft, postoffice or express money order, or registered letter, payable to the publishers, The C. V. Mosby Co.

Change of Address.—The publishers should be advised of change of subscriber's address about fifteen days before the date of issue, with both new and old addresses given.

Nonreceipt of Copies.—Complaints for nonreceipt of copies or requests for extra numbers must be received on or before the fifteenth of the month of publication; otherwise the supply is apt to be exhausted.

Advertisements.—The advertising policy of the Journal will conform to the standards set by the Council of Pharmacy and Chemistry of the American Medical Association. Only articles of known scientific value will be given space. Forms close first of month preceding date of issue. Advertising rates and page sizes on application.

CPSIA information can be obtained
at www.ICGtesting.com
Printed in the USA
LVHW080704280922
729462LV00004B/70